CHRONIC OBSTRUCTIVE PULMONARY DISEASE

This book is dedicated to George William Tatam who faced this terrible disease with such dignity and courage.

CHRONIC OBSTRUCTIVE PULMONARY DISEASE

Edited by

P.M.A. Calverley

Consultant Physician, Aintree Chest Centre, Fazakerley Hospital, Liverpool, UK
Senior Fellow, Department of Medicine, University of Liverpool, UK

and

N.B. Pride

Consultant Physician, Hammersmith Hospital, London, UK
Professor of Respiratory Medicine, Royal Postgraduate Medical School, London, UK

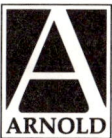

A
ARNOLD

A member of the Hodder Headline Group
LONDON • SYDNEY • AUCKLAND
Copublished in the USA by
Oxford University Press, Inc., New York

First published in Great Britain in 1995
Reprinted in 1999 by Arnold,
a member of the Hodder Headline Group,
338 Euston Road, London NW1 3BH

http://www.arnoldpublishers.com

Co-published in the USA by
Oxford University Press Inc.,
198 Madison Avenue, New York, NY 10016
Oxford is a registered trademark of Oxford University Press

Whilst the advice and information in this book are believed to be true and
accurate at the date of going to press, neither the authors nor the publisher
can accept any legal responsibility or liability for any errors or omissions
that may be made. In particular (but without limiting the generality of the
preceding disclaimer) every effort has been made to check drug dosages;
however, it is still possible that errors have been missed. Furthermore,
dosage schedules are constantly being revised and new side-effects
recognized. For these reasons the reader is strongly urged to consult the
drug companies' printed instructions before administering any of the drugs
recommended in this book.

British Library Cataloguing in Publication Data
A catalogue record for this book is available from the British Library

Library of Congress Cataloging-in-Publication Data
A catalog record for this book is available from the Library of Congress

ISBN 0 412 46450 0 (hb)

Typeset in 10/12pt Palatino by EXPO Holdings, Malaysia
Printed and bound in Great Britain by print in black, Midsomer Norton, Bath

What do you think about this book? Or any other Arnold title?
Please send your comments to feedback.arnold@hodder.co.uk

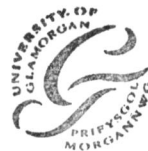

CONTENTS

CONTRIBUTORS

P.J. BARNES
Professor
National Heart and Lung Institute,
Dover Street,
London SW3 6LR,
UK.

B. BURROWS
Chalfant-Moore Professor of Respiratory
  Medicine,
University of Arizona,
College of Medicine,
AHSC, 1501 N Campbell Avenue,
Tuscon AZ 85724,
USA.

P.M.A. CALVERLEY
Aintree Chest Clinic,
Regional Thoracic Unit,
Fazakerley Hospital,
Longmoor Lane,
Liverpool L9 7AL,
UK.

C.J. CLARK
Consultant Physician
Hairmyrers Hospital,
East Kilbride,
Glasgow,
UK.

C.B. COOPER
Associate Professor of Medicine and
  Physiology,
UCLA School of Medicine,
10833 Le Conte Avenue, 37–131 CHS,
Los Angeles CA 90024,
USA.

P. CORRIS
Consultant Physician
Freeman Hospital,
High Heaton,
Newcastle-upon-Tyne NE7 7DN,
UK.

N.J. DOUGLAS
Reader in Medicine,
Respiratory Medicine Unit,
Royal Infirmary of Edinburgh,
Lauriston Place,
Edinburgh EH3 9YW,
UK.

J. FOULDS
Health Behaviour Unit,
Institute of Psychiatry,
4 Windsor Walk,
London SE5 8AF,
UK.

J. GIBSON
Professor,
Department of Respiratory Medicine,
Freeman Hospital,
High Heaton,
Newcastle-upon-Tyne NE7 7DN,
UK.

J.C. HOGG
Professor,
Department of Pathology,
University of British Columbia,
St Paul's Hospital,
1081 Burrard Street,
Vancouver BC,
Canada V6Z 1Y6.

M.J. JARVIS
Health Behaviour Unit,
Institute of Psychiatry,
4 Windsor Walk,
London SE5 8AF,
UK.

D. LAMB
Reader in Pathology,
Department of Pathology,
University of Edinburgh Medical School,
Teviot Place,
Edinburgh EH8 9AG,
UK.

W. MACNEE
Reader in Medicine,
Department of Medicine,
Royal Infirmary of Edinburgh,
Lauriston Place,
Edinburgh EH3 9YW,
UK.

M.J. MADOR
Associate Professor
Pulmonary Division,
School of Medicine,
University at Buffalo,
Veterans Administration Medical Center,
3495 Bailey Avenue,
Buffalo NY 14215,
USA.

J. MILIC-EMILI
Professor of Physiology,
Director,
Meakins-Christie Laboratory,
3626 St Urbin Street,
Montreal,
Quebec H2X 2E2,
Canada.

M.D.L. MORGAN
Consultant Physician in Respiratory
   Medicine,
The Glenfield Hospital,
Groby Road,
Leicester LE3 9QP,
UK.

P.D. PARÉ
Professor
Department of Medicine,
University of British Columbia,
St Paul's Hospital,
1081 Burrard Street,
Vancouver BC,
Canada V6Z 1Y6.

M.G. PEARSON
Consultant Physician
Aintree Chest Clinic,
Regional Thoracic Unit,
Fazakerley Hospital,
Longmoor Lane,
Liverpool L9 7AL,
UK.

D.S. POSTMA
Professor
Department of Pulmonary Diseases,
University Hospital,
Oostersingel 59,
9713 EZ Groningen,
The Netherlands.

N.B. PRIDE
Professor
Department of Medicine,
(Respiratory Division),
Hammersmith Hospital,
Du Cane Road,
London W12 0NN,
UK.

T.E.J. RENKEMA
Department of Pulmonology,
University Hospital,
Oostersingel 59,
9713 EZ Groningen,
The Netherlands.

J. ROCA
Associate Professor of Medicine,
Chief of Section,
Hospital Clinic-Servei de Pneumologia,
Villarroel 170,
08036 Barcelona,
Spain.

R. RODRIGUEZ-ROISIN
Professor of Medicine,
Chief of Service,
Hospital Clinic-Servei de Pneumologia,
Villarroel 170,
08036 Barcelona,
Spain.

G.L. SNIDER
Professor of Medicine,
Boston University School of Medicine,
150 South Huntington Avenue,
Boston MA 02130,
USA.

R.A. STOCKLEY
Reader in Respiratory Medicine,
Lung Immunobiochemical Research
    Laboratory,
Clinical Teaching Block,
General Hospital,
Steelhouse Lane,
Birmingham B4 6NH,
UK.

D.P. STRACHAN
Senior Lecturer in Epidemiology,
Department of Public Health Sciences,
St George's Hospital Medical School,
Cranmer Terrace,
London SW17 0RE,
UK.

M.J. TOBIN
Professor of Medicine,
Loyola University of Chicago,
Stricht School of Medicine,
Edward Hines Jr Veterans Administration
    Hospital,
Hines IL 60141,
USA.

A.G. WILSON
Consultant Radiologist,
St George's Hospital,
Blackshaw Road,
London SW17 0QT,
UK.

FOREWORD

Historically, the recognition of pulmonary emphysema and, less certainly, of chronic bronchitis can probably be attributed to Laennec. The two conditions became coupled and the relationship confused throughout the latter part of the last century and the first part of this. In the 1940s, the common story was as follows. Acute bronchitis is a bacterial infection, usually following viral upper respiratory infection. In some people, this acute bronchitis invariably followed such upper respiratory infections and persisted for increasingly long periods until, for most of the winter, they had cough and sputum. They were then said to have chronic bronchitis. This went on for years until they began to have troublesome breathlessness. At which time, it was thought that their lungs were destroyed by emphysema. This put a strain on the right heart and they became edematous and were said to have cor pulmonale. Usually, they died during an acute infection, and probably in respiratory failure but blood gases were not, of course, measurable until the 1960s. Throughout the 1930s, 1940s and 1950s, the situation was complicated by a difference in verbal habits on the two sides of the Atlantic. In Britain, many patients were said to have chronic bronchitis who, in the United States, were said to have emphysema. The situation was greatly clarified by the CIBA Symposium in 1958 which gave a sound basis for the discrimination of chronic bronchitis, emphysema and asthma, and led to the adoption of terms such as chronic airflow obstruction or chronic obstructive lung disease. Recognition of the common factor of chronic airflow obstruction or limitation can fairly be attributed to the Bellevue group in the late 1930s, and of emphysema and its subtypes to Gough.

In the late 1950s, it was recognized that bronchitis and emphysema did not necessarily follow each other in the order outlined above. Some patients died with little evidence of emphysema; some patients with emphysema had little bronchitis. With the advent of methods for measuring blood gases, it also became recognized that the hypoxaemia which was quite profound during acute infections required careful management; otherwise the patient died in CO_2 narcosis. It is to be wondered that until the 1950s cigarette smoking was not linked as an important factor in either chronic bronchitis or emphysema.

The chapters in this book fill out this sketch, give authoritative accounts of recent developments, point out the areas of ignorance and thus indicate the likely paths of future research.

When I was a student and houseman, chronic bronchitis and emphysema were unfashionable diseases, not generally seen in teaching hospitals and the vestige of this neglect is perhaps the fact that this is one of the few books devoted to the subject of chronic airflow obstruction.

E.J.M. Campbell

PREFACE

Chronic obstructive pulmonary disease (COPD) is one of the commonest respiratory diseases of the developed world. It kills many more people each year than does bronchial asthma and has a similar prevalence in adults but has not attracted an equivalent amount of attention from either research funding agencies or textbook writers. This surprising state of affairs is likely to have several causes. COPD is perceived as being a 'dull' chronic illness with undramatic physical signs which result from largely irreversible lung damage. As a result prognosis cannot usually be radically altered and is often the patient's own fault for having smoked. We reject this view and this book is an attempt to redress this unduly pessimistic perception. It cannot hope to be comprehensive given the wide range of disciplines needed to understand all aspects of COPD but we hope that the reader will find insights into the scientific basis of this illness and some guidance on the practical care of these patients.

Much of the scientific basis of COPD which is the subject of the first chapters is far from settled. Even the definition, particularly the borderlands between COPD and persistent asthma, remains controversial (indeed the remaining chapters diverge from Chapter 1 in *not* following the recommendation to include incompletely reversible asthma as a sub-category of COPD). Readers coming fresh to the field may be surprised that it is still unclear whether airway disease (Chapter 3) or emphysema (Chapter 2) is the more important factor determining obstruction; perhaps we are on the edge of some quan-

titative morphology of airways and airspace with increasing concentration on the microscopic rather than the macroscopic changes in lung structure ('the doughnut, not the hole'). Epidemiologic studies not only perform their traditional role of defining the scale of the problem, but have been important in defining the 'preclinical' course of the disease. The proteolytic theory of emphysema has provided a rational biochemical basis for the disease but remains a reasonable theory rather than an established fact, a point stressed in Chapter 6. Apart from their intellectual value these differing pathologic, etiologic and biochemical approaches have identified areas where intervention may modify the natural history. The most familiar is smoking cessation but modifications of small airways 'inflammation' by corticosteroids or even enhancement of antiprotease activity by appropriate supplementations are all under active investigation.

Physiologic abnormalities in lung mechanics, gas exchange and ventilatory control have been exhaustively studied and explain most of the clinical features with which the COPD patient presents. Even here new data are still emerging to challenge previous orthodoxy. The role of pulmonary hyperinflation especially in acute and chronic respiratory failure in COPD, the new understanding of ventilation–perfusion abnormalities using the multiple inert gas elimination technique and the importance of behavioral influences on the control of breathing are all relatively recent themes under-represented in most textbooks. The activities of the respiratory muscles and how they cope with the altered geometry of advanced COPD now merits separate consideration. Much of the research which led to long-term domiciliary oxygen treatment was based on studies of pulmonary circulation and its effects on cardiac function and fluid retention. This is reviewed in detail in Chapter 11 where some of the contradictions and misconceptions of the terms cor pulmonale and right heart failure are highlighted with the aid of more current investigational methods. Finally, the role of sleep and sleep-disordered breathing in the genesis of the daytime complications of COPD are authoritatively addressed in Chapter 12.

The remaining chapters look at the diagnosis, investigation and management of the COPD patient, hopefully in an equally critical fashion. They stress the importance of physiologic assessment for both the diagnosis and treatment selection and the range of imaging techniques available as well as their limitations. In considering management a graded approach seems reasonable. Thus all continuing smokers will need advice about nicotine withdrawal (Chapter 15) whilst many will benefit from symptomatic bronchodilator therapy although the exact choice of dose and type of drug may vary with the circumstance as indicated in Chapter 17. At present guidelines for routine corticosteroid prescription are lacking and the evidence of the benefits of this treatment are reviewed in Chapter 18. Many patients will present for the first time to hospital in an acute exacerbation and the modern approach to diagnosis and management is comprehensively addressed in Chapter 19. The more severe patient will need more specialized rehabilitation which will certainly include assessment for domiciliary oxygen (Chapters 20 and 21) as well as exclusion of surgically resectable bullous disease (Chapter 22). For the younger patient single or double lung transplantation may offer an escape from otherwise inevitable early death. Whether this treatment will be widely used is as likely to depend on the availability of donor organs as on technical considerations as pointed out in Chapter 23.

Although this book considers many aspects of COPD we have not specifically addressed the politics of its principal cause, tobacco smoking. Others better qualified than ourselves have already done so and we feel that to do so here would merely be to preach to the converted. Yet the global impact of tobacco is enormous and as the pressures increase within the developed world to restrict its consumption so the commercial energies of the relevant multinationals have switched their merchandising to the easier markets of the developing world and in particular the rapidly expanding economies of the Pacific rim. Given this depressing development it is likely that COPD will continue to be an important component of the work of all respiratory physicians. Moreover, since many patients who stop smoking in their fifties may still have done sufficient damage to develop physiologically important COPD in their seventies all responsible for the care of older patients are likely to be seeing new cases of this widespread illness.

This book would not have been completed without a great deal of effort by many people. We are especially grateful to our distinguished contributors who have borne the vagaries of our extended editing, resultant faxes and rewriting with great patience and understanding. It is a particular pleasure for us to have a forward by Professor Moran Campbell whose contributions to COPD through his insights into respiratory mechanics and breathlessness and his impact on patient care with the development of controlled oxygen therapy made him our obvious choice. Our secretaries have coped stoically with the further burden this project has produced in an already busy schedule whilst Ms Annalisa Page, the Commissioning Editor from Chapman & Hall, has shepherded us with patience and perseverance to the end of this project which has proven to be a greater task than either the Editors or she initially envisaged. The publishers hope the use of American spelling will make this book accessible to a wider market.

Finally, our wives and families have, as ever, had to put up with even more disruption than is their usual lot and for their sakes as well as that of our present and future patients we hope that you feel that the effort has been worthwhile.

Peter Calverley
Neil Pride

GLOSSARY OF ABBREVIATIONS

RESPIRATORY MECHANICS

STATIC LUNG VOLUMES

TLC	Total lung capacity
VC	(Slow) vital capacity
RV	Residual volume
FRC	Functional residual capacity (= end-expiratory volume)
Vr	Relaxation volume of the respiratory system

SINGLE BREATH N_2 TEST

SBN_2	Single breath nitrogen test
CV	Closing volume
CC	Closing capacity (sum of residual volume and closing volume)

CONTROL OF BREATHING

V_T	Tidal volume
T_I	Inspiratory time
T_E	Expiratory time
T_{TOT}	Total respiratory cycle time
$\dot{V}_E$	Expired minute ventilation
$P_{0.1}$	Mouth occlusion pressure 0.1 s after onset of inspiration

FORCED VITAL CAPACITY MANEUVRES

FEV_1	Forced expiratory volume in one second
FVC	Forced vital capacity
MEFV	Maximum expiratory flow-volume

MIFV	Maximum inspiratory flow-volume
MBC	Maximum breathing capacity
PEF	Peak expiratory flow
PIF	Peak inspiratory flow
$\dot{V}_E$ max	Maximum expiratory flow
$\Delta\dot{V}max_{50}$	Difference between maximum expiratory flow at 50% vital capacity breathing air and breathing a helium–oxygen mixture
$Viso\dot{V}$	Volume at which maximum expiratory flow is same breathing air and a helium–oxygen mixture
IVPF	iso-volume pressure-flow

MECHANICS OF BREATHING

Pressure measurements

P_L	Static transpulmonary pressure (syn. lung recoil pressure)
P_L max	P_L at TLC
Palv	Alveolar pressure
Ppl	Pleural pressure
Ppl min	Lowest Ppl during a maximum inspiratory effort
P_I max	Lowest mouth pressure during a maximum inspiratory effort
P_E max	Highest mouth pressure during a maximum expiratory effort
Pab	Abdominal pressure
Pdi	Transdiaphragmatic pressure (= Pab – Ppl)
Pdi max	Pdi during a maximum inspiratory effort

Pao	Pressure at airway opening (mouth, nose or tracheotomy)
PEEPi	Intrinsic positive end-expiratory pressure
TTdi	Tension–time index of diaphragm
CPAP	Continuous positive airway pressure

Resistance and compliance

Raw	Airways resistance
SGaw	Specific airway conductance
Rrs	Total respiratory resistance
ΔRrs	Additional total respiratory resistance
Est,rs	Static elastance of respiratory system
Edyn,L	Dynamic elastance of lungs
Cdyn,L	Dynamic compliance of lungs
PV	Static pressure–volume curve of the lungs
k	Shape factor of PV curve
Gus	Upstream conductance (ratio of maximum expiratory flow/P_L)

Work of breathing

W_I,rs	Total inspiratory work (static and dynamic) on the respiratory system
W_Ist,rs	Static component of total inspiratory work
$W_I,PEEPi$	Static work required to overcome PEEPi
W_Idyn,rs	Dynamic component of total inspiratory work
W_I,aw	Dynamic work to overcome subject's airway resistance
W_I,L	Dynamic work due to time constant inequality and viscoelastic pressure dissipation
W_I,w	Dynamic work to overcome chest wall tissue resistance

BLOOD AND ALVEOLAR GAS EXCHANGE AND PULMONARY CIRCULATION

BLOOD AND ALVEOLAR O_2 AND CO_2

SaO_2	arterial O_2 saturation
CaO_2	arterial O_2 content
DO_2	O_2 delivery
PaO_2	Arterial O_2 tension
$PaCO_2$	Arterial CO_2 tension
PAO_2	Alveolar O_2 tension
PAO_2–PaO_2	Alveolar–arterial PO_2 difference
$P\bar{v}O_2$	Mixed venous O_2 tension
$PtcO_2$	Transcutaneous O_2 tension
$PACO_2$	Alveolar CO_2 tension
$PetCO_2$	End tidal CO_2 tension
$\dot{V}O_2$	O_2 consumption
$\dot{V}O_2$ max	maximum O_2 consumption
$\dot{V}CO_2$	CO_2 production
RQ	Respiratory quotient
RE	Respiratory exchange ratio
FIO_2	Fractional concentration of O_2 in inspired air
$\dot{Q}$	Cardiac output
$\dot{V}A$	Alveolar ventilation
$\dot{V}A/\dot{Q}$	Ventilation–perfusion ratio
VD	Dead space
VD/VT	Dead space as a proportion of tidal volume
$\dot{Q}s/\dot{Q}t$	Proportion of shunt to total cardiac output

CARBON MONOXIDE TRANSFER

$TLCO$	Carbon monoxide transfer factor (syn. diffusing capacity for CO, $DLCO$)
$TLCO/VA$	TLCO per unit alveolar volume (VA) (syn. carbon monoxide transfer coefficient)
KCO	Krogh constant for CO, analogous to $TLCO/VA$

PULMONARY CIRCULATION

Ppa	Pulmonary artery pressure
Ppw	Pulmonary artery wedge pressure
Ppv	Pulmonary venous pressure

DEFINING CHRONIC OBSTRUCTIVE PULMONARY DISEASE

G.L. Snider

'Then you should say what you mean,' the March Hare went on.
'I do,' Alice hastily replied; 'at least – at least I mean what I say – that's the same thing, you know.'
'Not the same thing a bit!' said the Hatter. 'You might just as well say that "I see what I eat" is the same thing as "I eat what I see"!'

A Mad Tea Party
Alice's Adventures in Wonderland
Lewis Carroll [1]

That the initial chapter of this book is on the definition of chronic obstructive pulmonary disease (COPD) reflects not only the confusion that exists in the field of the obstructive airflow diseases [2], but also the confusion in nosology and definitions that has historically pervaded all of medicine. There is not even a generally accepted definition of the widely used term 'disease'. In this essay, I shall first deal with the concept and definition of the term 'disease' and how it is generally used in medical discourse. I shall then turn to a treatment of the issues associated with the definition and use of the term 'COPD'. Before proceeding, I would like to pay tribute to J.G. Scadding, whose thoughtful, rigorous work on the meaning of terms used in medicine, published over the last 3 decades, has helped enormously to clarify my thinking in this area [3–8].

1.1 THE CONCEPT OF DISEASE

1.1.1 HISTORICAL OVERVIEW

In the era of Hippocrates, disease was considered to be a purely clinical phenomenon; terms such as fever, dropsy or cyanosis were used as names of diseases. During the 17th century, Thomas Sydenham founded the discipline of nosology by insisting that diseases had their own natural history and could be described and classified on the basis of their specific characteristics [9]. This concept did not have a major impact until the latter part of the 19th century, when the observational techniques of physical examination – percussion, auscultation, sphygmomanometry and thermometry had been developed [9,10]. The correlation of first the gross and later the microscopic findings at necropsy with the clinical history and physical examination completely changed the concepts and names of diseases. This process accelerated in the 20th century as a result of a torrent of new information coming from radiography, ultrasonography and other biophysical techniques of imaging, and from epidemiology,

Chronic Obstructive Pulmonary Disease. Edited by Dr P. Calverley and Professor N. Pride. Published in 1995 by Chapman & Hall, London. ISBN 0 412 46450 0

microbiology, immunology, biochemistry, electron microscopy and molecular genetics.

1.1.2 DEFINITION OF DISEASE

It is important in nosology that the names of diseases not be used as if they were independent morbid entities with external existences that are causing the patient's illness. In the terms of philosophy, this approach represents a realist or essentialist definition [8,11,12]. An example of such usage would be to say that a patient was ill because of COPD. Such usage has inappropriate implications for therapy and also implies that there is a finite number of diseases in the universe.

The names of diseases should be considered verbal symbols designed to refer to an area of interest. In the terms of philosophy, this approach represents a nominalist definition. An example of such usage would be to say that the patient's diagnosis was COPD. This usage implies that diseases are due to interactions between the host and one or more causes of disease, thus permitting a potentially infinite number of interactions. The name of a disease is a relatively arbitrary way of referring to a particular patient's illness that is useful in communication. It is an abbreviated way of referring to groups of patients who have some common features to their illness.

Scadding [8] has provided a useful definition, which may be paraphrased as follows:

> The name of a disease should refer to the abnormal phenomena displayed by a group of persons who have a specified characteristic by which they differ from the norm in a way that is biologically disadvantageous.

The name of a disease should be as brief and descriptive as possible. It may be used in the title of an investigative report and it provides a convenient means of communication between patient and health-care givers. It is almost never possible to formulate a proper treatment plan simply from the name of a disease used as a diagnosis. The name of a disease need give no indication of its cause. Even when a disease is defined in terms of etiology, using the name of the disease as the patient's diagnosis gives only limited information as to its manifestations in the sick person. The diagnosis of tuberculosis reveals that a disease is present that is caused by *Mycobacterium tuberculosis*, but gives little indication of the exact nature of the patient's illness or even whether an illness is overtly manifest.

1.1.3 THE DEFINING CHARACTERISTICS

Concise definitions of the names of diseases can be developed using as the defining characteristics the common properties specifying the group of abnormal persons upon whom the description of a disease is based [4]. The characteristics specifying the population of interest may have different origins. The specifying characteristic may be a consistent syndrome (a set of clinical findings) whose etiology is unknown; it may be a specified disorder of structure or function of unknown etiology; or it may be the effects in persons of a particular etiologic agent [4,8]. These three levels indicate increasing knowledge of the disease, and they therefore acquire a progressively higher priority as a defining characteristic. The clinical features of a disease have the lowest priority, altered structure or function are intermediate, and etiology has the highest priority. It is apparent that according to this scheme, the name and the definition of a disease may change as new knowledge is acquired. However, the current definition should leave no doubt about the field of study from which the defining characteristic is drawn.

1.1.4 COMPOUND DEFINITIONS

A group of patients selected because they have a common characteristic in one field of study, will not necessarily share common characteristics in another field. Compound definitions, which utilize defining characteristics from two or more fields of study, may define subsets of patients with overlapping characteristics [8]. For example, pneumococcal pneumonia represents an overlapping subset of patients with pneumonia (defined in pathologic terms) and infection with *S. pneumoniae* (defined in etiologic terms).

1.1.5 DESCRIPTION OF A DISEASE

Once a disease has been defined, the next step is to study subjects with the defining characteristics by all available means, thus determining all ascertainable features. In this way the description of the disease is established, including features that are of frequent as well as of infrequent occurrence. If the population studied is large enough, the frequency of inconstant features can be estimated, although we do not usually redefine the disease in order to include the inconstant features.

1.1.6 DIAGNOSTIC CRITERIA

From the description of the disease, diagnostic criteria can be chosen, which are found in practice to best distinguish the disease from other diseases that resemble it. The diagnostic criteria may or may not include features of the defining criteria. When the defining characteristic is clinically based the diagnostic criteria must perforce include them. However, when the diagnostic criteria are based on etiology, the diagnostic criteria may not include the defining characteristics. For example, the diagnosis of viral diseases is regularly made without directly demonstrating the presence of the virus in the patient. The diagnosis of mitral stenosis may be made with considerable confidence from the characteristic heart murmur, and with more confidence by echocardiography or physiologic data from heart catheterization.

Although echocardiography comes closest as a surrogate, none of these methods actually demonstrate the pathology that is the defining characteristic of mitral stenosis. The validity of the diagnostic criteria should be established by appropriate correlative studies.

1.2 OBSTRUCTIVE AIRWAY DISEASES

1.2..1 HISTORICAL OVERVIEW

The occurrence of diseases characterized by cough, expectoration, wheezing, dyspnea, first on exercise, and later at rest has been known at least since the time of Hippocrates [13]. Floyer gave us the first clear description of asthma in the early part of the 18th century [14]. Through the early 19th century, the term asthma was used synonymously with dyspnea. Percussion was invented by Leopold Auenbrugger about 1751 but his 1761 report of his findings was given little notice by physicians until the publication in 1808 of Corvisart's translation into French of Auenbrugger's work [15]. The interest of the Parisian school in pathologic–clinical correlation, and the addition of the stethoscope to the tools of physical diagnosis by Laennec [16,17], began attempts to classify patients with obstructive airway diseases. Laennec used the term pulmonary or bronchial catarrh, from the Greek word meaning 'to flow down' for excessive production of bronchopulmonary secretion, and he defined emphysema as we know it today. Charles Badham introduced the term bronchitis into medicine in 1808 [18].

In the mid-20th century, as tuberculosis came under control, the increasing morbidity and mortality from chronic obstructive respiratory diseases was recognized [19]. Studies were undertaken to determine the nature, frequency and causes of these disorders. In 1958, a Ciba Foundation Guest Symposium was convened and subsequently published the first attempt to achieve a consensus on definitions of disorders associated with chronic airflow obstruction [20]. In 1962 definitions that were similar to those of the Ciba Symposium were published by the American Thoracic Society [21]. The subsequent history of definitions of these diseases has been reviewed recently by Samet [22].

1.2.2 CHRONIC BRONCHITIS

Chronic bronchitis is defined for epidemiologic purposes as the presence of chronic productive cough for three months in each of two successive years in a patient in whom other causes of chronic cough, such as infection with *Mycobacterium tuberculosis*, carcinoma of the lung, and chronic congestive heart failure, have been excluded [20,21]. It is practical for clinical purposes to define chronic bronchitis more simply as chronic productive cough, without a medically discernible cause, present for more than half the time for two years. This definition, based on symptoms, reflects our current state of knowledge regarding this condition.

Pathologic changes in the large and small airways have been described in chronic bronchitis, but the changes are non-specific, reflecting the relatively limited ways in which the airways can respond to injury [23] (Chapter 2). Tobacco smoking has been identified as the major risk factor for the development of chronic bronchitis and a number of other factors have been identified as less important risk factors [24–27] (Chapters 4 and 5). However, the risk factors are multiple and the proportion of individuals exposed to these agents who develop chronic bronchitis is relatively small – 15–20% [28]. The combination of multiple risk factors, and incomplete knowledge of etiology makes it impossible to use etiology as a defining characteristic for chronic bronchitis.

1.2.3 ASTHMA

Asthma was defined by the American Thoracic Society [21] as a disease character-ized by an increased responsiveness of the trachea and bronchi to various stimuli and manifested by a widespread narrowing of the airways that changes in severity either spontaneously or as a result of therapy. Subsequent official groups [29,30] have not substantially changed this definition.

1.2.4 EMPHYSEMA

Emphysema has been defined in morphologic terms since the Ciba symposium [20]. There have been clarifications from time to time [21,29,30,31]. In the latest of these [31], respiratory airspace enlargement was classified into three categories.

- Simple airspace enlargement is defined as enlargement of the respiratory airspaces without destruction. It may be congenital, as in Down's syndrome, or acquired, as in the overdistention of the contralateral lung that follows pneumonectomy.
- Emphysema is defined as a condition of the lung characterized by abnormal permanent enlargement of the airspaces distal to the terminal bronchioles accompanied by destruction of their walls and without obvious fibrosis. Destruction is defined as non-uniformity in the pattern of respiratory airspace enlargement; the orderly appearance of the acinus and its components is disturbed and may be lost.
- Airspace enlargement with fibrosis occurs with obvious fibrosis, such as associated with infectious granulomatous disease such as tuberculosis, noninfectious granulomatous disease such as sarcoidosis, or fibrosis of undetermined etiology. The scarring is readily evident in the chest radiograph, or in the inflation-fixed lung specimen, and is apparent to the naked eye. This form of airspace enlargement with fibrosis was formerly termed irregular or paracicatricial emphysema [21]. It is not included under the umbrella of COPD. The separation of airspace enlargement

with fibrosis and emphysema is not as clean as at first appears. In a recent review [19] I suggested that emphysema is multi-factorial in its pathogenesis and respiratory airspace enlargement is a stereotyped response of the lungs to a variety of injuries. Fibrosis may be part of the healing process after some injuries. Microscopic fibrosis is observed in the microbullae of centriacinar emphysema and these lesions may represent focal airspace enlargement with fibrosis. In the light of current thinking, the older term 'paracicatricial emphysema' seems more apropos than the current term 'airspace enlargement with fibrosis'.

1.2.5 CHRONIC OBSTRUCTIVE PULMONARY DISEASE

Chronic bronchitis [27] and emphysema [32] occur with or without airflow obstruction. Asthma, by definition [8,21] is associated at some time in its course with discernible airflow obstruction, although in variant asthma, special maneuvers may be necessary to make it evident. The diagnosis of mild or even moderate emphysema is not readily made during life except with computerized tomography (Chapter 14). Furthermore, chronic bronchitis and emphysema usually occur together [33]. Asthmatic individuals exposed to chronic irritation, as from cigarette smoke, may develop chronic productive cough, a feature of chronic bronchitis. Asthmatics may develop non-remitting airflow obstruction. Emphysema and asthma may coexist by coincidence. Patients without evidence of atopy who develop chronic bronchitis and emphysema as a result of long-standing cigarette smoking may develop increased reactivity of the airways that is responsive to bronchodilator drugs [34]; airways hyper-reactivity is an important feature of asthma.

Accordingly, precise classification of the disease of a patient with chronic productive cough with airflow obstruction may be difficult. A variety of terms have come into common usage to identify patients who have evidence of one or more of chronic bronchitis, asthma or emphysema with airflow obstruction. These terms, used synonymously, are chronic obstructive lung disease, chronic obstructive airways disease and the term used in this book, chronic obstructive pulmonary disease. The terms chronic non-specific lung disease and generalized obstructive lung disease [25] and chronic generalized airways obstruction [30] have never come into wide use.

The term COPD has been applied to patients who have airflow obstruction, manifested either clinically or by an abnormality in a standard spirometric index such as the FEV_1 [29,33]. The profession has not developed a generally agreed upon definition of COPD.

We can deal with the combination of chronic bronchitis defined in clinical terms, emphysema in anatomic terms, and airflow obstruction representing a physiologic state by using a compound definition.

> Chronic obstructive pulmonary disease is defined as a disease state characterized by the presence of chronic bronchitis and/or emphysema associated with airflow obstruction; the airflow obstruction may be accompanied by airways hyper-reactivity and may be partially reversible.

Figure 1.1 is a non-proportional Venn diagram, which shows the relations among chronic bronchitis, emphysema, asthma and airflow obstruction; the shaded band encloses the subsets comprising COPD. Patients who have features of chronic bronchitis or emphysema without airflow obstruction (subsets 1 and 2) are not considered to have COPD. The largest subset of patients with COPD is subset 5, patients who have features of both chronic bronchitis and emphysema. Patients who have completely reversible airways obstruction without features of chronic bronchitis or emphysema are classified as having asthma

CHRONIC OBSTRUCTIVE PULMONARY DISEASE

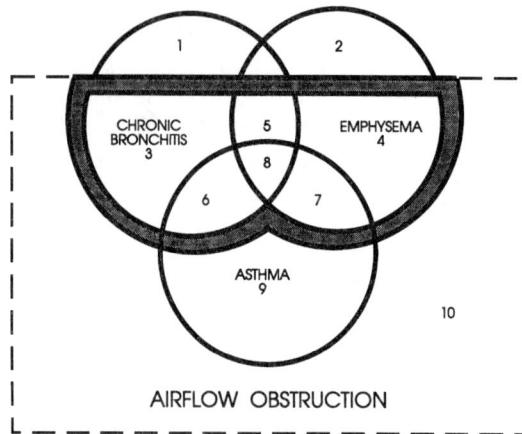

Fig. 1.1 Schema of chronic obstructive pulmonary disease. A non-proportional Venn diagram shows subsets of patients with chronic bronchitis, emphysema, and asthma in three overlapping circles; the shaded band encloses the subsets comprising COPD. Subsets of patients lying within the rectangle have airway obstruction. Subset 10 includes patients with airflow limitation that is not considered to be COPD such as cystic fibrosis and obliterative bronchiolitis. Patients in subset 1 and 2 have clinical or radiographic features of chronic bronchitis or emphysema; since they do not have airways obstruction as determined by an index such as the FEV_1, they are not classified as having COPD. Patients with unequivocal asthma (subset 9) defined as having completely reversible airways obstruction, are not classified as having COPD. Patients in subsets 6 and 7 have partially reversible airways obstruction with chronic productive cough or emphysema, respectively; since it is difficult to be certain whether such patients have asthma or whether they have developed bronchial hyper-reactivity as a complication of chronic bronchitis or emphysema they are included within COPD. Patients in subset 8 have features of all 3 disorders. Patients in subset 3 have chronic productive cough with airways obstruction but no emphysema; it is not known how large this subset is, since only limited epidemiologic studies using computerized tomography to diagnose emphysema are available. It is much easier to identify patients with emphysema in the chest radiograph who do not have chronic bronchitis (subset 4). Many patients who require medical care for their disease have features of both chronic bronchitis and emphysema and fall into subset 5.

(subset 9) and are not included within COPD. As a practical matter, patients whose asthma is characterized by incomplete remission of airways obstruction have been included as a subset of COPD (subsets 6–8) because it is often not possible to differentiate these individuals from persons with chronic bronchitis and emphysema who have partly reversible airways obstruction. It is apparent that those who use airflow obstruction as the sole defining characteristic of COPD would include all patients with asthma under this rubric. Although some authors have done so [35], patients with airways obstruction due to diseases with known etiology or specific pathology, such as cystic fibrosis or obliterative bronchiolitis, are not included in this definition.

In epidemiology, precise diagnostic criteria, and questionnaires that reflect them, have been developed for chronic productive cough and for features such as dyspnea on effort, which are descriptors of the disease [22]. Until the disease is severe, emphysema can only be diagnosed accurately by an imaging technique. The diagnosis of a patient's illness as COPD does not provide sufficient information to plan therapy and to make a prognosis; these are based on the physician's assessment of the nature of the pathology and pathophysiology, the history of response to previous treatment and other factors that cannot be epitomized in the name of a disease.

How should one deal with exceptions, for example, the smoker with bronchiolar inflammation and airflow obstruction but without productive cough or emphysema? Such patients are sometimes referred to as small airway disease and do not fit the diagnostic criteria of COPD. The diagnosis is readily recorded as airflow obstruction due to bronchiolitis (subset 10, Fig. 1.1).

Exceptions are to be expected, given the concept that there is a potentially infinite number of interactions between different hosts and an etiologic agent of disease. It is not possible to develop a definition of a disease that will encompass every exception.

Since the introduction of a code for COPD into the Ninth International Classification of Diseases, there has been a progressive shift of causes of death into this category from those for chronic bronchitis and emphysema [36]. This reflects clinical pathologic correlations showing that airflow obstruction can be due to both airway disease and emphysema and the difficulty of accurately diagnosing emphysema in life, until it is severe [28,32]. One approach to defining COPD is offered here. It is my hope that this presentation will initiate discussions in the pulmonary community that will lead to a widely accepted definition of the commonly used term 'COPD'.

REFERENCES

1. Carroll, Lewis (pseudonym of C.L. Dodgson) (1865) *Alice's Adventures in Wonderland*, R. Clay, Son, and Taylor, London, pp. 98.
2. Pride, N.B., Vermiere, P. and Allegra, L. (1989) Diagnostic labels applied to model case histories of chronic airflow obstruction. Responses to a questionnaire in 11 North American and Western European countries. *Eur. Resp. J.*, **2**, 702–9.
3. Scadding, J.G. (1959) Principles of definition in medicine. *Lancet*, **1**, 323–5.
4. Scadding, J.G. (1963) Meaning of diagnostic terms in bronchopulmonary disease. *Br. Med. J.*, **2**, 1425–30.
5. Scadding, J.G. (1972) The semantics of medical diagnosis. *Biomedical Computing*, **3**, 83–90.
6. Scadding, J.G. (1981) Talking clearly about bronchopulmonary diseases, in *Scientific Foundations of Respiratory Medicine* (eds J.G. Scadding and G. Cummings), Heinemann Medical Books, London, pp. 727–34.
7. Scadding, J.G. (1988) Health and disease: what can medicine do for philosophy? *J. Med. Ethics*, **14**, 118–24.
8. Scadding, J.G. (1993) Definition of asthma, in *Bronchial Asthma, Mechanisms and Therapeutics*, 3rd edn (eds E.B. Weiss and M. Stein), Little Brown, Boston, pp. 1–13.
9. Garrison, F.H. (1929) *An Introduction to the History of Medicine*, Saunders, Philadelphia, pp. 269–71.
10. Feinstein, A.R. (1973) An analysis of diagnostic reasoning; 1. The domains and disorders of clinical macrobiology. *Yale J. Biol. Med.*, **46**, 212–32.
11. Allbutt, T.C. (1896) Introduction, in *A System of Medicine* (ed. T.C. Allbutt), Macmillan, New York, pp. xxi–xxxix.
12. Crookshank, F.G. (1956) The importance of a theory of signs and a critique of language in the study of medicine, in *The Meaning of Meaning* (first published in 1923) (eds C.K. Ogden and I.A. Richards), Harcourt Brace Jovanovich, New York, pp. 327–55.
13. Adams, F. (1849) *The Genuine Works of Hippocrates, Translated from the Greek, With a Preliminary Discourse and Annotations, Vol. II, Aphorisms iii – 12 and 31*, Sydenham Society, London, pp. 717–772.
14. Floyer, J. (1726) *A Treatise of the Asthma*, 3rd edn, Wilkin, London, pp. 201–2.
15. Garrison, F.H. (1929) *History of Medicine*, Saunders, Philadelphia, pp. 352–3.
16. Laennec, R.T.H. (1819) *De L'Auscultation Médiate, ou Traité du Diagnostic des Maladies des Poumons et du Coeur*, Tome Premier, J.-A Brosson et J.-S. Chaudé, Paris.
17. Laennec, R.T.H. (1835) *A Treatise on the Diseases of the Chest and on Mediate Auscultation*. Translated by John Forbes. From

the Fourth London Edition, Desilver, Thomas & Co, Philadelphia, pp. 135–63.

18. Badham, C. (1814) *An Essay on Bronchitis with a Supplement Containing Remarks on Simple Pulmonary Abscess*, 2nd edn, Callow, London, pp. 25–45.

19. Snider, G.L. (1992) Emphysema: the first two centuries – and beyond; a historical overview, with suggestions for future research. *Am. Rev. Respir. Dis.*, **146**, Part 1, 1334–44; Part 2, 1613–14.

20. Ciba Foundation Guest Symposium (1959) Terminology, definitions and classification of chronic pulmonary emphysema and related conditions. *Thorax*, **14**, 286–99.

21. American Thoracic Society (1962) Chronic bronchitis, asthma and pulmonary emphysema. A statement by the Committee on Diagnostic Standards for Nontuberculous Respiratory Diseases. *Am. Rev. Respir. Dis.*, **85**, 762–8.

22. Samet, J.M. (1989) Definitions and methodology in COPD research, in *Clinical Epidemiology of Chronic Obstructive Pulmonary Disease* (eds M.J. Hensley and N.A. Saunders), Marcel Dekker, New York, pp. 1–22.

23. Jeffery, P.K. (1991) Morphology of the airway wall in asthma and in chronic obstructive pulmonary disease. *Am. Rev. Respir. Dis.*, **143**, 1152–8.

24. US Surgeon General (1984) The Health Consequences of Smoking: Chronic Obstructive Lung Disease. USDHHS Publ No 84–50205, US Department of Human Services, Washington DC.

25. Hensley, M.J. and Saunders, N.A. (1989) *Clinical Epidemiology of Chronic Obstructive Pulmonary Disease*, Marcel Dekker, New York.

26. Sherrill, D.L., Lebowitz, M.D. and Burrows, B. (1990) Epidemiology of chronic obstructive pulmonary disease. *Clin. Chest Med.*, **11**, 375–88.

27. Higgins, M. (1991) Risk factors associated with chronic obstructive lung disease. *Ann. N.Y. Acad. Sci.*, **624**, 7–17.

28. Snider, G.L. (1989) Chronic obstructive pulmonary disease: a definition and implications of structural determinants of airflow obstruction for epidemiology. *Am. Rev. Resp. Dis.*, **140**, S3–S8.

29. American College of Chest Physicians/ American Thoracic Society (1975) Pulmonary terms and symbols. *Chest*, **67**, 583–93.

30. World Health Organization (1975) Epidemiology of chronic non-specific lung diseases. *Bull. WHO*, **52**, 251–60.

31. Snider, G.L., Kleinerman, J., Thurlbeck, W.M. and Bengali, Z.K. (1985) The definition of emphysema: Report of a National Heart, Lung and Blood Institute, Division of Lung Diseases, Workshop. *Am. Rev. Respir. Dis.*, **132**, 182–5.

32. Petty, T.L.. Silvers, W. and Stanford, R.E. (1987) Mild emphysema is associated with reduced elastic recoil and increased lung size, but not with airflow limitation. *Am. Rev. Respir. Dis.*, **136**, 867–76.

33. Burrows, B. (1990) Airways obstructive diseases: pathogenetic mechanisms and natural histories of the disorders. *Med. Clin. North Am.*, **74**, 547–60.

34. Dosman, J.A., Gomez, S.R. and Zhou, C. (1990) Relationship between airways responsiveness and the development of chronic obstructive pulmonary disease. *Med. Clin. North Am.*, **74**, 561–9.

35. Cherniack, N.S. (1991) Introduction, in *Chronic Obstructive Pulmonary Disease* (ed. N.S. Cherniack), Saunders, Philadelphia, pp. ix.

36. Feinlieb, M., Rosenberg, H.M., Collins, J.G. *et al.* (1989) Trends in COPD morbidity and mortality in the United States. *Am. Rev. Respir. Dis.*, **140**, S9–S18.

PATHOLOGY

D. Lamb

2.1 INTRODUCTION

The pathologic changes found in the lungs of patients with COPD and in particular those who progress to respiratory failure and death are complex and show poor correlation with the clinical patterns of functional abnormalities in life [1,2].

All patients with COPD show a fixed airflow limitation. As a pathologist I can imagine only two patterns of change which could give rise to fixed airway obstruction. These are narrowing of the airway lumen due to inflammatory scarring or due to loss of alveolar support to an airway wall (with or without associated scarring). In both cases the proposed basis of the airway obstruction is irreversible. Despite the apparent simplicity of these two alternatives there is no clear consensus among pathologists as to what is the structural basis of the functional abnormalities in COPD.

This lack of a clear consensus is due to several factors:

1. Clinical studies, of necessity, describe features pertaining to the patient as a whole whereas pathologic study may involve a single lung lobe or even a small biopsy.
2. Pathologic material does not allow recognition of purely functional abnormalities such as bronchoconstriction or the effects of variation in respiratory chemosensitivity and drive.
3. Most pathologic studies attempting to identify the structural basis of functional abnormalities in COPD have been based on either surgically resected material (lobes or lungs) for which preoperative pulmonary function data were available or autopsy material on end-stage COPD. Such studies have allowed a cross-sectional analysis at two moments in the natural history of COPD, without any longitudinal information to relate the changes identified in the early disease to those seen in the end-stage disease. That this may be an important problem can be seen by the current interest and emphasis on the importance of airway wall inflammation in 'early' or mild disease and the apparent emphasis given to gross structural abnormalities such as centri- and pan-acinar emphysema found in most autopsy studies.
4. A confusing element in any attempt to elucidate the relation between histologic or structural abnormality and function, is the common factor of smoking. Smoking is associated with a wide range of what may be considered epiphenomena, e.g. mucus gland hypertrophy, which in themselves may not be associated with the development of functional abnormality. We must be clear that any structural change which is proposed as a basis for airflow limitation must show not just a

Chronic Obstructive Pulmonary Disease. Edited by Dr P. Calverley and Professor N. Pride. Published in 1995 by Chapman & Hall, London. ISBN 0 412 46450 0

general relationship with function but a clear quantitative relationship between severity of the structural abnormality and the severity of airflow limitation or other functional abnormality, by bivariate analysis and, if possible, a better relationship than other possible proposed causes using a multivariate analysis. Any proposed structural cause must relate to the airflow limitation and explain the airflow limitation in mechanistic terms.

5. Many of the techniques described by pathologists to assess structure have in fact not been true measurements but 'grading', 'scoring' or 'picture matching' which do not provide a true quantitative measure of structure and have often been inappropriate to the statistical analyses carried out.

2.2 PULMONARY ANATOMY

The airway develops during intrauterine life and provides about 25 generations along the longest axial path between the hilum and diaphragm with a decrease in this number through childhood associated with de-differentiation into respiratory bronchioles. Airways can be divided into bronchi and bronchioli, the bronchi containing cartilage and mucus glands in their walls while bronchioles have no cartilage or glands. The bronchi can be further subdivided into large and small bronchi, the large bronchi have numerous cartilage plates which surround the lumen whereas the smaller bronchi have smaller and more infrequent cartilage plates which do not provide circumferential support. The more peripheral bronchi have such scanty and widely separated cartilage plates that a histologic cross-section may fall between small islands of cartilage.

The bronchioli extend from the last plate of cartilage to the terminal bronchiole, which is defined as the last bronchiole to have a complete wall and which precedes the respiratory bronchioles which have alveoli forming part of their walls. The respiratory bronchioles therefore fulfil both a gas transfer and a conducting role. The terminal bronchiole, apart from its position immediately preceding respiratory bronchioles is structurally identical to the preceding generations of bronchioles. Both the more peripheral bronchi lacking integral cartilage support, and bronchioles, depend on the surrounding lung for their integrity as conducting airways.

Alveoli adjacent to the airways are attached to the outer aspect of the walls (Fig. 2.1) and this support is essential for their conducting function. In cross-sections of airways the alveolar wall attachments appear as guy ropes attached to a single point but in three dimensions the attachments form an interconnecting linear support called by Linhartova 'the alveolar footprints' [3].

The term 'small airway' describes a concept rather than a specific anatomic group of airways. It is a term widely used to describe the site of the increased resistance in COPD and dates from the pioneer work of Hogg, Macklem and Thurlbeck [4]. The 'small airways' are often defined as being those airways less than 3 mm, or less than 2 mm, in diameter depending on the publication. These do not conform to any specific structural type of airways (small bronchi and/or bronchioli) or a particular generation number but rather reflect the original catheter size used in the in vitro experiments [5]. As airways vary in diameter related to body stature, defining a group of peripheral airways on size criteria only will identify different airway populations in those of small, and those of large body stature. It is important to realize that the many smaller bronchi lacking cartilage support and all non-respiratory bronchioles probably behave in a similar manner with regard to their need for support from the surrounding parenchyma.

2.3.1 THE ACINAR UNIT

The portion of the lung supplied by the terminal bronchiole is the functional unit of the

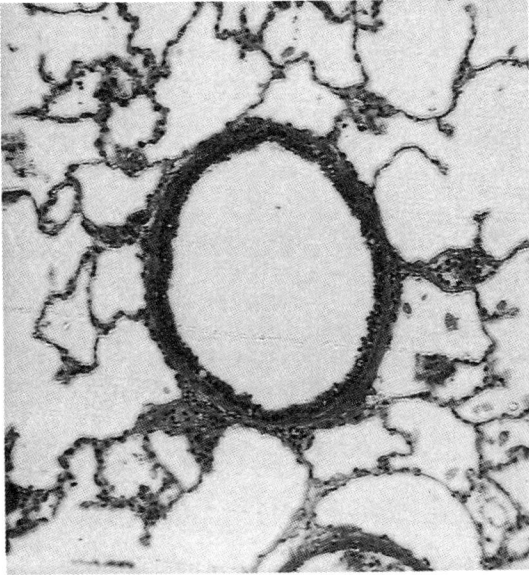

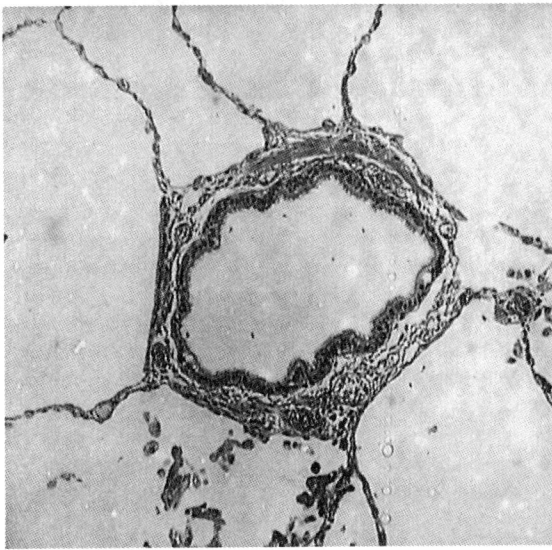

Fig. 2.1 Photomicrographs of two small airways cut in cross-section. (a) shows a small bronchiole from a normal non-smoking patient. The airway has a circular outline and the support provided by the adjacent alveolar walls in maintaining this is evident. (b) shows a small airway from a smoker with mild panacinar emphysema. The reduction in the alveolar walls and the number of their attachments to the airway are clearly seen. The airway has a mildly elliptical profile.

lung and this volume of lung tissue has had different terms applied to it: the primary lobule of Miller [6], the terminal respiratory unit [7] or the acinus [8]. Miller in fact described two lobules, the primary lobule being that volume of lung distal to the terminal bronchiole and the secondary lobule for the group of primary lobules arising from a common stem 'lobular bronchiole'. The supplying terminal bronchioles of the secondary lobule arise relatively close to one another and form the millimetre pattern seen on bronchograms in contrast to the 'lobular bronchioles' which form the centimetre pattern. It should be clear that there is no structural difference between these bronchioles but merely a difference in their arrangements. The adjacency of the terminal bronchioles within the secondary lobule explains the 'bunch of grapes' pattern of disease processes seen on the cut surface of a lung when the disease process involves the proximal parts of the acinar unit, e.g. centriacinar emphysema or bronchopneumonia (Fig. 2.2). There is much confusion, particularly among clinicians, between the primary and secondary lobules and for this reason the term acinus or acinar unit will be used in this text. It should, however, be clear that in the context of the definition and classification of emphysema the terms acinus, centriacinar emphysema and panacinar emphysema, are entirely and completely synonymous with lobule, centrilobular and panlobular emphysema. In man neither the acinar unit nor the secondary lobule of Miller is regularly demarcated by fibrous tissue septa, though septa are commoner at the periphery and margins of the lung and almost non-existent centrally. As a consequence there is the possibility of collateral drift via the pores of Kohn [9]. The importance of this has been questioned by in vivo studies of collateral ventilation during bronchoscopy in normal young adults [10]. The pathologists find no difficulty at autopsy in moving air around within a lobe in patients with panacinar emphysema and, to a lesser

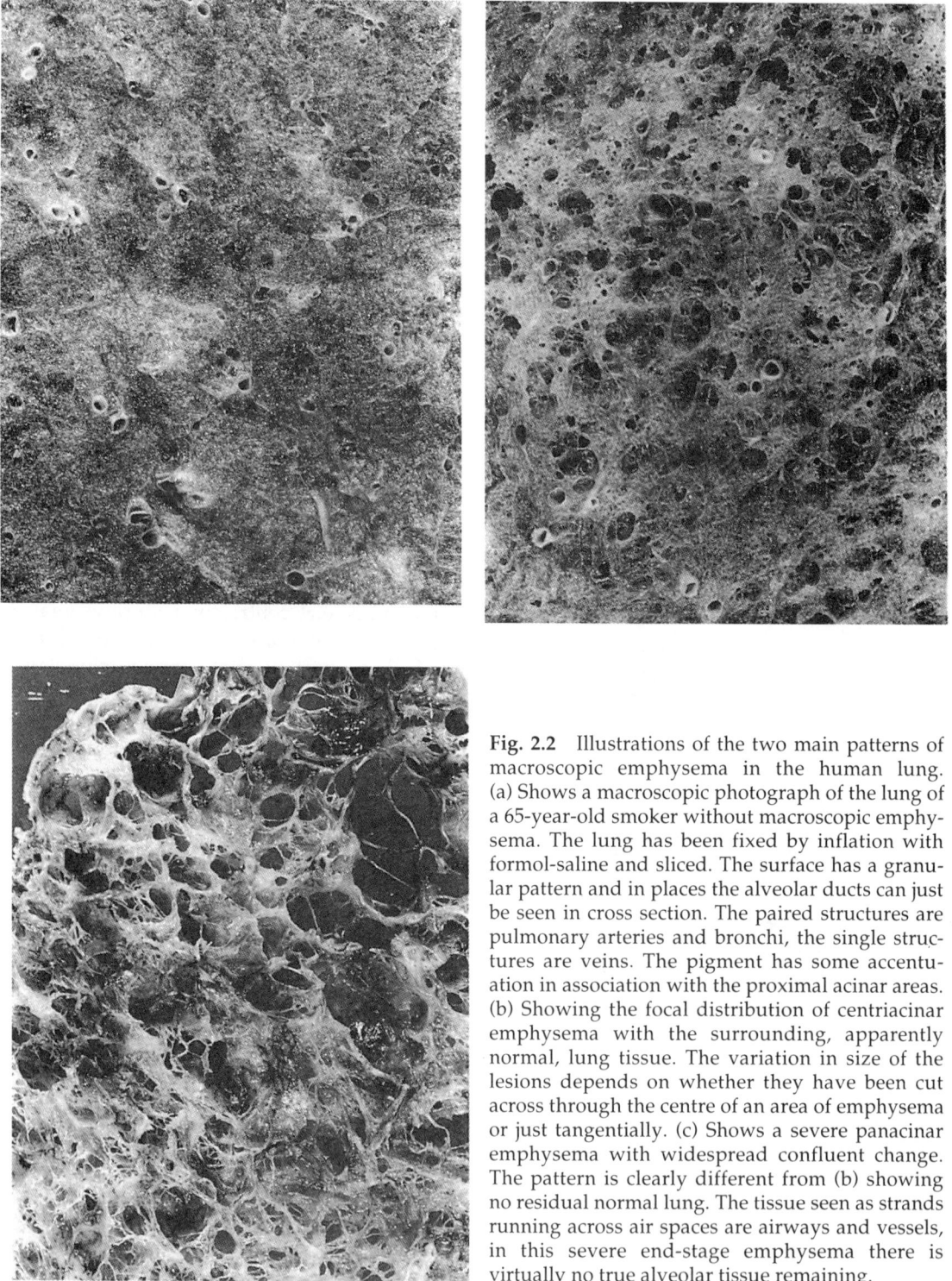

Fig. 2.2 Illustrations of the two main patterns of macroscopic emphysema in the human lung. (a) Shows a macroscopic photograph of the lung of a 65-year-old smoker without macroscopic emphysema. The lung has been fixed by inflation with formol-saline and sliced. The surface has a granular pattern and in places the alveolar ducts can just be seen in cross section. The paired structures are pulmonary arteries and bronchi, the single structures are veins. The pigment has some accentuation in association with the proximal acinar areas. (b) Showing the focal distribution of centriacinar emphysema with the surrounding, apparently normal, lung tissue. The variation in size of the lesions depends on whether they have been cut across through the centre of an area of emphysema or just tangentially. (c) Shows a severe panacinar emphysema with widespread confluent change. The pattern is clearly different from (b) showing no residual normal lung. The tissue seen as strands running across air spaces are airways and vessels, in this severe end-stage emphysema there is virtually no true alveolar tissue remaining.

degree, in the elderly lung but the gross inter-communication present in a severely emphy-sematous lung may not reflect any useful ventilatory function for such collateral drift.

The number of acinar units appears to be defined by the intrauterine development of the airways. With the increase in lung volume during childhood and adolescence the alveoli increase in number and as the size of alveoli in adult life appears to be fairly constant despite variation in body stature, it is the size of acinar units and the number of alveoli which vary with body size [8,10,11].

2.3 PATHOLOGY OF COPD

COPD is a complex clinical situation having as a common factor smoking-related, fixed airflow limitation. The clinical spectrum extends from a simple physiologic deficit through to acute and chronic respiratory failure, cor pulmonale and death in respira-tory or in cardiorespiratory failure. There are three clinicopathologic entities which have been considered as playing a role in the pathogenesis of the airflow limitation. These conditions are chronic bronchitis, emphysema and 'small airways disease'. These three con-ditions will be considered separately before proceeding to the correlation of structure with function and the pathologic findings in end-stage COPD.

2.4 CHRONIC BRONCHITIS

The term chronic bronchitis was originally defined clinically in terms of cough and spu-tum [12] production and effectively describes hypersecretion of mucus by the respiratory tract. The pathologic basis of this is an increase in the volume of submucosal glands and an increase in the number and distribution of goblet cells in the surface epithelium.

The bronchial submucosal glands are mixed glands formed of mucus and serous acini; they are found only in the bronchi and have a similar frequency distribution to the cartilage, being greatest in amount in large bronchi and diminishing markedly in the smaller and more peripheral bronchi. Submucosal glands are not present in bron-chioli. The submucosal glands increased markedly in mass in chronic bronchitis [14], largely as a consequence of cigarette smoking but other irritants may be involved. Animal experiments have shown that an increase in number of goblet cells and glands can occur in response to simple chemical stimuli such as sulfur dioxide [15,16], and infection is not a prerequisite. Increased submucosal glands may also be found in asthma.

Goblet cells are plentiful in the proximal airways in normal non-smokers but decrease in numbers more peripherally and normally there are no goblet cells in the more periph-eral generations of bronchioli. In smokers the goblet cells increase in number and their peripheral extent [17]. In the proximal airways there may be either an increase in goblet cells or a decrease due to squamous metaplastic and/or dysplastic changes induced by smoking, replacing the goblet cells of the normal respiratory epithelium.

As the mass of submucosal glands is much greater than that of the goblet cells most of the airway secretions are produced by the glands. There is a relationship between the amount of submucosal glands and the volume of sputum production [18].

Early studies were concerned about the role of infection and inflammation in the pro-gression of airflow limitation in patients with chronic bronchitis. The MRC subclassified chronic bronchitis depending on the presence or absence of pus in the sputum or of airways obstruction [13]. It soon became clear that even with adequate antibiotic treatment patients who had a reduction in the number of respiratory tract infections did not have an improved survival or a decrease in their rate of deterioration. Peto, *et al.* [19] in their epi-demiologic studies showed that there was clearly no relationship between cough and sputum and the rate of decline of FEV_1.

...ronchitis as defined by ... clearly related to smoking ... same population of patients ...velop airflow limitation the ...ersecretion is not related to the ...mitation (Chapter 4).

2.5 EMPHYSEMA

2.5.1 DEFINITION

Emphysema was first defined at the Ciba Foundation Guest Symposium [12] as 'a condition of the lung characterized by increase beyond the normal in size of the airspaces distal to the terminal bronchiole either from dilatation or from destruction of their walls'. This is an anatomical, or structural, definition and defines emphysema in terms of the acinus, that portion of the lung supplied by the terminal bronchiole. This original definition did not distinguish between over-inflation and the disruption of the lung architecture which occurs in smoking-related emphysema. Since then the definition has been modified on two occasions to emphasize the destructive process which is part of our concept of smoking-related emphysema. In 1962 the American Thoracic Society [20] suggested that emphysema should be defined as 'a condition of the lung characterised by abnormal, permanent enlargement of airspaces distal to the terminal bronchiole accompanied by destruction of their walls.' This was further modified by Snider, Kleinerman and Thurlbeck in 1985 [21] who added '... accompanied by destruction of their walls and *without obvious fibrosis*'.

None of the definitions was accompanied by criteria which allowed the concept of 'normal airspace size' to be defined and similarly in the 1985 definition the term 'without obvious fibrosis' is clearly a conceptual statement and may give rise to problems in relationship to the presence of smoking-related fibrosis in the lung (see below).

2.5.2 DIAGNOSIS AND CLASSIFICATION OF EMPHYSEMA

Emphysema is defined in structural or pathologic terms, therefore the diagnosis, classification and assessment of emphysema is primarily a pathologist's responsibility and limits opportunities for the study of emphysema to those situations where tissue is available. Although attempts to identify radiologic or physiologic criteria which identify the presence and severity of emphysema are constantly sought, it must be recognized that any such radiologic or functional criteria are indirect and must be clearly anchored to pathologic assessment.

To fulfil the definition of emphysema the pathologist might be expected to take the three points of the definition into account when identifying the presence of emphysema, i.e. the size of airspace, evidence for a destructive process, and an assessment that fibrosis is minimal. In practice, pathologists rely almost entirely on the size of the airspaces in the assessment of severity and the classification of the subtypes of emphysema.

The inclusion of the amount of fibrosis in the definition in 1985 [21] was not based on any actual knowledge of the fibrous tissue in emphysema compared with the normal lung, but rather to exclude certain pathologic conditions where enlarged airspaces are accompanied by gross fibrosis such as the honeycomb lung of cryptogenic fibrosing alveolitis, that the unwary and unsophisticated pathologist might try to diagnosis as emphysema.

In the context of COPD and smoking-related emphysema the concept that emphysema should only be considered when there has been a destructive process associated with the enlargement of airspaces is of value as it excludes those conditions where overinflation is present, such as post-pneumonectomy cases or the hyperinflation of asthma or when an atrophic process may be concerned, such as the aged lung. However, this aspect of the definition also excludes certain pediatric conditions previously included under the heading emphysema where the pathogenetic mechanism is an abnormality of intrauterine or postnatal development [22]. The pathologist has a problem when looking at an established example of emphysema to state that the airspace walls which are no longer present were removed by a destructive process. This is a conceptual rather than a practical aspect of the definition at this stage of the disease. However, in the very early stages of emphysema the concept that a destructive process (breaks in the alveolar walls attached to airways) is involved may be valuable in that at a stage when airspaces show little or no abnormality there may be evidence of the destructive process; this was the basis of the development of the Destructive Index by Cosio *et al.* in 1985 [23,24] (Section 2.5.7).

Accepting that pathologists depend largely on the increased size of airspaces to diagnose and classify emphysema, there remains the problem of the definition of normality of airspace size. The problem of defining accurately normality was avoided by early workers who looked at the cut surface of lungs inflated with formol saline and noted that the fine granular appearance did not allow the normal airspaces to be identified as such, but that in abnormal lungs the airspaces could be seen at a time when their diameter reached 1 mm. Such lungs were considered as having emphysema. Such macroscopic examination of the lung surface also allowed a classification of types of emphysema in relationship to the position of the abnormal airspaces within the acinar unit.

The classification of emphysema into three major types – panacinar (syn. panlobular), centriacinar (syn. preacinar, proximal acinar, centrilobular) and paraseptal (syn. periacinar, distal acinar) emphysema [12] has stood the test of time and is still in current use (Fig. 2.3).

Panacinar Emphysema (PAE): where the abnormally large airspaces are found evenly distributed across the acinar unit. Adja. acinar units are usually involved to a similai degree giving a confluent appearance to the cut surface of the lung with extensive areas being involved.

Centriacinar Emphysema (CAE): where the abnormal airspaces are found initially in association with respiratory bronchioles though in more severe cases virtually the whole acinar unit may be involved. In centriacinar emphysema the focal nature of the lesions stand out against often apparently normal lung and quite small lesions can be identified. However, when centriacinar and panacinar emphysema coexist and the panacinar emphysema is of some severity it may be very difficult to identify the presence of associated centriacinar emphysema.

Paraseptal Emphysema: where the abnormal airspaces run along the edge of the acinar unit but only where it abuts against a fixed structure such as the pleura, a vessel or a septum.

Two other types of emphysematous change are:

Scar, or irregular emphysema where the emphysematous spaces are found around the margins of a scar. As the scar itself may not be related to the anatomy of the acinar unit this type of emphysema is not classified in relationship to the acinus.

Bullae (Chapter 22). Bullae are areas of emphysema which locally overdistend to produce a lesion which, if superficial, stands proud of the pleural surface. By convention, only lesions of more than 1 cm in diameter justify the description of bullae [12]. Bullae are easily identified by pathologists, but they are much less easy to identify in life by radiologic techniques. They have been classified into 3 subtypes [22]. Type i has a narrow neck and is overdistention of a small portion of lung. Type ii has a broad base and is over-

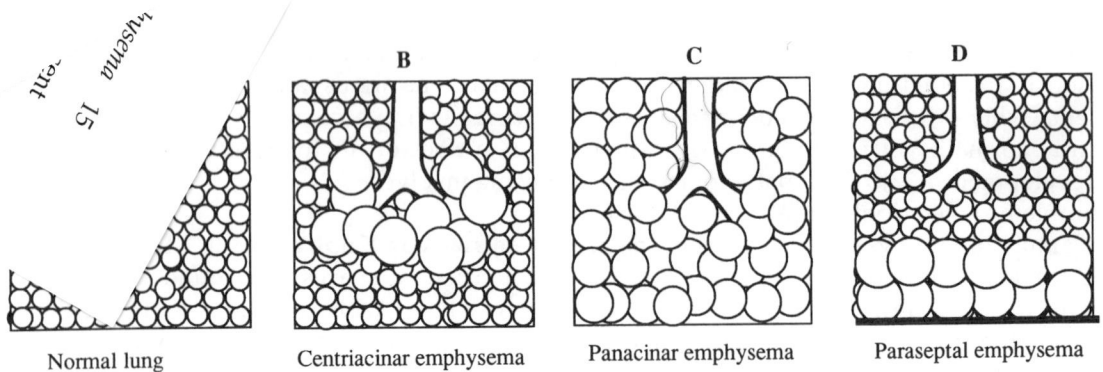

Normal lung	Centriacinar emphysema	Panacinar emphysema	Paraseptal emphysema

Fig. 2.3 A diagrammatic representation of the distribution of the abnormal airspaces within the acinar unit in the three major types of emphysema. (a) represents the acinar unit from a normal lung, though illustrated as a clearly defined area for the purposes of this diagram it must be remembered that, in the lung adjacent acinar units inter-communicate and are not necessarily demarcated by septa. (b) shows the focal enlargement of the airspaces around the respiratory bronchioles in centriacinar emphysema. (c) shows the confluent even involvement of the acinar unit in panacinar emphysema, and (d) shows the peripherally distributed enlarged airspaces where that portion of the acinar unit butts up against a fixed structure such as the pleura in paraseptal emphysema.

distention of a moderate area of emphysema and type iii is relative overdistention of part of a lobe or lung due to severe emphysema in it. Types ii and iii are complications of severe panacinar emphysema, type iii is only really seen in end-stage emphysematous change. Type i arising on a narrow neck is pushed by the chest wall back into the lung, where it is surrounded by a double layer of pleura which may be clearly seen radiologically. The pathogenesis of the type i bulla is uncertain, but is probably overdistention arising from damage in an area of scarred lung. There is no evidence for the bulla being congenital in origin.

The two common types of emphysema, panacinar and centriacinar, have differing distributions within the lung. Panacinar involving confluent areas of lung tissue may be found in the upper or lower lobe but particularly in α_1-antitrypsin (α_1-AT) deficiency it is characteristically maximal at the base. Centriacinar emphysema has a very clear preference for the upper zones of both the upper and lower lobes [25] and centriacinar emphysema only involves acinar units from apex to base in end-stage COPD and in coal-workers' pneumoconiosis. The differing types of emphysema are not exclusive and may occur alone in a lung or together and a major problem to the pathologist is the separate identification of the different types and their severity in a lung with more than one pattern of emphysema.

There has been some debate as to whether centriacinar and panacinar emphysema are different disease processes [24,25] and it has been suggested by some workers that panacinar emphysema is a natural progression of centriacinar emphysema [26,27,28]. However, the original workers who defined these conditions clearly recognized in the early stages a difference in position within the acinar unit and also described differences in distribution within the lung [25,29]. Centriacinar emphysema has a closer relationship to cigarette smoking than panacinar emphysema [30]. It has been shown that the presence of centriacinar lesions is independent of the occurrence of microscopic panacinar emphysema in surgically resected lungs [31,32]. These differences suggest a difference in the pathogenetic mechanisms giving rise to the two forms of emphysema and emphasize the importance of trying to keep the patterns of emphysema separate in assessing the severity of emphysema.

2.5.3 MACROSCOPIC ASSESSMENT OF SEVERITY

The macroscopic examination of inflated lung tissue allowed the presence or absence of emphysema to be identified easily but it was more difficult to give a truly quantitative assessment. Dunnill [33] described the value of the point counting technique for the assessment of the extent of macroscopic emphysema but it was difficult to combine assessment of the extent of lung involvement with an assessment of the severity of the emphysematous process. Heard [34] described a grading method whereby the lung cut surface was divided into six zones and each zone subdivided into fields where the presence or absence of emphysema was recorded, giving an estimate of the amount of lung involved by emphysema. This was not truly quantitative and there were difficulties when trying to record the different types of emphysema. Thurlbeck *et al.* [35,36] simplified the grading of emphysema by using a series of paper mounted cross-sections, ranking these from 0 to 100, where 0 was a normal lung and 100 the worst case of emphysema encountered in a series of 500 paper-mounted sections. They produced a series of standard pictures for comparison as a general standard. A problem with this grading system was that there was no measured quantitative relationship between the various grades such that a grade of 25 was not necessarily half as severe or as extensive as grade 50. Neither the point counting technique nor the picture matching technique could separately assess the different patterns of emphysema. Thurlbeck has gone so far as to say such separation of types of emphysema is unnecessary [37]. Though

this may be so in true end-stage disease when confluent centriacinar emphysema becomes, *de facto*, panacinar emphysema this is certainly not the case in early disease where one wishes to study the pathogenesis or possible functional effects of the separate types of emphysema.

With macroscopic techniques the criterion for recognition of emphysema was visible airspaces with an airspace size of approximately 1 mm as the cut-off point, so ignoring early stages of emphysema which could only be identified microscopically.

2.5.4 MICROSCOPIC ASSESSMENT OF SEVERITY

The normal alveolus is approximately 250 μm in diameter and thus by the time the airspaces in panacinar emphysema have reached 1 mm, approximately three-quarters of the alveolar surface area has been destroyed (Fig. 2.4). If one is to study early emphysema and its relationship to pathogenesis or to function, then it is obviously important to study it at the microscopic stage. Dunnill [38] and Thurlbeck [39] both used microscopic techniques to identify early abnormalities using the linear intercept technique which gave an estimate of the diameter of the airspaces. This technique was moderately tedious and time-consuming to apply but when combined with careful lung sampling gave a good estimate for the airspace size of a lung. However, to produce sufficient data for different areas of the lung to be compared one with another, a very large number of measurements had to be made. With the introduction of image analysis systems it has become easier to make accurate estimate of the alveolated portion of the lung and recently a fast fully automatic method based on the linear intercept technique has been developed [40] which allows a detailed analysis of large numbers of lung samples, almost as a routine. These microscopic techniques produce data which can be

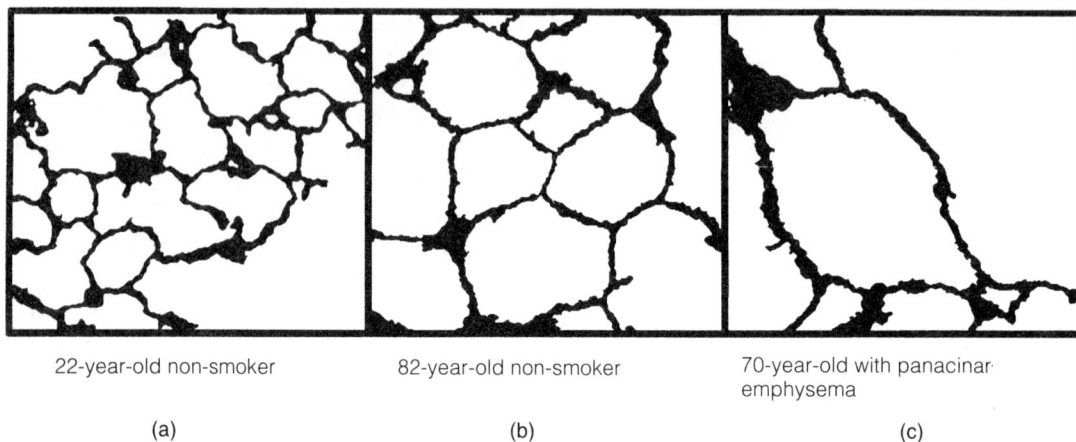

22-year-old non-smoker   82-year-old non-smoker   70-year-old with panacinar
                                                                emphysema

(a)   (b)   (c)

Fig. 2.4 This figure represents three binary images from the image analysis estimation of emphysema. Each square represents a 1 mm square of tissue. (a) is derived from a 22-year-old non-smoker. (b) is from an 82-year-old non-smoker, and (c) is from a 70-year-old patient with mild panacinar emphysema. The difference between (a) and (b) is not macroscopically recognizable, (c) would show as a mild macroscopic panacinar change. It is clear from this that if only macroscopic techniques are used, large changes in alveolar surface area will be missed. Magnification × 40.

expressed in terms of airspace size [38] e.g. mean linear intercept (Lm) or in terms of surface area of alveolar or airspace wall which surround the enlarged air spaces.* There are advantages in expressing the data in terms of surface area of airspace wall per unit volume (AWUV)[†] [41,42,43] when comparing the results with CT scan which provides the radiologic tissue density, and with tests for pulmonary function in which the function is related more to the airspace wall than to the hole in the middle.

Having measured accurately either airspace size or alveolar surface area there remains a problem: what is normal and what

is abnormal? Thurlbeck [39] investigated the Lm of groups of cases described as 'normal' and 'emphysematous', but these terms refer to the presence or absence of macroscopically recognized emphysema and the normal group included smokers. More recently Gillooly and Lamb [44] have studied a group of non-smokers between the ages of 23 and 93 and defined a normal range for AWUV (Fig. 2.5). These authors suggest defining normality as those values lying outside the 95% confidence limits of their measurements, or one can normalize the data for age by calculating a percentage of the predicted value. This change in mean AWUV identified an

---

*Mean linear intercept (Lm) is calculated as the total length of graticule test-line divided by the total number of intercepts between the test-line and alveolar walls [41]. The values obtained for Lm depend on the number of intercepts counted for each alveolar wall. Ideally, 2 intercepts should be counted for each, as both sides of the alveolar wall are involved in the gas exchange process. From the literature it is obvious that some workers have counted only 1 intercept, with the result that they quote Lm values which are twice as large as Lm obtained by counting 2 intercepts per wall.

[†]AWUV is directly related to Lm using the formula:

Surface area = $2V / Lm$ (in the case of AWUV $V = 1$ mm^3, so this becomes AWUV = $2/Lm$ [40]. It is therefore possible to derive AWUV from Lm values, and vice versa, provided care is taken with the formula used (the formula $2V/Lm$ applied only if *two* intercepts have been counted for each alveolar wall. If only *one* intercept has been counted, the appropriate formula to use is $4V/Lm$.

Mean AWUV plotted against age in 38 non-smokers

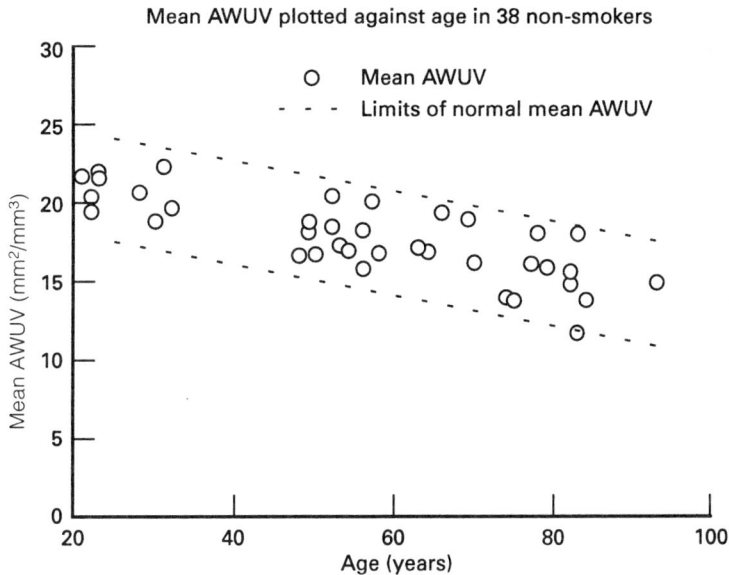

Fig. 2.5 This figures shows the mean AWUV (expressed as mm^2/mm^3 lung tissue). The mean value varies with the age of the patient in a linear manner. The dotted lines indicate the 95% prediction limits and indicate the limits of the normal mean AWUV values.

overall change in the whole lung and is probably appropriate for the identification of early panacinar emphysema as this appears to affect the whole lung.

Gillooly and Lamb [45] have studied a population of smokers and compared the mean AWUV values for the smokers with a population of non-smokers (Fig. 2.6). The large majority of smokers lie within the normal range with only about 30% having evidence of developing PAE (a larger proportion had CAE). There was no dose relationship between the number of cigarettes smoked and the risk of having an abnormally low AWUV value. These authors raised the possibility that there was a group who had a genetic predisposition to developing PAE, independent of the risk of developing CAE.

However, focal types of emphysema such as centriacinar emphysema may not affect the overall mean AWUV or Lm value as they only involve a small proportion of the total lung volume [31,32]. There are two ways of identifying early centriacinar emphysema; by the examination of tissue sections and observing qualitatively the presence of focal abnormalities of centriacinar type or looking at the frequency distribution of the actual measurements looking for evidence of focal abnormality [31,32]. Using such techniques these authors have emphasized that the two patterns of emphysema (PAE and CAE) are clearly separate in their clinical associations and development. This raises the important point that if there are two independent smoking-related patterns of emphysema there should be two pathogenetic mechanisms involved in their production.

The point of using a microscopic technique to assess the severity of emphysematous change is to ensure a quantitative linear measurement covering normality through to

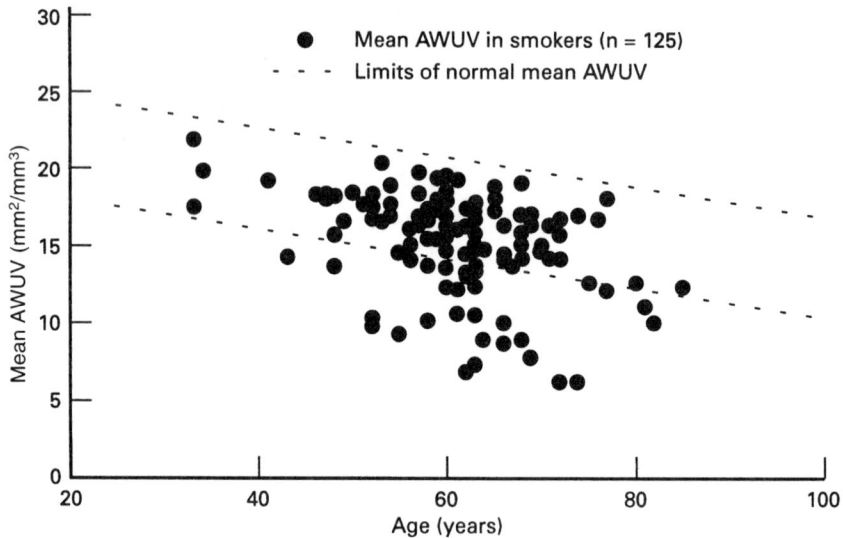

Fig. 2.6 The effect of smoking on the mean AWUV values. The dotted lines indicate the normal range derived from a population of non-smokers. It is clear that not all smokers show an abnormal mean AWUV value and, interestingly, those that fall outside of the normal range have a similar smoking history to those lying within. The reason for the development of this microscopically assessed panacinar emphysema does not appear to be smoking-dose related.

emphysema. It is not limited to the assessment of early emphysema. To get a linear quantitative measurement covering normality through early emphysema to end-stage disease means it is necessary to measure all degrees of severity on histological material using the same technique. One must not confuse the 'microscopic measurement' with emphysema that is only identifiable by a histological technique.

2.5.5 LOSS OF ALVEOLAR WALL ATTACHMENTS TO AIRWAYS IN EMPHYSEMA

Bronchioles and small bronchi are supported by, and owe their tubular integrity to, the attachment of adjacent alveolar walls to the outer aspect of their airway wall. It has been suggested [46,47,48] that loss of such attachments may lead to distortion and irregularity of airways and consequent functional effects,

possibly airflow limitation. Any loss of attachments of alveolar walls to airways will fulfil the criteria of the definition of emphysema as there must be an increase in size of the airspaces adjacent to airways associated with the loss (destruction ?) of alveolar walls. Airways run between acinar units and those alveoli that abut against the bronchiolar walls would be those that are at the periphery or distal aspects of the acinar unit. These areas will be affected by a panacinar or paraseptal pattern of emphysema. It is possible that our current classification of emphysema based on observations of macroscopic emphysema may not include all patterns of abnormality found at a microscopic level and, in particular the selective loss or retention of alveolar walls adjacent to airways has not been so far studied. The integrity of the alveolar wall supports can be assessed by measuring the linear distance between the junction of the alveolar walls with the outside of the airways walls.

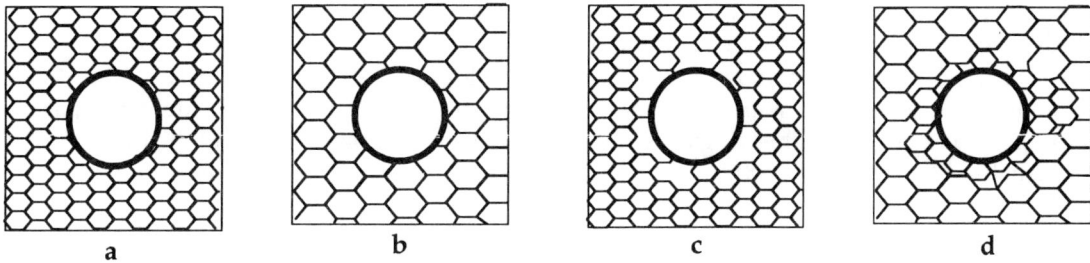

Fig.2.7 The diagrammatic representation of how variation in the interalveolar attachment distance (IAAD) may arise. (a) represents a normal lung with airway cut in cross-section. The alveoli are represented by the hexagons. In (b) showing panacinar emphysema the hexagons are larger and it is clear that the distance between alveolar walls attached to the outer aspect of the airway is increased. In (c) there is selective loss of alveolar wall attachments adjacent to the airway despite the presence of normal alveoli a short distance away, this might occur in paraseptal emphysema. (d) shows an appearance which is occasionally seen in what otherwise appears to be macroscopically panacinar emphysema. At the microscopic level this does not extend right up to the airway, leaving a narrow band of maintained alveoli giving a normal IAAD despite the loss of surface area elsewhere. Such a situation may conserve function.

The actual measured distance is proportional to the diameter of the alveolar spaces which abut on the airways. The possible situations giving rise to an increase in the interalveolar wall attachment distance (IAAD) are shown in Fig. 2.7. The situation seen in Fig. 2.7(d) where there is selective retention of attachments around airways in panacinar emphysema certainly does occasionally occur and may preserve pulmonary function. Whether or not there is a pure loss of alveolar walls adjacent to airways as in Fig. 2.7(c) is unproven but if so this would probably be a variation on paraseptal emphysema with selective loss of alveolar walls occurring at the periphery of the acinar unit. Such a selective loss could be caused by local inflammatory changes in the airway wall and might link those who feel that airway inflammation is an important pathogenetic mechanism in airway obstruction with those who believe the obstruction is a consequence of emphysema.

2.5.6 FIBROSIS AND EMPHYSEMA

The current definition of emphysema defines emphysema 'as being without obvious fibrosis' [21]. Most pathologists would agree that it is characteristic of an emphysematous lung that when it is fixed by inflation with formol saline and sliced, the slices collapse down upon themselves due to the lack of substance associated with the loss of alveolar walls. If the protease/antiprotease theory of pathogenesis of emphysema is correct one might expect a reduced collagen and elastin in emphysematous pulmonary parenchyma. Histologically there is clearly fibrosis in the region of terminal and respiratory bronchioles, the respiratory bronchiolitis described by Niewoehner, and this may occasionally produce a true interstitial lung disease [49,50]. However, it is difficult to actually measure the amount of collagen within the parenchyma of the lung in relationship to the alveolar walls. A large amount of the total collagen framework of the lung is associated with the bronchovascular bundles, the pleura and septa and not in the alveolar walls themselves. When sensitive techniques are applied and levels of collagen and elastin in the samples of lung of smokers and nonsmokers consisting predominantly of alveolar walls are measured an increase in collagen can be identified in the parenchyma of the smokers [51]. When emphysematous lungs are examined the amount of collagen is also increased in relationship to less emphysematous areas or to non-emphysematous lungs [52,53]. The fibrosis in association with end-stage emphysema is clearly seen in histological sections or visualized by scanning electron microscopy [54]. One must be careful in interpretation of such results because there is a condensation or concentration of the connective tissue framework around the mouths of alveolar spaces in the alveolar ducts and it is possible that a loss of alveolar wall with a relative retention of the architectural framework of the lung could give an increase in collagen and elastin associated with a loss of alveolar wall surface area. However the work of Lang *et al.* [52] suggests that whether collagen and elastin data are expressed per unit volume of lung or per alveolar wall surface area there is an increase in emphysema. This is a timely reminder that in our discussion of the role of emphysema in affecting pulmonary function we have assumed that the quality of the lung is constant, but that the quantity is altered. It is possible that both the quality and quantity of alveolar walls may change and both may affect elastic recoil and the support to small airway walls. So far no consideration of such qualitative changes in the function of the pulmonary parenchyma have been included in structure function studies.

2.5.7 DESTRUCTION OF AIR SPACE WALLS

In an attempt to combine an estimate of airspace size with the element of destruction of alveolar walls included in the 1985 definition of emphysema Saetta *et al.* [23] described a Destructive Index (DI) which used a point-counting technique to identify the proportion of airspaces surrounded by walls showing evidence of destruction, or conforming to a subjective assessment of 'classic emphysematous lesion'. Using this technique it has been possible to identify smoking-related alveolar wall damage in the absence of measurable emphysema [23,24].

There is no proof that such damage to alveolar walls is a necessary stage in the development of either CAE or PAE. Such evidence of destruction may identify a pathogenetic mechanism and fulfil the definition of emphysema. It does not reflect outcome, the severity of emphysema, and therefore is unlikely to correlate with any functional variable.

2.5.8 EMPHYSEMA AND CT ASSESSMENT (SEE ALSO CHAPTER 14)

In 1978 Thurlbeck and Simon [55] described criteria for the diagnosis of emphysema using the chest radiograph. These were based on indications of overinflation and vascular pruning and showed only a moderate correlation with macroscopic emphysema as assessed by the picture matching technique. When CT scans became available it became possible to extract quantitative data on lung density. When quantitative histologic assessment is compared with quantitative CT density a good correlation is found even within the range of those showing normal age change and early emphysema [42]. Quantitative CT gives directly comparable data to quantitative histological assessment, as Gould *et al.* [42,56] found when they compared AWUV measurements to CT volume values for 1 mm cubes of lung tissue. Those using quantitative CT scans to identify and assess the severity of emphysema must still take into account whether a decrease in density is due to hyperinflation or true emphysema, and what are age-related normal values. Changes in mean values are likely to reflect panacinar emphysema whereas the focal lesions of CAE can only be identified by careful examination of frequency distributions of density measurement or qualitative assessment in the identification of individual lesions [56]. It is a pity that many attempts to use CT to identify emphysema have compared CT and lung using qualitative grading, scoring or picture matching techniques which have a poor correlation with pulmonary function (Section 2.7) rather than actual quantitative measurements. Those groups who have used true density measurements have shown better correlation of their lung density measurements ('emphysema') with pulmonary functional changes including carbon monoxide transfer coefficient and FEV_1 [42,56,58,59].

2.6 SMALL AIRWAYS DISEASE

The concept of small airways disease is based on the work of Hogg, Macklem and Thurlbeck who showed that the increased airflow resistance in COPD lies in the peripheral airways [4]. Whatever the pathogenesis of the fixed increase in resistance to airflow which develops in the airways of some smokers the actual mechanism for the final airway obstruction, if this is due to changes in the airways, must be scarring with distortion and narrowing of the lumen. Such histological changes are clearly seen in patients who develop bronchiolitis obliterans or constrictive bronchiolitis [60] as a sequela of severe acute insult [60,61] such as the inhalation of toxic fumes [62] or part of an ongoing acute or chronic inflammatory state involving the airways such as extrinsic allergic alveolitis, rheumatoid arthritis [66] or in post-transplant cases [63,65] or as part of severe post-inflammatory damage in chronically infected lung, those with severe bronchiectasis or in cystic fibrosis [63,64,65,67]. In these cases the pathologist easily identifies the airway changes at a subjective level. He looks, sees the abnormality and suggests a diagnosis. He does not need to make careful quantitative measurements to identify the changes from normal. In COPD the small airways do not appear to show such severe changes and researchers are driven to make detailed and time-consuming measurements on the airways to try and identify a cause for the increased airways resistance.

Airways are a set of tapering tubes and measurement of the size of small airways on histologic sections may differ depending on sampling site in the lung. Thus it is likely that the samples from the midsagittal site will provide a set of values rather higher than that from the subpleural position. The smallest non-respiratory bronchioles in a large person will be larger than those from a smaller person, therefore both selection of the population to be studied and sample site within the lung can provide a variation of small airway size. The ideal would be to study the patient's values against a known normal range, normalized for body size. Unfortunately no such data are available.

What measurement of a cross-sectioned airway should be made? Figure 2.8 shows some of the potential problems involved. Ideally measurements can be made on airways cut in true cross-section (Figs. 2.1 and 2.8(a)) but in reality most airways are tangentially sectioned (Fig. 2.8(b)). These two have in common the measurement of the minimal diameter which is easily measured by an eye piece graticule or simple image analysis system. However, there are two problems which affect the minimum diameter of a cross-sectioned airway. First the degree of 'tone' provided by the bronchial muscle in resected specimens results in varying degrees of crenated outline (Fig. 2.8(d)) which give apparently smaller diameter airways. Measurements of either diameter or lumen area made on such an airway would be unrepresentative of its true dimensions. Secondly even truly cross-sectioned airways may have an elliptical profile which may be produced by inadequate distending pressure during fixation, but may also be seen in association with lack of support to the airway wall by adjacent alveoli in emphysema, in particular, in the loss of the alveolar wall attachments to the outer aspect of the small airway. If more sophisticated measurements, using image analysis, are made it is possible to measure the circumference, the lumen area and to derive a theoretical lumen area from the measured circumference. This problem of

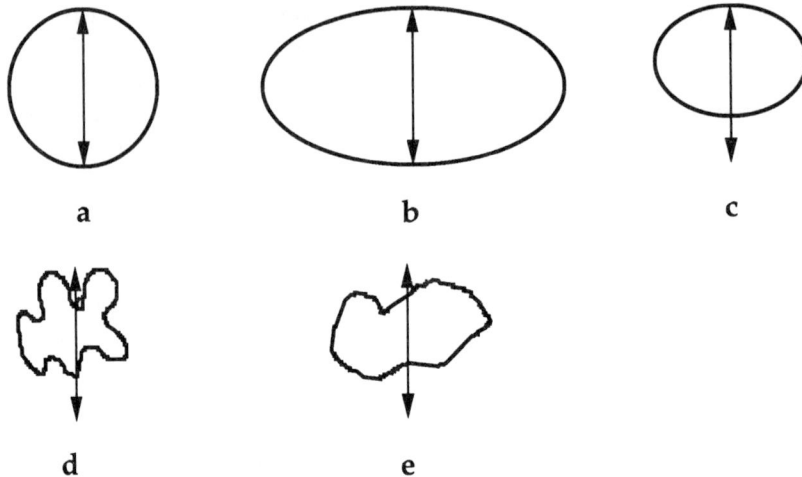

Fig. 2.8   Five diagrams of cross-sections of small airways in lung. (a) a perfect cross-section of an airway with a rounded outline. The vertical line indicates the diameter. (b) a tangential section across an airway of the same minimum diameter as (a). (c) a cross-section of a similar sized airway to (a) but with compression due to technical artefact or poor inflation during fixation. The minimum diameter is decreased. (d) a crenated outline of an airway showing increased muscle tone, the original airway size similar to that in (a) measured in the crenated position shows a significant diminution in minimum diameter. (e) shows an airway lacking alveolar wall support with partial collapse, its minimal diameter is significantly decreased, though the lumen area available if the outline is circular is the same as for (a).

elliptical airways is important because it is possible to imagine a population of such elliptical airways being measured to provide evidence of decreased minimum diameter (despite no change in the true lumen area) on the one hand, or the degree of ellipticality being used for evidence of lack of support to the airways by the pulmonary parenchyma in emphysema. These two approaches provide evidence for entirely different pathogenesis for any functional abnormality!

Apart from measurement of small airway dimensions the commonest series of 'measurements' in the literature are those relating to the smoking-related effects in the airway wall. These were originally described by Niewhoener [49] and extended by Cosio *et al.* in 1978 [68]. Eight aspects were included by Cosio in his assessment:

1. Occlusion of the lumen by mucus and cells.
2. Presence or absence of mucosal ulceration.
3. Goblet cell hyperplasia.
4. Squamous cell metaplasia.
5. Inflammatory infiltrate of the airway wall.
6. Amount of fibrosis in the airway wall.
7. Amount of muscle.
8. Degree of pigmentation.

The first two of these were directly assessed as a percentage of airways involved; the remaining six were scored 0–3 qualitatively and the score expressed as % of maximum possible score of 18. The total of the three individual % scores were added to provide an overall small airway disease score (SAD) (maximum 300).

The assessment of each of these variables is 'semi-quantitative' by a subjective grading which became refined by a use of a set of standard illustrations of the various grades of abnormality [69]. The main problem about the SAD score of Cosio was the fact that the scores for each variable provided a ranking of severity. However, the overall score which was a sum of the individual rankings of several variables is not a true quantitative figure and is unsuited for parametric statistical analysis.

2.7 STRUCTURAL BASIS FOR ABNORMALITIES IN PULMONARY FUNCTION IN COPD

Historically there have been three phases in attempts to identify the structural basis of pulmonary function tests. In the 1960s and early 1970s most interest was in end-stage COPD with autopsy studies largely relating to patterns and severity of emphysema. This phase was well summarized by Thurlbeck in 1976 [25]. There was then a reappraisal of the complexities of studying end-stage disease and a recognition of the importance of small airways disease and the next phase was a study of early disease using surgically resected lungs and lobes with an emphasis on small airways as well as emphysema assessed both macroscopically and microscopically. More recently there has been a recognition that as emphysema with its increased airspace size and decreased alveolar walls represents a fall in tissue density, CT scanning can be used to quantify emphysema [42]. Clinicians tried to bypass the complexities of pathologic assessments of autopsy material and studied pulmonary function in relationship to CT-assessed emphysema in living patients.

At autopsy on patients dying of COPD emphysema is commonly widespread and severe [2,22,25,70]. When the amount of emphysema in COPD patients is compared with randomly selected smoking populations, there is more severe emphysema in the COPD cases [1,25,71]. This is not an absolute relationship, for there are patients with moderate or even severe emphysema, as assessed macroscopically, without clinically identified COPD in this series. Despite this it has been the custom to ascribe a major causative role to emphysema in producing the complex patho-

physiologic abnormalities found in end-stage COPD.

Quantitative correlations of the severity of emphysema with the severity of airway obstruction have appeared to confirm a causative relationship [1,2,70,71,72]. There does not appear to be any marked changes in the small airways in parallel with the severity of the emphysema to offer an alternative explanation for the severe airway obstruction [1,2,70,72,73,74]. It is unfortunate that much of the work referred to was based on assessment of emphysema which was semi-quantitative involving grading or picture matching. These techniques did not separately identify the different patterns of emphysema. It may seem surprising that there is no clear information on the physiologic consequences of CAE itself, PAE or a combination of the two. One might expect differences in the physiologic effects of two such different patterns of alveolar wall destruction. The discrete focal lesions of CAE lying in the proximal part of the acinus have a predominant effect on diffusion in the gas phase, but not directly affecting support to airways which lie at the periphery of the acinar unit. PAE on the other hand may be the basis for changes in lung elasticity and affect measurements of pressure volume curves or of the constant k, and be the basis of the loss of alveolar wall attachments to small airways with consequent decrease in support to small airways on expiration. It is perhaps relevant that at autopsy on patients with end-stage COPD, it is usual for both patterns of emphysema to be present and usually both in a severe form.

The one clearly measurable aspect of emphysema which may affect airway resistance is the assessment of the support provided to small airways by the adjacent alveolar walls by measuring the distance between the alveolar wall attachments to the airways.

The work of Anderson and Foraker and Linhartova and co-workers [46,48,75] has stressed the importance of peribronchial alveolar attachments in maintaining airway shape. These authors proposed that airway distortion due to loss of such attachments may be related to airflow limitation. A relationship between loss of alveolar attachments and a decrease in FEV_1 has been shown in patients with COPD coming to necropsy [76] and in early disease [77,78]. Nagai et al. [79] measured the distance between alveolar attachments and also quantitatively assessed emphysema in a series of autopsied patients with COPD. They could not identify a relationship between the inter-attachment distance and changes in FEV_1, believing that all such changes were more closely related to their assessments of emphysema. In early or mild disease we have shown clearly a relationship with an increased IAAD and the percent predicted FEV_1; the relationship between alveolar wall attachments and the percent predicted FEV_1 were closer than for measurement of alveolar surface area [78].

The findings of Nagai [79] and Lamb et al. [78] raise the possibility that the changes in FEV_1 associated with loss of support to the airways in emphysema may be associated with two aspects of the loss of alveolar walls. In early disease the loss of immediate support as represented by the changes in the inter-alveolar attachment distances may be more important than the more distal generalized effect provided by panacinar emphysema though this may be more important in end-stage disease.

The measurements of alveolar wall attachments have been made usually on the most peripheral bronchioles. The fact that a change in the support of the most peripheral bronchioles may be associated with the loss of FEV_1 in COPD may seem surprising. Several studies have reported, however, that the major site of increased resistance to airflow in COPD is the peripheral airways and therefore the FEV_1 might be expected to reflect abnormalities of peripheral airways [4,5,9,78]. Although the alveolar attachments are meas-

ured in relationship to the small peripheral bronchioles, the effect of any lack of support associated with such changes is not confined to such airways. It is probable that all bronchioles and small peripheral bronchioli in which the cartilage plates are widely separated, depend on support from adjacent alveolar walls for their functional integrity. It might be argued that a measure of the largest gaps between alveolar attachments supporting a bronchiole would be more important in providing an opportunity for premature airway closure than a change in the mean values. This may be the case, but in our experience the relationship between the largest gaps and the mean values of the IAAD measured are mathematically so related that it is not possible to identify a preferential role for the widest gaps or for the mean value [78].

If the changes in alveolar wall attachments to bronchioli are the prime cause of the increased airway resistance in COPD, then it might be expected that there would be a relationship between measurement of the alveolar wall attachments and other tests of small airway function. There is a positive relation between the distance between the alveolar wall attachments and the slope of the single N_2 test (SBN_2) [78,79]: thus loss of attachments leads to increased lack of homogeneity in the distribution of ventilation in the lungs [80]. There was no direct relationship between CV/VC% and IAAD as might be predicted if loss of attachments allowed airway closure to occur at a higher lung volume. There was a negative relation between CV/VC% and measurements of alveolar surface area reflecting a reduction in general support for the airways, thus allowing premature collapse. These results, although requiring confirmation, do suggest a certain complexity in the relationship between emphysema in its various patterns and its physiologic effects.

Though airway obstruction and changes in the FEV_1 may be the prime abnormality in COPD, there are other physiologic abnormalities which are more clearly related to emphysema. Both single breath and steady state carbon monoxide transfer (transfer factor) measurements show a significant decrease with increasing degree of emphysema [42,43,72,79, 81,82,87]. The relation of transfer factor values to a macroscopic assessment of emphysema was not close enough to be of major clinical importance; however, if microscopic measurements of emphysema, either Lm or surface area, are used, there was a very close and linear correlation between the loss of alveolar surface area and the transfer factor [42,43].

An even better predictor of the presence and severity of emphysema are changes in lung elastic recoil [72,82,83,84,85]. Changes in the static deflation pressure volume curve and in particular, the constant k used in describing the shape of the curve are the single best predictor of emphysema [72,82]. The constant k is influenced mainly by surface tension forces within the lung, and hence relates directly to the alveolar surface to volume ratio. This should directly relate to the mean size of peripheral air spaces or the alveolar surface area [72]. If this is the case, one might expect some disparity between changes in k and changes in FEV_1, and the slope of the SBN_2 test which both appear to have a closer relationship to alveolar attachments [78,79].

2.8 SMALL AIRWAYS DISEASE AS A CAUSE OF SMOKING-RELATED AIRFLOW LIMITATION

In 1968 Hogg, Macklem and Thurlbeck [4] showed that the small airways (airways <2 mm in diameter) had a low resistance in normal lungs but that they were the major site of increased resistance in patients with COPD. These experiments suggested that the increase in resistance was due to structural changes in the small airways rather than a consequence of the elastic recoil changes found in emphysema. Based on this work Hogg developed the hypothesis that small airways disease as a cause of the airflow limi-

tation in COPD was a structural consequence of small airway inflammation.

Evidence for smoking-related inflammatory change in small airways has steadily accumulated [49,68,86,88,89], much based on the SAD score of Cosio *et al.* Using such scoring systems relationships between these inflammatory changes and reduced FEV_1 have been shown [77,86]. The significance of these findings is not straightforward, for the scoring system is a summation of several individual semi-quantitative gradings of histologic features representing inflammation or the consequences of inflammation and it is difficult to see how these particular features could be directly related, in a cause and effect sense, with airflow resistance unless there is an associated decrease in airway lumen.

It is possible that the evidence of inflammation may be related to later structural changes and a relationship between inflammation and airway scarring and loss of alveolar attachments has been reported [76,77].

Structural narrowing of small airways in smokers has been related to functional changes of airflow limitation [90,91], but while the changes have been statistically significant they are not great in absolute terms. For example Bosken *et al.* [90] showed that 70% of membranous bronchioles were <0.85 mm in internal diameter in patients with measured air flow obstruction compared with 55% in groups of patients with FEV_1 within normal limits.

We have not been able to confirm the relationship between a decreased small airway lumen size and the FEV_1 [78] and, in fact, in our study there was a trend for the small airways to be increased in their lumen size in patients with a decreased % predicted FEV_1.

Epidemiologic studies of decline in FEV_1 in patients with COPD [92,17] have shown that this accelerated decline appears to affect only some 20% of heavy smokers. Studies of inflammatory change in small airways and changes in bronchiolar diameter have not identified a susceptible group among the smokers which would account for these epidemiologic findings, though there may be a group of smokers who are susceptible to developing PAE [45].

Attempts to work out the structural basis for the physiologic abnormalities in COPD have not produced clear-cut definitive answers. In particular there is no universally accepted explanation for the structural basis of the fixed airway obstruction. There is certainly no obvious narrowing and scarring of the small airways as seen in bronchiolitis iobliterans. There is a group of smoking related changes in small airways, associated with which are minor changes in airway diameter, but there is no evidence that these changes progress and are of sufficient severity to explain the severe fixed airway obstruction in late stage COPD.

It is possible that such changes found in studies using material resected from lung cancer was from an older age range, or represent a mild smoking-related abnormality independent from early COPD, which was the aim of the investigations.

Personally, I believe that the airway obstruction in COPD is largely, if not entirely, due to the consequences of emphysema, if one accepts that changes in alveolar wall attachments to airway walls is one aspect of emphysema. However, the physiologic significance of the different patterns of emphysema still require elucidation.

The main confounding feature in understanding the pathophysiology of COPD is the co-correlation of our measures of histologic and structural change with smoking and aging. The smoking-related problems are well recognized [72]. The problem of co-correlation of structural changes with aging is just being recognized. Studies of life-long non-smokers has shown that there is a clear linear fall in alveolar surface area with age [39,44] and a rise in the inter-alveolar attachment distance [93]. The FEV_1 has also an age-related fall in its value. If we believe that smoking may exaggerate the loss of alveolar surface area, the increase in alveolar wall attachments and the decrease in FEV_1, we have a situation where the structural and functional variables all vary

with age and smoking. To identify the functional significance of such structural changes requires a normalization of the structural data against standard values for a non-smoking population: such values are only just becoming available [45]. It may be that the commonly used measure of smoking dose 'pack years' is inappropriate in the context of COPD when both components, time, and the number smoked, are independently related to change in structure.

2.9 AUTOPSY FINDINGS IN PATIENTS WITH COPD

All those changes described earlier in this chapter under the heading of 'Pathology of COPD' section 2.3 may be found at autopsy. However, the most prominent abnormality seen in the lungs at post-mortem in a patient with COPD is the presence of severe macroscopically evident emphysema [1,2,25,70,71,94]. The emphysema may be predominantly centriacinar or panacinar or a mixture with recognizable focality of lesions with an overlying panacinar pattern. It is characteristic of the centriacinar emphysema in end-stage COPD that the lesions are larger and more extensive than found in smokers without COPD and it is common for the lesions which are normally distributed in the upper parts of the upper and lower lobes to extend throughout the lung from apex to diaphragm surface. Such a wide distribution of centriacinar emphysema lesions is only seen in end-stage COPD or in coal-workers' pneumoconiosis. The panacinar emphysema may be widespread throughout the lung, or predominantly upper or lower in its distribution. There appears to be no clear reason for such variation in pattern of distribution. It has been suggested that the variation and severity of emphysema may be related to clinical patterns of COPD (the 'pink puffer' and 'blue bloater') [95], but more recent studies have shown no correlation between the amount or type of macroscopic emphysema and chronic hypoxemia [96].

At autopsy it is common to see bullae of type ii or type iii [22] particularly at the apex or the diaphragmatic surface of the lower lobe.

The airways at autopsy often contain mucus and many of the peripheral bronchioles may be plugged, but these plugs of mucus are never as frequent or as inspissated with cellular debris as is the case in asthma. Because a terminal chest infection is common, this may exaggerate the problems of mucus plugging of airways and also the degree of inflammatory change in airway walls. It is usual to find areas of bronchopneumonia or more confluent lower lobe consolidation in such patients. As with all heavy smokers lung cancer is not uncommon but there is epidemiologic evidence that even taking smoking history into account, lung cancer is more common in patients with COPD than one would expect [97,98] Fig. 2.9.

Some patients dying with COPD have a history of chronic hypoxemia and this group of patients characteristically shows changes of pulmonary hypertension and right ventricular hypertrophy of cor pulmonale. Alveolar hypoxia is associated with an increase in pulmonary vascular resistance, both in the acute and chronic states, although the mechanisms for this response is still uncertain [99,100] (Chapter 11).

Morphologic changes in the pulmonary blood vessels are characteristically those of an increase in medial muscle, an extension of the medial muscle distally to involve small 'arterial' vessels which in normal subjects have no muscle in their wall [101,102,103,104]. The intima shows fibrous thickening and bands of longitudinal muscle develop within the intima and also external to the elastica lamina. The significance of the fibrous thickening is uncertain, because it is clearly present in smokers without COPD [104,105]. The large pulmonary arteries show intimal atheroma and the main pulmonary trunks may show an aneurysmal dilatation often containing laminated thrombus.

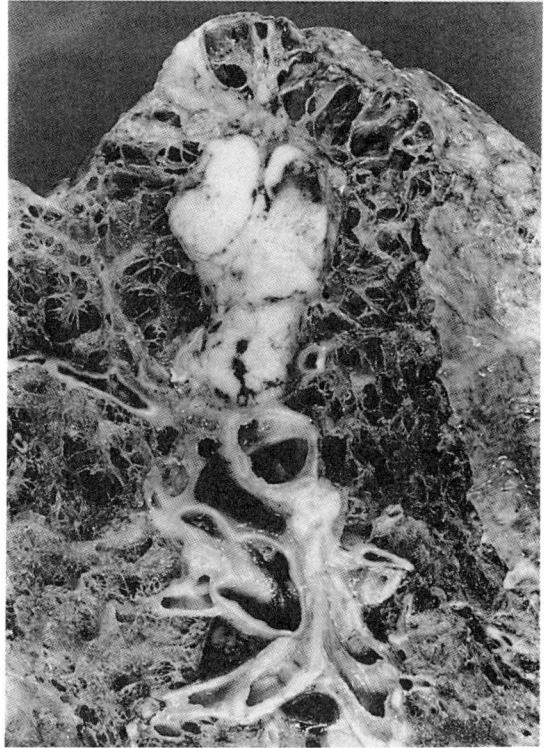

Fig. 2.9 Lung from an autopsy of a 58-year-old patient with a history of many years COPD and three years' domiciliary oxygen treatment. The patient died in what appeared to be a typical exacerbation of his COPD. At autopsy the lung showed severe widespread emphysema with some scarring and there was an undiagnosed upper lobe carcinoma on the left. The picture illustrates a primary squamous carcinoma arising in relationship to the apical segment of the upper lobe. Hilar nodes are involved. The lung shows severe, widespread panacinar emphysema; the pulmonary artery is atheromatous.

Attempts to quantify structural abnormalities in the pulmonary vasculature in relationship to the degree of pulmonary hypertension and the right ventricular hypertrophy are as complex as the problems associated with the assessment of small airways disease! Much work in the literature is based on relatively crude techniques in which the muscle hypertrophy is assessed by comparing the thickening of the muscle to the diameter of the artery as seen in cross-section. Unfortunately, this takes no account of the vasoconstriction which is clearly seen even in post-mortem material. Improved measurement techniques which allow more accurate assessment of medial muscle and intima are available [106,107]. As with airways disease, the blood vessels may show changes produced by cigarette smoking which may or may not be part of the pathophysiology of vascular disease in COPD, in particular, marked intimal changes may be seen without evidence of significant airways obstruction [105,106].

Right ventricular hypertrophy is characteristically found in patients with a history of chronic hypoxemia [94] and is best assessed at autopsy by dissection of the heart and separate weighing of the free wall of the right ventricle, left ventricle and septum by the technique of Fulton [109]. There is a wide variation in ventricular weight due to the variation of body size and physical activity and this makes the assessment of minimal degrees of right ventricular hypertrophy difficult. The most sensitive method is to compare the ratio between the weight of the left ventricle and septum to that of the right ventricle. This ratio is normally greater than 2.2, but values as low as 1, associated with the weight of the free wall of the right ventricle as high as 160 g, can be seen in hypoxic cor pulmonale due to COPD. Simple measurements of the thickness of ventricular wall at post-mortem are of little value in the assessment of right ventricular hypertrophy, owing to the complicating effects of ventricular dilatation in heart failure [110].

Several other extrapulmonary abnormalities have been described in hypoxemic COPD including carotid body enlargement [111,112] and enlargement of the renal glomeruli [113].

REFERENCES

1. Mitchell, R.S., Stanford, R., Johnson, J.M. *et al.* (1976) The morphologic features of the bronchi, bronchioles, and alveoli in chronic airway obstruction. A clinicopathological study. *Am. Rev. Respir. Dis.*, **114**, 137–45.
2. Nagai, A., West, W.M. and Thurlbeck, W.M. (1985). The National Institutes of Health Intermittent Positive-Pressure Breathing Trial: Pathology Studies. II. Correlations between morphologic findings, clinical findings and evidence of expiratory airflow obstruction. *Am. Rev. Respir. Dis.*, **132**, 946–53.
3. Linhartova, A., Anderson, A.E. and Foraker, A.G. (1974) Topology of nonrespiratory bronchioles of normal and emphysematous lungs. *Hum. Pathol.*, **5**, 729–35.
4. Hogg, J.C., Macklem, P.T. and Thurlbeck, W.M. (1968) Site and nature of airway obstruction in chronic obstructive lung disease. *N. Engl. J. Med.*, **278**, 1355–60.
5. Gelb, A.F., Gobel, P.H., Fairshter, R. and Zamel, N. (1981) Predominant site of airway resistance in chronic obstructive pulmonary disease. *Chest*, **79**, 273–6.
6. Miller, W.S. (1937) *The Lung*. Thomas, Springfield, Ill. pp. 27–37.
7. Murray, J.F. (1986) *The Normal Lung. The Basis for Diagnosis and Treatment of Pulmonary Disease* 2nd edn, Saunders, Philadelphia, pp. 43–6
8. Dunnill, M.S. (1962) Post natal growth of the lung. *Thorax*, **17**, 329–33.
9. Macklem, P.T. (1971) Airway obstruction and collateral ventilation. *Physiol. Rev.*, **51**, 368–436.
10. Thurlbeck, W.M. (1975) Post natal growth and development of the lung. *Am. Rev. Respir. Dis.*, **111**, 803–44.
11. Thurlbeck, W.M. and Angus, G.E. (1975) Growth and aging of the normal human lung. *Chest*, **67** (suppl): 3s–6s.
12. Ciba Foundation Guest Symposium (1959) Terminology, definitions and classification of chronic pulmonary emphysema and related conditions. *Thorax*, **14**, 286–99.
13. Medical Research Council (1965) Definition and classification of chronic bronchitis for clinical and epidemiological purposes. A report to the Medical Research Council by their Committee on the aetiology of chronic bronchitis. *Lancet*, **i**, 775–9.
14. Thurlbeck, W.M. and Angus, G.E. (1964) A distribution curve for chronic bronchitis. *Thorax*, **19**, 436–42.
15. Lamb, D. and Reid, L. (1968) Mitotic rates, goblet cell increase and histochemical changes in mucus in rat bronchial epithelium

during exposure to sulphur dioxide. *J. Pathol. Bacteriol.*, **96**, 97–111.

16. Lamb, D. and Reid, L. (1969) Goblet cell increase in rat bronchiolar epithelium after exposure to cigarette and cigar smoke. *Br. Med. J.*, **i**, 33–5.

17. Lumsden, A.B., McLean, A. and Lamb, D. (1984) Goblet and Clara cells of human distal airways: Evidence for smoking induced changes in their numbers. *Thorax*, **39**, 844–9.

18. Reid, L. (1960) Measurements of the bronchial mucous gland layer: a diagnostic yardstick in chronic bronchitis. *Thorax*, **15**, 132–41.

19. Peto, R., Speizer, F.E., Moore, C.F. *et al.* (1983) The relevance in adults of airflow obstruction, but not of mucous hypersecretion to mortality from chronic lung disease. *Am. Rev. Respir. Dis.*, **128**, 491–500.

20. American Thoracic Society (1962) Chronic bronchitis, asthma and pulmonary emphysema. A statement by the committee on diagnostic standards for non-tuberculous respiratory diseases. *Am. Rev. Respir. Dis.*, **85**, 762–8.

21. Snider, G.L., Kleinerman, J. and Thurlbeck, W.M. (1985) The definition of emphysema. Report of a National Heart, Lung and Blood Institute, Division of Lung Diseases Workshop. *Am. Rev. Respir. Dis.*, **132**, 182–5.

22. Reid, L. (1967) *The Pathology of Emphysema.* Lloyd-Luke, London, pp. 1–21.

23. Saetta, M., Shiner, R.J., Angus, G.E. *et al.* (1985) Destructive Index: A measurement of lung parenchymal destruction in smokers. *Am. Rev. Respir. Dis.*, **131**, 764–9.

24. Eidelman, D.H., Ghezzo, H., Kim, W.D. and Cosio, M.G. (1991) The destructive index and early lung destruction in smokers. *Am. Rev. Respir. Dis.*, **144**, 156–9.

25. Thurlbeck, W.M. (1976) Chronic airflow obstruction in lung disease. In *Major Problems in Pathology. Series No. 5*, (ed. J.L. Bennington) Saunders, Philadelphia.

26. Mitchell, R.S., Silvers, G.W., Goodman, N. *et al.* (1970) Are centrilobular and panlobular emphysema two different diseases? *Hum. Pathol.*, **1**, 433–41.

27. Pratt, P.C. and Kilburn, K.H. (1970) A modern concept of the emphysemas based on correlations of structure and function. *Hum. Pathol.*, **1**, 443–53.

28. Anderson, A.E. and Foraker, A.G. (1973) Centrilobular and panlobular emphysema: two different diseases. *Thorax*, **28**, 547–50.

29. Thurlbeck, W.M. (1963) The incidence of pulmonary emphysema with observations on the relative incidence and spatial distribution of various types of emphysema. *Am. Rev. Respir. Dis.*, **87**, 206–15.

30. Gillooly, M. and Lamb, D. (1993) Cigarette smoking and the susceptibility to microscopic emphysema. *Thorax*, **48**, 445.

31. Gillooly, M. and Lamb, D. (1993) The relationship between centriacinar emphysema and microscopically assessed emphysema. *Am. Rev. Respir. Dis.*, **147** (suppl.), A864.

32. Kim, W.D., Eidelman, D.H., Izquierdo, J.L. *et al.* (1991) Centrilobular and panlobular emphysema in smokers. Two distinct morphologic and functional entities. *Am. Rev. Respir. Dis.*, **144**, 1385–90.

33. Dunnill, M.S. (1962) Quantitative methods in the study of pulmonary pathology. *Thorax*, **17**, 320–9.

34. Heard, B.E. (1960) Pathology of pulmonary emphysema. Methods of study. *Am. Rev. Respir. Dis.*, **82**, 792–99.

35. Thurlbeck, W.M., Horowitz, I., Siemiatycki, J. *et al.* (1969) Intra- and interobserver variations in the assessment of emphysema. *Arch. Environ. Health*, **18**, 646–59.

36. Thurlbeck, W.M., Dunnill, M.S., Hartung, W. *et al.* (1970) A comparison of three methods of measuring emphysema. *Hum. Pathol.*, **1**, 215–26.

37. Thurlbeck, W.M. (1988) Chronic airflow obstruction. In *Pathology of the Lung* (ed. W.M. Thurlbeck) Thieme, New York, pp. 538–75.

38. Dunnill, M.S. (1970) The recognition and measurement of pulmonary emphysema. *Path. Microbiol.*, **35**, 138–45.

39. Thurlbeck, W.M. (1967) The internal surface area of non-emphysematous lungs. *Am. Rev. Respir. Dis.*, **95**, 765–73.

40. Gillooly, M., Lamb, D. and Farrow, A.S.J. (1991) A new automated technique for the assessment of emphysema on histological sections. *J. Clin. Pathol.*, **44**, 1007–11.

41. Aherne, W.A. and Dunnill, M.S. (1982) *Morphometry*, Arnold, London.

42. Gould, G.A., MacNee, W.M., McLean, A. *et al.* (1988) CT measurements of lung density in life can quantitate distal air space enlargement – an essential defining feature of human emphysema. *Am. Rev. Respir. Dis.*, **137**, 380–92.

43. McLean, A., Warren, P.M., Gillooly, M. *et al.* (1992) Microscopic and macroscopic meas-

urements of emphysema: relation to carbon monoxide gas transfer. *Thorax*, **47**, 144–9.

44. Gillooly, M. and Lamb, D. (1993) Airspace size in lungs of life long non-smokers: effect of age and sex. *Thorax*, **48**, 39–43.

45. Gillooly, M. and Lamb, D. (1993) Microscopic emphysema in relation to age and smoking habit. *Thorax*, **48**, 491–5.

46. Linhartova, A., Anderson, A.E. and Foraker, A.G. (1971) Radial traction and bronchiolar obstruction in pulmonary emphysema. *Arch. Pathol.*, **92**, 384–91.

47. Linhartova, A., Anderson, A.E. and Foraker, A.G. (1974) Topology of nonrespiratory bronchioles of normal and emphysematous lungs. *Hum. Pathol.*, **5**, 729–35.

48. Linhartova, A., Anderson, A.E. and Foraker, A.G. (1982) Affixment arrangements of perbronchiolar alveoli in normal and emphysematous lungs. *Arch. Pathol. Lab. Med.*, **106**, 499–502.

49. Niewoehner, D.E., Kleinerman, J. and Rice, D.B. (1974) Pathologic changes in the peripheral airways of young cigarette smokers. *N. Engl. J. Med.*, **291**, 755–8.

50. Myers, J.L., Weil, C.F., Shin, M.S. *et al.* (1987) Respiratory bronchiolitis causing interstitial lung disease: a clinicopathological study of 6 cases. *Am. Rev. Resp. Dis.*, **135**, 880–4.

51. Lang, M.R., Fiaux, G.W., Hulmes, D.J.S. *et al.* (1993) Quantitative studies of human lung airspace wall in relation to collagen and elastin content. *Matrix*, **13**, 471–80.

52. Lang, M.R., Fiaux, G.W., Gillooly, M. *et al.* (1993) Alveolar collagen in non-emphysematous and emphysematous lungs. *Am. Rev. Respir. Dis.*, **147** (suppl.), A864.

53. Cardoso, W.V., Sekhon, H.S., Hyde, D.M. and Thurlbeck, W.M. (1993) Collagen and elastin in human pulmonary emphysema. *Am. Rev. Respir. Dis.*, **147**, 975–81.

54. Nagai, A. and Thurlbeck, W.M. (1991) Scanning electron microscopic observations of emphysema in humans. *Am. Rev. Respir. Dis.*, **144**, 901–8.

55. Thurlbeck, W.M. and Simon, G. (1978) Radiographic appearance of the chest in emphysema. *Am. J. Radiol.*, **130**, 429–40.

56. MacNee, W., Gould, G. and Lamb, D. (1991) Quantifying emphysema by CT scanning. Clinicopathologic correlations. *Ann. N.Y. Acad. Sci.*, **624**, 179–94.

57. Murata, K., Itoh, H., Todo, G. *et al.* (1986) Centrilobular lesions of the lung. Demonstration by high resolution CT and pathologic correlation. *Radiology*, **161**, 641–5.

58. Moudgil, H., Morrison, D., Skevarski, K. *et al.* (1993) Change in CT lung density. Measurement of microscopic emphysema with age. *Thorax*, **48**, 1075.

59. Heremans, A., Verschakelen, J.A., Fraeyenhoven, L. and van Demedts, M. (1992) Measurement of lung density by means of quantitative CT scanning. A study of correlations with pulmonary function tests. *Chest*, **102**, 805–11.

60. Colby, T.V. and Myers, J.L. (1992) The clinical and histological spectrum of bronchiolitis obliterans including bronchiolitis obliterans organising pneumonia (BOOP). *Semin. Respir. Med.*, **13**, 119–33.

61. Wright, J.L., Cargel, P., Churg, A. *et al.* (1992) State of the art. Diseases of the small airway. *Am. Rev. Respir. Dis.*, **140**, 240–62.

62. Woodford, D.M., Coutu, R.E. and Gaensler, E.A. (1979) Obstructive lung disease from acute sulphur dioxide exposure. *Respiration*, **38**, 238–45.

63. Burke, C.M., Theodore, J., Dawkins, K.D. *et al.* (1984) Post transplant obliterative bronchiolitis and other late lung sequelae in human heart lung transplantation. *Chest*, **86**, 824–9.

64. Theodore, J., Starnes, B.A. and Lewiston, N.J. (1990) Obliterative bronchiolitis. *Clin. Chest Med.*, **11**, 309–21.

65. Epler, G.R. (1988) Bronchiolitis obliterans and airways obstruction associated with graft versus host disease. *Clin. Chest Med.*, **9**, 551–6.

66. Geddes, D.M., Webley, M. and Emerson, P.A. (1979) Airways obstruction in rheumatoid arthritis. *Ann. Rheum. Dis.*, **38**, 222–5.

67. Reid, L.M. (1950) Reduction in bronchiolar subdivision in bronchiectasis. *Thorax*, **5**, 233–47.

68. Cosio, M.G., Ghezzo, H., Hogg, J.C. *et al.* (1978) The relations between structural changes in small airways and pulmonary function tests. *N. Engl. J. Med.*, **298**, 1277–81.

69. Wright, J.L., Cosio, M., Wiggs, B. and Hogg, J.C. (1985) A morphologic grading scheme for membranous and respiratory bronchioles. *Arch. Pathol. Lab. Med.*, **109**, 163–5.

70. Nagai, A., West, W.W., Paul, J.L. and Thurlbeck, W.M. (1985) The National Institutes of Health Positive Pressure

Breathing Trial: Pathology studies. 1. Inter-relationship between morphologic lesions. *Am. Rev. Respir. Dis.*, **132**, 937–45.

71. Ryder, R., Dunnill, M.S. and Anderson, J.A. (1971) A quantitative study of bronchial mucous gland volume, emphysema and smoking in a necropsy population. *J. Pathol.*, **104**, 59–71.

72. Greaves, I.A. and Colebatch, H.J.H. (1986) Observations on the pathogenesis of chronic airflow obstruction in smokers: implications for the detection of 'early' lung disease. *Thorax*, **41**, 81–7.

73. Matsuba, K. and Thurlbeck, W.M. (1971) The number and dimensions of small airways in non-emphysematous lungs. *Am. Rev. Respir. Dis.*, **104**, 516–24.

74. Matsuba, K. and Thurlbeck, W.M. (1972) The number and dimensions of small airways in emphysematous lungs. *Am. J. Pathol.*, **67**, 265–75.

75. Linhartova, A., Anderson, A.E. and Foraker, A.G. (1973) Non-respiratory bronchiolar deformities. *Arch. Pathol.*, **95**, 45–8.

76. Petty, T.L. Silvers, G.W. and Stanford, R.E. (1986) Radial traction and small airways disease in excised human lungs. *Am. Rev. Respir. Dis.*, **133**, 132–5.

77. Saetta, M., Ghezzo, H., Kim, W.D. *et al.* (1985) Loss of alveolar attachments in smokers. A morphometric correlate of lung function impairment. *Am. Rev. Respir. Dis.*, **132**, 894–900.

78. Lamb, D., McLean, A., Gillooly, M. *et al.* (1993) Relation between distal airspace size, bronchiolar attachments and lung function. *Thorax*, **48**, 1012–7.

79. Nagai, A., Yamawaki, I., Takizawa, T. and Thurlbeck, W.M. (1991) Alveolar attachments in emphysema of human lungs. *Am. Rev. Respir. Dis.*, **144**, 888–91.

80. Buist, A.S. and Ross, B.B. (1973) Quantitative analysis of the alveolar plateau in the diagnosis of early airway obstruction. *Am. Rev. Respir. Dis.*, **108**, 1078–87.

81. Thurlbeck, W.M., Henderson, J.A., Fraser, R.G. and Bates, D.V. (1970) Chronic obstructive lung disease. *Medicine*, **49**, 81–145.

82. Paré, P.D., Brooks, L.A., Bates, J. *et al.* (1982) Experimental analysis of the lung pressure-volume curve as a predictor of pulmonary emphysema. *Am. Rev. Respir. Dis.*, **126**, 54–61.

83. Berend, N., Skoog, C. and Thurlbeck, W.M. (1980) Pressure-volume characteristics of excised human lungs: effects of sex, age and emphysema. *J. Appl. Physiol., Respirat. Environ. Exercise Physiol.*, **49**, 558–65.

84. Silvers, G.W., Petty, T.L. and Stanford, R.E. (1980) Elastic recoil changes in early emphysema. *Thorax*, **35**, 490–5.

85. Petty, T.L., Silvers, G.W. and Stanford, R.E. (1981) Functional correlations with mild and moderate emphysema in excised human lung. *Am. Rev. Respir. Dis.*, **124**, 700–4.

86. Wright, J.L., Wiggs, B.J. and Hogg, J.C. (1984) Airway disease in upper and lower lobes in lungs of patients with and without emphysema. *Thorax*, **39**, 282–5.

87. Berend, N., Woolcock, A.J. and Martin, G.E. (1978) Correlation between the function and structure of the lung in smokers. *Am. Rev. Respir. Dis.*, **119**, 695–705.

88. Wright, J.L., Hobson, J., Wiggs, B.R. *et al.* (1987) Effect of cigarette smoking on structure of the small airways. *Lung*, **165**, 91–100.

89. Cosio, M.G., Hale, K.A. and Niewoehner, D.E. (1980) Morphologic and morphometric effects of prolonged cigarette smoking on the small airways. *Am. Rev. Respir. Dis.*, **122**, 265–71.

90. Bosken, C.H., Wiggs, B.R., Paré, P.D. and Hogg, J.C. (1990) Small airway dimensions in smokers with obstruction to airflow. *Am. Rev. Respir. Dis.*, **142**, 563–70.

91. Matsuba, K., Wright, J.L., Wiggs, B.R. *et al.* (1989) The changes in airways structure associated with reduced forced expiratory volume in one second. *Eur. Respir. J.*, **2**, 834–9.

92. Fletcher, C.M., Peto, R., Tinker, C.M. *et al.* (1976) *The Natural History of Chronic Bronchitis and Emphysema*. Oxford University Press, Oxford.

93. Gillooly, M. and Lamb, D. (1993) The effect of age on the alveolar support of peripheral bronchioles in non-smokers. *Am. Rev. Respir. Dis.*, **147** (suppl), A864.

94. Calverley, P.M., Howatson, R., Flenley, D.C. and Lamb, D. (1992) Clinicopathological correlations in cor pulmonale. *Thorax*, **47**, 494–8.

95. Burrows, B., Fletcher, C.M., Heard, B.E. *et al.* (1966). The emphysematous and bronchial types of chronic airways obstruction. *Lancet*, i, 830–5.

96. Flenley, D.C. (1986) Long term oxygen therapy and the pulmonary circulation. In: *Aspects of Hypoxia* (ed. D. Heath), Liverpool University Press, Liverpool, pp. 45–59.

97. Samet, J.M., Humble, C.G. and Pathak, D.R. (1986) Personal and family history of respiratory disease and lung cancer risk. *Am. Rev. Respir. Dis.*, **134**, 466–70.

98. Skillrid, D.M., Offord, K.P. and Miller R.D. (1986) Higher risk of lung cancer in chronic pulmonary disease: a prospective matched case-control study. *Ann. Intern. Med.*, **105**, 503–7.

99. Fishman, A.P. (1976) Hypoxia on the pulmonary circulation: how and where it acts. *Circ. Res.*, **38**, 221–31.

100. Sylvester, J.T., Gottlieb, J.E., Rock, P. and Wetzel, R.C. (1986) Acute hypoxic responses. In: *Abnormal Pulmonary Circulation* (ed. E.H. Bergofsky), Churchill Livingstone, Edinburgh, pp. 127–65.

101. Hazelton, P.S., Heath, D. and Brewer, D.B. (1968) Hypertensive pulmonary vascular disease in states of chronic hypoxia. *J. Pathol. Bacteriol.*, **95**, 431–40.

102. Hicken, P., Heath, D., Brewer, D.B. and Whitaker, W. (1965) The small pulmonary arteries in emphysema. *J. Pathol. Bacteriol.*, **90**, 107–14.

103. Wagenvoort, C.A. and Wagenvoort, N. (1973) Hypoxic pulmonary vascular lesion in man at high altitude and in patients with chronic respiratory diseases. *Pathol. Microbiol.*, **39**, 276.

104. Hale, K.A., Niewoehner, D.E. and Cosio, M.G. (1980) Morphologic changes in the muscular pulmonary arteries: Relationship to cigarette smoking, airway disease and emphysema. *Am. Rev. Respir. Dis.*, **122**, 273–8.

105. Fernie, J.M., McLean, A. and Lamb, D. (1988) Significant intimal abnormalities in muscular pulmonary arteries of patients with early obstructive lung disease. *J. Clin. Pathol.*, **41**, 730–3.

106. Fernie, J.M. and Lamb, D. (1985) New method for quantitating the medial component of pulmonary arteries. *Arch. Pathol. Lab. Med.*, **109**, 843–8.

107. Fernie, J.M. and Lamb, D. (1985) New method for measuring intimal component of pulmonary arteries. *J. Clin. Pathol.*, **38**, 1374–9.

108. Fernie, J.M. and Lamb, D. (1988) Assessment of the effects of age and smoking on the media of the muscular pulmonary arteries. *J. Pathol.*, **155**, 241–6.

109. Fulton, R.M., Hutchinson, E.C. and Jones, A.M. (1952) Ventricular weight in cardiac hypertrophy. *Br. Heart J.*, **14**, 413–20.

110. Lamb, D. (1973) Heart weight and assessment of ventricular hypertrophy. In: *Recent Advances in Clinical Pathology, Series 6* (ed. S.C. Dyke), Churchill Livingstone, Edinburgh, pp. 133–48.

111. Heath, D., Smith, P. and Jago, R. (1982) Hyperplasia of the carotid body. *J. Pathol.*, **138**, 115–27.

112. Bee, D. and Howard, P. (1993) The carotid body: a review of its anatomy, physiology and clinical importance. *Monaldi Arch. Chest. Dis.*, **48**, 48–53.

113. Campbell, J.L., Calverley, P.M.A., Lamb, D. and Flenley, D.C. (1982) The renal glomerulus in hypoxic cor pulmonale. *Thorax*, **37**, 607–11.

LUNG STRUCTURE–FUNCTION RELATIONSHIPS

P.D. Paré and J.C. Hogg

3.1 INTRODUCTION

The characteristic physiologic abnormality that defines chronic obstructive pulmonary disease (COPD) is a decrease in the maximal expiratory flow. Mead and his associates [1] developed the concept that during forced expiration lateral pressures at points within the airways become equal to pleural pressure and that the pressure driving flow from the alveoli to these equal pressure points approximates the static recoil pressure of the lung. This means that forced expiratory flow can be reduced by (1) a loss of lung elasticity, (2) an increase in resistance of the airways upstream from the equal pressure points, and/or (3) an increase in the compliance of airways downstream from equal pressure points. Over the past 15 years we have collected data on lung function and structure on more than 400 patients who have had a surgical resection of a lung or lobe. Despite a remarkably uniform smoking duration and intensity and a narrow age distribution these patients show a wide variation in the degree of airway obstruction. The purpose of this chapter is to examine the factors that determine maximal expiratory flow in an attempt to define the relative importance of loss of lung elastic recoil and peripheral airways obstruction to the reduction in forced expiratory flow.

3.2 RELATIONSHIP OF LUNG RECOIL PRESSURES TO LUNG STRUCTURE

It is often assumed that changes in lung elastic recoil can be equated with the morphologic lesions of emphysema. Elastin is a major component of the lung interstitium and an important contributor to the elastic recoil properties of the lung parenchyma. Destruction of the connective tissue framework of the lung by the emphysematous process disrupts the elastic tissue network of the lung and this is assumed to account for the physiologic decrease in elastic recoil pressure.

Figure 3.1 shows a pressure–volume curve obtained in a patient with COPD prior to resectional surgery. Multiple volume and static lung recoil points are recorded by measuring transpulmonary pressure (the difference between mouth pressure and pleural pressure determined using the esophageal balloon technique) at lung volumes between FRC and TLC. Quantitative data concerning lung elasticity can be obtained from this relationship by fitting an exponential equation of the form $V = A - Be^{-kp}$ [2] to the deflation curve. The constant k describes the shape of the pressure–volume curve: increased values for k are associated with loss of lung elastic recoil and decreased values indicate lung stiffening.

Chronic Obstructive Pulmonary Disease. Edited by Dr P. Calverley and Professor N. Pride. Published in 1995 by Chapman & Hall, London. ISBN 0 412 46450 0

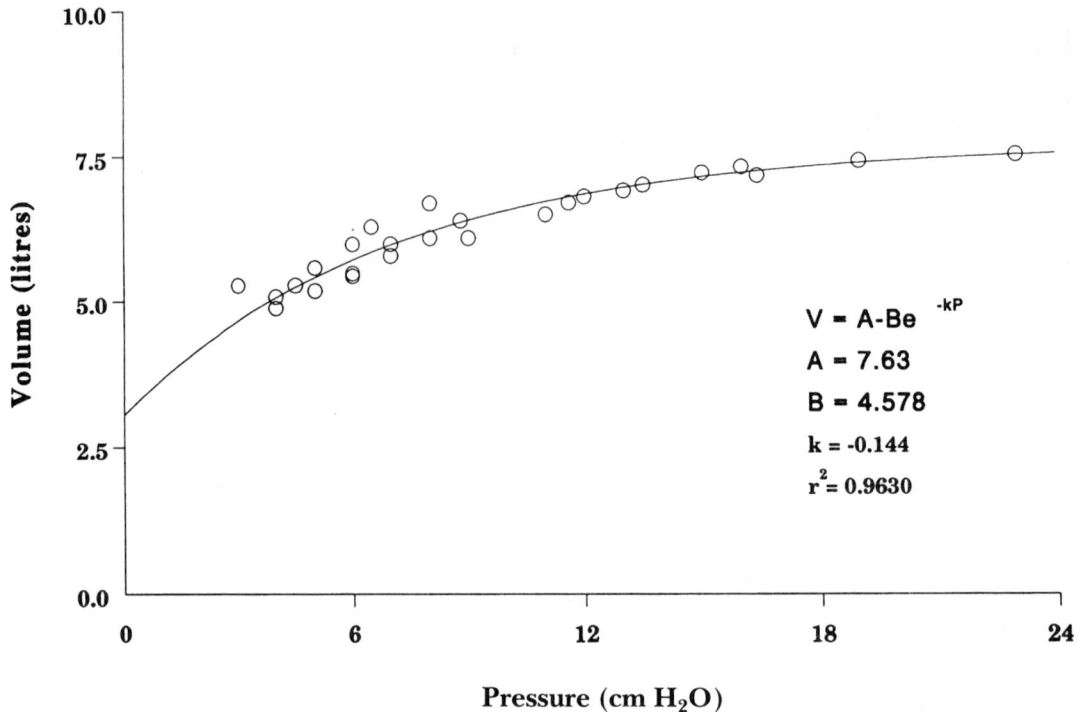

$$V = A - Be^{-kP}$$
$$A = 7.63$$
$$B = 4.578$$
$$k = -0.144$$
$$r^2 = 0.9630$$

Fig. 3.1 Relation between lung recoil pressure (PL) and lung volume (pressure–volume data) in a patient with COPD. Multiple transpulmonary pressure and volume points are obtained using an esophageal balloon technique and a body plethysmograph. The pressure–volume data are best described by an exponential function in which A = the theoretical maximal lung volume at infinite transpulmonary pressure, B = the volume difference between A and the volume at 0 transpulmonary pressure and *k* is a description of the PV curve. Increased *k* indicates loss of lung recoil.

In addition to fitting the pressure–volume relationship to an exponential function, discrete pressure volume points representing the elastic recoil pressure at TLC (PL max) or at 90%, 80%, 70%, or 60% of TLC can be used to characterize the pressure–volume behavior of the lung.

Emphysema was quantitated in these resected lung specimens using a modification of the pictorial grading system originally developed by Thurlbeck *et al.* [3,4]. This requires that the lung or lobe is inflated with a fixative at a constant pressure and sliced in a predetermined manner after it is fixed. A grade of emphysema is then assigned to the specimen by comparing the cut surface of the lung to a standard set of pictures. This technique

allows the emphysematous lung destruction visible to the naked eye to be quantitated on a scale of 0 to 100 and it provides values for emphysematous destruction that are in reasonably good agreement with the extent of emphysema detected on CT scans [5].

It is also possible to quantify the destruction of the alveolar surface by measuring airspace dimensions on histologic preparations of the lung using the light microscope. This is accomplished by projecting a grid of lines of known length on the microscopic image and calculating mean linear intercept or the average distance between alveolar walls (Lm). Although it is true that areas of emphysema will result in an increased average alveolar size it is not necessarily true that lungs in which there is an increase in average alveolar size will have the macroscopic characteristics of emphysema. It is our contention that changes in average alveolar size represented by an increase in Lm provide a more precise morphologic counterpart of loss of lung elasticity than macroscopic emphysematous lesions [6]. In fact, over the range of volumes between FRC and TLC the pressure–volume relationship of macroscopic emphysematous spaces have a value of *k* that is substantially *lower* than the lung parenchyma surrounding it [7]. In addition, fully developed emphysematous lesions change very little in volume as the lung is deflated and so they contribute very little to the expired lung volume or to the pressure–volume relationship of the whole lung.

Studies on a group of 163 patients showed no significant relationship between the preop-

erative measurement of the exponential constant K and the emphysema score determined macroscopically on their resected lungs (Fig. 3.2). Since lung recoil is one of the major determinants of maximal expiratory flow, a corollary of this observation is that one would not predict a close relationship between macroscopically determined emphysematous destruction of the lung and decreased maximal expiratory flow. Figure 3.3 shows that this prediction was confirmed in the same group of patients where some individuals had severe airflow obstruction but no emphysema and others had marked emphysema but no decrease in maximal expiratory flow.

The airspace size (Lm) away from the emphysematous spaces was examined in a separate group of 44 patients to test the hypothesis that the PV curve of the lung reflects the behavior of the lung parenchyma

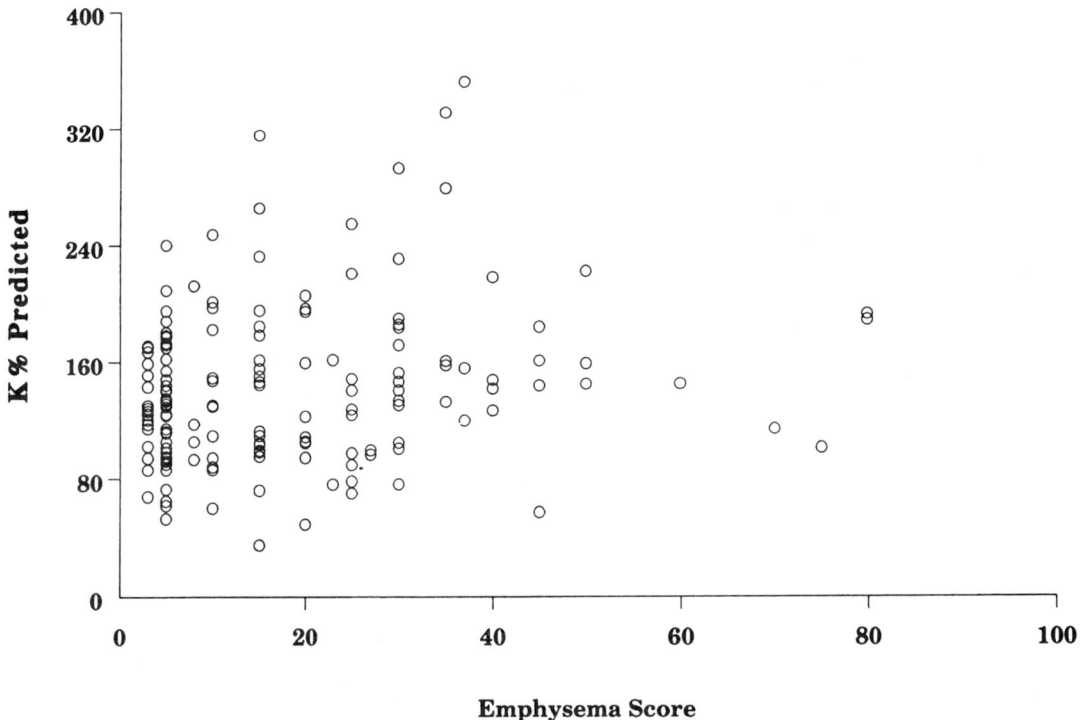

Fig. 3.2 Emphysema score plotted against the exponential constant *k*. There is no significant relationship (N = 163).

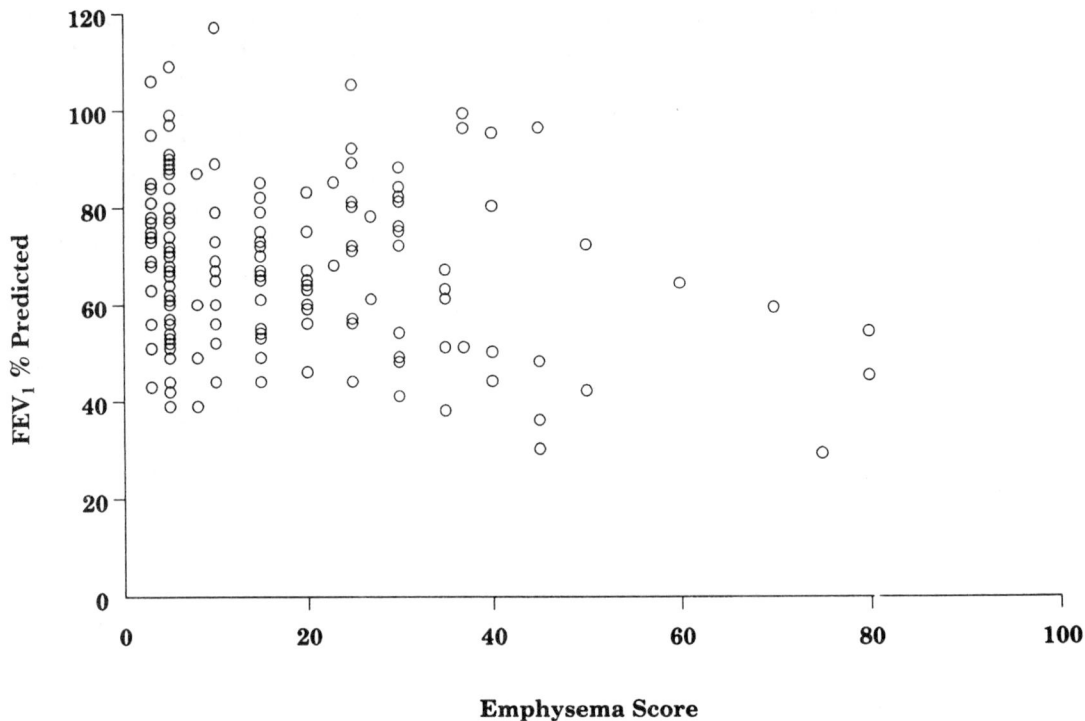

Fig. 3.3 Emphysema score versus $FEV_1\%$ predicted (N = 163). There is no significant relationship. Patients who have mild emphysema may be severely obstructed and vice versa.

away from these lesions. This analysis showed (Table 3.1) that the patients who had decreased lung elastic recoil (i.e. increased k) had increased values for Lm irrespective of the absence (Group 2) or presence (Group 4) of macroscopic emphysema. This suggests that k reflects the structure of the lung *apart* from the grossly visible emphysematous

lesions and indicates an increased mean alveolar size in these regions. Airspace size is an important determinant of lung elastic recoil because of the contribution of surface tension. The Laplace relationship shows that the pressure (P) generated across a spherical structure is related to the surface tension (T) and the radius of curvature (r) of the structure (P =

Table 3.1

	Group 2 No significant emphysema		Group 4 Significant emphysema	
	Normal k	*Increased k*	*Normal k*	*Increased k*
Emphysema score	2±4	2±3	26±17	29±11
k %P	107±21	176±26	107±9	180±19
Lm (μm)	188±38[a]	251±74	239±50	260±75
PL max%P	91±35	73±18	79±33	66±15

Mean ± standard deviation; %P, percent predicted.
[a]Significantly different from Group 2 or 4.

2T/r). This means that the larger the radius of curvature of the airspace units the lower transmural (tranpulmonary) pressure and that increasing airspace size will reduce lung elastic recoil pressure if surface tension remains the same.

A similar conclusion regarding the relationship between lung structure and recoil was reached by Kim *et al.* [8] using a different approach. They used a microscopic scoring procedure to characterize emphysema into its centrilobular form, where the respiratory bronchioles and alveolar ducts of the primary lobule are grossly dilated and the alveolar sacs adjacent to interlobular septa are of normal size, and the panlobular form of emphysema where all airspaces are enlarged. When they measured mean linear intercept in two groups, one with predominant centrilobular and the other with predominant panlobular emphysema they found no significant difference in the average value for Lm but those with centrilobular emphysema had a significantly increased value for the standard deviation of Lm. The lungs with the panacinar type of emphysema on the other hand had a narrow standard deviation for Lm (i.e. indicating uniformly increased alveolar size). Despite similar average values for Lm the subjects who showed panlobular emphysema had more loss of lung recoil ($\uparrow k$, $\uparrow$ compliance and $\downarrow$ values for P_{L90} and P_{L60}). They concluded that the pressure–volume behavior of the lung was influenced by the distribution of alveolar destruction where homogeneous alveolar destruction results in an increase in Lm with little variation in mean alveolar size, increased K, and decreased elastic recoil.

These results indicate that the loss of lung recoil in COPD correlates with an increase in airspace size in the lung parenchyma away from centrilobular emphysematous spaces. During the process of emphysematous destruction there is presumably a phase when individual alveolar walls are disrupted; the resulting moderately enlarged alveolar airspaces continue to empty during lung deflation and so they contribute to the pressure–volume behavior of the lung. When these enlarged airspaces coalesce into gross emphysematous lesions which tend to remain inflated during expiration [7], they stop making a contribution to expired lung volume. When this occurs the pressure–volume behavior is determined by the remaining airspaces and if their average size is normal, a relatively normal PV curve is the result. However, if the alveolar wall destruction is homogeneous throughout the lung parenchyma and the average alveolar size of contributing airspaces increases, lung elastic recoil will decrease irrespective of whether or not gross morphologic emphysematous spaces can be detected.

3.3 MAXIMUM EXPIRATORY FLOW AND SMALL AIRWAY PATHOLOGY

In the early part of this century Rohrer [9] calculated the resistance of central and peripheral airways based on measurements made from lung casts and predicted that the small airways were the major site of resistance in normal lungs. This concept was not challenged until Macklem and Mead [10] developed a retrograde catheter technique that allowed total airway resistance to be partitioned into its peripheral and central components. Direct measurements with the retrograde catheter, on post-mortem lungs [11,12] and more recent measurements with a new technique in living patients [13] have confirmed that the peripheral airways are not the major site of resistance in normal human lungs. Verbeken *et al.* [14] have recently shown that much of the peripheral resistance in normal human lungs is tissue resistance rather than airway resistance. However, direct measurements in both post-mortem lungs and in living patients have now confirmed that the peripheral lung is the major site of obstruction in disease and that it is peripheral airways, not tissue resistance, that is increased [14]. These studies showed that the contribution of the peripheral airways to total resistance increases from 20–30% of the total in normals to as much as 80% of the increased value of resistance in patients who have moderate COPD. The concept that the peripheral airways represent a relatively silent zone in the healthy lung, but becomes a major site of increased resistance in disease led to a series of investigations attempting to identify the earliest structural and functional abnormalities in these airways [15,16].

Possible causes of peripheral airway narrowing are listed below:

Loss of alveolar attachments
Decreased lung recoil
Altered surface tension in the airway lumen
Occlusion of the lumen by exudate
Edema, cellular infiltration, fibrosis and scarring of the wall
Airway smooth muscle contraction

In addition to the loss of elastic recoil and destruction of alveolar support which are part of the emphysematous destruction of the lung parenchyma, the airways are also changed by the inflammatory process. These changes include those produced by an inflammatory exudate into the lumen as well as those which occur deeper in the airway wall. Furthermore, functional events such as airway smooth muscle shortening may act in conjunction with the changes in the wall and lumen to narrow the caliber of the airway.

Some years ago Macklem, Proctor and Hogg [17] showed that the peripheral airways were lined by surfactant which has a surface tension of 3 dynes/cm. If this was replaced by an exudate of plasma which has a surface tension of 50 dynes/cm it would increase transmural pressure of a 1 mm diameter airway by approximately 1.0 cm H_2O. This would decrease the stability of the peripheral airways particularly at low lung volumes and markedly reduce the total cross-sectional area in this region. Since in virtually all studies of

peripheral airway morphology the lungs have been inflated with a fixative the potential contribution of surface tension differences to airway diameter cannot be assessed.

In 1977 Cosio, Ghezzo and Hogg [18] showed that decreased maximal expiratory flow correlated with morphologic evidence of a chronic inflammatory process in the walls of the peripheral airways. Surprisingly, the occlusion of the lumen by an inflammatory exudate that formed a mucus plug appeared to have little effect on total airway function. This suggests that peripheral airway plugging is scattered and has little effect on total airways cross-section or that mucous plugs are lost during fixation. The findings of Cosio *et al.* were confirmed and extended in several laboratories [19,20] but in many of these studies, including the original one by Cosio *et al.*, the groups with the best lung function were younger and had smoked less than those with the worst lung function. More recent evaluations are beginning to show that in patients who are correctly matched for age and smoking history there is little difference in the semiquantitative estimate of the inflammatory process in those with or without reduced FEV_1. This suggests that the functional abnormality in the peripheral airways in COPD may be related to increased airway wall thickness in the same way as has been demonstrated in asthma. To test this hypothesis Bosken *et al.* [21] compared the airways from 30 subjects with mild to moderate airways obstruction to those from 30 non-obstructed patients selected from our patient group (Tables 3.2 and 3.3). They examined 189 and 175 membranous airways per group with at least 5 bronchioles per patient. There was no difference in the frequency distribution of the airway internal perimeter in the non-alveolated, non-cartilaginous airways examined, suggesting that smaller membranous bronchioles were not systematically selected in patients with airways obstruction ($P>0.05$ for internal perimeter). The airways of the obstructed individuals had a smaller luminal

Table 3.2

	Non-obstructed	Obstructed
N	30	30
Age	65±9	64±8
Pack years	45±36	70±42[a]
$FEV_1/FVC\%$	77±4	55±6[a]
PL max (cmH$_2$O)	25±8	18±5[a]
Membranous bronchiolar pathology score	126±49	154±45[a]

[a]Significantly different obstructed vs non-obstructed (*P*<0.05).

Table 3.3

	Non-obstructed	Obstructed
Membranous airways	189	175
Luminal diameter (mm)	0.74±0.5	0.61±0.4[a]
Luminal perimeter (mm)	3.77±2.21	3.47±2.2
Wall thickness (mm)	0.106±0.06	0.132±0.08[a]

[a]Significantly different obstructed vs non-obstructed (*P*<0.05).

area and thicker walls than the non-obstructed patients and the relationship between internal perimeter and wall thickness was significantly different from the non-obstructed subjects. In addition, quantitative study of the components of the airways based on point counting showed that all three layers of the airway wall (submucosa, muscle, and adventitia) were significantly increased in thickness in the obstructed subjects. The obstructed individuals also had significantly greater inflammation scores in membranous bronchioles as judged semi-quantitatively; however, there were subjects who had thick airways with low inflammation scores and vice versa. The fact that there was better separation of obstructed and non-obstructed individuals based on airway wall thickness than on inflammation scores suggests that the presence of an inflammatory process as

judged by a visual grading system provides only part of the answer as to why the peripheral airways are obstructed. It also suggests that the structural consequences of chronic inflammation as represented by the thickness of the airway wall may be a better way to estimate the long-term effect of the inflammatory process on airway function. However, the differences in small airway dimensions between the obstructed and non-obstructed individuals is not as great as might be expected for the differences in flows. It is possible that it is not the average peripheral airway dimensions that are important but rather the existence of short critically narrowed segments that could be missed during random sampling.

During forced expiration the maximal expiratory airflow at each lung volume is determined by the behavior of the airways upstream and downstream from the equal pressure point. With relatively normal lungs the equal pressure point occurs in cartilaginous central airways and it is the dynamic pressure–area behaviour of these airways which is an important determinant of maximal expiratory flow. With peripheral airway narrowing and decrease in lung recoil the equal pressure points and therefore flow limiting segments move toward the alveoli during forced expiration. Under these circumstances the dynamic behaviour of the peripheral airways will determine airway cross-sectional area and maximal expiratory flow. Unfortunately, examination of the airway morphometry in a fixed specimen cannot determine the mechanical behavior of the airway wall as it is stressed during forced expiration. Deposition of connective tissue in the airway walls could either stiffen the peripheral airways and prevent their cross-section from decreasing during forced expiration or, alternatively, make them more compliant so that their cross-section would be obliterated as the lung is forcibly emptied.

We have recently examined the structural differences in the lungs and airways of smokers with and without airway hyper-responsiveness. Airway hyper-responsiveness was correlated most closely with baseline values for FEV_1, but when this was corrected for peripheral airway wall thickness and lung recoil provided separate contributions to the prediction of airway responsiveness [22].

The relative contribution of loss of lung elasticity and increase in peripheral airway resistance to expiratory air flow obstruction can be appreciated by constructing maximal expiratory flow–static recoil plots, the slope of which is upstream conductance (Fig. 3.4). Patients can have decreased flow purely related to loss of recoil, purely related to increased upstream resistance, or due to a combination of these changes. In a patient in whom decreased flow is due only to loss of recoil, the relationship between maximal flow and recoil will be normal; the flows are decreased simply because the recoil forces during flow are decreased. Those who have decreased flow due only to an increase in airway resistance will have a normal range of recoil pressures but a decreased slope of the maximal flow–recoil relationship.

The normal range for this relationship illustrated in Figs 3.4 and 3.5 was constructed by using the range of normal maximal flow and recoil pressures from data of Morris, Koski and Johnson, [23] and Colebatch, Greaves and Ng [24] respectively. The maximal flows and recoil pressures from the effort-independent portion of the patients' flow–volume curves and pressure–volume curves between 25 and 75% of VC were used to construct individual maximal flow–static recoil plots. The curves represent the slope between the pressure and flow points at 25 and 75% of measured vital capacity. A mean curve for each group of sub-

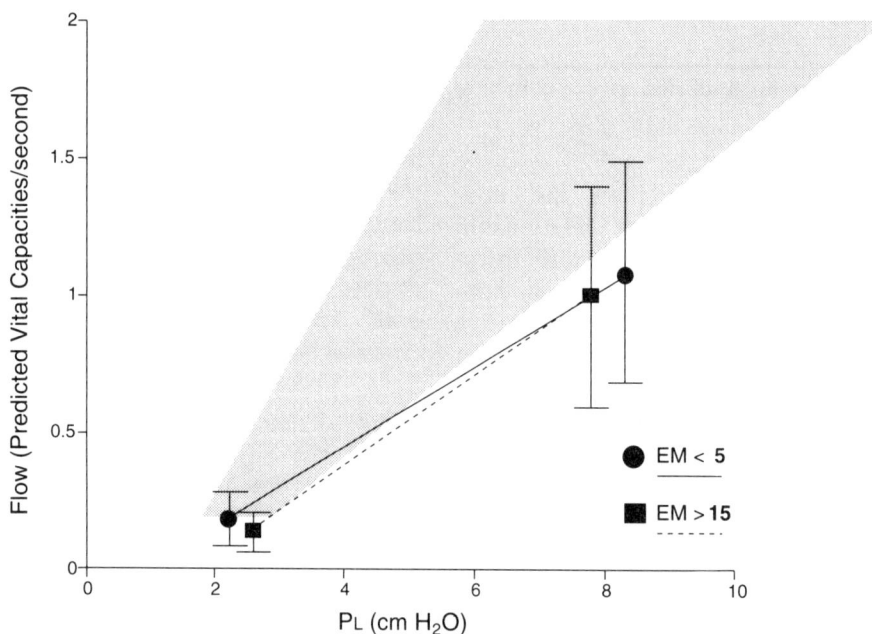

Fig. 3.4 Mean maximal flow–static recoil plots in the 26 patients who had significant emphysema (EM>15) and those who did not (EM<5). The normal range for the relationship between maximal flow and recoil is shown in the shaded area and is expressed as predicted vital capacities/sec/cmH$_2$O (Table 3.4). The slope of the relationship is upstream conductance (Gus). Dividing patients on the basis of emphysema does not separate a group with normal and decreased upstream conductance.

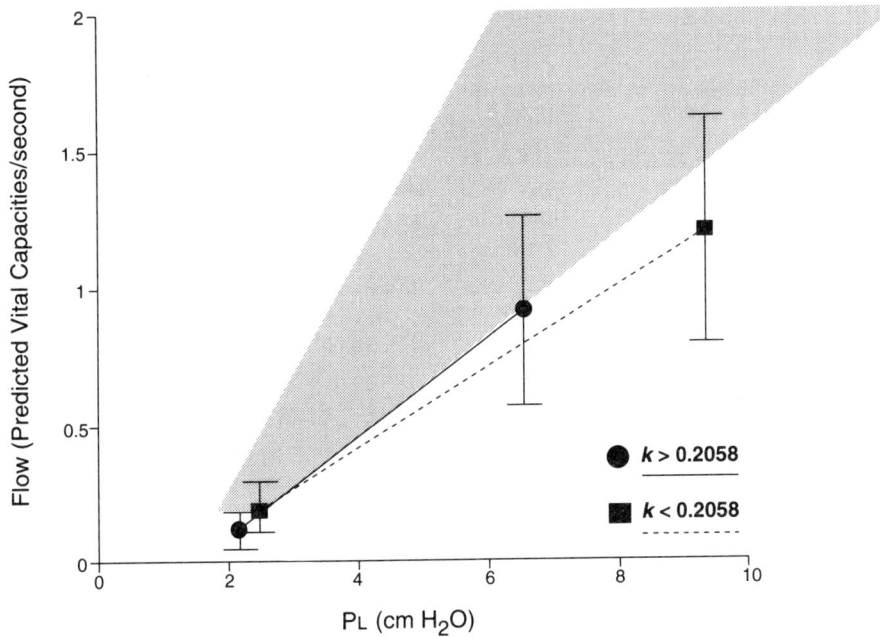

Fig. 3.5   The mean maximal flow–static plots in the 26 subjects with the lowest and the highest values for *k* (Table 3.5). Dividing subjects on the basis of recoil separates those whose obstruction is primarily related to decreased recoil (normal upstream conductance) and those whose obstruction is primarily related to peripheral airway narrowing (decreased upstream conductance).

jects was determined and expressed as predicted VC/sec to normalize for lung size. Table 3.4 shows data from 52 patients with evidence of mild to moderate airflow obstruction, 26 of whom had either no or minimal emphysema (score <5) and 26 of whom had mild to moderate emphysema (score of >15). It is apparent that those who have no or minimal emphysema have FEV_1/FVC and $FEV_1\%$ predicted values that are comparable to those who have moderate emphysema. Figure 3.4 shows the mean maximal flow–static recoil plot for these two groups. The data show that there was no difference in the slope for subjects with or without emphysema but both groups had mean curves which fall below the normal range. Some patients in both groups had slopes which were well within the normal range. However, when the subjects were divided into two equally sized groups based on lung recoil (*k* <0.2058 and >0.2058) (Table

Table 3.4   Anthropometric and physiologic data: subjects divided on basis of emphysema score

	Emphysema <5	Emphysema >15
N	26	26
Emphysema score	0.7±1.3	31±15[a]
Males/females	20/6	22/4
$FEV_1\%P$	85±10	89±9
$FEV_1/FVC\%$	67±5	66±4
PL max %P	81±25	78±26
k%P	125±30	131±38
Gus VC/sec/cmH₂O	0.15±0.07	0.16±0.05

%P, percent predicted; Gus, upstream conductance.
[a]Significantly different (*P*<0.05).

3.5) those subjects who had high values for *k* have a mean slope of maximal flow vs recoil which falls within the normal range. On the other hand, those subjects who were equally obstructed but had a more normal *k* had a significant reduction in upstream conductance.

Table 3.5 Anthropometric and physiologic data: subjects divided on basis of exponential constant *k*

	k<0.2058	*k>0.2058*
N	26	26
Emphysema score	13±15	18±16
Males/females	21/5	21/5
FEV_1%P	88±9	86±11
FEV_1/FVC%	68±6	66±5
PL max %P	86±22	76±30
k%P	107±14	148±24[a]
Gus VC/sec/cmH$_2$O	0.12±0.03	0.19±0.05[a]

%P, percent predicted; Gus, upstream conductance.
[a]$P<0.05$.

This analysis illustrates that dividing subjects on the basis of either the presence of macroscopic emphysematous lesions (Table 3.4) or on lung elasticity (Table 3.5) does not identify a group in whom there is a greater reduction in FEV_1, or FEV_1/ FVC. Separation of patients on the basis of emphysema (Table 3.4 and Fig. 3.4) shows that upstream conductance was decreased irrespective of the severity of emphysema. However, separation of patients on the basis of the lung pressure–volume behavior does result in identification of groups who have normal and decreased upstream conductance.

In summary, structure–function comparison supports the hypothesis that the decrease in maximal expiratory flow in chronic smokers develops because of both decreased lung elasticity and increased peripheral airway resistance. A combination of these processes occurs in most patients with COPD and separation of a group who have gross emphysema does not select those in whom loss of recoil is more important than increased resistance. Conversely, loss of recoil contributes equally to decreased flow in individuals who do not have gross emphysema. The closest morphologic counterpart of decreased lung recoil is increased mean alveolar size in parenchyma away from emphysematous spaces and the closest correlate of decreased peripheral airway conductance is the thickening of the membranous bronchioles produced by the inflammatory process.

REFERENCES

1. Mead, J., Turner, J.M., Macklem, P.T. and Little, J.B. (1967) Significance of the relationship between lung recoil and maximum expiratory flow. *J. Appl. Physiol.*, **22**, 95–108.
2. Colebatch, H.J.H., Ng, C.K.Y. and Nikov, N. (1979) Use of an exponential function for elastic recoil. *J. Appl. Physiol.*, **46**, 387–93.
3. Wright, J. L., Wiggs, B., Paré, P.D. and Hogg, J.C. (1986) Ranking the severity of emphysema on whole lung slices. *Am. Rev. Respir. Dis.*, **133**, 930–1.
4. Thurlbeck, W.M., Dunnill, M.S., Hartung, W. *et al.* (1970) A comparison of three methods of measuring emphysema. *Hum. Pathol.*, **1**, 215–26.
5. Bergen, C., Müller, M., Nicholls, D.M. *et al.* (1986) The diagnosis of emphysema. *Am. Rev. Respir. Dis.*, **133**, 541–6.
6. Osborne, S., Hogg, J.C., Wright, J.L. *et al.* (1988). Exponential analysis of the pressure volume curve. *Am. Rev. Respir. Dis.*, **137**, 1083–8.
7. Hogg, J.C., Nepszy, S., Macklem, P.T. and Thurlbeck, W.M. (1969) The elastic properties of the centrilobular emphysematous space. *J. Clin. Invest.*, **48**, 1306–12.
8. Kim, W.D., Eidelman, D.H., Izquierdo, J.L. *et al.* (1991) Centrilobular and panlobular emphysema in smokers. *Am. Rev. Respir. Dis.*, **144**, 1385–90.
9. Rohrer, F. (1915) Der Stromungswiderstand in den menschlichen Atemwegen und der Eimflub der unregelmassgen Verzweigung des bronchialsystems auf den Atmungsverlauf in vershiedenen Lungenbezirken. *Arch. Ges. Physiol.*, **162**, 225–9.
10. Macklem, P.T. and Mead, J. (1967). Resistance of central and peripheral airways measured by a retrograde catheter. *J. Appl. Physiol.*, **22**, 395–401.
11. Hogg, J.C., Macklem, P.T. and Thurlbeck, W.M. (1968). Site and nature of airways obstruction in chronic obstructive lung disease. *N. Engl. J. Med.*, **278**, 1355–60.
12. Van Brabandt, H., Cauberghs, M., Verbeken, E. *et al.* (1983). Partitioning of pulmonary impe-

dence in excised human and canine lungs. *J. Appl. Physiol.*, **55**, 1733–42.

13. Yanai, M., Sekizawa, K., Ohru, P. *et al.* (1992) Site of airway obstruction in pulmonary disease: direct measure of intrabronchial pressure. *J. Appl. Physiol.*, **72**, 1016–23.

14. Verbeken, E.K., Cauberghs, M., Mertens, I. *et al.* (1992) Tissue and airway impedence of excised normal senile, and emphysematous lungs. *J. Appl. Physiol.*, **72**, 2343–53.

15. Mead, J. (1970) The lung's 'quiet zone'. *N. Engl. J. Med.*, **282**, 1318–19.

16. Macklem, P.T. and Permutt, S. (eds) (1979) The lung in the transition between health and disease In: *Lung Biology in Health and Disease,* (Executive Editor Claude Lenfant) Marcel Dekker.

17. Macklem, P.T., Proctor, D.F. and Hogg, J.C. (1970). The stability of peripheral airways, *Resp. Physiol.*, **8**, 191–203.

18. Cosio, M., Ghezzo, H. and Hogg, J.C. *et al.* (1977) The relationship between structural changes in small airways and pulmonary function tests. *N. Engl. J. Med.*, **298**, 1277–81.

19. Berend, N., Wright, J.L., Thurlbeck, W.M. *et al.* (1981). Small airways disease: reproducibility of measurements and correlation with lung function. *Chest*, **79**, 263–8.

20. Petty, T.L., Silvers, G.W., Stanford, R.E. *et al.* (1980). Small airway pathology as related to increased closing capacity and abnormal slope of Phase 3 in excised human lungs. *Am. Rev. Respir. Dis*, **121**, 449–56.

21. Bosken, C.H., Wiggs, B.R., Paré, P.D. and Hogg, J.C. (1990) Small airway dimensions in smokers with obstruction to airflow. *Am. Rev. Respir. Dis.*, **142**, 563–70.

22. Riess, A., Wiggs, B., Wright, J.L. *et al.* Morphologic determinants of airway responsiveness in chronic smokers. *Am. Rev. Respir. Dis.* Submitted.

23. Morris, J.R., Koski, A. and Johnson, L.C. (1971) Spirometric standards for healthy non-smoking adults. *Am. Rev. Respir. Dis.*, **133**, 132–5.

24. Colebatch, H.J.H., Greaves, I.A. and Ng, C.K.Y. (1979). Exponential analysis of elastic recoil and aging in healthy males and females. *J. Appl. Physiol.*, **47**, 683–91.

EPIDEMIOLOGY: A BRITISH PERSPECTIVE

4

D.P. Strachan

4.1 INTRODUCTION

Bronchitis has been recognized as a disease with a high prevalence in Great Britain since the early years of this century, even before smoking became a habit of mass appeal [1]. The 'English disease' (from which the Scots, Welsh and Irish are by no means immune!) became the focus of epidemiologic interest following the demonstration of the acute toxic effects of smoke and sulfur dioxide air pollution during the London smog of 1952 [2]. This led to the development of a standardized definition of the disease that would be suitable for clinical and epidemiologic purposes. The outcome of early studies [3] was the recommendation by the Medical Research Council's Committee on the Aetiology of Chronic Bronchitis [4] of a standardized questionnaire [5] and diagnostic criteria [6]. Chronic bronchitis thus became one of the first diseases to be defined for the purposes of epidemiologic research.

The MRC Committee defined chronic bronchitis as chronic productive cough for at least three months of the year in two successive years [6]. Breathlessness on exertion was used to distinguish between 'simple' and 'obstructive' bronchitis. Their discussions reflected the prevailing 'British' hypothesis that individuals reporting chronic phlegm production would later become disabled by chronic airflow obstruction. Longitudinal studies of

working men in the fourth to sixth decades of life [7] later demonstrated that mucus hypersecretion and progressive airflow obstruction were independent disorders, each related to smoking, but with distinct natural histories. A subsequent overview of mortality in a number of early cohort studies of chronic respiratory disease showed that airflow obstruction, but not chronic cough and phlegm, was related to future mortality certified as due to chronic bronchitis or emphysema [8]. This led to the recommendation that the term 'chronic bronchitis' should be used only to denote chronic or recurrent mucus hypersecretion [9].

Over time there has been substantial variation in the diagnostic label applied to patients with chronic respiratory symptoms, and even in recent years there may be considerable similarities in the clinical characteristics of patients labelled as asthmatic and those labelled as having chronic bronchitis [10]. Routine statistics relating to specific diagnoses (bronchitis, chronic bronchitis, emphysema, asthma, or chronic obstructive airways disease) are likely to be misleading unless they are grouped together to minimize the effects of diagnostic transfer. In the subsequent sections, the term 'chronic respiratory disease' is used to denote these groups in combination (i.e. ICD9 codes 490–493 and 496).

While the symptomatic definition of chronic bronchitis derived from the MRC

Chronic Obstructive Pulmonary Disease. Edited by Dr P. Calverley and Professor N. Pride. Published in 1995 by Chapman & Hall, London. ISBN 0 412 46450 0

questionnaire may not adequately distinguish those at most risk of severe disability and death, it remains a useful tool for studying recurrent morbidity. Early studies, using clinical or sickness absence records, suggested that those who suffered from bronchitis in middle age often had a history of recurrent chest illness dating back to early adulthood [11,12]. On the other hand, when the MRC questionnaire has been administered on repeated occasions, there have been substantial numbers of those with chronic cough or phlegm who deny these symptoms on follow-up. Sharp *et al.* [13] found that half of their middle-aged men who reported chronic symptoms had 'recovered' seven years later. Symptoms were more likely to persist in smokers than in non-smokers. Among a national sample of young adults studied by Kiernan *et al.* [14], less than half of those reporting chronic winter cough at age 20 did so five years later. This was so even after removing from the comparison subjects who had changed their smoking habits. Thus, simple questions about persistent cough and phlegm do not appear to identify a universally 'chronic' tendency to mucus hypersecretion.

Although complete absence of a mortality risk from simple mucus hypersecretion has been questioned [15,16], the occurrence of severe disability and death in chronic lung disease is related most closely to symptoms of breathlessness [17,18] and to levels of ventilatory function measured up to 20 years previously [8,18]. Spirometric indices measured in middle and old age depend upon the level achieved in early adult life (determined by lung growth in childhood) and the rate of decline during adult life (determined by the pathology leading to progressive airflow limitation), superimposed upon which may be episodes of reversible airflow obstruction (the hallmark of asthma). The etiological factors influencing these three processes may be very different. Thus, cross-sectional surveys of ventilatory function are a blunt tool for investigating the causes of chronic airflow limita-

tion. On the other hand, longitudinal studies of lung function decline which specifically address the progression of disease in adult life cannot investigate the determinants of lung growth in childhood.

4.2 BURDEN OF DISEASE

4.2.1 PREVALENCE

Table 4.1 summarizes the prevalence of symptoms of mucus hypersecretion as reported in surveys of general population samples in Great Britain over the past forty years. The prevalence of chronic cough and phlegm in men appears to have declined in line with a decreasing proportion of active smokers, although there has been little change in women. In the late 1980s, 15–20% of middle-aged men and about 8% of middle-aged women in Britain reported chronic cough and phlegm (Table 4.1).

There has been only one national study of ventilatory function among British adults of a broad age range. The Health and Lifestyle Survey assessed a representative sample of 2484 men and 3063 women aged 18–65 years by turbine spirometry in the home [29]. Overall, 10% of men and 11% of women performed two or more standard deviations below the predicted value for their age and height. This proportion with 'poor' ventilatory function increased with age, particularly among smokers. At ages 18–39, 11% of currently smoking men and 9% of lifetime non-smoking men had 'poor' FEV_1, whereas at ages 40–65 the equivalent figures were 18% and 7%. Among women at ages 18–39, 12% of smokers and 11% of lifetime non-smokers had 'poor' function, whereas at ages 40–65, the figures were 14% and 6% respectively. Although these are cross-sectional findings, they are consistent with what is known of the natural history of lung function change in smokers and non-smokers. A follow-up study of the original sample was completed in 1992 and the results should prove of considerable

Table 4.1 Prevalence of chronic cough and phlegm in population-based studies in Great Britain 1950–1990

Area surveyed	Date	Ref.	Age of subjects	Percentage of men					Number of women	Percentage of women			
				Number of men	Chronic cough	Chronic phlegm	Persistent cough and phlegm	Current smokers		Chronic cough	Chronic phlegm	Persistent cough and phlegm	Current smokers
Leigh (urban England)	1954	19	55–64	84	30	33	18	87					
Glamorgan (rural Wales)	1955	20	55–64	86	31	28	26	74	92	13	13	8	24
Annandale (rural Scotland)	1956	21	55–64	87	29	23	20	80	92	15	14	11	22
Rhondda Fach[a] (industrial Wales)	1958	22	55–64	88	42	35	29	73	173	16	16	10	17
Great Britain (selected practices)	1958	17	45–54	422	43	34		77	346	20	15		37
			55–64	420	53	49		73	344	22	21		26
Great Britain (general population)	1965	23	35–54	2936			17	57	3115			9	44
			55–64	1355			25	56	1591			9	25
Great Britain (general population)	1972	24	37–54	3610	28		17		3716	18		12	
			40–59	3832	29		19		4031	20		13	
			55–64	1836	32		24		2045	21		14	
Great Britain (selected towns)	1978	25	40–59	7735			16	41					
London (suburban practice)	1985	10	40–59	414	20	18			482	12	8		
			55–64	197	27	27	21		245	15	12	9	
Scotland (selected areas)	1987	26	40–59	4114	16	17		39	5220	12	11		38
Southern England (rural population)	1990	27	35–54	1123	16		8		1241	11		7	
			55–64	539	19		15	29	716	13		8	23

Modified and updated from Cullinan (1992) [27] and Anderson et al. (1992) [28].
[a]Non-miners only.

interest in distinguishing true age-related changes in lung function from generational (cohort-related) variations in level of FEV_1.

Information from three national surveys of consultations in British general practice [30–32] indicate the prevalence of clinically diagnosed chronic bronchitis, asthma, emphysema and COPD in different age and sex groups over the past forty years (Table 4.2). Overall, there has been a modest decline in the proportion of middle-aged men consulting for chronic respiratory disease, whereas there has been a slight increase among middle-aged women. Among both men and women over 65 years of age the proportion consulting for any of the four diagnoses has changed little over the 25-year period. However, there is evidence of larger shifts in diagnostic preference, away from the label of chronic bronchitis towards other diagnostic terms (Table 4.2). The extent to which these shifts reflect true alterations in the nature of disease presenting to clinicians, as opposed to changes in diagnostic fashion, is unclear. Considerable overlap between the characteristics of patients with different respiratory diagnoses has been documented in recent years [10].

4.2.2 MORTALITY

The interpretation of mortality statistics relating to chronic respiratory disease is not straightforward. Symptoms of mucus hypersecretion or airflow limitation are common in most populations, particularly at advanced ages. A substantial proportion of people therefore die 'with' chronic respiratory disease. However it is the decision of the certifying doctor whether a patient with (for example) a terminal respiratory infection died 'of' chronic respiratory disease (i.e. with chronic bronchitis, emphysema, asthma or chronic airways obstruction as an underlying cause).

Recent changes in the rules for coding the underlying cause of death (WHO Rule 3)

Table 4.2 Proportion of persons consulting a general practitioner annually for chronic respiratory disease by age and sex, Great Britain: 1955–6, 1970–1, 1981–2

Diagnosis	Age	Men (per 1000)			Women (per 1000)		
		1955–6	1970–1	1981–2	1955–6	1970–1	1981–2
Chronic	45–64	32.7	29.6	12.3	12.9	12.0	6.7
bronchitis[a]	65–74		73.8	37.9		23.5	13.6
	75+		70.7	47.5		23.2	12.3
	65+	72.0			32.3		
Emphysema	45–64	3.1	3.4	6.5	0.2	0.5	3.0
and COPD[b]	65–74		11.1	26.2		1.5	7.8
	75+		5.0	31.2		0.4	7.2
	65+	4.4			0.8		
Asthma	45–64	9.0	8.1	13.9	10.6	9.7	18.1
	65–74		10.7	21.5		9.1	18.7
	75+		6.6	16.2		5.7	12.9
	65+	7.9			8.9		
Chronic	45–64	44.8	41.1	32.7	23.7	22.2	27.8
bronchitis,	65–74		95.6	85.6		34.1	40.1
emphysema,	75+		82.3	94.9		29.3	32.4
COPD and asthma	65+	84.3			42.0		

Sources: National Morbidity Surveys in General Practice [30–32].
[a]Excludes bronchitis unspecified but includes bronchitis with mention of emphysema (in 1955–6).
[b]Emphysema without mention of bronchitis in 1955–6; includes chronic obstructive pulmonary disease in 1981–2 only.

ensure that where pneumonia is certified as the underlying cause of death (in Part 1 of the death certificate), a range of diseases (including the four mentioned above) may be coded as the underlying cause of death if they appear in Part II of the certificate (contributory causes). This convention only partly rectifies the problem as full information may not be provided in Part II of the certificate.

Several recent studies have demonstrated that reduced levels of FEV_1 predict subsequent mortality from a range of non-respiratory diseases, particularly coronary heart disease [33,34] and stroke [35]. These associations are independent of smoking habit and are apparent in lifelong non-smokers [36]. It seems highly probable, therefore, that rates of death certified as chronic bronchitis, emphysema, asthma or chronic airways obstruction underestimate the mortality due to COPD. Indeed, it is arguable that the greater part of the burden of mortality attributable to these conditions is concealed among deaths certified to other causes.

Comparisons of mortality rates over time and between countries are complicated by the use of different diagnostic labels to describe fatal chronic respiratory disease. Historically, chronic bronchitis (ICD8&9 491) was the cause certified in the majority of such deaths in Britain. Emphysema (ICD8&9 492), asthma (ICD8&9 493) and bronchitis unspecified (ICD8&9 490) were each coded in a small proportion of cases. A separate ICD code for 'chronic airways obstruction not elsewhere classified' (hereafter termed COAD) was introduced in 1978 (ICD8 519.8, ICD9 496) and since then it has been used increasingly. Over the same period, there has been a substantial decline in mortality attributable to chronic bronchitis, suggesting diagnostic transfer, rather than a recent epidemic of fatal COPD (Figs 4.1 and 4.2).

In England and Wales in 1992, the latest year for which national figures are available, there were 3873 deaths certified as due to chronic bronchitis, 251 due to bronchitis not

specified as acute or chronic, 1946 due to emphysema, 1791 due to asthma, and 19 963 due to chronic obstructive airways disease. Together, these accounted for 6.4% of all deaths in males and 3.9% of all deaths in females [37].

4.2.3 IMPACT ON HEALTH SERVICES AND EMPLOYMENT

Information available on hospital admissions and general practice consultations indicates the utilization of health services for chronic respiratory disease in the United Kingdom. As with mortality, these figures refer to consequences directly attributable to bronchitis, emphysema, asthma or COPD, and do not take account of their role as co-morbid conditions which may influence the occurrence or severity of other respiratory or non-respiratory illness. Table 4.3 summarizes the estimated workload currently attributable to chronic respiratory disease in an average UK health district serving 250 000 people.

Chronic respiratory disease is also an important cause of lost working time. Changes in the regulations for sick pay have resulted in exclusion of many short periods of sickness absence from official UK statistics since 1983. Before these changes were introduced, bronchitis, emphysema, asthma and COPD accounted for 24.4 million lost working days annually (9% of all certified sickness absence) among men, and 3.1 million days (3.5% of the total) among women [38].

4.3 TIME, PLACE AND PERSON

4.3.1 TIME TRENDS

Figures 4.2 and 4.3 show recent trends in mortality from chronic respiratory disease in England and Wales. These broadly correspond to the changes in disease prevalence as indicated by prevalence surveys and general practitioner consultations (Tables 4.1 and 4.2), with declining rates among older

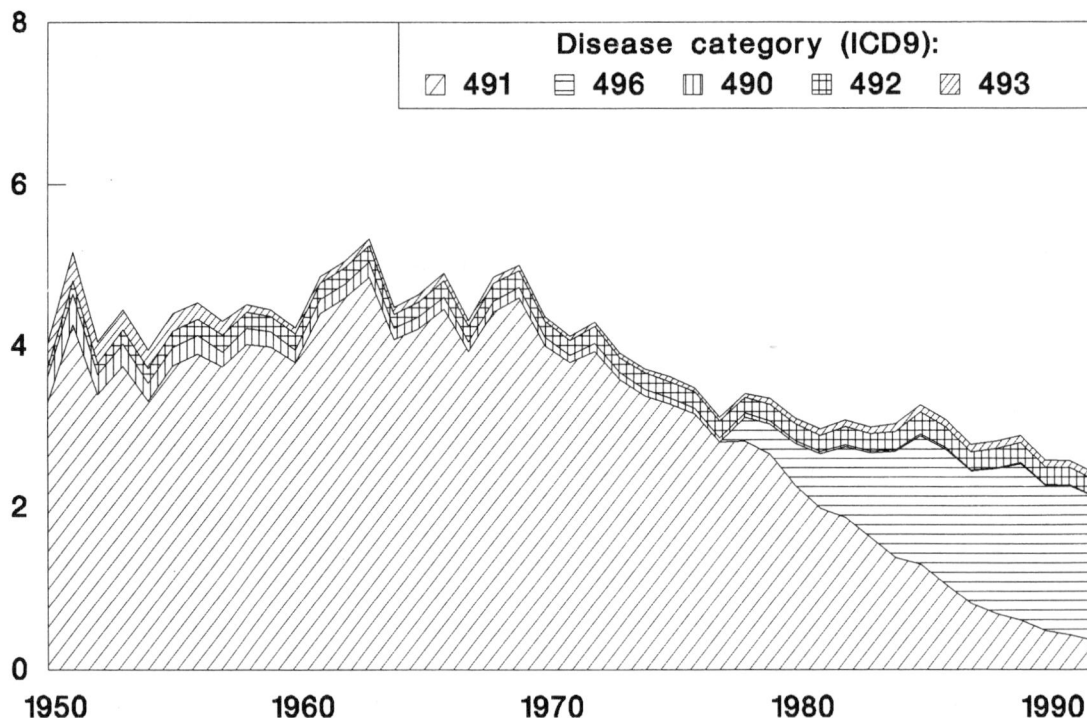

Fig. 4.1 Age-standardized mortality rates (per 1000 per year) for chronic respiratory diseases (ICD9 490–493 and 496) by diagnosis, males aged 55–84, England and Wales 1950–1992. (Source: Office of Population Censuses and Surveys and Lung and Asthma Information Agency.)

women in the 1950s and 1960s and among middle-aged men in the 1970s and 1980s.

Age- and sex-specific mortality rates from chronic respiratory disease can be described simply in terms of the combined effects of age, period of death and cohort (generation, or year of birth) on the risk of death for each sex. Two such age-period–cohort analyses have been published [39,40]. Each shows a marked generation effect, with a peak for men born around 1900 and for women born around 1925. These non-linear cohort effects closely follow those for lung cancer mortality and correspond to what is known of inter-generational differences in lifetime cigarette consumption at various ages [40].

The analyses differ in the effect shown for period of death on chronic respiratory disease mortality. This is because there has been a very substantial downward 'drift' in age-specific mortality rates since the Second World War and it is statistically impossible to assign this with confidence to a generation or to a period of death effect, or to some combination of the two. However, the downward drift started in the late nineteenth century in all age-groups simultaneously [41] and therefore is perhaps more likely to be a period of death effect. It continued throughout the 1970s, a period during which there were substantial reductions in urban smoke and sulfur dioxide air pollution in Britain [42].

4.3.2. INTERNATIONAL VARIATIONS

International comparisons of chronic respiratory disease based on figures published annually [43] are difficult to interpret because

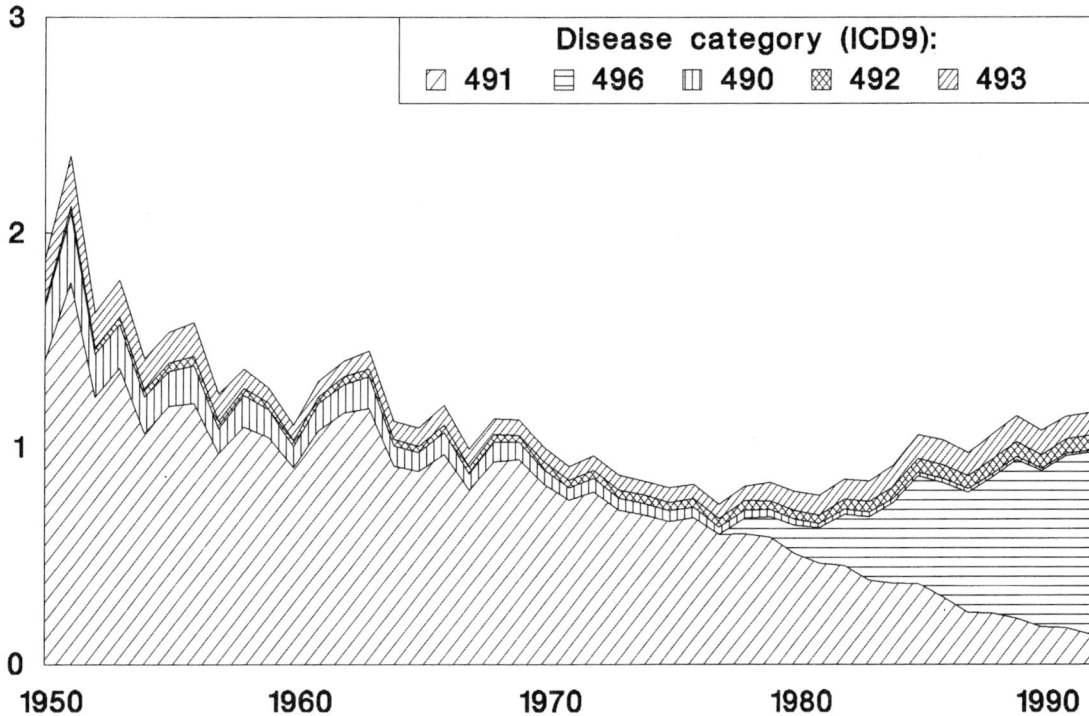

Fig. 4.2 Age-standardized mortality rates (per 1000 per year) for chronic respiratory diseases (ICD9 490–493 and 496) by diagnosis, females aged 55–84, England and Wales 1950–1992. (Source: Office of Population Censuses and Surveys and Lung and Asthma Information agency.)

Table 4.3 Estimated annual health service workload due to chronic respiratory disease in an average UK health district serving 250 000 persons

	Hospital admissions	In-patient bed-days	General practice consultations
Chronic bronchitis[a]	100	1500	4400
Emphysema and COPD	240	3300	2700
Asthma	410	1800	11900
Chronic bronchitis, emphysema, asthma and COPD	750	6600	19000

Modified from Anderson *et al.* [28].
[a]Includes bronchitis unspecified for hospital use but not for GP consultations.

deaths attributed to COAD (ICD9 496) are not included. A special study among men and women aged 65–74 in 26 countries during 1984 showed considerable variation between countries in the proportion of all chronic respiratory deaths attributed to COAD, rather than bronchitis, emphysema or asthma. The proportion certified as COAD varied from almost none in Poland to about two-thirds in the USA [44].

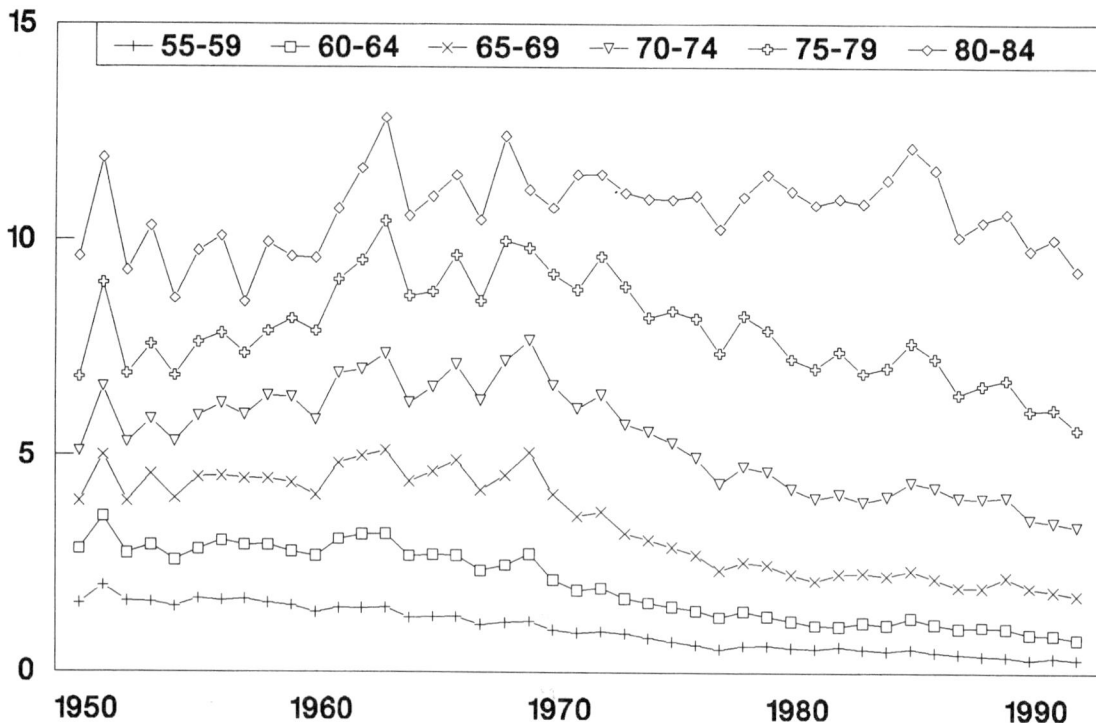

Fig. 4.3   Age-specific mortality rates (per 1000 per year) for chronic obstructive lung diseases (ICD9 490–493 and 496), all diagnoses combined, for males aged 55–84, England and Wales 1950–1992. (Source: Office of Population Censuses and Surveys and Lung and Asthma Information Agency.)

The general pattern of mortality from all chronic respiratory disease (ICD9 490–496) among 31 developed countries is of high rates in Great Britain, Eastern Europe and Australasia, intermediate rates in Western Europe and North America, and low rates in Southern Europe, Scandinavia, Israel and Japan [44]. Romania had the highest death rates from all chronic respiratory diseases (ICD9 490–496) amongst both men and women aged 65–74 in 1984. Countries of the British Isles had the next highest rates, with Ireland and Scotland slightly higher than England and Wales. British rates were exceeded only by Romania (in both sexes), the German Democratic Republic (in men) and New Zealand (in women).

The high rates of mortality from chronic respiratory disease in Britain have been rec-

ognized for several decades and cannot be attributed solely to diagnostic variations, although the specific labels used to describe chronic respiratory illness do vary between Great Britain, Europe and the United States [45]. There have been few standardized international comparisons of symptom prevalence or ventilatory function, but those which have been conducted, mainly between Great Britain, Norway and the USA, suggest that international differences in smoking habits largely explain variations in the prevalence of chronic phlegm, whereas British men have lower ventilatory function than their American and Norwegian counterparts, after controlling for smoking [45]. On the other hand, studies of respiratory symptoms among middle-aged migrants from the British Isles to the United States of America and

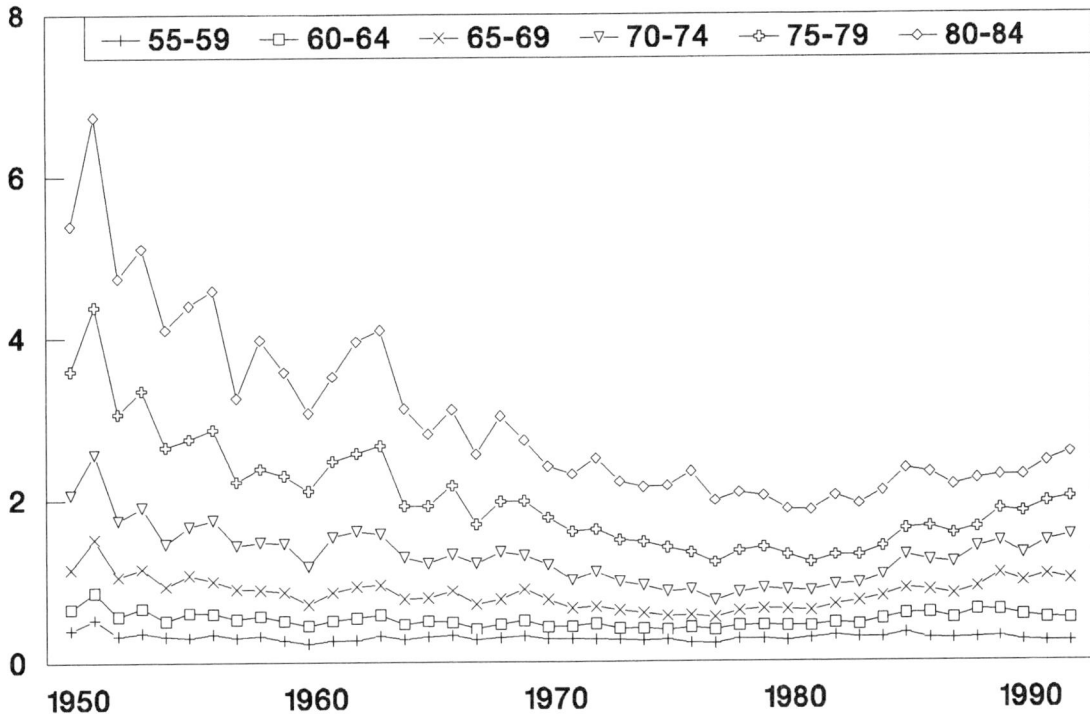

Fig. 4.4 Age-specific mortality rates (per 1000 per year) for chronic obstructive lung diseases (ICD9 490–493 and 496), all diagnoses combined, for females aged 55–84, England and Wales 1950–1992. (Source: Office of Population Censuses and Surveys and Lung and Asthma Information Agency.)

among indigenous Americans with similar smoking habits suggested that a high-risk 'British factor' was carried with migrants when they moved elsewhere [46].

4.3.3 GEOGRAPHIC VARIATIONS WITHIN ENGLAND AND WALES

Age-adjusted death rates from chronic respiratory disease vary by a factor of more than 5 (in men) and more than 10 (in women) between small areas of Great Britain [39]. There are two major underlying trends: a tendency for higher mortality rates in the towns and particularly in major conurbations; and a regional trend, independent of urbanization, from south-east (low) to north-west (high), with high rates in South Wales and Scotland [47].

Early prevalence surveys showed considerable variation in morbidity from chronic bronchitis which broadly followed the pattern described for bronchitis mortality [23,24,48]. This contrasts with the finding that in studies of individuals, symptoms of mucus hypersecretion are poor predictors of mortality from chronic respiratory disease [8]. Fewer studies have assessed ventilatory function in different areas of the United Kingdom, but there is the expected pattern of lower ventilatory function in towns [49] and in the more northerly regions [29]. The high level of mortality in South Wales is accompanied by low levels of ventilatory function, independent of smoking habits [50].

Reid [51] hypothesized that the geographic distribution of chronic respiratory disease might be determined in childhood. Mortality rates from chronic bronchitis in adults during 1968–78 in small areas of England and Wales were highly correlated with rates of mortality from bronchitis and pneumonia in infancy in the same areas during earlier years of this century [39], suggesting that some aspect of the environment in early childhood, possibly early episodes of chest infection, might be responsible for the geographic distribution of disease in adults. However, they were also correlated with the current prevalence of cough and phlegm among children in the same areas [52]. Thus, a continuation of the adverse environmental influence could not be excluded.

Studies of migrants are required to clarify the critical age at which area differences in disease occurrence are determined. Rosenbaum [53] found that military recruits from industrial areas carried an increased risk of episodes of respiratory disease compared with those from rural areas, regardless of the region to which they were posted. This would favour the hypothesis of an influence in early life. On the other hand, a study of proportional mortality (the proportion of all deaths due to chronic bronchitis) in 153 areas of England and Wales found that the area of death had a much greater influence than place of birth, although a statistically significant birthplace effect could be discerned [54].

4.3.4 SOCIAL CLASS

It has long been recognized that there is a strong association between poor socio-economic status and chronic respiratory disease in Great Britain [55]. Table 4.4 shows the extent of social class variations in mortality and general practitioner consultations for chronic respiratory disease around the 1981 census. Marked social class trends are apparent in women (classified by their husband's occupation) as well as men, suggesting that specific occupational exposures play only a small part in explaining socio-economic differentials. There are intriguing differences between the sexes in the relationship of social class to consultations for asthma. One explanation would be that practitioners more readily apply the diagnostic label of chronic bronchitis to a man with a manual occupation than to his wife.

Table 4.4 Social class variations in general practice consultations and mortality due to chronic respiratory disease in Great Britain, 1979–83

			Registrar-General's social class					
			I	II	IIIN	IIIM	IV	V
Standardized mortality ratio for bronchitis, emphysema and asthma	Men	20–64	34	48	85	110	133	211
	Married women[a]	20–59	41	61	70	122	144	222
Standardized mortality ratio for cancer of trachea, bronchus and lung	Men	20–64	43	63	80	120	126	178
	Married women[a]	20–59	50	73	81	122	138	170
Consultation ratio for chronic bronchitis	Men	45–64		48	77	123	161	
		65–74		53	95	113	141	
	All women[a]	45–64		69	72	140	177	
		65–74		56	64	150	127	
Consultation ratio[b] for asthma	Men	45–64		97	94	106	98	
		65–74		90	93	91	126	
	All women[a]	45–64		71	81	109	147	
		65–74		69	112	113	114	

Sources: Registrar-General's decennial supplement, occupational mortality 1979–80, 1982–83 [57]
Morbidity statistics from general practice 1981–82, socio-economic analyses [58].
[a]Married women classified by their husband's occupation.
[b]Proportion of patients consulting annually relative to the proportion in all social classes combined (=100).

The social class gradient in mortality from lung cancer, among both men and women, is of comparable magnitude, suggesting that much of the variation in chronic respiratory disease is attributable to social class differences in lifetime smoking habits. On the other hand, population surveys have shown associations of socio-economic status with symptoms of mucus hypersecretion [24,56] and measures of ventilatory function [29], independent of current smoking habit. Furthermore, bronchitis mortality showed a strong social class gradient long before there was any substantial variation in smoking behaviour by social class [55]. Thus, it seems likely that smoking offers only a partial explanation for the observed trends in mortality and consultations by socio-economic status in Britain.

An important and topical issue is the extent to which such gradient reflect upbringing and living conditions in childhood or lifestyle and environment in adult life. Among a national cohort followed from birth in 1946 to adult life, strong associations have been demonstrated between indices of socio-economic deprivation in childhood (particularly domestic crowding) and adult ventilatory function [59]. However, chronic cough and peak flow rate were also related to current socio-economic circumstances, as indicated by housing tenure [60]. More specific studies of socially mobile individuals are required to distinguish reliably between influences in childhood and later life.

4.4 CAUSES

4.4.1 ACTIVE SMOKING

Tobacco smoking is undoubtedly the most important influence on the development of chronic respiratory disease in adults in developed countries. The evidence implicating smoking and the benefits of smoking cessation have been extensively reviewed [61,62] and only the salient points will be reiterated here.

Smoking is a cause of both mucus hypersecretion and progressive airflow limitation. Symptoms of cough, phlegm, wheeze and breathlessness are much more common among individuals and populations who smoke and are reduced when they quit the habit [25]. Although ventilatory function does not improve substantially on stopping smoking, the subsequent rate of decline in FEV_1 is slower [7]. The benefits of smoking cessation have been determined largely from observational studies. Two randomized controlled trials of antismoking advice which have been conducted tend to support these conclusions, although they have lacked statistical power to conclusively demonstrate the benefits of stopping smoking, particularly in terms of respiratory mortality [63,64].

The tar content of cigarettes is an important determinant of mucus hypersecretion, but not of impaired ventilatory function. For a given amount smoked, high tar cigarettes are more likely to cause mucus hypersecretion, the effect being more marked at lower cigarette consumption [65]. However, a randomized controlled trial of different types of cigarette was unable to demonstrate any symptomatic benefit from switching to lower tar preparations [66].

4.4.2 PASSIVE SMOKING

Quantitative overviews have demonstrated a weak but statistically significant association between environmental tobacco smoke exposure and lung cancer among non-smokers, with a pooled relative risk of the order of 1.2–1.3 [67,68]. Given that active smoking is as strongly related to death from chronic respiratory disease as it is to fatal lung cancer, in a dose-dependent fashion [69], a similar weak relationship might be expected between passive smoking and development of chronic airflow limitation.

Three case-control studies [70–72] and one cohort study [73] have investigated the relationship of chronic bronchitis, asthma or emphysema among non-smokers to passive smoke exposure in the home or workplace. The findings would be consistent with a relative risk of the same magnitude as for lung cancer, although none of these studies, either individually or pooled, are powerful enough to demonstrate such a weak effect as statistically significant. As with the lung cancer studies, residual confounding by unmeasured active smoking may account for some of the observed association [68].

Studies of the effects of passive smoking on lung function in middle-aged adults have yielded inconsistent findings [74,75]. However, a study of young adult non-smokers suggested that cumulative lifetime exposure to tobacco during childhood was associated with significantly poorer lung function, suggesting that the peak level of ventilatory function attained during life might be impaired by parental smoking [76]. Only four studies have investigated the relationship of parental smoking to rates of lung growth in childhood. These, too, are inconsistent; two found little effect [77,78], one showed a highly significant adverse effect [79], while in the fourth and largest study the effect of maternal smoking on initial FEV_1 was more convincing than the effect on lung growth [80].

Maternal smoking is an important determinant of low birth weight [81] and smoking by either parent is associated with an increased incidence of respiratory illnesses in the first three years of life [75]. These may be mechanisms whereby passive smoke exposure in childhood may influence the future development of chronic respiratory disease in adult life.

4.4.3 AIR POLLUTION

A major stimulus to epidemiologic investigation of chronic respiratory disease in Great Britain was the occurrence of some 4000 excess deaths during the London smog of December 1952 [2]. Concentrations of smoke and sulfur dioxide in central London during this 5-day period were about 100 times higher than those recorded in urban areas of Great Britain nowadays. The excess deaths were mainly due to cardiorespiratory disease and occurred principally among the elderly and chronic sick, suggesting that their demise was precipitated earlier than would otherwisehave been the case by the irritant air pollution.

Similar analyses of short-term (usually daily) variations in mortality, hospital admissions and symptoms experienced by panels of bronchitic patients were conducted in London during the 1950s and 1960s [82]. These suggested that, as smoke and sulfur dioxide levels declined and became less variable during the 1960s, temporal relationships with respiratory outcomes diminished. The winter of 1962–63 was the last in which readily discernible peaks of pollution-related morbidity and mortality occurred in Greater London.

An expert group meeting under the auspices of WHO in 1990 [83] concluded that acute effects on health of sulfur dioxide and particulate air pollution (as indicated by measures of black smoke) could be expected at concentrations of about 250 μg/m^3 SO$_2$, or similar concentrations of black smoke, with an increase in respiratory morbidity among adult patients with chronic bronchitis. At levels in excess of 500 μg/m^3 SO$_2$ or black smoke an increase in mortality among elderly and chronically sick persons could be expected.

More recent application of complex statistical modelling to daily deaths data from Greater London and elsewhere has challenged these conclusions, and suggested that a temporal correlation between particulate air pollution and total mortality may extend into the range 0–100 μg/m^3 (black smoke) currently experienced in many urban areas of the UK and other developed countries [84]. Whether this effect is due to pollution or to the confounding effects of meterologic variables, operating either directly or through behavioral changes, remains unclear.

While smoke and sulfur dioxide ('winter pollutants') have been of greatest interest in the past, attention is now turning to the possible hazards of 'summer' (photochemical) pollutants such as nitrogen oxides, ozone and acid aerosols. Time–series analyses addressing the acute effects of photochemical 'smogs' have been confined to asthmatic patients and there are no reports of panel studies of the effects of ozone on chronic obstructive lung disease, nor of the association of ozone episodes with mortality [85]. Natural fluctuations in nitrogen dioxide exposure were not associated with short-term effects on symptoms or lung function in a combined laboratory and community-based study of patients with chronic respiratory illness [86].

Studies of the chronic effects of air pollution rely upon geographic variations in prevalence of symptoms, ventilatory function or mortality. Such studies are highly prone to confounding by broader urban–rural and regional effects, even if they control for risk factors at the individual level such as smoking and occupation. A number of extensive reviews have commented on the literature relating to smoke and sulfur dioxide pollution [42,87–89]. Many of these studies relate to children, or to mortality data. Few have studied adults, possibly because chronic lung disease in adults may be attributable to delayed consequences of past (e.g. childhood) exposure to air pollution. However, longitudinal studies of a British cohort born in 1946 (and therefore potentially exposed to high urban levels of smoke and SO_2 throughout childhood) have failed to demonstrate a major influence of early pollution exposure on chronic phlegm or peak expiratory flow rate at age 36 years, after controlling for other factors [59].

Although historically there has been a geographic relationship between particulate pollution and chronic respiratory disease mortality in Great Britain [90], this became less marked after control of pollution in the 1960s [91]. Whereas early prevalence studies suggested relationships of British urban pollution with chronic phlegm [23] and reduced levels of FEV_1 [49], more recent studies of lower levels of pollution in the USA have yielded conflicting results. Repeated prevalence studies and longitudinal investigations have generally not shown improvement in respiratory health of populations when smoke and sulfur dioxide levels decline. Nevertheless, a recent review concluded that the possibility of chronic effects on respiratory health at levels of particulates below 100 $\mu g/m^3$ annual average could not be excluded [42].

Prevalence studies investigating the chronic health effects of photochemical air pollution in North America have found a higher prevalence of respiratory symptoms and reduced lung function in more polluted areas, but the specific pollutant responsible could not be identified [92]. Nitrogen dioxide is found at higher levels indoors than outdoors, particularly in homes with unvented gas or paraffin appliances. Few studies have investigated the effects of indoor NO_2 on respiratory health in adults. The findings with respect to chronic cough and phlegm and lung function are inconsistent, possibly because the presence of a gas cooker has been used as a crude surrogate for personal NO_2 exposure [74]. In one small study where NO_2 exposure was measured in adult non-smoking women, there was a significant association with measurements of lung function at entry to the study, but not with the rate of subsequent decline [93].

4.4.4 OCCUPATIONAL EXPOSURES

While a causal link between occupational dust exposure and mucus hypersecretion is generally acknowledged [24,94], the role of dust and fumes in the etiology of progressive airflow obstruction remains controversial.

The best evidence for the latter comes from longitudinal studies of workers in specific occupations, where the exposure can be characterized in detail, longitudinal measurements of ventilatory function can be obtained, and confounding by smoking and socio-economic status can be controlled. Becklake [94] reviewed ten such workforce studies, including six where the exposure was primarily to dusts, two to gases only, and two to a combination of dusts and fumes. Exposures to a variety of inorganic dusts and to sulfur dioxide were consistently related to more rapid decline in FEV_1, whereas exposure to chlorine was not.

Cross-sectional studies of the general population are less easy to interpret. They are usually constrained to a single measurement of ventilatory function and to questionnaire reports of occupational exposures. Past changes in occupation may be difficult to deal with analytically and confounding by smoking and socio-economic status may not be adequately controlled. Nevertheless, they are broadly consistent with longitudinal studies in that the relationship of ventilatory function impairment to mineral dusts is clearer than its association with exposure to fumes and chemicals [95].

Mortality from chronic respiratory disease in Britain is significantly raised in only a few occupational groups, after adjustment for age, social class and region of residence (Table 4.5). In some groups e.g. artists, hotel managers, butchers, steel erectors and boatmen), the increased risks appears to be due to a high prevalence of smoking, as indicated by a similarly raised risk of lung cancer. In others (e.g. clerks, painters, lorry and crane drivers), a moderately raised risk is statistically significant because of the large size of the occupational group. Few of the remaining occupations are obviously associated with exposure to dusts or fumes.

Among coal miners and general labourers there is known to be a degree 'numerator–denominator bias' in occupational mortality statistics, because the sources of information on occupation on death certificates and census returns are not strictly comparable. On the other hand, there is evidence that these occupations may pose a true risk of chronic respiratory disease. Construction work has emerged as a significant exposure in some cross-sectional studies [96] and longitudinal studies of British coal miners support a relationship between dust exposure and the development of progressive airflow obstruction [97] and related mortality [98].

4.4.5 CHILDHOOD CHEST INFECTION

The association between chest illness in childhood and both chronic respiratory morbidity and impaired ventilatory function is well documented [99]. However, it remains unclear whether this reflects lung damage due to early episodes of chest infection or a longstanding susceptibility to all forms of chest illness [100]. Investigation of this issue raised serious methodologic problems because of the long timescale between early childhood and the development of clinically significant mucus hypersecretion or chronic airflow limitation in late middle age.

A recent study of Hertfordshire men born 1911–30 overcame this difficulty by using historic records compiled by health visitors of illnesses in early childhood. Records of illnesses labelled as whooping cough, bronchitis or pneumonia in the first year of life were associated with a significant reduction in FEV_1 measured at age 59–70 [101]. These same illnesses at age 1–4 years were not associated with significant deficits in lung function. Somewhat surprisingly, none of the illnesses were associated with father's social class, which in turn was not related to adult lung function.

Studies of the British 1946 cohort provide the most comprehensive prospective data linking early chest illness with adult symptoms and lung function. Chronic cough and phlegm were more commonly reported at ages

Table 4.5 Occupations with significantly raised standardized mortality ratios for chronic respiratory disease among men aged 20–64, after adjustment for social class and region of residence, Great Britain 1979–83

Group number	Brief description of occupations included in the group	Bronchitis, emphysema and asthma SMR (deaths)	Cancer of trachea, bronchus and lung SMR (deaths)
001	Judges, barristers, solicitors	189 (12)	82 (25)
016	Nurses	192 (23)	132 (76)
019	Authors, writers, journalists	166 (16)	99 (48)
020	Artists, designers	172 (14)	151 (59)
021	Actors, musicians, entertainers	221 (14)	118 (36)
027	Electrical and electronic engineers	172 (17)	142 (65)
039	Hotel and club managers	219 (151)	185 (559)
044	Managers not elsewhere classified	170 (68)	187 (344)
046	Clerks	110 (486)	95 (1488)
055	Salesmen, shop assistants	147 (71)	119 (196)
064	Chefs, cooks	155 (36)	103 (100)
069	Travel attendants, porters	138 (59)	114 (180)
077	Farm workers	137 (101)	100 (274)
085	Tannery and leather workers	164 (30)	113 (88)
089	Chemical, gas, petroleum plants	134 (87)	132 (308)
091	Bakers	193 (85)	108 (83)
092	Butchers	170 (42)	157 (159)
096	Glass and ceramics workers	165 (26)	103 (64)
110	Metal drawers, moulders, casters	154 (58)	134 (193)
126	Sheet metal workers, platers	125 (91)	134 (192)
127	Steel erecters, benders, fixers	208 (46)	192 (168)
133	Painters, decorators, polishers	123 (192)	121 (779)
145	Face-trained coalminers	172 (125)	97 (273)
148	Bargemen, boatmen	271 (42)	239 (136)
152	Bus, coach and lorry drivers	121 (561)	118 (2310)
153	Bus conductors, drivers' mates	147 (27)	103 (65)
155	Plant, truck and crane drivers	122 (155)	97 (508)
160	General and unskilled labourers	170 (1264)	141 (3347)

Source: Registrar-General's decennial supplement, occupational mortality 1979–80, 1982–83 [57].

20–36 by subjects with a history of chest illness in childhood [59,60,102,103]. After adjustment for smoking and socio-economic status both in childhood and adult life, there was no significant effect of bronchitis, bronchiolitis or pneumonia before age 2 years on peak expiratory flow rate at age 36 years [59]. However, when all respiratory illnesses up to 10 years were considered, a significant effect on peak flow was found for bronchitis and pneumonia [60], but not for whooping cough [103].

The findings with respect to ventilatory function contrast with the results of the Hertfordshire study and suggest that recurrent episodes of bronchitis, which might nowadays receive a diagnosis of childhood asthma, may be the respiratory illnesses more strongly associated with adult lung function. This would be consistent with a retrospective study of Burrows, Knudsen and Lebowitz [104] which suggested that the respiratory problems in childhood which were associated with adult obstructive airways disease were those in the category of 'chronic or recurrent airway disease' rather than 'severe acute respiratory illness'.

Asthma is a possible link between respiratory problems in childhood and adult life.

Two long-term follow-up studies confirm that although the majority of wheezy children apparently grow out of their asthma, those that do not are at increased risk of chronic cough and phlegm in their twenties [105,106]. Asthmatic children often have a history of early episodes of chest illnesses labelled as bronchitis, bronchiolitis or pneumonia, but the direction of cause and effect is a matter of debate. Abnormalities of lung function have been described in newborn infants who subsequently develop recurrent wheezing [107], suggesting that susceptibility to chest illnesses may exist from birth. Reports of an association of birth weight with adult lung function [101] may be evidence that such susceptibility continues into adult life.

4.4.6 GROWTH AND NUTRITION

Until recently, there was little evidence to implicate diet and nutrition as causes of chronic respiratory disease. However, the results of several recent studies suggest that both the growth and decline of ventilatory function may be affected by nutritional factors.

Among men born in Hertfordshire during 1911–30, mortality from chronic respiratory disease (ICD9 491–493 and 496) was significantly and inversely related to weight at birth and at one year of age [101]. Deaths from lung cancer did not show this pattern, suggesting that confounding by smoking habit was unlikely. Although these trends were not adjusted for socio-economic status in childhood or in adult life, they raise the possibility that impaired growth *in utero* or in the early postnatal period may be a risk factor for the later development of fatal chronic respiratory disease.

A subsequent field study among a sample of this historic cohort showed that birth weight was positively correlated with FEV_1 at ages 59–70, though not with FVC nor with persistent cough and phlegm [101]. These effects were independent of smoking habit and of social class at birth and in adult life.

The effect of weight at one year on FEV_1 (after adjustment for birth weight) was weak and non-significant, but the study lacked statistical power to discriminate conclusively between prenatal and postnatal growth as influences on adult lung function. Further long-term cohort studies are required to further investigate these intriguing observations.

Consideration of the role of proteases and antiproteases in the pathogenesis of emphysema suggests that tissue levels of dietary antioxidants, such as the vitamins A, C and E might protect against destruction of alveolar tissue. A cross-sectional study of British adults showed a correlation between frequent fresh fruit consumption (reported by food frequency questionnaire) and levels of ventilatory function [108]. This relationship was found among both current smokers and lifelong non-smokers and was independent of a wide range of possible confounding variables. Nevertheless, the possibility of uncontrolled confounding persists, and because of the crude nature of the dietary information the role of specific nutrients could not be investigated.

A possible protective effect of high vitamin C intake was also suggested by an analysis of data from US National Health and Nutrition Examination Survey [109]. This found a relationship between physician-diagnosed bronchitis and both dietary and plasma levels of ascorbic acid. In contrast, symptomatic chest disease was unrelated to fruit intake in the study of British adults [108].

Heavy alcohol consumption has been suggested as a risk factor for impaired ventilatory function [110]. However, this finding may be due to inadequate control of the effects of smoking, which is very closely associated with alcohol consumption.

4.5 CONCLUSIONS

Tobacco smoking has proved a most effective method of delivering toxic particles and gases to the lungs. There have been few epidemiologic tools as powerful as the cigarette, due to the wide variations in its use both within and between populations. The volume, strength and consistency of epidemiologic evidence implicating active smoking as a cause of both mucus hypersecretion and progressive airflow limitation is overwhelming. The distributions of both forms of chronic respiratory disease with respect to time, place and person are heavily influenced by smoking and it is here that any programme of disease prevention must start.

Mucus hypersecretion appears to be a largely reversible response of the bronchial epithelium to airborne irritants, including tobacco smoke, urban air pollution and occupational dust exposures. Arguably, this represents the body's natural defensive reaction to mucosal irritation. The development of disabling airflow obstruction is probably a more complex process, influenced by the growth of the lung from an early age, as well as by the rate of functional decline in adult life.

The focus of respiratory epidemiologic research in recent years has been upon pathophysiologic indicators of the smoker at risk of more rapid lung function decline. There has been a relative neglect of more promising targets for prevention, such as the promotion of lung growth in childhood and protection of lung tissue against the toxic effects of cigarette smoke. Future epidemiologic studies need to take a broad etiological perspective and encompass a wide age range if our understanding of the causes and natural history of chronic obstructive airways disease is to be better understood.

ACKNOWLEDGEMENTS

My thanks are due to Katie Paine and Jen Hollowell for assistance with data collection and production of graphics.

REFERENCES

1. Collis, E.L. (1923) The general and occupational prevalence of bronchitis and its relation to other respiratory diseases. *J. Ind. Hyg. Toxicol.*, **5**, 264.
2. Ministry of Health (1954) *Mortality and morbidity during the London fog of December 1952.* HMSO, London.
3. Fletcher, C.M., Elmes, P.C., Fairburn, A.S. and Wood, C.H. (1959) The significance of respiratory symptoms and the diagnosis of chronic bronchitis in a working population. *Br. Med. J.*, **2**, 259–73.
4. Medical Research Council Committee on the Aetiology of Chronic Bronchitis (1960) Standardised questionnaire for respiratory symptoms. *Br. Med. J.*, **2**, 1665.
5. Medical Research Council (1966) *Questionnaire on respiratory symptoms.* Medical Research Council, London.
6. Medical Research Council Committee on the Aetiology of Chronic Bronchitis (1965) Definition and classification of chronic bronchitis for clinical and epidemiological purposes. *Lancet*, **i**, 775–9.
7. Fletcher, C.M., Peto, R., Tinker, C, and Speizer, F.E. (1976) *The natural history of chronic bronchitis and emphysema. An 8-year study of working men in London.* Oxford University Press, Oxford.
8. Peto, R., Speizer, F.E., Cochrane, A.L. *et al.* (1983). The relevance in adults of airflow obstruction, but not of mucus hypersecretion, to mortality from chronic lung disease. *Am. Rev. Respir. Dis.*, **128**, 491–500.
9. Fletcher, C.M. and Pride, N.B. (1984) Definitions of emphysema, chronic bronchitis, asthma and airflow obstruction: 25 years on from the CIBA symposium. *Thorax*, **39**, 81–5.
10. Littlejohns, P., Ebrahim, S. and Anderson, R. (1989) Prevalence and diagnosis of chronic respiratory symptoms in adults. *Br. Med. J.*, **298**, 1556–60.
11. Oswald, N.C., Harold, J.T., and Martin, W.J. (1953) Clinical pattern of chronic bronchitis. *Lancet*, **ii**, 639–45.
12. Reid, D.D. and Fairburn, A.S. (1958) The natural history of chronic bronchitis. *Lancet*, **i**, 1147–52.
13. Sharp, J.T., Paul, O., McKean, H. and Best, W.R. (1973) A longitudinal study of bronchitic symptoms and spirometry in a middle-aged male industrial population. *Am. Rev. Respir. Dis.*, **108**, 1066–77.
14. Kiernan, K.E., Colley, J.R.T., Douglas, J.W.B. and Reid, D.D. (1976) Chronic cough in

young adults in relation to smoking habits, childhood environment and chest illness. *Respiration*, **33**, 236–44.

15. Annesi, I, and Kaufmann, F. (1986) Is respiratory mucus hypersecretion really an innocent disorder? *Am. Rev. Respir. Dis.*, **134**, 688–93.

16. Lange, P., Nyboe, J., Appleyard, M. *et al.* (1990) The relation of ventilatory function impairment and of chronic mucus hypersecretion to mortality from obstructive lung disease and from all causes. *Thorax*, **45**, 579–85.

17. Carpenter, L., Beral, V., Strachan, D. *et al.* (1989) Respiratory symptoms as predictors of 27-year mortality in a representative sample of British adults. *Br. Med. J.*, **299**; 357–61.

18. Ebi-Kryston, K.L. (1989) Predicting 15-year chronic bronchitis mortality in the Whitehall study. *J. Epidemiol. Community Health*, **43**, 168–72.

19. Higgins, I.T.T., Oldham, P.D., Cochrane, A.L. and Gilson, J.C. (1956) Respiratory symptoms and pulmonary disability in an industrial town: survey of a random sample of the population. *Br. Med. J.*, **ii**, 904–9.

20. Higgins, I.T.T. (1957) Respiratory symptoms, bronchitis and ventilatory capacity in a random sample of an agricultural population. *Br. Med. J.*, **ii**, 1198–203.

21. Higgins, I.T.T. and Cochran, J.B. (1958) Respiratory symptoms, bronchitis and disability in a random sample of an agricultural community in Dumfriesshire. *Tubercle*, **39**, 296–301.

22. Higgins, I.T.T. and Cochrane, A.L. (1961) Chronic respiratory symptoms in a random sample of men and women in the Rhondda Fach in 1958. *Br. J. Ind. Med.*, **18**, 93–102.

23. Lambert, P.M., and Reid, D.D. (1970) Smoking, air pollution and bronchitis in Britain. *Lancet*, **i**, 853–7.

24. Dean, G., Lee, P.N., Todd, G.F., Wicken, A.J. and Sparks D.N. (1978) Factors related to respiratory and cardiovascular symptoms in the United Kingdom. *J. Epidemiol. Community Health*, **32**, 86–96.

25. Cook, D.G., Kussick, S.J. and Shaper, A.G. (1990) The respiratory benefits of stopping smoking. *J. Smoking Related Disorders*, **1**, 45–58.

26. Brown, C.A., Crombie, I.K., Smith, W.C.S. and Tunstall-Pedoe, H. (1991). The impact of quitting smoking on symptoms of chronic bronchitis: results of the Scottish Heart Health Study. *Thorax*, **46**, 112–6.

27. Cullinan, P. (1992) Persistent cough and phlegm: prevalence and clinical characteristics in south-east England. *Respir. Med.*, **86**, 143–6.

28. Anderson, H.R., Esmail, A., Hollowell, J. *et al.* (1994) *Epidemiologically based needs assessment: lower respiratory disease.* Department of Health, London.

29. Cox, B.D. (1987) Blood pressure and respiratory function. In: *The health and lifestyle survey. Preliminary report of a nationwide survey of the physical and mental health, attitudes and lifestyle of a random sample of 9003 British adults.* Health Promotion Research Trust, London, pp. 17–33.

30. General Register Office (1958) *Morbidity statistics from General Practice 1955–56.* SMPS no. 14. HMSO, London.

31. Royal College of General Practitioners, Office of Population Censuses and Surveys, Department of Health and Social Security (1974) *Morbidity Statistics from General Practice, 1970–71. Second national study.* SMPS no. 26. HMSO, London.

32. Royal College of General Practitioners, Office of Population Censuses and Surveys, Department of Health (1986) *Morbidity statistics from General Practice, 1981–82. Third national study.* Series MB5 no. 1. HMSO, London.

33. Cook, D.G. and Shaper, A.G. (1988) Breathlessness, lung function and risk of a heart attack. *Eur. Heart J.*, **9**, 1215–22.

34. Ebi-Kryston, K.L. (1986) Respiratory symptoms and pulmonary function as predictors of 10-year mortality from respiratory disease, cardiovascular disease and all causes in the Whitehall study. *J. Epidemiol. Community Health*, **41**, 251–60.

35. Strachan, D.P. (1991) Ventilatory function as a predictor of fatal stroke. *Br. Med. J.*, **302**, 84–7.

36. Strachan, D.P. (1992) Ventilatory function, height and mortality among lifelong non-smokers. *J. Epidemiol. Community Health*, **46**, 66–70.

37. Office of Population Censuses and Surveys (1993) *Mortality statistics, cause: England and Wales 1992.* Series DH2 no. 19. HMSO, London.

38. Department of Social Security (1983) *Sickness and invalidity benefit statistics 1982–83.* HMSO, London.

39. Barker, D.J.P, and Osmond, C. (1986) Childhood respiratory infection and chronic

bronchitis in England and Wales. *Br. Med. J.*, **293**, 1271–5.

40. Lee, P.N., Fry, J.S. and Forey, B.A. (1990) Trends in lung cancer, chronic obstructive lung disease and emphysema death rates for England and Wales 1941–85 and their relation to trends in cigarette smoking. *Thorax*, **45**, 657–65.

41. Strachan, D.P. (1991) Trends in respiratory mortality in England and Wales (letter). *Thorax*, **46**, 149–52.

42. Department of Health Advisory Group on the Medical Aspects of Air Pollution Episodes (1992). *Second report: sulphur dioxide, acid aerosols and particulates.* HMSO, London.

43. World Health Organization (1992) *World Health Statistics Annual 1991.* WHO, Geneva.

44. Thom, T.J. (1989) International comparisons in COPD mortality. *Am. Rev. Respir. Dis.*, **140**, S27–S34.

45. Reid, D.D. and Fletcher, C.M. (1971) International studies in chronic respiratory disease. *Br. Med. Bull.*, **27**, 59–64.

46. Reid, D.D., Cornfield, J., Markush, R.E. *et al.* (1966) *Studies of disease among migrants and native populations in Great Britain, Norway and United States. III: Prevalence of cardiorespiratory symptoms among migrants and native-born in the United States.* National Cancer Institute Monograph no 19. Government Printing Office, Washington DC. pp. 321–46.

47. Gardner, M.J., Winter, P.D. and Barker, D.J.P. (1984) *Atlas of mortality from selected diseases in England and Wales 1968–78.* Wiley, Chichester.

48. Reid, D.D. and Fairburn, A.S. (1958) Air pollution and other local factors in respiratory disease. *Br. J. Prev. Soc. Med.*, **12**, 94–103.

49. Holland, W.W., and Reid, D.D. (1965) The urban factor in chronic bronchitis. *Lancet*, **i**, 445–6.

50. Burr, M.L. and Halliday, R.M. (1987) Why is chest disease so common in south Wales? Smoking, social class and lung function: a survey of elderly men in two areas. *J. Epidemiol. Community Health*, **41**, 140–4.

51. Reid, D.D. (1969) The beginnings of bronchitis. *Proc. R. Soc. Med.*, **62**, 311–6.

52. Colley, J.R.T., and Reid, D.D. (1970) The urban and social origins of childhood bronchitis in England and Wales. *Br. Med. J.*, **2**, 213–6.

53. Rosenbaum, S. (1961) Home localities of national servicemen with respiratory disease. *Br. J. Prev. Soc. Med.*, **15**, 61–7.

54. Osmond, C., Slattery, J.M. and Barker, D.J.P. (1990) Mortality by place of birth. In: *Mortality and Geography. A review in the mid-1980s. The Registrar-General's Decennial Supplement for England and Wales* (ed. M. Britton), HMSO, London (Series DS no. 9): 96–100.

55. *Registrar-General's Decennial Supplement for England and Wales 1921. Occupational Mortality* (1931) HMSO, London.

56. Respiratory Diseases Study Group of the College of General Practitioners (1961). Chronic bronchitis in Great Britain. *Br. Med. J.*, **ii**, 973–8.

57. Office of Population Censuses and Surveys (1986) *Occupational mortality: The Registrar-General's decennial supplement for Great Britain 1979–80, 1982–83.* Series DS no. 6. Part II: Microfiche tables. HMSO, London.

58. Royal College of General Practitioners, Office of Population Censuses and Surveys, Department of Health (1990) *Morbidity statistics from general practice, 1981–82. Third national study, socio-economic analyses.* Series MB5 no. 2. HMSO, London.

59. Mann, S.L., Wadsworth, M.E.J., and Colley, J.R.T. (1992) Accumulation of factors influencing respiratory illness in members of a national birth cohort and their offspring. *J. Epidemiol. Community Health*, **46**, 286–92.

60. Britten, N., Davies, J.M.C. and Colley, J.R.T. (1987) Early respiratory experience and subsequent cough and peak expiratory flow rate in 36 year old men and women. *Br. Med. J.*, **294**, 1317–20.

61. United States Department of Health and Human Services, Public Health Service (1984) *The health consequences of smoking: chronic obstructive lung disease. A report of the Surgeon General.* US Government Printing Office, Washington, DC.

62. United States Department of Health and Human Services, Public Health Service (1990). *The health benefits of smoking cessation. A report of the Surgeon General.* US Government Printing Office, Washington, D.C.

63. Rose, G. and Hamilton, P.J.S (1978) A randomised controlled trial of the effect on middle-aged men of advice to stop smoking. *J. Epidemiol Community Health*, **32**, 275–81.

64. Kuller, L.H., Ockene, J.K., Townsend, M. *et al.* (1989) The epidemiology of pulmonary function and COPD mortality in the Multiple Risk Factor Intervention Trial. *Am. Rev. Respir. Dis.*, **140**, S76–S81.

65. Higenbottam, T., Clark, T.J.H., Shipley, M.J. and Rose, G. (1980) Lung function and symptoms of cigarette smokers related to tar yield and number of cigarettes smoked. *Lancet*, **i**, 409–12.

66. Withey, C.H., Papacosta, O., Swan, A.V. *et al.* (1992) Respiratory effects of lowering tar and nicotine levels of cigarettes smoked by young male middle tar smokers. II: Results of a randomised controlled trial. *J. Epidemiol. Community Health*, **46**, 281–5.

67. Wald, N.J., Nanchahal, K., Thompson, S.G. and Cuckle, H.S. (1986). Does breathing other people's tobacco smoke cause lung cancer? *Br. Med. J.*, **293**, 1216–22.

68. Lee, P.N. (1992) *Environmental Tobacco Smoke and Mortality.* Karger, Basel.

69. Doll, R. and Peto, R. (1976) Mortality in relation to smoking. 20 years observation on male British doctors. *Br. Med. J.*, **ii**, 1525–36.

70. Kalandidi, A., Trichopoulos, D., Hatzakis, A. and Tzannes, A. (1987) Passive smoking and chronic obstructive lung disease. *Lancet*, **ii**, 1325–6.

71. Lee, P.N. Chamberlain, J. and Alderson, M.R. (1986) Relationship of passive smoking to risk of lung cancer and other smoking-associated diseases. *Br. J. Cancer*, **54**, 97–105.

72. Sandler, D.P., Comstock, G.W., Helsing, K.J. and Shore, D.L. (1989) Deaths from all causes in non-smokers who lived with smokers. *Am. J. Public Health*, **79**, 163–7.

73. Hirayama, T. (1981) Non-smoking wives of heavy smokers have a higher risk of lung cancer. *Br. Med. J.*, **282**, 183–5.

74. Samet, J.M., Marbury, M.C. and Spengler, J.D. (1987) Health effects and sources of indoor air pollution. Part 1. *Am. Rev. Respir. Dis.*, **136**, 1486–1508.

75. Fielding, J.E. and Phenow, K.J. (1988) Health effects of involuntary smoking *N. Engl. J. Med.*, **319**, 1452–60.

76. Masi, M.A., Hanley, J.A., Ernst, P. and Becklake, M.R. (1988) Environmental exposure to tobacco smoke and lung function in young adults. *Am. Rev. Respir. Dis.*, **138**, 296–9.

77. Dodge, R. (1982) The effects of indoor pollution on Arizona children. *Arch. Environ. Health*, **37**, 151–5.

78. Lebowitz, M.D., Holberg, C.J., Knudson. R.J. and Burrows, B. (1987) Longitudinal study of pulmonary function development in childhood, adolescence and early adulthood. *Am. Rev. Respir. Dis.*, **136**, 69–75.

79. Tager, I.B., Weiss, S.T., Munoz, A. *et al.* (1983) Longitudinal study of the effects of maternal cigarette smoking on pulmonary function development in children. *N. Engl. J. Med.*, **309**, 699–703.

80. Berkey, C.S., Ware, J.H., Dockery, D.W. *et al.* (1986) Indoor air pollution and pulmonary function growth in preadolescent children. *Am. J. Epidemiol.*, **123**, 250–60.

81. Brooke, O.G., Anderson, H.R., Bland, J.M. *et al.* (1989) The effects on birthweight of smoking, alcohol, caffeine, socio-economic factors and psycho-social stress. *Br. Med. J.*, **298**, 795–801.

82. Waller, R.E. (1978) Control of air pollution: present success and future prospect. In *Recent Advances in Community Medicine I* (ed. A.E. Bennett) Churchill Livingstone, Edinburgh. pp. 59–72.

83. World Health Organization (1992) *Acute effects on health of smog episodes.* WHO Regional Publications, European Series no. 43. WHO, Copenhagen.

84. Schwartz, J. and Marcus, A. (1990) Mortality and air pollution in London: a time series analysis. *Am. J. Epidemiol*, **131**, 185–94.

85. Department of Health Advisory Group on the Medical Aspects of Air Pollution Episodes (1991) *First report: ozone.* HMSO, London.

86. Hackney, J.D., Linn, W.S., Avol, E.L. *et al.* (1992) Exposures of older adults with chronic respiratory illness to nitrogen dioxide. A combined laboratory and field study. *Am. Rev. Respir. Dis.*, **146**, 1480–6.

87. World Health Organization (1979) *Sulfur oxides and suspended particulate matter. Environmental Health Criteria no. 8.* WHO, Geneva.

88. United States Environmental Protection Agency (1982) *Air quality criteria for particulate matter and sulfur oxides. Vol 1. Report no. EPA-600/8-82-029a.* USEPA, Triangle Park, NC.

89. World Health Organization (1987) *Air quality guidelines for Europe.* WHO Regional Publications, European Series no. 23. WHO, Copenhagen.

90. Gardner, M.J., Crawford, M.D. and Morris, J.N. (1969) Patterns of mortality in middle and old age in the county boroughs of

England and Wales. *Br. J. Prev. Soc. Med.*, **23**, 133–40.

91. Chinn, S., Florey, C.D.V., Baldwin, I.G. and Gorgol, M. (1981) The relationship of mortality in England and Wales 1969–73 to measurements of air pollution. *J. Epidemiol. Community Health*, **35**, 174–9.

92. Detels, R., Sayre, J.W., Coulson, A.H. *et al.* (1981) The UCLA population studies of chronic obstructive respiratory disease. IV: Respiratory effects of long-term exposure to photochemical oxidants, nitrogen dioxide and sulfates on current and never smokers. *Am. Rev. Respir. Dis.*, **124**, 673–80.

93. Fischer, P., Remjin, B., Brunekreef, B. *et al.* (1985) Indoor air pollution and its effect on pulmonary function of adult non-smoking women. II: Associations between nitrogen dioxide and pulmonary function. *Int. J. Epidemiol*, **14**, 221–6.

94. Becklake, M.R. (1989) Occupational exposures: evidence for a causal association with chronic obstructive pulmonary disease. *Am. Rev. Respir. Dis.*, **140**, S85–S89.

95. Morgan, W.K.C. (1978) Industrial bronchitis. *Br. J. Ind. Med.*, **35**, 285–91.

96. Lebowitz, M. (1977) Occupational exposures in relation to symptomatology and lung function in a community population. *Environ. Res.*, **44**, 59–67.

97. Love, R.G. and Miller, B.G. (1982) Longitudinal study of lung function in coal miners. *Thorax*, **37**, 193–7

98. Miller, B.G. and Jacobsen, M. (1985) Dust exposure, pneumoconiosis and mortality of coal miners. *Br. J. Ind. Med.*, **42**, 723–33.

99. Samet, J.M., Tager, I.B., and Speizer, F.E. (1983) The relationship between respiratory illness in childhood and chronic air-flow obstruction in adults. *Am. Rev. Respir. Dis.*, **127**, 508–23.

100. Strachan, D.P. (1990) Do chesty children become chesty adults? *Arch. Dis. Child.*, **65**, 161–62.

101. Barker, D.J.P., Godfrey, K.M., Fall, C. *et al.* (1991) Relation of birth weight and childhood respiratory infection to adult lung function and death from chronic obstructive lung disease. *Br. Med. J.*, **303**, 671–5.

102. Colley, J.R.T., Douglas, J.W.B., and Reid, D.D. (1973) Respiratory disease in young adults: influence of early childhood lower respiratory tract illness, social class, air pollution and smoking. *Br. Med. J.*, *iii*, 195–8.

103. Britten, N, and Wadsworth, J. (1986) Long term sequelae of whooping cough in a nationally representative sample. *Br. Med. J.*, **292**, 441–4.

104. Burrows, B. Knudson, R.J. and Lebowitz, M.D. (1977) The relationship of childhood respiratory illness to adult obstructive lung disease. *Am. Rev. Respir. Dis.*, **115**, 751–60.

105. Martin, A.J., Landau, L.I. and Phelan, P.D. (1982) Asthma from childhood at age 21: the patient and his disease. *Br. Med. J.*, **284**, 380–2.

106. Strachan, D.P., Anderson, H.R,. Bland, J.M. and Peckham, C. (1988). Asthma as a link between chest illness in childhood and chronic cough and phlegm in young adults. *Br. Med. J.*, **296**, 890–3.

107. Martinez, F.D., Morgan, W.J., Wright, A.L. *et al.* (1991) Initial airway function is a risk factor for recurrent wheezing respiratory illnesses during the first three years of life. *Am. Rev. Respir. Dis.*, **143**, 312–6.

108. Strachan, D.P., Cox, B.D., Erzinclioglu, S.W. *et al.* (1991) Ventilatory function and winter fresh fruit consumption in a random sample of British adults. *Thorax*, **46**, 624–9.

109. Schwartz, J. and Weiss, S.T. (1990) Dietary factors and their relation to respiratory symptoms. *Am. J. Epidemiol.*, **132**, 67–76.

110. Lange, P., Groth, S., Mortensen, J. *et al.* (1988) Pulmonary function is influenced by heavy alcohol consumption. *Am. Rev. Respir. Dis.*, **137**, 1119–23.

N.B. Pride and B. Burrows

5.1 INTRODUCTION

The definition of COPD adopted in this chapter is that proposed by Burrows [1]:

> 'A chronic, slowly progressive airway obstruction disorder resulting from some combination of pulmonary emphysema and irreversible reduction in the calibre of small airways of the lung'.

There are three important consequences; first, COPD will be used solely to refer to persistent airway obstruction; second, asthma and COPD are regarded as distinct conditions even when asthma leads to persistent airways obstruction; third, a patient with fixed obstruction of the peripheral airways without chronic cough and expectoration ('chronic bronchitis') and without destruction of alveolar ducts and walls ('emphysema') can still be accepted as having COPD, even although the obstructive bronchiolitis (and accompanying obstruction of small bronchi) in smokers is not readily differentiated from other causes of persistent bronchiolitis. This is supported in practice by the studies of Fletcher, Peto and colleagues [2,3] which suggested that while both chronic mucus hypersecretion ('chronic bronchitis') and progressive airway obstruction were related to inhaling cigarette smoke the two conditions were relatively distinct. Chronic mucus hypersecretion, which resulted in persistent cough and phlegm, was largely the result of pathologic changes in the central conducting airways. In contrast the progressive airways obstruction of smokers (COPD) originated chiefly in the peripheral airways and air spaces of the lung, was responsible for breathlessness on exertion and ultimately led to disability and death. In support of this dissociation Fletcher and colleagues [3] showed that about 20% of male smokers with chronic bronchitis had a completely normal FEV_1 at age 50 years, while a further 25% of smokers with definitely reduced FEV_1 denied chronic productive cough. Further studies investigating the relative independence of the two conditions are considered in Section 5.3.4.

5.2 DEVELOPMENT OF IMPAIRMENT IN LUNG FUNCTION

The development of severe impairment in spirometry in COPD is believed to result from many years of moderately accelerated decline in lung function. This was first suggested by the modest increase in rates of decline in FEV_1 observed in symptomatic patients with COPD (Table 5.1). Subsequently Fletcher, Peto and colleagues [3] obtained direct evidence of the early change in FEV_1 in working men in London; because they found a relationship between the annual rate of decline in FEV_1 over 8 years ('slope') and the level of FEV_1, they suggested susceptible smokers

Chronic Obstructive Pulmonary Disease. Edited by Dr P. Calverley and Professor N. Pride. Published in 1995 by Chapman & Hall, London. ISBN 0 412 46450 0

Table 5.1 Some reported rates of change in FEV$_1$ in chronic obstructive pulmonary disease

	Mean change in FEV$_1$ (ml/year)
Pre-clinical OLD	
Tucson population, smokers	−91
Relatively mild clinical illness	
British chronic bronchitis	−83[a]
Chicago emphysema FEV$_1$ >1.24 l	−72
Salt Lake City chronic OLD	−69
More severe clinical illness	
Chicago emphysema, all patients	−56
Houston VA Hosp. COPD	−52
Groningen CNSLD	−54
IPPB study of COPD	−48

Reprinted from Burrows [8].
[a]Studied FEV$_{0.75}$ rather than FEV$_1$.
OLD, obstructive lung disease; COPD, chronic obstructive pulmonary disease; CNSLD, chronic non-specific lung disease; IPPB, intermittent positive pressure breathing.

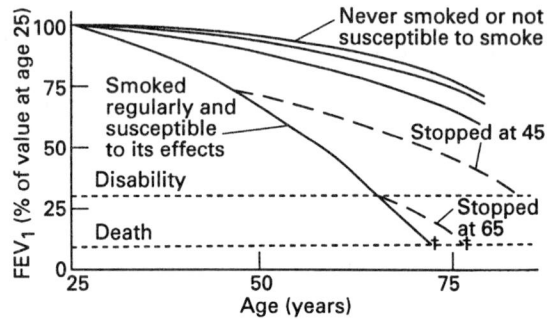

Fig. 5.1 Hypothetical model of development of impairment of FEV$_1$ in a susceptible smoker according to Fletcher and Peto [2]. Annual decline in FEV$_1$ is assumed to slightly accelerate with increasing age. In practice there will be a range of rates of decline in FEV$_1$ in susceptible smokers. On stopping smoking there no improvement in FEV$_1$ but subsequent loss of FEV$_1$ is similar to that in healthy never-smokers. (Reproduced from Fletcher and Peto [2] with permission.)

could be identified by reduction in FEV$_1$ by early middle age (Fig. 5.1). This assumes that individuals in the highest or lowest percentiles with regard to FEV$_1$ stay in the same percentile over many subsequent years, so showing 'horse-racing' or 'tracking', as has been described in longitudinal studies of blood pressure. An alternative hypothesis has been proposed: because the initial stages of smoking-related lung damage are characterized by inflammatory and obstructive changes in the peripheral airways, which have an enormous functional reserve, these pathologic changes might cause few symptoms and negligible decline in tests of overall lung function such as the FEV$_1$ until they become very severe and widespread. Susceptible smokers might only declare themselves by accelerated decline of FEV$_1$ in late middle age, while earlier in their smoking years their FEV$_1$, although slightly lower than in most non-smokers, might be indistinguishable from FEV$_1$ in the general population of smokers. If this was the usual course it would be difficult to study risk factors by following annual decline in lung

function, as studies early in the smoking lifetime would not be predictive of later disability, whilst studies in symptomatic subjects are complicated by exclusions due to severe disease and 'survivor' effects. A few long-term studies of individual smokers are available; most individuals appear to show a moderately accelerated decline but occasional examples of a rapid decline in middle age have been observed (Fig. 5.2). More systematic support for the strength of tracking comes from a 20-year follow-up study of 2718 working men whose pulmonary function was assessed between 1954 and 1961, in whom the risk of death from chronic airflow obstruction was more than 50 times greater in men whose initial FEV$_1$ was more than two standard deviations below average values than in men whose initial FEV$_1$ was above average [4] (Fig. 5.3). Most of these men were studied initially in middle age during their working life at a time when there were only minor abnormalities in FEV$_1$. Further population studies of men and women in Copenhagen [5] and North

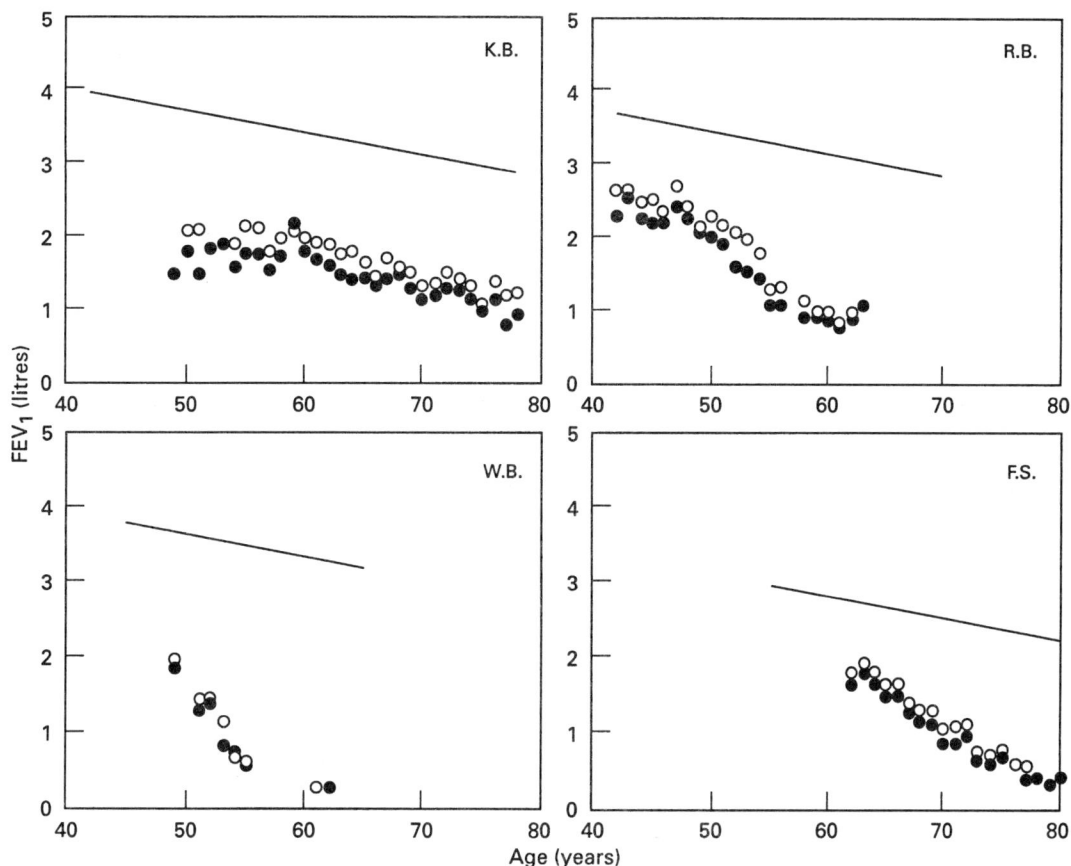

Fig. 5.2 Examples of long-term changes in FEV_1 (● pre-, ○ post-bronchodilator) in 4 men identified when FEV_1 was about 2 l. The continuous line indicates the predicted values of FEV_1. The top left panel shows a man in whom observed decline in FEV_1 parallels the predicted fall, while the three remaining men show accelerated decline, particularly fast in WB (lower left panel) in whom decline may have commenced in his mid-forties.

America [6] with follow-up of 10–12 years have confirmed similar high risk rates for death from COPD associated with a moderately lowered FEV_1. Studies in Tucson, Arizona have suggested a limited period of rapid decline in some individuals but overall confirmed the presence of tracking for decline in FEV_1 in middle-aged males, but not in women smokers [7].

As reviewed by Burrows [8], there is a tendency for annual rates of decline in FEV_1 to be slower in advanced than in milder disease (Table 5.1). This trend is in apparent disagree-

ment with earlier proposals that the rate of decline of FEV_1 in an individual may accelerate as disease advances. The findings in advanced disease may be due to loss of the most rapid decliners by death, but undoubtedly individuals who earlier in their life have shown rapid decline may subsequently show a prolonged survival and relative stability of FEV_1.

All longitudinal studies of decline in FEV_1 show considerable differences in rate between individuals. If the follow-up period is short this is largely due to a large signal–noise ratio with spirometry; 95% confidence limits for

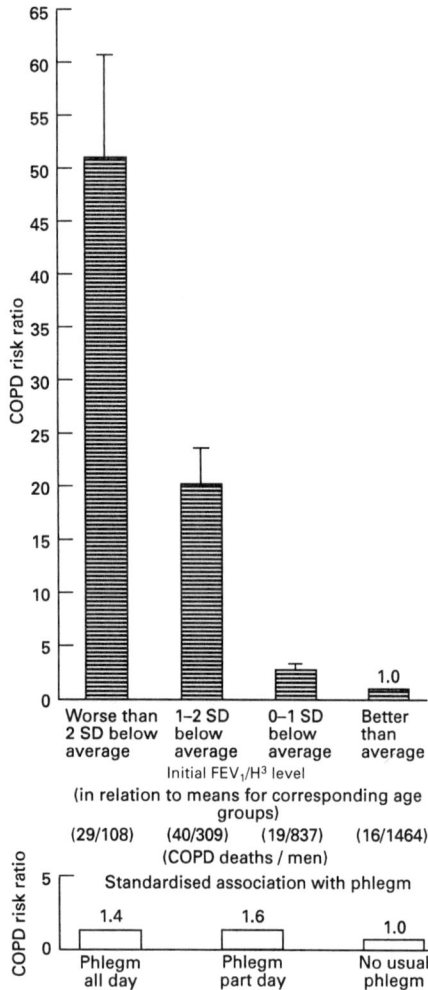

Fig. 5.3 Risk ratios for death from COPD (top) according to initial value of height corrected FEV_1/H^3 (where H is height in metres) at survey 20–25 years before (bars indicate standard errors). (bottom) according to presence of phlegm after standardization for FEV_1/H^3. (Reproduced from Peto *et al.* [4] with permission.)

short-term repeatability of FEV_1 in an individual is 190 ml [9] which is several years' annual decline in FEV_1 even in smokers. But the range of annual decline in FEV_1 between individuals is still considerable when follow-up is for 10 years or more and is found in healthy never-smokers although over a narrower range than in subjects with identified

risk factors such as cigarette smoking or severe α_1-AT deficiency (Fig. 5.4) Presumably patients destined to develop severe ventilatory impairment emerge from the tail of fast-declining subjects observed in population studies.

Most information on the natural history of COPD comes from sequential measurement of FEV_1 which can be applied over the whole range from health to advanced disease. Attempts have been made to amplify this information in the early stages of disease, because 'low normal' values of FEV_1 are derived from a mixture of subjects whose lungs are structurally normal but smaller than average and others in whom disease has started to cause a decline in lung function from initial average or even above average values. Tests of lung function which are more sensitive to minor changes in the peripheral airways and airspaces, such as the single breath nitrogen (SBN_2) test or the later part of the maximum expiratory flow-volume curve, should therefore aid in interpretation of slightly reduced values in FEV_1. Six to ten year follow-up of subjects in whom the SBN_2 test has been measured at a time FEV_1 is normal confirms that the SBN_2 is abnormal in almost all subjects who subsequently develop a reduced FEV_1 [10]; but many subjects with an abnormal SBN_2 test do not develop a reduced FEV_1 over this period so the predictive value of the test has not yet proved as strong as originally hoped.

Many smokers also show a small reduction in CO transfer coefficient ($TLCO/VA$) (which cannot be explained by CO back pressure in the blood) at an early stage in their natural history [11]. Although moderate or severe reductions in $TLCO/VA$ are associated with the presence of emphysema [12,13], mild reductions in $TLCO/VA$ are reversed on quitting smoking, suggesting removal of a pulmonary vascular response [11]. Therefore allowance has to be made for current smoking habit to estimate irreversible reduction in $TLCO/VA$ [14]. Nevertheless occasional patients with

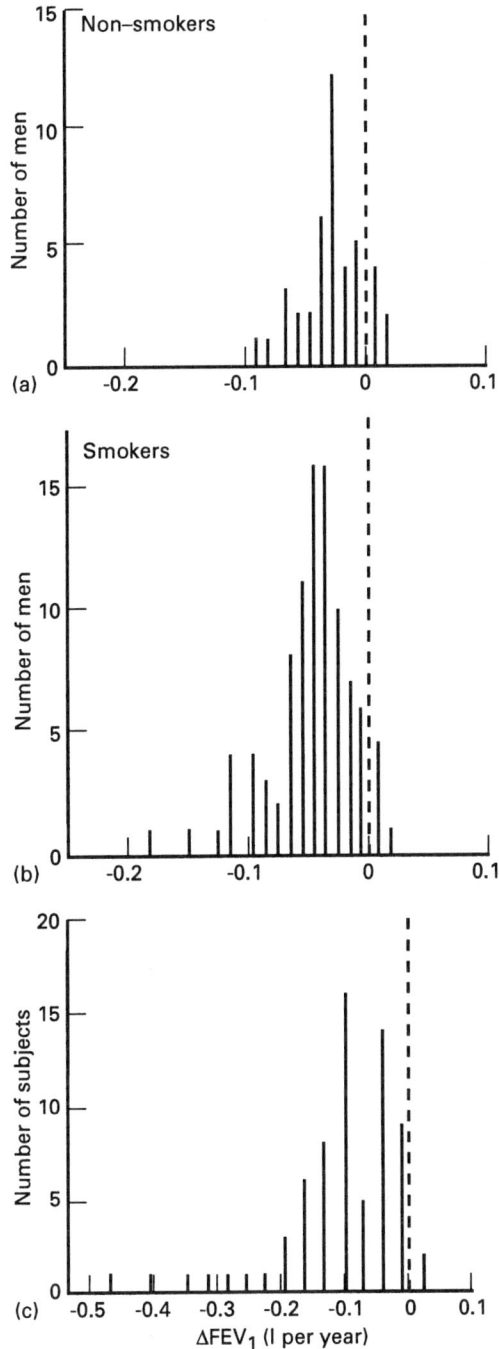

Fig. 5.4 Distribution of rates of annual decline in FEV_1 in (a) 42 middle-aged male never smokers, average decline 26 ml per year, (b) 97 middle-aged men who were continuing cigarette smokers, average decline 47 ml per year, (c) in 71 subjects with homozygous α_1-AT deficiency (PiZ) identified in studies in the USA and Sweden. Rates of decline are very variable, but usually faster than in non-deficient subjects (note difference in scale from two upper panels). (Panel (c) modified from Buist *et al.* [51] with permission.)

COPD have considerable reduction in T_{LCO}/V_A at a time when spirometry is relatively well preserved [15]. Sequential studies of change in T_{LCO}/V_A are sparse. In an unpublished 19-year follow-up of 17 men first identified at a mean age of 54 years with FEV_1 56% of predicted there was a wide range of initial T_{LCO}/V_A. In the 10 men in whom T_{LCO}/V_A was >80% predicted value at recruitment, T_{LCO}/V_A remained within the normal range during follow-up despite considerable falls in FEV_1; subjects in whom T_{LCO}/V_A was reduced at recruitment showed further falls in T_{LCO}/V_A and a faster decline in FEV_1. These results support separation between the development of predominant emphysema and predominant intrinsic airway disease occurring before severe airways obstruction has developed. Loss of lung recoil pressure has also been described at an early stage in the evolution of airways obstruction [15,16], but again there is very limited longitudinal information [16]. Sequential use of CT of the thorax should improve knowledge of the natural history of emphysema in the future.

With advanced disease severe hypoxemia and a high pulmonary artery pressure develop and worsen prognosis [8,17]. Sequential studies of mean pulmonary artery pressure show increases which average 0.5–0.6 mmHg/year [18].

5.3 RISK FACTORS

Only a small part, probably less than 20%, of the varying susceptibility of a cigarette smoker to develop progressive airflow obstruction is explained by current research. Even with the strongest genetic risk factor (homozygous α-antitrypsin deficiency) there is a very wide variation in FEV_1 between individuals (Fig. 5.4). Hence small differences in mean rates of decline in lung function may conceal a much greater susceptibility in an important subgroup of subjects; although this has been evident in many studies of smokers

over the last two decades, there is very little information on variations in susceptibility to other external agents.

Because morbidity and mortality in COPD are very strongly linked to the development of ventilatory impairment, in particular a low FEV_1, risk factors are usually investigated either by studying related mortality or by seeking evidence of accelerated annual decline in FEV_1. A further risk factor may be impaired childhood lung growth and development, so that subjects enter adult life either with reduced FEV_1 or with lungs particularly susceptible to damage by smoking or other unfavorable influences.

Risk factors have been identified by two main routes – large-scale epidemiologic studies using simple measurements and end-points and more detailed clinical studies of proposed risk factors. Intervention studies aimed at specific risk factors provide further information. As discussed in Chapter 4 epidemiologic studies have usually been cross-sectional and have used end-points such as impairment of lung function, symptoms of cough, phlegm, wheeze and breathlessness, morbidity and mortality to detect the effects of age, gender, smoking habit, urban living, environmental pollution, occupation, diet and socio-economic status (Table 5.2). In this section some additional evidence concerning smoking, occupation, the protease–antiprotease hypothesis, recurrent bronchopulmonary infections ('British' hypothesis) and allergy and airway hyper-responsiveness ('Dutch' hypothesis) will be reviewed.

5.3.1 CIGARETTE SMOKING

Although not formally included in the definition of COPD, in Western countries cigarette smoking is usually regarded as the dominant risk factor and much of our knowledge of the natural history comes from studies in smokers. Indeed many clinicians are reluctant to make the diagnosis except in a smoker or ex-smoker, but clearly COPD can

Table 5.2 Proposed risk factors for COPD

Risk factor	Comments
Increasing age	Ventilatory impairment predominantly reflects cumulative life-time smoking history
Gender	After standardizing for smoking, males more at risk than females
Smoking habit	Some relation to number of cigarettes smoked per day and cumulative pack-years
Environmental pollution	Large differences in urban and rural death rates. Particulates more important than photochemical pollutants
Occupation	Many dusts cause mucus hypersecretion. Persistent obstruction develops in coal and gold miners, farmers, grain handlers, cement and cotton workers. Cadmium workers have increased risk of emphysema
Socio-economic status	More common in individuals of low socio-economic status
Diet	High fish intake may reduce risk in smokers
Genetic factors	Homozygous α_1-antitrypsin deficiency is strongest single risk
Birthweight and childhood respiratory illness	Low birthweight predicts low FEV_1 and high COPD mortality in later life. Chronic childhood disease predisposes to chronic adult disease
Recurrent bronchopulmonary infections	Cause short-term decline in lung function, but not shown to accelerate long-term decline in otherwise healthy smokers
Allergy and airway hyper-responsiveness	Increased blood IgE and eosinophils and hyper-responsiveness found in smokers but significance as risk factors may be confined to a subgroup of smokers

See text and Chapter 4 for further details.

occur in non-smokers (for instance with α_1-antitrypsin deficiency [19]) while chronic bronchitis is found in about 4% of never-smokers without other obvious respiratory disease. Equally it is accepted that only a minority of smokers develop disabling airway obstruction. On average current cigarette smokers show rather less than double the annual decline of FEV_1 found in non-smokers – about 50 compared to 30 ml per year – but this average value conceals a considerable range of decline in FEV_1 in individuals, in particular a tail of smokers showing unusually rapid decline (Fig. 5.4). Annual decline in

FEV_1 in smokers probably begins at a younger age than in healthy never-smokers, who show a plateau of FEV_1 in early adult life until 30–35 years of age [20].

An obvious possible cause for the differing susceptibility of smokers is variation in exposure to tobacco smoke. When smokers are subdivided according to reported daily number of cigarettes smoked, some relation between cigarette numbers and annual decline in FEV_1 is found, but a wide variation in annual rate of decline in FEV_1 persists among smokers of similar numbers of cigarettes. Nevertheless there is a more than two-fold difference in mortality from COPD between smokers of <15 and >25 cigarettes a day [21]. Characterization of smoking habit solely by current daily cigarette consumption – or even cumulative pack-years – does not allow for many other factors which influence the individual's exposure to cigarette smoke, such as the extent to which smoke is taken from the burning cigarette and inhaled deep into the lungs and the yield of tar, nicotine and other constituents of the cigarette. Because a smoker's own assessment of depth of inhalation is unreliable, smoking pattern (or chemical markers of smoking intensity) must be measured directly. Small studies of smoking pattern in men showing rapid and normal rates of decline in FEV_1 have failed to show significant differences. Reduction in the tar content of the cigarettes smoked reduces mucus hypersecretion [22,23] but it has been difficult to determine if the progression of airflow obstruction is slowed [22,24–26]. One large scale study of mortality and smoking habit found fewer deaths ascribed to emphysema in smokers of lower tar cigarettes than in smokers of medium or high tar cigarettes [27]. Undoubtedly any benefit is modest; potential benefit may be counteracted by more intense smoking of low-tar cigarettes [28]. Because there are so many potentially toxic constituents of tobacco smoke, it is impossible to exclude the possibility that some particular component of smoke, which might not be inhaled in parallel with any of the established markers, might be of overwhelming importance. But despite inevitable deficiencies in quantifying smoke exposure, there is probably a true wide difference in susceptibility between smokers which is not explained by variation in dose of tobacco smoke. As discussed below, there is clear evidence that smoking adds to the risk attached to α_1-antitrypsin deficiency and dusty occupations; interactions between smoking and other currently unidentified risk factors could account for this difference in susceptibility between smokers.

5.3.2 OCCUPATION

There are considerable difficulties in identifying occupational risks from simple epidemiologic data, because even such obvious factors as quantification of occupational exposure or smoking are often not known. Studies of the general population usually include a greater proportion of workers with low exposure, while long-term workplace follow-up may exclude some of those at most risk, but allows quantification of exposure and change in FEV_1. The distinction between hypersecretory and obstructive disease is particularly important in considering the effects of dust and irritant fume inhalation at work. Workers in many of the most dusty occupations are frequently heavy smokers, and in the past often lived in polluted general environments. Furthermore it is necessary to distinguish between the effects of dust in causing relatively transient bronchoconstriction during and shortly after exposure and the development of persistent airway obstruction when removed from exposure.

There is no doubt that many dusty occupations are associated with the development of mucus hypersecretion [29,30]: this has been established by simple cross-sectional studies and general population surveys [30,31,32]. Many such studies also show reduced FEV_1 in workers exposed to dust, but it has been more difficult to determine whether persistent airway obstruction develops to a greater extent than predicted from smoking history and socio-economic factors. In urban population studies occupational dust exposure is associated with a higher risk of reduced FEV_1 than exposure to gas or fumes [30,31,22]. Recent longitudinal studies of decline in FEV_1 together with quantification of dust exposure in coal [33,34] and gold miners have established a small additive effect of dust exposure and smoking in accelerating decline in FEV_1, previously the source of much controversy [34,35]. Accelerated decline of FEV_1 is also found in cotton workers even with improved dust control [36,37] and in grain handlers [38]; cement workers and farmers also appear to be at risk of progressive airways obstruction [30]. As with other risk factors, there may well be considerable differences in susceptibility between individuals. The role of fumes and gases such as ammonia and SO_2 in causing chronic symptoms after acute exposure is more controversial. The prevalence of emphysema has been claimed to be greater following chronic low dose exposure to cadmium fumes and to oxides of nitrogen. Recent evidence supports an increased risk of developing emphysema in cadmium workers [39], although this could be by increasing the effects of cigarette smoke rather than by an independent effect which would also be found in non-smokers. The evidence incriminating oxides of nitrogen is so far inconclusive.

Because of the long natural history of COPD and the overriding importance of smoking it is difficult to establish subtle occupational effects; probably these are currently under-estimated.

5.3.3 α_1-ANTITRYPSIN DEFICIENCY

The genetic and biochemical background and clinical presentation with chronic airways obstruction and basal emphysema is discussed in Chapter 6. Although the genetics have turned out to be relatively complex with over 75 biochemical variants of the protease inhibitor (Pi) system described, the situation is simplified by the belief that the risk of developing airflow obstruction is indicated by serum levels of α_1-AT measured in the basal state.

This is particularly convenient because there is considerable separation between the serum α_1-AT levels with different alleles [40]. 'Normal' values for the population are derived from subjects with the PiMM allele, which is found in 85–90% of the population in Britain. The next two commonest alleles, PiMZ and PiMS, are associated with serum α_1-AT levels 50–75% of mean levels of PiMM subjects, as is the much less common PiSS

allele. Most of the subjects with the lowest serum levels are homozygous for the Z allele (PiZZ) and have blood levels <20% of the basal levels in PiMM subjects; a few rare variants, some of which result in complete functional absence of circulating α_1-AT, account for the remainder of severely deficient patients. The most important other Pi type is PiSZ where basal serum levels are 35–40% of the levels in PiMM subjects; PiSZ subjects are about 7 times more common than PiZZ subjects.

Overall clinical evidence supports a very strong relation of disabling emphysema and PiZZ, possibly some increased risk with PiSZ, while other variants with serum levels 50% or more of those in PiMM subjects are not definitely associated with increased risk of developing COPD. PiSZ subjects have significantly lower serum α_1-AT levels than other heterozygotes and so would be expected to be at greater risk. Nevertheless increased risk has been shown only in one [41] of three studies [42,43]. More information is available on the risk of emphysema and airways obstruction in PiMZ subjects, which was extensively investigated in the 1970s. These studies typically showed a two to five-fold excess of PiMZ subjects in hospital based studies of COPD patients [40,44,45] and mild abnormalities of lung function in PiMZ subjects, identified by studying relatives of PiZZ subjects with COPD [40]. In contrast it has proved difficult to show impairment in spirometry in PiMZ subjects identified in epidemiologic surveys [45]; subtle change in other tests of lung function and elasticity have been suggested [46] but the most comprehensive study failed to confirm any significant changes in a wide range of tests [47]. One longitudinal study has shown a slightly accelerated annual decline in FEV_1 in PiMZ subjects who smoked [48]. Overall therefore there may be a small increased risk associated with the PiMZ allele; in contrast more limited studies have failed to show any risk in PiMS subjects [40].

Early studies in Sweden indicated a very poor prognosis for subjects with PiZZ, especially in men who smoked. Few identified male smokers lived beyond 60 years and COPD developed even in life-long never-smokers [19]. Nevertheless there is a suspicion that a considerable proportion of PiZZ subjects must escape disability. Cross-sectional studies of PiZZ relatives of identified patients show considerable variations in spirometry, beyond that expected from age and smoking history [49] and longitudinal studies of the rates of decline in lung function in PiZZ subjects also show a very wide variation (Fig. 5.4) [50,51]. How many PiZZ subjects escape severe COPD is unknown; screening of adult blood donors in the USA has identified a 1/2700 prevalence of PiZZ subjects, most of whom had normal spirometry and had not been suspected of any abnormality [52].

5.3.4 RECURRENT BRONCHOPULMONARY INFECTIONS

The relations between chronic mucus hypersecretion, airways obstruction and mortality of smokers are still disputed. In the 1950s it was realized that the normal bacterial sterility of the bronchi was lost in the presence of mucus hypersecretion [53] and the 'British' hypothesis arose that chronic bronchitis, although often a trivial symptom, could sometimes predispose to infections which in turn damaged the airways and/or alveoli leading to progressive airflow obstruction. This led to a great deal of emphasis being placed on the history of chronic cough and expectoration and the overall diagnosis 'chronic bronchitis' was commonly used, contrasting with the emphasis on 'emphysema' in North America. The British Medical Research Council report in 1965 [54] which recommended dividing chronic bronchitis into simple mucus hypersecretion, purulent hypersecretion and 'chronic obstructive bronchitis' – the last being the combination of hypersecretion and persis-

tent airway narrowing – suggested a single progressive process.

There is no dispute that the frequency of bronchopulmonary infective episodes increases with increase in severity of airways obstruction and that infection is the commonest precipitant of acute-on-chronic respiratory failure and is often finally responsible for death in advanced disease. There is considerable evidence that smokers have chronic inflammation of the airways, irrespective of the presence of exacerbation of infections. Nevertheless despite its inherent plausibility, little experimental support has been obtained for the hypothesis that bronchopulmonary infections initiate the progressive decline in airway function by causing irreversible damage to alveolar and airway walls in smokers. Trials of continuous winter antibiotic prophylaxis and treatment over several years (admittedly often in low dose) in men with chronic bronchitis in the 1960s found no significant slowing of decline in lung function [55–57]. Also in the 1960s Fletcher, Peto and colleagues [3] set up an 8-year prospective study in working men in West London expecting to establish the effects of mucus hypersecretion and bronchopulmonary infections on rate of decline in FEV_1. They found that acute bronchopulmonary infection caused declines in lung function which sometimes lasted for several weeks but that recovery was usually complete. Although they found the usual associations between mucus hypersecretion, increased frequency of infection and lower absolute levels of FEV_1, they concluded that neither mucus hypersecretion nor bronchial infection caused FEV_1 to decline more rapidly because after adjusting for age, smoking and FEV_1 level, there was no independent correlation between indices of mucus hypersecretion or bronchial infection and annual decline in FEV_1. This led them to suggest that the hypersecretory and obstructive components of smoking-induced chronic lung disease should be regarded as 'largely unrelated conditions, chronic phlegm production being much less important'. With the known potential of infection to cause tissue damage, these results were, and remain, extremely surprising.

A number of subsequent studies have re-examined this important question. No relation between frequency of respiratory infections and decline in FEV_1 or FVC was found in members of the Belgian Air Force [58], obviously an unusually young and fit group of men. In compiling the Tecumseh index of risk of chronic obstructive pulmonary disease (COPD), Higgins and colleagues [59] found no additional predictive value from the presence of cough or phlegm after allowing for age, smoking habit and FEV_1. Peto, Speizer and colleagues [4] analysed mortality from chronic lung disease in a large number of men who had been studied in surveys in the UK between 1954 and 1961; after adjustment for initial lung function, the relative risk of chronic phlegm production for mortality was only 1.4 and not statistically significant (Fig. 5.3). This compares with a risk ratio of over 50 for the correlation between reduction in FEV_1 and COPD mortality. A similar relative risk factor for phlegm (1.35) contributing to total mortality in a 22 year follow-up has also been found in Paris men [60]. Negative studies have been published from follow-up of men in the Whitehall study [61] and in Cracow (relative risk 1.1) [62]; the latter study did show a marginally significant association of mucus hypersecretion and mortality (relative risk 1.56) in women. These studies, therefore, generally support the conclusions of the original West London Study that any risk associated with mucus hypersecretion was small. In contrast, Kanner in Salt Lake City found that frequent lower respiratory tract illnesses were associated with accelerated decline in FEV_1 and FVC in a group of patients who already had COPD at recruitment [63]. (In this study annual decline in FEV_1 was examined without allowing for FEV_1 at the time of recruitment.) The major source of the positive association was a group of 15 patients with intermediate or severe α-antitrypsin deficiency. Two other studies [5,6] have found 3 or 4-fold increases in risk ratios for death from COPD associated with chronic mucus hypersecretion, still an order less important than for a reduced FEV_1. In the study from Copenhagen [5] hypersecretion was associated with a relative risk of death from COPD of 1.2 if FEV_1 was 80% predicted and of 4.2 if FEV_1 was 40% predicted. Thus, once obstruction has developed, hypersecretion and/or infections may accelerate further decline in FEV_1 and even precipitate respiratory failure. Apart from the Salt Lake City [63] and Copenhagen [5] studies, there are indications of this in the more obstructed subgroups of men in both West London [3, p. 256] and Paris [60] studies.

Certainly when there are additional mechanical or immune defects in lung defence mechanisms, such as in cystic fibrosis [64] and complete [65] or subclass [66] hypogamma-globulinemia, frequency of infections does appear to be related to sustained decline in FEV_1. Childhood infections may be more immediately damaging or may subtly impair the subsequent ability of the adult lung to handle irritants [67]. Infection both in children and adults may be more important in communities with poor socio-economic conditions where infections are particularly common and severe, nutritional status is poor and antibiotics are less available. Hence the conclusions reached about the apparent lack of effect of mucus hypersecretion and bronchial infections in causing progressive airway obstruction in the general population of smokers with mild or moderate impairment of lung function should not be extended beyond the relatively healthy adult populations in which they were obtained.

5.3.5 ALLERGY AND AIRWAY HYPER-RESPONSIVENESS

In contrast to most British and North American doctors, some doctors in the Netherlands have regarded asthma and

COPD as two aspects of the same basic process, proposing that smokers with chronic and largely irreversible airflow obstruction shared with asthmatic subjects a common allergic constitution and increased airway responsiveness [68]. This theory was termed the 'Dutch' hypothesis by Fletcher and colleagues [3] whose own investigation failed to find any relation between increased airway responsiveness to inhaled histamine (or evidence of allergy) and accelerated annual decline of FEV_1 in smokers. However, subsequent studies of middle-aged smokers with some impairment of lung function have consistently shown a positive relation between increased airway responsiveness to inhaled methacholine or histamine and accelerated annual decline in FEV_1 over the preceding years [69,70]. In addition smokers show a slight elevation of total serum IgE which is independent of atopic status as defined by positive skin tests to common inhaled allergens [70–73]. These findings will be described in more detail in the next two sections before considering their importance as risk factors for progressive airways obstruction.

(a) Airway hyper-responsiveness

Investigation of airway hyper-responsiveness (AHR) in smokers and patients with COPD in the last 15 years has centered on two main questions: (1) is the AHR found in these subjects similar to that found in atopic or asth-matic subjects, or is it directly related to smoking?; (2) is AHR in smokers important for the development of progressive airways obstruction?

Some qualitative differences between AHR in smokers or COPD and asthma have been described (Table 5.3). Thus cross-sectional studies show that AHR is more common in middle-aged than young non-atopic smokers [69,74] and is almost invariably present when there is reduction in baseline FEV_1 [75,76] (Fig. 5.5). In contrast, in asthma AHR may be found with normal baseline lung function. The intensity of AHR tends to be greater in asthma than COPD, patients with COPD having AHR in the range of mild to moderate asthma as defined by the McMaster group [77]. The intensity of AHR in asthma is related to the eosinophil count in the peripheral blood but this is not the case in COPD [68]. In normal subjects a plateau of airway narrowing restricting constriction is found as the dose of inhaled histamine or methacholine is increased [78,79]. No limits are found in symptomatic asthmatic subjects [78], but smokers with COPD show limited bronchial narrowing to inhaled methacholine but not to histamine [80]. Some, but not all, studies suggest that patients with COPD are significantly less responsive to methacholine than histamine [80,81]. For a given intensity of AHR diurnal variation in peak expiratory flow is greater in asthma than in COPD [82].

Table 5.3 Contrasts between airway hyper-responsiveness to inhaled histamine in subjects with asthma and smokers

	Asthma	Smokers
Relation to		
baseline FEV_1	Weak	Strong
diurnal variation in PEF	Strong	Weak
blood eosinophil count	Present	Absent
Slope of dose–response curve	Steep	Shallow
Plateau of response when symptomatic	Absent	Sometimes present
Response to indirect stimuli	Consistently present	Weaker but present

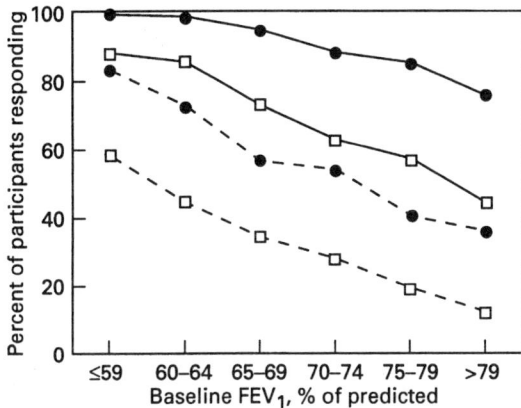

Fig. 5.5 Percentages of men and women responding to <5 and <25 mg/ml concentrations of methacholine with a >20% decline in FEV_1 from baseline, by baseline FEV_1, percent predicted. –•– = women, <25 mg/ml; –□– = men, <25 mg/ml; – -•- - = women, <5 mg/ml; – -□- - = men, <5 mg/ml. Data of Lung Health Study: tests were made in 3572 men and 2074 women; mean age 48 years and smoking on average 30 cigarettes/day. (Reproduced from Tashkin *et al.* 1992 [76] with permission.)

In the studies reviewed so far, AHR tests were performed with directly acting bronchoconstrictor drugs such as histamine or methacholine. These drugs may be expected to give enhanced airways responses when there is airway wall thickening [83] as is found both in asthma and to a more limited extent in COPD [84]. Investigators have therefore searched for a specific constrictor challenge which might depend on release of mediators from mast cells and be present in asthma but not in COPD. Many stimuli which do not act by directly contracting airway smooth muscle have been investigated in asthma; these 'indirect' stimuli are believed to act by stimulating neural pathways or by cellular activation (or both) which then results in contraction of airway smooth muscle. The most specific challenge appears to be with inhaled adenosine monophosphate (AMP), which slightly dilates the airways in normal, non-atopic individuals but causes airway narrowing in asthma. Inhaled AMP is believed to stimulate mast cells in the airway lumen/wall to release histamine and other mediators and its bronchoconstrictor effect is inhibited by treatment with H_1-antagonists in subjects with asthma [85]. Smokers with mild airways obstruction, however, also develop airway narrowing after inhaling adenosine, although they are less sensitive than subjects with asthma. Similarly all other 'indirect' stimuli that have been examined so far in smokers and/or patients with COPD cause some airway narrowing although in general the stimulus has to be stronger and the response is weaker than in subjects with asthma.

Numerous studies of the short-term effects of drugs in attenuating AHR in asthma and in smokers have also been made. In asthma beta-adrenoceptor agonists have a considerably larger short-term effect on attenuating AHR to histamine or methacholine (up to 4 doubling dilutions increase in provocation concentrations) than anti-muscarinic drugs (up to 1.5 doubling dilutions) [86]. Similar results are found in smokers with mild airflow obstruction, which is slightly surprising in view of the emphasis given to the usefulness of muscarinic antagonists in smoking-related airways obstruction. Short-term studies of aspirin and other non-steroidal anti-inflammatory drugs have shown no effect on AHR in smokers [87]. The most striking difference between the AHR of asthma and smokers is the response to 2–3 months treatment with inhaled corticosteroids, which is very effective in attenuating AHR in asthma but is usually ineffective in smokers with mild airways obstruction. (Chapter 18).

Thus no test for distinguishing the AHR of smokers from that of asthma been established but the increase in prevalence of AHR with length of smoking history and reduction in baseline FEV_1 have led to the hypothesis that in many smokers AHR may be acquired. There is a variety of possible geometric explanations for increased responsiveness [69] which include (a) airways obstruction resulting in more central deposition of aerosols,

(b) a given absolute shortening of airway smooth muscle resulting in a proportionately bigger rise in resistance in a narrowed airway, (c) loss of airway wall support due to emphysema [88], (d) increased thickening of airway walls [83].

(b) Allergy

Non-asthmatic smokers show modestly raised serum IgE, greater sensitization to certain rare occupational allergens, and increased blood eosinophil counts compared to healthy never-smokers. The increase in total IgE is independent of the presence of positive skin tests to common aero-allergens [71–73], does not follow the usual pattern of seasonal variation [71] and is not related to allergic rhinitis. Furthermore the prevalence of a personal or family history of allergic disease or positive skin tests to common aero-allergens is not increased in smokers [70,75]. In contrast the increase in IgE is related to age and pack-years smoked, and occurs at an age when IgE is decreasing in cross-sectional population surveys of never-smokers; the level of IgE in groups of ex-smokers declines over the years following stopping smoking [71]. This has prompted study of whether the raised IgE is specifically related to allergy to tobacco [70] or to colonization by *Strep. pneumoniae* [89], but no conclusive results have been obtained. Another hypothesis has been that the airway inflammation induced by smoking may increase mucosal permeability allowing non-specific sensitization to inhaled allergens. This has been supported by finding that smokers develop specific IgE more readily than non-smokers to a variety of unusual occupational antigens [70,90,91]; this finding conflicts with the lack of evidence that the general population of smokers show increased skin sensitization to common aero-allergens.

Total eosinophil counts in venous blood are higher in non-asthmatic smokers than never smokers but it is less certain whether the increase is disproportionate to the approxi-

mately 30% rise in total leucocyte count found in smokers [73,92,93]. An increase in eosinophils (>5% of total leucocytes) is associated with ventilatory impairment [94], but the strength of this association at least in subjects without a diagnosis of asthma is rather weak and probably stronger in never and ex-smokers than in current smokers [75,93]. Indeed Burrows' group in Tucson, who have been impressed with the general importance of allergic indicators as predictors of symptoms and reduced lung function in their population studies [94], find that once subjects with diagnosed asthma are removed, there is no evidence that these allergic indicators are important in smokers [95].

(c) Relevance as risk factors for progression of COPD

Atopy and cigarette smoking both involve about one-third of the population. Because there is a clear relationship between total IgE, positive skin tests to aero-allergens and airway hyper-responsiveness in asthmatic and atopic subgroups of the population, these relationships will be found also in large population studies which include smokers unless the adverse effects of smoking are so strong as to make smoking a rarity among asthmatic subjects. Despite the presumption that adolescents with asthma would be particularly discouraged from taking up smoking, smoking is not rare among asthmatic subjects [96] and the onset of asthma in middle-age has been found to be no more common in smokers than non-smokers [97]. Indeed there is a contrary strand of reports of asthma first emerging after quitting smoking [98].

Recent results of the Lung Health Study in North America confirm the importance of AHR as a risk factor for subsequent decline in FEV_1 in smokers. Some of the difficulty in determining the importance of hyper-responsiveness in the pathogenesis of accelerated decline in FEV_1 (see review in [70]) could be explained if increases in airway responsive-

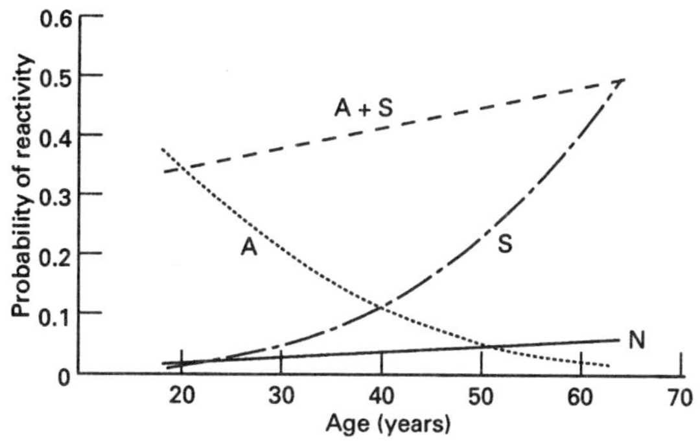

Fig. 5.6 Probability of airway hyper-responsiveness to inhaled histamine in a community survey in South of England in subjects 18–64 years according to current smokings and atopic (A) status (mean weal size to 3 common aero-allergens >4 mm). (Slightly modified from Burney *et al.* [74] with permission.)

ness (and to a lesser extent increase in total IgE) could result either from an allergic or a smoking related mechanism. Community surveys provide some evidence supporting this (Fig. 5.6) [74] and also for some interaction between smoking and atopy [74,92]. Because at present there is no way to distinguish these two types of pathogenesis in epidemiologic studies, the results of such studies will be heavily influenced by the rates and strength of smoking habit and the age, gender and atopy profile in the community studied. Indeed Burrows and co-workers have suggested that it is useful to consider two major causes of persistent airflow obstruction in middle-aged and elderly subjects. One type is associated with an asthmatic predisposition, and may be associated with childhood respiratory problems, atopy, blood eosinophilia and high levels of serum IgE. The second type occurs primarily in male smokers, has a more insidious progression of airways obstruction, a much worse prognosis and has no obvious relation to eosinophilia or elevated serum IgE. Burrows has suggested calling the first type 'chronic asthmatic bronchitis' in contrast to the more emphysematous type of COPD

[99]. In this schema allergy and AHR would be important for the pathogenesis of airway disease in the first type of persistent airways obstruction (as proposed by the 'Dutch' hypothesis), but be without any pathogenic role in the second type, where the AHR may be acquired following structural and geometric changes which are the consequence rather than the cause of accelerated decline in lung function. This does not mean AHR in smokers with the latter type of obstruction is without clinical significance; AHR may be responsible for some of the overlapping symptoms between asthma and COPD, for the increased susceptibility to exposure to smog episodes and cold air, perhaps play a part in the reduction in lung function which persists for some weeks after acute infections, and may be responsible for the improvement after bronchodilator drugs in acute exacerbations.

5.3.6 INTERACTION OF RISK FACTORS

A clear interaction between homozygous α_1-antitrypsin deficiency and smoking habit has been demonstrated for rate of decline in FEV_1 [50] and mortality [19]. Some studies of occupational dust exposure also find an additive effect in smokers and a very much smaller attributed effect in never-smokers. There are also suggestions that women are less likely to develop chronic mucus hypersecretion [100] and impaired lung function [102] for a given smoking history.

5.4 MODIFICATION OF RISK FACTORS

Few controlled long-term intervention studies have been made in COPD. Some non-systematic information is available on the results of bullectomy (Chapter 22) and lung transplantation (Chapter 23); undoubtedly these surgical procedures can improve radically the prognosis for a few patients with COPD, but the number of patients so treated is small. Two controlled studies have been made of the improved prognosis associated with long-term home oxygen in patients with advanced disease and chronic hypoxemia (Chapter 20). Trials of replacement therapy in α_1-antitrypsin deficiency in North America are proceeding but without control groups.

Several long-term studies of inhaled drug treatment are in progress: The Lung Health Study in North America in which the effects of quitting smoking and of regular use of an inhaled muscarinic antagonist were studied over 5 years [76] has shown AHR to be an important risk factor for accelerated decline in FEV_1 in smokers, although this decline was not slowed by treatment with the muscarinic antagonist, perhaps because these agents only weakly attenuate AHR [86]. One three-year study of inhaled glucocorticosteroids has been published [101] and three large studies are in progress in Europe.

At present, most information is available on the effects of quitting smoking; there are no studies following removal of any environmental or occupational risk.

5.4.1 EFFECTS OF STOPPING SMOKING

In younger subjects with relatively minor loss of lung function short-term studies have shown small improvements in some aspects of lung function (SBN_2 test, frequency dependence of compliance) on stopping smoking but changes in spirometry or maximum expiratory flow–volume curves have been inconsistent [103]. In middle-aged or older subjects with mild airways obstruction, rates of decline in FEV_1 after quitting smoking approach those found in never-smokers [2,3,101,104]. There is also a small early improvement in FEV_1. When cigarette consumption is assessed in terms of total 'pack-years' (average daily consumption in packs of 20 cigarettes × years of smoking) some, but not all, cross-sectional studies have shown slightly higher mean FEV_1 in ex-smokers than current smokers [105–107].

Longitudinal measurements in the Lung Health Study show an improvement in FEV_1

in the first months after quitting and, indeed, a decrement if smoking is resumed, confirming the presence of a reversible element in spirometry in smokers. Nevertheless, at any given time in an individual the cumulative total smoking history is the major determinant of lung function. There is very little direct information on the short-term and long-term effects on FEV_1 of quitting smoking in individuals with more advanced COPD. It has been difficult to find an improved prognosis in ex-smokers with advanced disease [8,17]; indeed the British doctors' study showed increased mortality during the first 9 years after quitting [21].

As discussed in the earlier section on impairment of lung function, mild reductions in T_{LCO}/V_A are reversed fully on quitting smoking, so that ex-smokers as a group are indistinguishable from never-smokers [11]. But as disease progresses an irreversible reduction in T_{LCO}/V_A develops in a proportion of subjects who develop impaired FEV_1 [14].

5.5 PROGNOSIS

Overall, age and baseline FEV_1 are the strongest predictors of mortality [8,17]. Fewer than 50% of patients with FEV_1 <30% predicted survive 5 years, and the prognosis is still poor in patients with higher initial FEV_1 (Fig. 5.7) [17]. Survival is more closely related to post- than pre-bronchodilator FEV_1. Mortality is related to reduced body weight, but because this in turn is related to reduced FEV_1, it is not clear if it has an independent effect on survival in COPD.

Concealed in these group trends there are great variations between individuals and variations within individuals in the rate of progression with time (and possibly treatment). Survival for 10 years or more has been observed in individuals with advanced disease and very low FEV_1 (even in individuals who have continued smoking) yet such individuals must have had accelerated decline in FEV_1 at some earlier period.

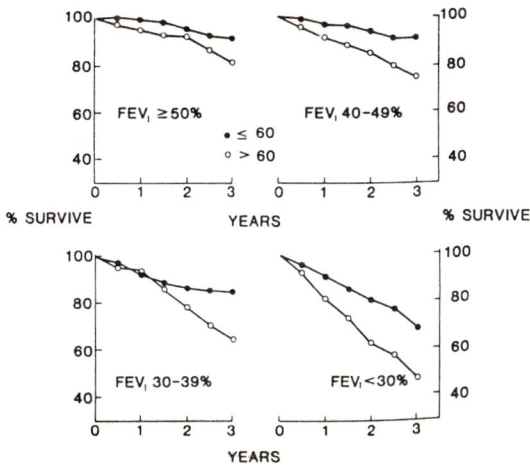

Fig. 5.7 Three-year survival of patients with COPD in the intermittent positive-pressure breathing (IPPB) trial in North America according to post-bronchodilator FEV_1 at entry. As IPPB treatment had no effect, results for IPPB and control group are combined. ● ≤60, ○ >60 years at entry. (Reproduced from Anthonisen [17] with permission.)

The dominant role of FEV_1 in predicting outcome is in part because it can be applied across the full spectrum of disease from initial health to advanced disease, and in part because the amount of data available on FEV_1 is much greater than that on other potential prognostic factors. Particularly when patients with more advanced disease and a more limited range of FEV_1 are studied, other important prognostic factors can be identified [8,17]. Unfavorable factors include severe hypoxemia, high pulmonary artery pressure and low carbon monoxide transfer. Favorable factors presumably include stopping smoking (at least when this is achieved before COPD is too advanced) and a large bronchodilator response.

There is very little information on the extent to which the 'natural history' can be modified by current treatment. The only treatment so far shown to improve long-term prognosis is home O_2 for 15 hours or more a day in patients with advanced disease (Chapter 20). The use of intermittent positive-pressure breathing as an addition to a standard regimen failed to improve survival [108]. A large controlled trial of regular inhaled muscarinic antagonists in North America failed to slow the 5-year decline in FEV_1. Ongoing trials of inhaled glucocorticosteroids in Europe should clarify whether this widely used treatment slows decline in FEV_1. Prognosis in a small number of individuals can be radically improve by lung transplantation or bullectomy.

As originally shown in the Framingham study [109], a modestly reduced FEV_1 is a significant predictor of later cardiovascular mortality, even after adjustment for cumulative smoking habit and other associated factors [61,110]. Airways obstruction is also an important additional risk factor for lung cancer, independent of increasing age or smoking history [111].

5.6 DIFFERENT SUBGROUPS OF COPD

Most published surveys, and indeed trials of treatment such as that of intermittent positive-pressure breathing, assume that COPD can effectively be separated from asthma. While this is relatively easy in younger subjects with highly variable and fully reversible disease, in middle-aged and older subjects asthma often becomes incompletely reversible with persistent airway obstruction despite vigorous treatment. Analysis of the characteristics and prognosis of individuals with an initial FEV_1 of 45–59% of predicted value in a community survey in Tucson, USA showed that when individuals with a reported diagnosis of asthma, who also were non-smokers and/or atopic ('chronic asthmatic bronchitis') were separated from those with classic COPD (who were all non-atopic smokers or ex-smokers), there were large differences in 10-year survival (Fig. 5.8). Survival of the COPD group was no better than that of patients studied in Chicago 20 years earlier [112]. Average rates of decline in FEV_1 were 5 ml per year in the asthma group

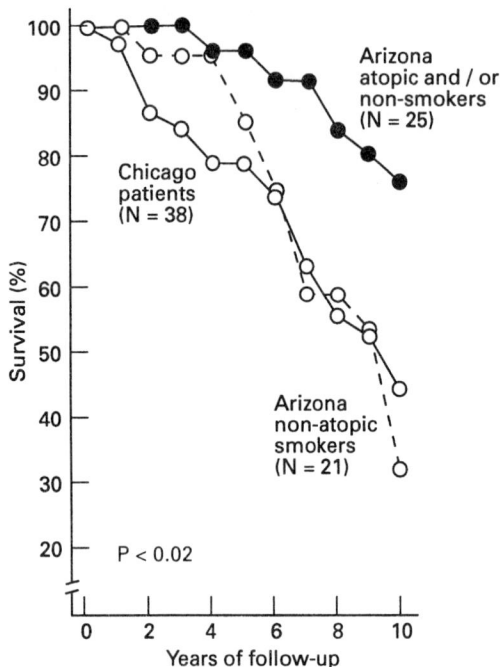

Fig. 5.8   Ten-year survival in three groups of subjects with initial FEV_1 45–59% of predicted value. Two groups of subjects identified in Arizona community survey (atopic and/or non-smokers ●–●; non-atopic smokers ○– -○) and followed in the 1980s are compared with an earlier group of patients with smoking-related COPD (○–○) followed in Chicago in the 1960s. (Reproduced from Burrows *et al.* [112] with permission.)

and 70 ml per year in the COPD group. In the Arizona community survey there were also many subjects who were difficult to place in the two polar groups. These subjects were predominantly men, had similar mean age and FEV_1 to the other two groups at enrolment and similar smoking histories to individuals in the classic COPD group but differed from the group with classic COPD in showing more asthmatic features such as positive allergy skin tests, increased blood eosinophils, raised serum IgE and wheezing. This group had annual rates of decline in FEV_1 and survival intermediate between the subjects classed as asthma and COPD, presumably because their

obstruction can be partially reversed by treatment.

As discussed in the section on allergy and airways hyper-responsiveness, these results support the relevance of the 'Dutch' hypothesis for a subgroup of subjects with persistent airways obstruction; they emphasize that COPD is a non-specific diagnosis of exclusion applied to subjects with persistent airways obstruction which is poorly responsive to treatment and cannot be ascribed to a lengthening list of identifiable specific causes which include cystic fibrosis, bronchiolitis following lung or bone marrow transplant and byssinosis. But no precise criteria have been developed for distinguishing individuals whose persistent airways obstruction is thought to be due to asthma. Because smoking, allergy and asthma are so common in the community, inevitably many individuals will have a combination of features attributed to COPD and to asthma, even if the pathogenesis of the two conditions was by entirely separate pathways. Because drug treatment at present aims to improve airway function and inflammation and is not directly aimed at preventing progression of emphysema, it is broadly similar for all forms of persistent airflow obstruction. As a consequence distinction between different subgroups of patients has not been of practical importance for management. But with such different prognoses and with apparently divergent trends in prevalence in Western countries (asthma rising, COPD falling, at least in men) clearer means of making a practical distinction are required.

REFERENCES

1. Burrows, B. (1985). Course and prognosis in advanced disease, in *Chronic Obstructive Pulmonary Disease*, (ed. T.L. Petty), Marcel Dekker Inc., New York, pp. 31–42.
2. Fletcher, C. and Peto, R. (1977). The natural history of chronic airflow obstruction. *Br. Med. J.*, i, 1645–8.
3. Fletcher, C.M., Peto, R., Tinker, C.M. and Speizer, F.E. (1976). *The Natural History of*

Chronic Bronchitis and Emphysema. Oxford University Press, Oxford.

4. Peto, R., Speizer, F.E., Cochrane, A.L. *et al.* (1983). The relevance in adults of air-flow obstruction, but not of mucus hypersecretion, to mortality from chronic lung disease. *Am. Rev. Respir. Dis.,* **128**, 491–500.

5. Lange, P., Nyboe, J., Appleyard, M. *et al.* (1990). The relation of ventilatory impairment and of chronic mucus hypersecretion to mortality from obstructive lung disease and from all causes. *Thorax,* **45**, 579–85.

6. Speizer, F.E., Fay, M.E., Dockery, D.W. and Ferris, B.G. Jr (1989). Chronic obstructive pulmonary disease mortality in six U.S. Cities. *Am. Rev. Respir. Dis.,* **140**, S49–S55.

7. Burrows, B., Knudson, R.J., Camilli, A.E. *et al.* (1987). The 'Horse-Racing effect' and predicting decline in forced expiratory volume in one second from screening spirometry. *Am. Rev. Respir. Dis.,* **135**, 788–93.

8. Burrows, B. (1991). Predictors of loss of lung function and mortality in obstructive lung diseases. *Eur. Respir. Rev.,* **1**, 340–5.

9. Tweeddale, P.M., Merchant, S., Leslie, M. *et al.* (1984). Short term variability in FEV_1: relation to pretest activity, levels of FEV_1, and smoking habits. *Thorax,* **39**, 928–32.

10. Buist, A.S., Vollmer, W.M., Johnson, L.R. and McCamant, L.E. (1988). Does the single-breath N_2 test identify the smoker who will develop chronic airflow limitation? *Am. Rev. Respir. Dis.,* **137**, 293–310.

11. Watson, A., Joyce, H., Hopper, L. and Pride, N.B. (1993). Influence of smoking habits on change in carbon monoxide transfer factor over 10 years in middle-aged men. *Thorax,* **48**, 119–24.

12. McLean, A., Warren, P.M., Gillooly, M. *et al.* (1992). Microscopic and macroscopic measurement of emphysema: relation to carbon monoxide gas transfer. *Thorax,* **47**, 144–9.

13. Gould, G.A., Macnee, W., Mclean, A. *et al.* (1988). CT measurements of lung density in life can quantitate distal airspace enlargement – an essential defining feature of human emphysema. *Am. Rev. Respir. Dis.,* **137**, 380–92.

14. Knudson, R.J., Kaltenborn, W.T. and Burrows, B. (1989) The effects of cigarette smoking and smoking cessation on the carbon monoxide diffusing capacity of the lung in asymptomatic subjects. *Am. Rev. Respir. Dis.,* **140**, 645–51.

15. Petrik Pereira R., Hunter, D. and Pride, N.B. (1981). Use of lung pressure–volume curves and helium-sulphur hexafluoride washout to detect emphysema in subjects with mild airflow obstruction. *Thorax,* **36**, 29–37.

16. Corbin, R.P., Loveland, M., Martin, R.R. and Macklem, P.T. (1979) A four-year follow-up study of lung mechanics in smokers. *Am. Rev. Respir. Dis.,* **120**, 293–304.

17. Anthonisen, N.R. (1989) Prognosis in chronic obstructive pulmonary disease: results from multicenter clinical trials. *Am. Rev. Respir. Dis.,* **140**, S95–S99.

18. Weitzenblum, E., Sautegeau, A., Ehrhart, M. *et al.* (1984). Long-term course of pulmonary arterial pressure in chronic obstructive pulmonary disease. *Am. Rev. Respir. Dis.,* **130**, 993–8.

19. Larsson, C. (1978) Natural history and life expectancy in severe alpha$_1$-antitrypsin deficiency, PiZ. *Acta Med. Scand.,* **204**, 345–51.

20. Tager, I.B., Segal, M.R., Speizer, F.E. and Weiss, S.T. (1988). The natural history of forced expiratory volumes. Effect of cigarette smoking and respiratory symptoms. *Am. Rev. Respir. Dis.,* **138**, 837–49.

21. Doll, R. and Peto, R. (1976) Mortality in relation to smoking: 20 years' observation on male British doctors. *Br. Med. J.,* **2**, 1525–36.

22. Higenbottam, J., Shipley, M.J., Clark, T.J.H. and Rose, G. (1980) Lung function and symptoms of cigarette smokers related to tar yield and number of cigarettes smoked, *Lancet,* **i**, 409–12.

23. Schenker, M.B., Samet, J.M. and Speizer, F.E. (1982) Effect of cigarette tar content and smoking habits on respiratory symptoms in women. *Am. Rev. Respir. Dis.,* **125**, 684–90.

24. US Department of Health and Human Services (1981). *Public Health Service, Office on Smoking and Health. The health consequences of smoking – the changing cigarette: a report of the Surgeon General.*

25. Royal College of Physicians of London (1983) *Health or Smoking?* Pitman, London.

26. Krzyanowski, M., Sherrill, D.L., Paoletti, P. and Lebowitz, M.D. (1991) Relationship of respiratory symptoms and pulmonary function to tar, nicotine, and carbon monoxide yield of cigarettes. *Am. Rev. Respir. Dis.,* **143**, 306–11.

27. Lee, P.N. and Garfinkel, L. (1981). Mortality and type of cigarette smoked. *J. Epidemiol. Community Health,* **35**, 16–22.

28. Withey, C.H., Papacosta, O., Swan, A.V. *et al.* (1992) Respiratory effects of lowering tar and nicotine levels of cigarettes smoked by young male middle tar smokers. II: Results of a randomised controlled trial. *J. Epidemiol. Comm. Health*, **46**, 281–5.

29. Becklake, M.R. (1989). Occupational exposures: evidence for a causal association with chronic obstructive pulmonary disease. *Am. Rev. Respir. Dis.*, **140**, S85–S89.

30. Speizer, F.E. (1994) Environmental lung disease, in: *Harrison's Principles of Internal Medicine* (eds J.D.Wilson *et al.*), 13th edn, McGraw-Hill, New York, pp. 1176–83.

31. Korn, R.J., Dockery, D.W., Speizer, F.E. *et al.* (1987). Occupational exposures and chronic respiratory symptoms. *Am. Rev. Respir. Dis.*, **136**, 296-304.

32. Xu, X., Christiani, D.C., Dockery, D.W. and Wang, L. (1992) Exposure–response relationships between occupational exposures and chronic respiratory illness: a community-based study. *Am. Rev. Respir. Dis.*, **146**, 413–8.

33. Love, R.G. and Miller, B.G. (1982). Longitudinal study of lung function in coalminers. *Thorax*, **37**, 193–7.

34. Marine, W.M., Gurr, D. and Jacobsen, M. (1988) Clinically important respiratory effects of dust exposure and smoking in British coal miners. *Am. Rev. Respir. Dis.*, **137**, 106-12.

35. Oxman, A.D., Muir, D.C., Shannon, H.S. *et al.* (1993). Occupational dust exposure and chronic obstructive pulmonary disease. A systematic overview of the evidence. *Am. Rev. Respir. Dis.*, **148**, 38–48.

36. Zuskin, E., Ivankovic, D., Schachter, E.N. and Witek, T.J. Jr (1991) A ten-year follow-up study of cotton textile workers. *Am. Rev. Respir. Dis.*, **143**, 301–5.

37. Glindmeyer, H.W., Lefante, J.J., Jones, R.N. *et al.* (1991) Exposure-related declines in the lung function of cotton textile workers. *Am. Rev. Respir. Dis.*, **144**, 675–83.

38. Enarson, D.A., Vedal, S. and Chan-Yeung, M. (1985) Rapid decline in FEV_1 in grain handlers. *Am. Rev. Respir. Dis.*, **132**, 814–7.

39. Davison, A.G., Fayers, P.M., Newman-Taylor, A.J. *et al.* (1988) Cadmium fume inhalation and emphysema. *Lancet*, **i**, 663–7.

40. Hutchison, D.C.S. (1988) Natural history of alpha-1-protease inhibitor deficiency. *Am. J. Med.*, **84** (Suppl. 6A), 3–12.

41. Bartmann, K., Fooke-Achterrath, M., Koch, G. *et al.* (1985) Heterozygosity in the Pi-system as a pathogenic cofactor in chronic obstructive pulmonary disease (COPD). *Eur. J. Respir. Dis.*, **66**, 284–96.

42. Lieberman, J., Winter, B. and Sastre, A. (1986) Alpha₁-antitrypsin Pi-types in 965 COPD patients. *Chest*, **89**, 370–3.

43. Hutchison, D.C.S., Tobin, M.J. and Cook, P.J.L. (1983). Alpha₁-antitrypsin deficiency: clinical and physiological features in heterozygotes of Pi type SZ. A survey by the British Thoracic Association. *Br. J. Dis. Chest*, **77**, 28–34.

44. Shigeoka, J.W., Hall, W.J., Hyde, R.W. *et al.* (1976) The prevalence of alpha₁-antitrypsin heterozygotes (PiMZ) in patients with obstructive pulmonary disease. *Am. Rev. Respir. Dis.*, **114**, 1077–84.

45. Morse, J.O., Lebowitz, M.D., Knudson, R.J. and Burrows, B. (1977) Relation of protease inhibitor phenotypes to obstructive lung diseases in a community. *N. Engl. J. Med.*, **296**, 1190-4.

46. Tattersall, S.F., Petrik Pereira, R., Hunter, D. *et al.* (1979). Lung distensibility and airway function in intermediate alpha₁-antitrypsin deficiency (Pi MZ). *Thorax*, **34**, 637–46.

47. Bruce, R.M., Cohen, B.H., Diamond, E.L. *et al.* (1984) Collaborative study to assess risk of lung disease in Pi MZ phenotype subjects. *Am. Rev. Respir. Dis.*, **130**, 386–90.

48. Eriksson, S., Lindell, S-E. and Wiberg, R. (1985). Effects of smoking and intermediate alpha₁-antitrypsin deficiency (PiMZ) on lung function. *Eur. J. Respir. Dis.*, **67**, 279–85.

49. Silverman, E.K., Pierce, J.A., Province, M.A. *et al.* (1989). Variability of pulmonary function in alpha₁-antitrypsin deficiency: clinical correlates. *Ann. Intern. Med.*, **111**, 982–91.

50. Janus, E.D., Phillips, N.T. and Carrell, R.W. (1985). Smoking, lung function and alpha₁-antitrypsin deficiency. *Lancet*, **1**, 152–4.

51. Buist, A.S., Burrows, B., Eriksson, S. *et al.* (1983). The natural history of air-flow obstruction in PiZ emphysema. *Am. Rev. Respir. Dis.*, **127**, S43–S45.

52. Troyer, B.E., Silverman, E.K., Wade, M.A. and Campbell, E.J. (1994). α_1-antitrypsin deficiency detected through blood donor screening: clinical features and natural history. *Am. J. Resp. Crit. Care Med.*, **149**, A1014.

53. Brumfitt, W., Willoughby, M.L.N. and Bromley, L.L. (1957) An evaluation of sputum examination in chronic bronchitis. *Lancet*, **ii**, 1306–9.

54. Medical Research Council (1965). Definition and classification of chronic bronchitis for clinical and epidemiological purposes. *Lancet*, i, 775–9.

55. Medical Research Council (1966) Value of chemoprophylaxis and chemotherapy in chronic bronchitis. *Br. Med. J.*, 1, 1317–22.

56. Johnston, R.N., McNeill, R.S., Smith, D.H. *et al.* (1969) Five-year winter prophylaxis for chronic bronchitis. *Br. Med. J.*, 4, 265–9.

57. Johnston, R.N., McNeill, R.S., Smith, D.H. *et al.* (1976) Chronic bronchitis – measurements and observations over 10 years. *Thorax*, 31, 25–9.

58. Clément, J. and Van de Woestijne, K.P. (1982) Rapidly decreasing forced expiratory volume in one second or vital capacity and development of chronic airflow obstruction. *Am. Rev. Respir. Dis.*, 125, 553–8.

59. Higgins, M.W., Keller, J.B., Becker, M. *et al.* (1982) An index of risk for obstructive airways disease. *Am. Rev. Respir. Dis.*, 125, 144–51.

60. Annesi, I. and Kauffman, F. (1986) Is respiratory mucus hypersecretion really an innocent disorder? *Am. Rev. Respir. Dis.*, 134, 688–93.

61. Ebi-Kryston, K.L. (1988). Respiratory symptoms and pulmonary function as predictors of 10-year mortality from respiratory disease, cardiovascular disease and all causes in the Whitehall study. *J. Clin. Epidemiol.*, 41, 251–60.

62. Kryzyzanowski, M. and Wysocki, M. (1986). The relation of thirteen-year mortality to ventilatory impairment and other respiratory symptoms. *Int. J. Epidemiol.*, 15, 56–64.

63. Kanner, R.S., Renzetti, A.D. Jr, Klauber, M.R. *et al.* (1979). Variables associated with changes in spirometry in patients with obstructive lung diseases. *Am. J. Med.*, 67, 44–50.

64. Wang, E.E.L., Prober, C.G., Mansion, B. *et al.* (1984). Association of respiratory viral infection with pulmonary deterioration in patients with cystic fibrosis. *N. Engl. J. Med.*, 311, 1653–8.

65. Björkander, J., Bake, B. and Hansion, L.A. (1984). Primary hypogammaglobulinaemia: impaired lung function and body growth with delayed diagnosis and inadequate treatment. *Eur. J. Respir. Dis.*, 65, 529–36.

66. Björkander, J., Bake, B., Oxelius, V.A. *et al.* (1985). Impaired lung function in patients with IgA deficiency and low levels of IgG2 or IgG3. *N. Engl. J. Med.*, 313, 720–4.

67. Samet, J.M., Tager, I.B. and Speizer, F.E. (1983) The relationship between respiratory illness in childhood and chronic air-flow obstruction in adulthood. *Am. Rev. Respir. Dis.*, 127, 508–23.

68. Orie, N.G.M., Sluiter, H.J., De Vries, K. *et al.* (1961). The host factor in bronchitis, in: *Bronchitis*, an International Symposium, 27–29 April 1960, University of Grönigen. Royal Van Gorcum, Assen, pp. 43–49.

69. Pride, N.B., Taylor, R.G., Lim, T.K. *et al.* (1987). Bronchial hyperresponsiveness as a risk factor for progressive airflow obstruction in smokers. *Bull. Eur. Physio-Pathol. Respir.*, 23, 369–75.

70. O'Connor, G.T., Sparrow, D. and Weiss, S.T. (1989) The role of allergy and nonspecific airway hyperresponsiveness in the pathogenesis of chronic obstructive pulmonary disease. *Am. Rev. Respir. Dis.*, 140, 225–52.

71. Burrows, B., Halonen, M., Barbee, R.A. and Lebowitz, M. (1981) The relationship of serum immunoglobulin E to cigarette smoking. *Am. Rev. Respir. Dis.*, 124, 523–5.

72. Warren, C.P., Holford-Strevens, V., Wong, C. and Manfreda, J. (1982). The relationship between smoking and total immunoglobulin E levels. *J. Allergy Clin. Immunol.*, 69, 370–5.

73. Taylor, R.G., Gross, E. Joyce, H. *et al.* (1985). Smoking, allergy and the differential white blood cell count. *Thorax*, 40, 17–22.

74. Burney, P.G.J., Britton, J.R., Chinn, S. *et al.* (1987) Descriptive epidemiology of bronchial reactivity in an adult population: results from a community study. *Thorax*, 42, 38-44.

75. Taylor, R.G., Joyce, H., Gross, E. *et al.* (1985). Bronchial reactivity to inhaled histamine and annual rate of decline in FEV_1 in male smokers and ex-smokers. *Thorax*, 40, 9–16.

76. Tashkin, D.P., Altose, M.D., Bleecker, E. *et al.*, (1992) The Lung Health Study: airway responsiveness to inhaled methacholine in smokers with mild to moderate airflow limitation. *Am. Rev. Respir. Dis.*, 145, 301–10.

77. Cockcroft, D.W., Killian, D.N., Mellon, J.A. and Hargreave, F.E. (1977). Bronchial reactivity to inhaled histamine: a method and clinical survey. *Clin. Allergy*, 7, 235–43.

78. Woolcock, A.J., Salome, C.M. and Yan, K. (1984). The shape of the dose-response curve to histamine in asthmatic and normal subjects. *Am. Rev. Respir. Dis.*, 130, 171–5.

79. Sterk, P.J., Daniel, E.E., Zamel, N. and Hargreave, F.E. (1985) Limited bronchoconstriction to methacholine using partial

flow-volume curves in nonasthmatic subjects. *Am. Rev. Respir. Dis.*, **132**, 272–7.

80. Du Toit, J.I., Woolcock, A.J., Salome, C.M. *et al.* (1986). Characteristics of bronchial hyper-responsiveness in smokers with chronic airflow limitation. *Am. Rev. Respir. Dis.*, **134**, 498–501.

81. Higgins, B.G., Britton, J.R., Chinn, S. *et al.* (1988) Comparison of histamine and methacholine for use in bronchial challenge tests in community studies. *Thorax*, **43**, 605–10.

82. Ramsdale, E.H., Morris, M.M. and Hargreave, F.E. (1986). Interpretation of the variability of peak flow rates in chronic bronchitis. *Thorax*, **41**, 771–6.

83. James, A.L., Paré, P.D. and Hogg, J.C. (1989). The mechanics of airway narrowing in asthma. *Am. Rev. Respir. Dis.*, **139**, 242–6.

84. Kuwano, K., Bosken, C.H., Paré, P.D. *et al.* (1993). Small airways dimensions in asthma and in chronic obstructive pulmonary disease. *Am. Rev. Respir. Dis.*, **148**, 1220–5.

85. Phillips, G.D., Rafferty, P., Beasley, R. and Holgate, S.T. (1987) Effect of oral terfenadine on the bronchoconstrictor response to inhaled histamine and adenosine 5′-monophosphate in non-atopic asthma. *Thorax*, **42**, 939–45.

86. Tattersfield, A.E. (1987). Effect of beta-agonists and anticholinergic drugs on bronchial reactivity. *Am. Rev. Respir. Dis.*, **136**, S64–S68.

87. Lim, T.K., Turner, N.C., Watson, A. *et al.* (1990). Effects of nonsteroidal anti-inflammatory drugs on the bronchial hyperresponsiveness of middle-aged male smokers. *Eur. Respir. J.*, **3**, 872–9.

88. Cheung, D., Merkenhof, W.M., Schot, R. *et al.* (1993) Relationship between indices of parenchymal destruction and maximal airway narrowing *in vivo* in humans with α_1-antitrypsin deficiency. *Am. Rev. Respir. Dis.*, **147**, A834.

89. Bloom, J.W., Halonen, M., Dunn, A.M. *et al.* (1986). *Pneumococcus*-specific immunoglobin E in cigarette smokers. *Clin. Allergy*, **16**, 25–32.

90. Zetterstrom, O., Osterman, K., Machado, L. and Johansson, S.G.O. (1981) Another smoking hazard: raised serum IgE concentration and increased risk of occupational allergy. *Br. Med. J.*, **283**, 1215–7.

91. Venables, K.M., Topping, M.D., Howe, W. *et al.* (1985). Interaction of smoking and atopy in producing specific IgE antibody against a hapten protein conjugate. *Br. Med. J*, **290**, 201–4.

92. O'Connor, G.T., Sparrow, D., Segal, M.R. and Weiss, S.T. (1989) Smoking, atopy, and methacholine airway responsiveness among middle-aged and elderly men. *Am. Rev. Respir. Dis.*, **140**, 1520–6.

93. Frette, C., Annesi, I., Korobaeff, M. *et al.* (1991) Blood eosinophilia and FEV_1. *Am. Rev. Respir. Dis.*, **143**, 987–92.

94. Burrows, B., Hasan, F.M., Barbee, R.A. *et al.* (1980) Epidemiologic observations on eosinophilia and its relation to respiratory disorders. *Am. Rev. Respir. Dis.*, **122**, 709–19.

95. Burrows, B., Knudson, R.J., Clinc, M.G. and Lebowitz, M.D. (1988) A re-examination of risk factors for ventilatory impairment. *Am. Rev. Respir. Dis.*, **138**, 829–36.

96. Higenbottam, T.W., Feyerabend, C. and Clark, T.J.H. (1980). Cigarette smoking in asthma. *Br. J. Dis. Chest*, **74**, 279–84.

97. Vesterinen, E., Kaprio, J. and Koskenvuo, M. (1988) Prospective study of asthma in relation to smoking habits among 14729 adults. *Thorax*, **43**, 534–9.

98. Hillerdahl, G. and Rylander, R. (1984) Asthma and cessation of smoking. *Clin. Allergy*, **14**, 45–7.

99. Burrows, B., Bloom, J.W., Traver, G.A. and Cline, M.G. (1987) The course and prognosis of different forms of chronic airways obstruction in a sample from the general population. *N. Engl. J. Med.*, **317**, 1309–14.

100. Tager, I. and Speizer, F.E. (1976) Risk estimates for chronic smokers – a study of male-female differences. *Am. Rev. Respir. Dis.*, **113**, 619–25.

101. Dompeling, E., Van Schayck, C.P, Van Grunsven, P.M. *et al.* (1993). Slowing the deterioration of asthma and COPD observed during bronchodilator therapy by adding inhaled corticosteroids. *Am. Intem. Med.*, **118**, 770–8.

102. Camilli, A.E., Burrows, B., Knudson, R.J. *et al.* (1987) Longitudinal changes in forced expiratory volume in one second in adults. Effects of smoking and smoking cessation. *Am. Rev. Respir. Dis.*, **135**, 794–9.

103. Cherniack, R.M. and McCarthy, D.S. (1979). Reversibility of abnormalities of pulmonary function, in *The Lung in the Transition Between Health and Disease*, (eds P.T. Macklem and S. Permutt), Vol. 12 Dekker, New York, pp. 329–42.

104. U.S. Department of Health and Human Services (1990) *The health benefits of smoking*

cessation – a report of the Surgeon General. Centers for Disease Control, Office on Smoking and Health, Rockville, Maryland. DHHS Publication No. CDC 90–8416.

105. Burrows, B., Knudson, R.J., Cline, M.C. and Lebowitz, M.D. (1977). Quantitative relationships between cigarette smoking and ventilatory function. *Am. Rev. Respir. Dis.*, **115**, 195–205.

106. Beck, G.J., Doyle, C.A. and Schachter, E.N. (1981) Smoking and lung function. *Am. Rev. Respir. Dis.*, **123**, 149–55.

107. Dockery, D.W., Speizer, F.E., Ferris, B.G. Jr *et al.* (1988). Cumulative and reversible effects of lifetime smoking on simple tests of lung function in adults. *Am. Rev. Respir. Dis.*, **137**, 286–92.

108. IPPB Trial Group (1983) Intermittent positive pressure breathing therapy of chronic obstructive pulmonary disease. *Ann. Intern. Med.*, **99**, 612–20.

109. Ashley, F., Kannel, W.B., Soolie, P. and Masson, R. (1975). Pulmonary function: relation to aging, cigarette habit, and mortality. The Framingham Study. *Ann. Intern. Med.*, **82**, 739–45.

110. Cook, D.G., and Shaper, A.G. (1988). Breathlessness, lung function and risk of a heart attack. *Eur. Heart J.*, **9**, 1215–22.

111. Tockman, M.S., Anthonisen, N.R., Wright, E.C. and Donithan, M.G. (1987) IPPB Trial Group, Johns Hopkins Lung Project. Airways obstruction and the risk for lung cancer. *Ann. Intern. Med.*, **106**, 512–8.

112. Burrows, B. (1989) The course and prognosis of different types of chronic airflow limitation in a general population sample from Arizona: comparison with the Chicago 'COPD' series. *Am. Rev. Respir. Dis.*, **140**, S92–S94.

BIOCHEMICAL AND CELLULAR MECHANISMS

R.A. Stockley

6.1 INTRODUCTION

At first sight it may seem an impossible task to cover the biochemical and cellular aspects of a variety of chronic destructive lung diseases encompassed by a term as broad as COPD. Indeed even if one assumes that the term is largely synonymous with emphysema, as suggested by Thurlbeck [1], it is clear that even this covers a variety of pathologically and anatomically distinct conditions. Whereas it is far from the scope of this chapter to argue the pros and cons of pathophysiologic similarities, it may well be that the basic processes that lead to COPD (whatever its pathologic features) have a common theme.

Chronic destructive lung diseases have well recognized associations, including risk factors such as smoking, pollution, infection and some clear genetic associations as in cystic fibrosis. However, it remains clear that even when the apparent risk factors are present there remains a 'susceptibility' that determines the presence and degree of lung disease. This was best demonstrated by the longitudinal studies of Fletcher and Peto [2] who suggested that within a population of smokers there is a subsection who develop accelerated evidence of airflow obstruction. Because cessation of smoking prevents this rapid decline, the evidence would suggest that events related to smoking are the direct cause of progressive destructive lung disease in this 'susceptible' group (Fig. 6.1).

Cigarette smoke is essentially a lung irritant and results in lung inflammation manifest by bronchitis and increased permeability to radio-tracers [3]. In addition, lung lavage has consistently demonstrated an increase in inflammatory cells including macrophages and neutrophils in the lungs of smokers. This continual and low grade 'inflammation' probably underlies the pathogenesis of emphysema in smokers but may also play a role in

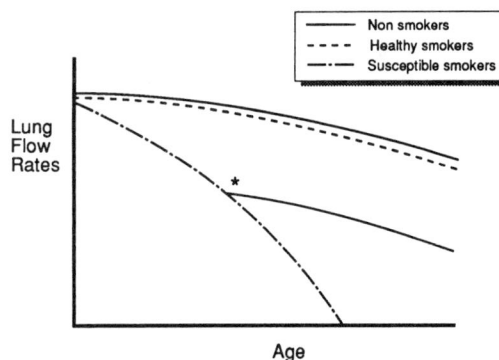

Fig. 6.1 The effect of age upon airflow obstruction is indicated for healthy subjects. The slow decline is similar to that seen for most regular smokers. The accelerated rate of decline is also shown for the 'susceptible smoker'. Cessation of smoking (*) returns the rate of decline to normal (adapted from reference [2].)

Chronic Obstructive Pulmonary Disease. Edited by Dr P. Calverley and Professor N. Pride. Published in 1995 by Chapman & Hall, London. ISBN 0 412 46450 0

other conditions including bronchiectasis and cystic fibrosis (see later).

The susceptibility of a small population at risk from cigarette smoke would probably have remained obscure but for two observations in the early 1960s. The most important observation was of the association between deficiency of alpha$_1$-antitrypsin (α_1-AT) and emphysema in 1963 [4]. In the same year Gross and his colleagues also described the first animal model of emphysema produced by the instillation of a proteolytic enzyme into the lungs [5]. Since α_1-AT is a major plasma inhibitor of proteolytic enzymes [6] and since such enzymes can induce experimental emphysema it seemed likely that the association of α_1-AT deficiency with emphysema represented cause and effect.

On the basis of these two observations the proteinase/antiproteinase theory of emphysema was founded. This hypothesis states that in health the lungs are protected from tissue degradation by inhibitors of proteolytic enzymes. However, when the inhibitors are deficient or the enzyme load is excessive the protective screen of inhibitors is no longer sufficient and the uncontrolled enzymes degrade lung tissues, leading to destructive lung disease.

This concept has now become central to our understanding of the pathogenesis of many lung diseases and has influenced thinking to such an extent that pharmaceutical agents have been developed to regulate the process. The remainder of this chapter examines the evidence to support this concept, explores the putative mechanisms and addresses the potential for determining susceptibility and modifying the disease process therapeutically.

6.2 ANIMAL MODELS

The development of animal models of emphysema has increased greatly our understanding of the pathogenic mechanisms of the disease process. There remain concerns,

however, over the validity of such emphysema models. In particular the pathologic changes of air space enlargement are often not typical of those seen in the human disease. In addition, many of the models depend upon single exposure to the relevant agent and rapid development of the changes, which does not mimic the chronic development of emphysema in man. Furthermore there has yet to be an animal model devised that develops emphysema purely as a result of cigarette smoke exposure. Nevertheless, with these reservations the relevance of animal models to human emphysema does have some foundation.

6.2.1 ELASTASE MODEL

By far the most extensively studied model of emphysema relates to the role of elastases. This is because of the association of α_1-AT deficiency with emphysema and the subsequent evolution of the proteinase/antiproteinase hypothesis. Only enzymes with the ability to degrade elastin (elastases) have the potential to cause experimental emphysema. The early experiments were carried out with porcine pancreatic elastase but studies rapidly progressed to identify and assess a human enzyme with the same capability.

In 1968 Janoff and Scherer first described an elastinolytic enzyme in the human neutrophil [7] and since the plasma of α_1-AT deficient subjects had a decreased ability to inhibit this enzyme [8] it became the most likely mediator of emphysema in these subjects. The poor neutrophil elastase (NE) inhibitory capacity of α_1-AT deficient serum is shown in Fig. 6.2 and studies confirm that α_1-AT is the most potent natural inhibitor of this enzyme [9]. In 1972 Lieberman demonstrated that leukocyte enzymes could digest α_1-AT deficient lungs and that this could be prevented by α_1-AT [10]. It was not until 1977 that purified NE was shown to produce emphysema in experimental animals [11] and that it was associated with decreased lung elastin [12]. The decrease in

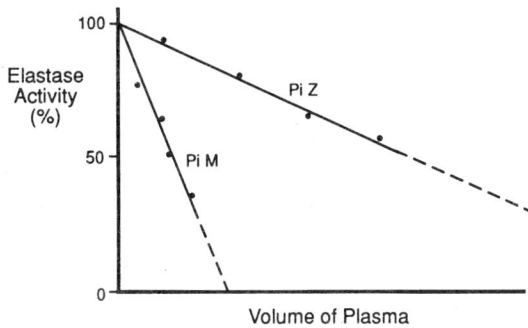

Fig. 6.2 Inhibition of neutrophil elastase is shown for increasing volumes of normal (PiM) plasma and α_1-antitrypsin deficient (PiZ) plasma. The latter requires greater volumes of plasma to inhibit the same amount of enzyme.

lung elastin was transient and after the initial exposure to elastase the lung elastin gradually returned to normal [12]. Despite this 'repair' process to the connective tissue the lung architecture remained abnormal and 'emphysema' developed [12].

The experiments summarized above are unphysiologic and involve the intratracheal instillation of single doses of neutrophil contents or purified enzymes. However, similar though milder lesions have been generated following intrapulmonary sequestration of neutrophils with endotoxin both in monkeys [13] and dogs [14]. Furthermore the generation of anti-elastase deficiency at the same time results in the development of a greater degree of emphysema [15].

These, and many other studies, confirm the potential of NE to cause 'emphysematous' lesions in the lungs of experimental animals. On the basis of these studies, the reduced plasma inhibitory activity against elastase and the susceptibility of patients with α_1-AT deficiency to develop emphysema, NE has been considered the most likely cause of this disease in man. Thus the proteinase/ antiproteinase theory has largely developed into an elastase/anti-elastase theory of the pathogenesis of emphysema with NE being the major enzyme implicated.

6.3 ALPHA₁-ANTITRYPSIN

Alpha₁-antitrypsin is a 52 KDa glycoprotein that is a potent inhibitor of serine proteinases. Although it has a broad spectrum of inhibitory activity against enzymes in this class its greatest affinity is for the enzyme neutrophil elastase and this is believed to be its major role [9]. It is made by hepatocytes [16] and its 'normal' plasma concentration is approximately 2 g/l although this can increase rapidly [17] as part of the 'acute phase' response.

The protein is readily identified in the lung secretions and its concentration is dependent upon its size, plasma concentration and the degree of lung inflammation [18–20]. Although monocytes and macrophages can also make α_1-AT it is generally believed that most of the lung α_1-AT is derived from the plasma.

The protein is coded for by a single 12.2 kilobase gene on chromosome 14 [21] and consists of seven exons (4 of which code for the mature protein) and 6 introns. The first 3 exons are not translated into protein and their transcription to mRNA is dependent upon the cell of origin [22]. The relevance of this difference is not known.

The mature protein consists of 394 amino acids with 3 carbohydrate side chains. The genes are pleomorphic with over 70 known alleles and these usually involve amino acid changes that do not alter protein structure, function or expression. Most such changes alter protein charge which is reflected in changes in electrophoretic mobility. These electrophoretic changes are responsible for the original classification of α_1-AT phenotypes (the Pi classification), some of which are related to deficiency states (see below). The protein is globular in structure but the enzyme inhibitory region protrudes and interacts with the active site of its target enzyme. In this respect the Met[358]-Ser[359] sequence at the active site is the crucial sequence that gives α_1-AT its specificity. This sequence has implications for both the function of α_1-AT and potential therapy in emphysema (see later).

6.3.1 ALPHA$_1$-ANTITRYPSIN DEFICIENCY

Our current concepts concerning the cellular and biochemical events underlying the pathogenesis of emphysema relate directly to the first description of α_1-AT deficiency in 1963. In the preliminary paper [4], Laurell and Eriksson first described 5 subjects in whom the α_1 band on paper electrophoresis was absent (Fig. 6.3). Three of the original subjects

had severe, early onset emphysema suggesting an association, which was confirmed in a subsequent study including the inherited nature of the deficiency [23].

(a) The Pi System

Isoelectric focusing showed that α_1-AT from normal subjects and those with deficiency could be distinguished (Fig. 6.4) and it became clear that the protein showed marked electrophoretic pleomorphism. This led to the protein being classified phenotypically by its isoelectric properties (Pi). Such studies clarified the genetic expression of the protein. The common Pi type was designated M and the deficient Pi type was designated Z. Studies confirmed that heterozygotes with a combination of both patterns (M and Z) also existed (Fig. 6.4). The phenotype related to the plasma concentrations of α_1-AT: M homozygote approximately 2 g/l;

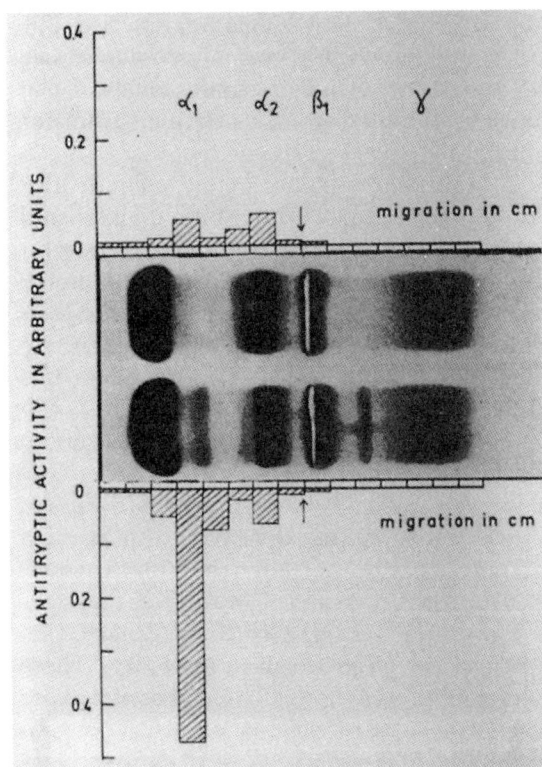

Fig. 6.3 Paper electrophoretic strips from normal (lower track) and α_1-AT deficient plasma (upper track). Note the absence of the α_1 protein band in the upper track. The trypsin inhibitory activity is shown for the respective bands (hatched columns). The major trypsin inhibition resides in the α_1 band (reproduced with permission from reference [6].)

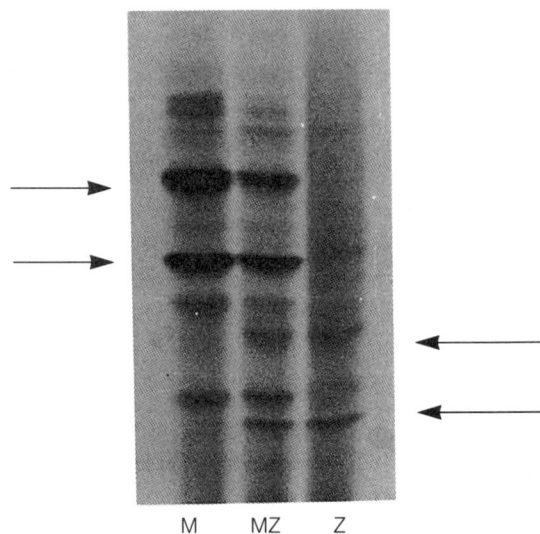

Fig. 6.4 Isoelectric focusing of α_1-AT M, MZ and Z phenotypes are shown. Note the heterozygote is a combination of patterns seen for the M and Z phenotypes (figure kindly supplied by E.J. Campbell, University of Utah, USA). M and Z specific bands are shown by arrows.

Table 6.1 Average plasma levels of α_1-antitrypsin for more common phenotypes

Phenotype	Average basal concentration	Risk factor for emphysema
MM	2 g/l	No
SS	1.2 g/l	No
MS	1.6 g/l	No
MZ	1.2 g/l	No
MNull	1.0 g/l	No ←
SZ	0.8 g/l	Yes
ZZ	0.4 g/l	Yes
ZNull	0.2 g/l	Yes
Null Null	–	Yes

Relationship of phenotype to average α_1-AT concentrations and risk for emphysema. Note, however, that the M and S phenotypes show acute phase responses and the range for these phenotypes is wide (MM normal range 1.4–2.8 g/l but may rise to 4–6 g/l). On the other hand the PiZ phenotype may only rise to 0.55 g/l. The arrow indicates threshold for risk.

MZ heterozygote approximately 1.2 g/l and Z homozygote approximately 0.3 g/l (Table 6.1). Thus it became apparent that the genome possessed 2 α_1-AT alleles that determined the plasma concentration with each M allele responsible for approximately 1 g/l and the Z allele for 0.1–0.15 g/l.

Since these early studies more than 75 different Pi types of α_1-AT have been identified and a complex system of nomenclature has evolved, some Pi types being associated with normal α_1-AT concentrations and some with low to absent concentrations. The Pi letter relates to the position on the isoelectric focusing gel (from A to Z) but even the PiM phenotype can be subdivided into those with normal α_1-AT concentrations (indicated by the amino acid variation): M1 (Ala²¹⁸), M1 (Val²¹⁸) and the rarer varieties with very low concentrations (indicated by the town of origin): M$_{Malton}$. Finally there are some alleles associated with no detectable α_1-AT at all: Null $_{Isola de Procida}$, and Null $_{Mattawa}$. In the null states no α_1-AT can be identified on isoelectric focusing and if the subject is heterozygous (M:Null) the pattern will reflect the α_1-AT positive allele alone (M). The clue to the presence of a null gene depends on the demonstration of a low α_1-AT concentration (approximately 50% normal) or a family including a homozygote null. Hence

identification of α_1-AT deficiency and its nature requires a combination of quantification, isoelectric focusing, familial studies and gene sequencing. Indeed it should be emphasized that simple quantitation of α_1-AT is insufficient to identify some of the deficiency states. The values given above are average results for a healthy population. The M and S phenotypes (commonly found in partial deficiencies) are regulatable and may rapidly double in concentration as part of the acute phase response. Thus the MZ, MNull and even SZ phenotypes may have concentrations in the 'normal' range at certain times. However, average concentrations for the more common phenotypes are shown in Table 6.1.

(b) Cause of deficiency states

In theory plasma α_1-AT deficiency can occur for many reasons. Like all secreted proteins it depends upon the presence of a gene that can be transcribed to form messenger RNA. This message has to be translated into the protein which is then transported from the rough endoplasmic reticulum of the cell, processed intracellularly and finally secreted. Defects at any step in this process can lead to decreased or absent plasma protein.

Although the Z deficiency state has been recognized for almost 30 years the mechanism has only recently been elucidated. One of the features of patients with the PiZ phenotype is the presence of PAS positive inclusion bodies in the liver (Fig. 6.5). These are accumulations of the α_1-AT protein at the rough endoplasmic reticulum suggesting blockage at this point. Indeed studies have shown that liver and mononuclear cells from PiZ patients make normal amounts of mRNA [16,24] and this can be translated into normal amounts of protein in a cell-free translation system [25]. However, if the mRNA is introduced into a cellular translation system the protein is made but little is secreted indicating that intracellular processing is impaired [26].

Genetic studies demonstrated that the Z α_1-AT gene was normal except for a single point mutation (change of a glycine nucleotide for adenine) in the DNA sequence that codes for the amino acid at position 342 on the molecule, resulting in a change from the normal glutamic acid to lysine [27]. It was originally believed that this single change interfered with protein folding because the normal glutamic acid at position 342 forms a salt bridge with lysine at position 290 [28]. The poorly folded protein would not pass through the endoplasmic reticulum to enter the secretory pathway. However, subsequent studies suggested this was not the case and the salt bridge was irrelevant but the charge of the amino acid at 342 was crucial [29]. Recent studies seem to have clarified the mechanism

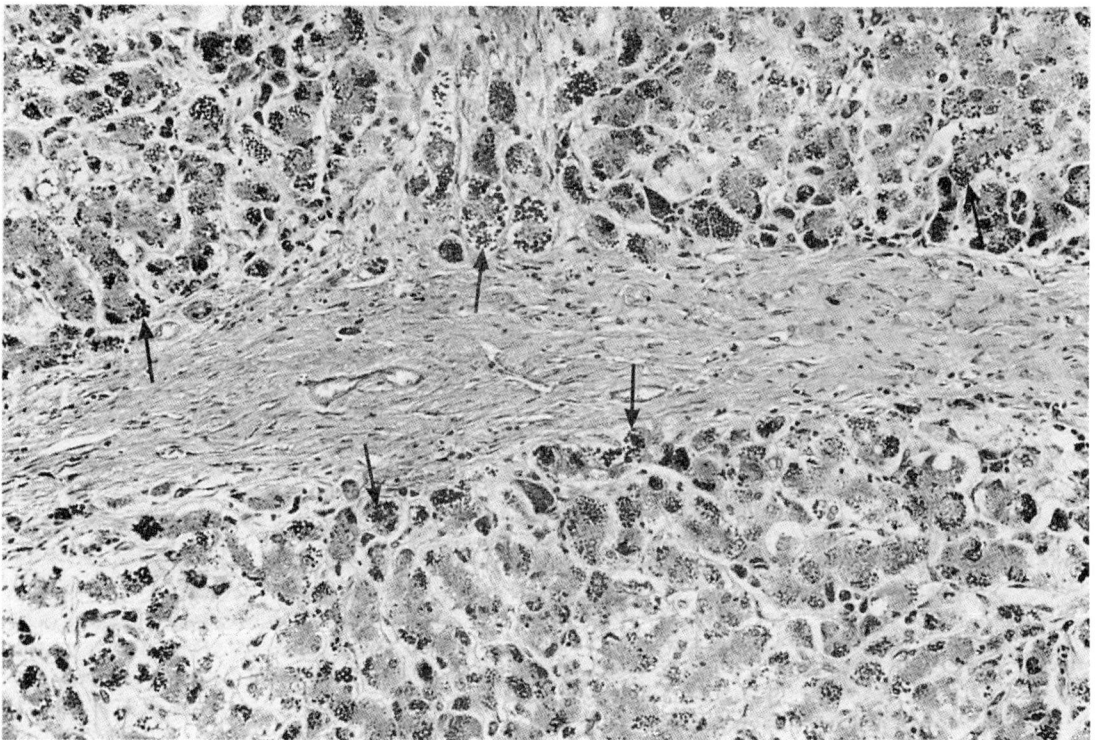

Fig. 6.5 Histology of liver from a patient with the PiZ phenotype showing the PAS-positive inclusion bodies in hepatocytes (arrowed). (The figure was kindly provided by Dr S. Hubscher, Department of Pathology, University of Birmingham.)

involved. The glutamic acid at position 342 is at the base of the inhibitory active site loop. When replaced by lysine the normal 'hinge' at this region is altered and the active site loop is extended. This loop then fits between the A sheets of a second molecule leading to spontaneous polymerization of the protein [30]. The net effect is large α_1-AT polymers (seen as PAS positive bodies, Fig. 6.5), which cannot pass through the rough endoplasmic reticulum and hence impair secretion.

The explanations for other deficiency states have taken less time. M$_{Malton}$ (deletion of phenyalanine at position 52 [31]) and S$_{iiyama}$ (serine^{53} changed to phenylalanine^{53} [32]) also result in accumulation at the endoplasmic reticulum. These defects affect the B helix which stabilizes the A sheets and is thought to make the space between the sheets more accessible for the normal active site loop [30], again leading to polymerization.

A multitude of other defects have been identified, characterized and explained by a series of molecular and biochemical studies. These are covered extensively elsewhere [33] but examples of other defects include:

1. gene deletion: Null $_{Isola\ De\ Procida}$ [34];
2. premature termination of gene transcription: Null$_{Bellingham}$ [35] and Null$_{Granite\ falls}$ [36];
3. production of a protein that is less stable and thus becomes degraded intracellularly: S[37] and P$_{lowell}$ [38];
4. normal secretion of α_1-AT that is non-functional as an inhibitor: M$_{Mineral\ springs}$ [39].

All these defects (with the exception of the S variant) have been associated with the presence of emphysema suggesting a causal relationship.

6.3.2 PATHOGENESIS OF EMPHYSEMA IN ALPHA$_1$-ANTITRYPSIN DEFICIENCY

The deficiency alleles are associated with decreased plasma concentrations of α_1-AT. The common deficiency state (PiZ) probably arose in Northern Europe and is confined to caucasians. In Britain approximately 86% of subjects have α_1-AT alleles associated with normal concentrations of α_1-AT (MM) whereas 9% have the MS phenotype; 3% – MZ; 0.25% – SS; 0.2% – SZ and 0.03% – ZZ [40]. Of these MS, MZ and SS are associated with partial deficiency and SZ and ZZ with severe deficiency. Emphysema is well recognized in association with severe deficiency of the SZ [41] and ZZ phenotype [42], as well as the rarer null phenotypes [43]. The incidence of the null phenotypes is unknown but is probably ten times less than the PiZ phenotype. However, the relationship to partial deficiency and in particular the MZ phenotype remains controversial. Large population studies of subjects with the MZ phenotype do not indicate that it is a significant risk factor [44]. On the other hand large studies of patients with established lung disease indicate that the MZ phenotype is over-represented suggesting some susceptibility [45]. In reality the effect of the MZ phenotype may be small, but it may, in the presence of other risk factors, tend to result in more severe disease [46].

The relationship of phenotypes with lower α_1-AT concentrations to emphysema is not controversial and this has led to concept of a threshold of α_1-AT concentration below which susceptibility to emphysema increases. This concept has implications for therapy (see later).

Serum deficiency of α_1-AT results in a comparable decrease in the plasma inhibitory capacity for the enzyme NE (Fig. 6.2). Since α_1-AT enters the lung largely by diffusion from plasma [18] the deficiency is also reflected in lung fluids [47,48]. Studies have suggested that α_1-AT is the only major inhibitor of NE in the lower airways [49,50] and hence protection of lung tissue from NE would be defective in α_1-AT deficiency. Indeed animal models have shown that generation of α_1-AT deficiency increases the severity of emphysema following neutrophil sequestration [15].

Thus it seems likely that the low α_1-AT levels in severe deficiency result in reduced anti-elastase protection for the lung. In addition, the lungs of α_1-AT deficient subjects contain more PMN [47] possibly due to the release of chemotactic factors such as LTB4 [51], thereby increasing the elastase load and highlighting the defective anti-elastase screen. The net result would be continued and poorly controlled degradation of lung elastin by the NE released from the recruited cells.

On the basis of these results and the elastase/anti-elastase theory of emphysema it is easy to understand the susceptibility of deficient subjects to disease. Indeed the life expectancy of α_1-AT deficient subjects is significantly reduced especially if they smoke [52] as indicated in Fig. 6.6. The additive effect of cigarette smoke may be complex (see later) but could influence disease progression merely by the increased recruitment of PMN (and hence NE) seen in the lungs of smokers [53].

Nevertheless although mortality is increased in early life in α_1-AT deficiency [52] the relationship of deficiency to disease is not entirely clear. Some patients live to old age with relatively well preserved lung function even if they smoke [54]. Furthermore our impression of the relative risks may be influenced by the methods of identification of deficiency. Patients are usually identified

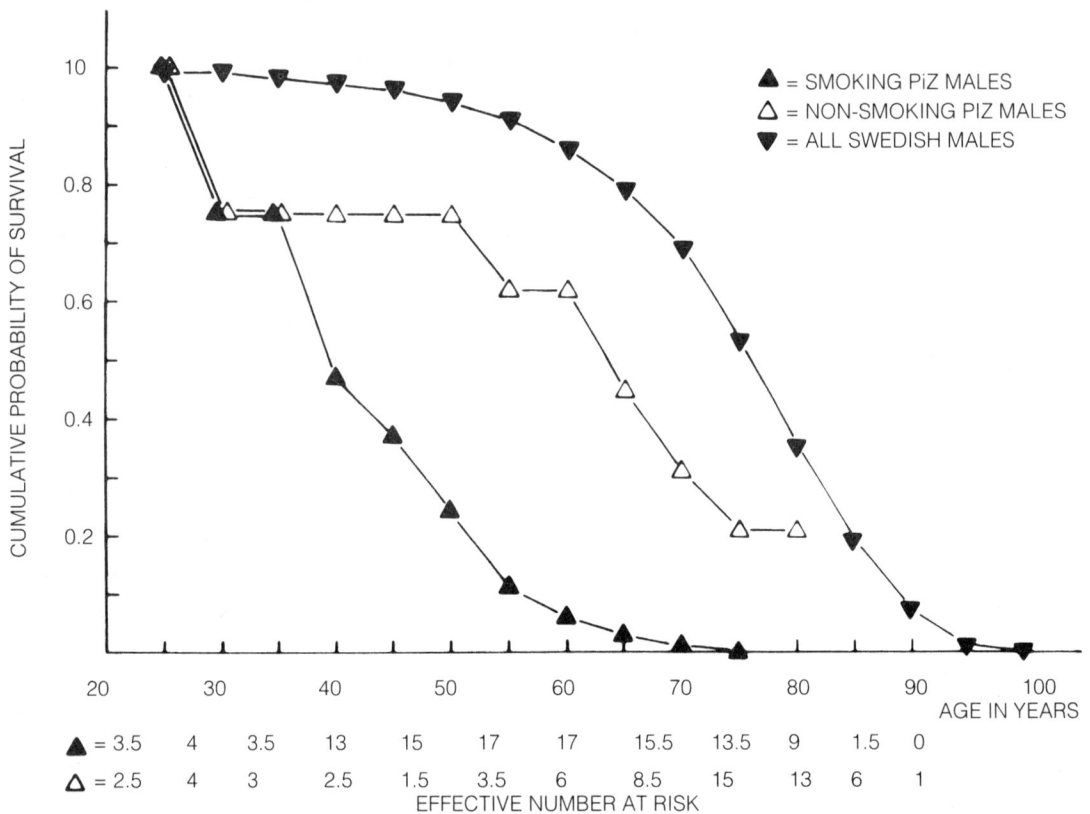

Fig. 6.6 Life expectancy curves for normal Swedish subjects and those with α_1-AT deficiency. (Reproduced with permission from reference [52].)

after presentation with disease and other members of the same family are then investigated. Thus most α_1-AT deficient subjects are identified because of established disease in themselves or a relative. Studies have shown that factors other than α_1-AT deficiency may play a role in these families [55,56]. Hence there may well be a selection bias leading to an over-estimation of risk and indeed population screening has identified more 'healthy' α_1-AT deficient subjects [57]. Perhaps the true risk in α_1-AT deficient subjects will only be determined with lengthy follow-up of subjects identified at birth [58]. In addition, an understanding of the disease process in these deficient subjects depends upon the assumption that α_1-AT is the major lung anti-elastase and NE is the enzyme which causes emphysema. Since both assumptions may be incorrect (see later) our concepts may also be, at least in part, incorrect.

6.3.3 REASONS FOR IDENTIFICATION OF DEFICIENCY

There are three potential strategies that can be employed to identify subjects with α_1-AT deficiency:

1. identification in a population of patients with established disease;
2. routine population screening;
3. identification in the perinatal period.

There are reasons for identifying subjects with any of these three approaches although each has different indications and implications.

The identification of subjects with established emphysema is most cost effective. The incidence is relatively high, ranging from 1–2% of all patients presenting with COPD [59] to greater than 50% for patients with severe disease who are less than 40 years of age [60]. The identification of these patients has several benefits. First, an explanation for their susceptibility can be imparted, thereby assisting their medical management. Second,

the presence of deficiency will affect prognosis and this will also help management and reinforce the introduction of preventative measures (smoking cessation). Third, family studies may identify other unrecognized members with deficiency who may be less severely affected permitting earlier intervention and genetic counselling. Finally, the suitability of the patients for replacement or other therapies can be addressed and this will be discussed in more detail later.

The second approach of routine population screening is difficult in practice and less cost effective, with an expected incidence of 1 in 3000 in the UK. The advantages of this approach would be to address the true prognosis of the deficiency in the general population without the added effects of other social, environmental and genetic factors that may influence the observations in family studies based upon index cases (see above). In addition screening may identify subjects with early disease where intervention may be more effective.

The final approach involves perinatal identification. This can be achieved by both postnatal [58] and prenatal diagnosis [61]. The advantage of postnatal screening is to identify subjects prior to the development of disease. Potentially this means that behavioral patterns can be impressed in childhood thereby preventing late sequelae. However, since the proportion of these subjects who will develop disease remains unknown, the true cost benefit may not be determined for 20 or 30 years. At present follow-up of such subjects has highlighted an increased incidence of asthmatic symptoms [62] and provided reassurance concerning possible psychological problems in other family members aware of the deficiency at this early stage [63]. The advantages of screening at primary and secondary school age may be similar to postnatal screening without the potential familial disadvantages although the cost-benefit will still await extensive long term non-interventionist studies.

The use of prenatal screening is very limited. Chorionic villus sampling has shown that it is possible to diagnose α_1-AT deficiency during early fetal development [61]. The only advantage to this approach is if therapeutic abortion were to be considered. Clearly this is not indicated for the lung consequences since it is unknown whether they will occur in an individual subject and advice on smoking may prevent most of the morbidity. Even if disease occurs it is compatible with a reasonable though reduced life expectancy: 40–50% survival to 50 years of age [52]. However, another major problem associated with α_1-AT deficiency is liver disease, including cirrhosis [64], primarily liver cancer [65] and neonatal jaundice [66]. The latter can be fatal and particularly if one such infant has been born the risk of a subsequent PiZ infant developing the same problem is greater than 75% [66]. Thus in this limited situation prenatal screening may be indicated and the possibility of therapeutic abortion can be discussed and possibly implemented.

6.3.4 TREATMENT

Once a diagnosis of α_1-AT deficiency has been made in patients with COPD the therapeutic strategies are largely similar to those used in non-deficient patients. These include counselling about the effects of smoking, bronchodilators if of proven efficacy and treatment for exacerbations and complications including cor pulmonale. However, on the assumption that the low levels of α_1-AT in the lung cannot protect the tissue from damage by NE, alternative strategies have been developed. This is based largely upon the unproven hypothesis that such approaches will alter the natural history of the disease process significantly.

(a) Increase natural α_1-AT production

Alpha$_1$-AT is an acute phase protein with an ability to double its plasma concentration within days and, although the exact mechan-

isms are unknown *in vivo*, interleukin 6 can increase gene transcription *in vitro* [67]. Based on the assumption that α_1-AT gene transcription is regulatable even in PiZ deficiency, several approaches have been investigated in an attempt to raise endogenous plasma α_1-AT levels.

Danazol (17 α-ethinyl testosterone) does result in moderate elevation of plasma levels in some subjects with the PiZ phenotype of about 37% on average, but not to levels considered to be above the 'at risk' threshold of 800 mg/l [68]. Thus together with the potential long term side effects, especially in females, this approach is not practical. An alternative agent is tamoxifen which binds to estrogen receptors and hence should mimic the rise in plasma α_1-AT found in pregnancy. This has also been shown to have little effect in PiZ patients [69]. Interestingly tamoxifen does increase the levels of α_1-AT alleles associated with increased cellular degradation of the mature protein such as the S variant [70]. Thus it may be that tamoxifen would be appropriate therapy in the SZ phenotype which does impart an increased risk of emphysema but is on the borderline of the 'at risk' threshold and is heterozygotic for the regulatable S allele.

It may be that other agents will be identified with greater potential to increase endogenous α_1-AT production. However, they will not be effective in the Pi null variants and may actually exaggerate the PiZ protein accumulation and polymerization at the rough endoplasmic reticulum and thereby worsen hepatocyte damage [30]. Thus this general approach is likely to prove impractical in the majority of deficient subjects.

(b) Replacement therapy

Because the lung disease is thought to relate directly to a deficiency state the most appropriate therapy would appear to be intravenous replacement to raise the circulating plasma levels above the 'at risk' threshold. This was first shown to be feasible in 1982 by Gadek and colleagues in a limited study [71]. In addition the authors demonstrated that the alveolar lining fluid responded in a similar manner with an increase in the anti-elastase protective screen. Subsequent studies confirmed that administering 60 mg/kg on a weekly basis maintained the plasma level above the protective threshold [72]. An alternative strategy based upon monthly administration of 250 mg/kg is also effective in maintaining 'protective' plasma concentrations of α_1-AT [73] but may prove more acceptable to patients.

These replacement strategies depend upon the availability of native α_1-AT purified from whole blood that has been collected for other purposes (transfusions, factor VIII, etc). The supply is finite and if replacement therapy becomes established an alternative source will be required. It is feasible to produce a_1-AT by recombinant DNA technology [74] and thus the demand could be met. However, recombinant α_1-AT ($r\alpha_1$-AT) lacks carbohydrate side chains and has a serum half life of approximately 90 min [75], suggesting that administration by this route would be impractical. The alternative is to deliver the $r\alpha_1$-AT directly into the airways. Studies have shown that aerosolization does not inactivate the $r\alpha_1$-AT and a single administration of 200 mg raises the levels in bronchial fluids above 'normal' for 12 hours or more [76]. In addition the $r\alpha_1$-AT enters the circulation, suggesting it has diffused into the lung interstitium where its major protective role is required [77]. Whether the concentrations achieved at this site are adequate and influence the course of the disease needs to be determined.

Clearly these strategies replenish α_1-AT levels in deficiency states. However, they are all expensive and have to be given for life. As yet it remains uncertain whether this approach will actually influence disease progression and it may prove more cost effective to instigate a successful no smoking programme. Both approaches assume that the progression can be altered once moderate to severe airflow obstruction has been established and that the lung disease itself does not become self perpetuating. These doubts can only be answered by a formal controlled trial although the numbers (more than 600) and the time (5 years) required make a worthwhile evaluable study highly unlikely. Thus at present each case will have to be taken on merit with the understanding that this form of therapy could be a very expensive placebo.

(c) Gene therapy

The severe deficiency states (with the exception of the Z allele) are caused by defects of gene transcription or translation. Thus potentially the introduction of a normal gene into the cell of origin or cells in the lung could 'cure' the deficiency. Although the prospect of gene therapy in humans still has a long way to go the methodology is being developed. Initial studies showed it was possible to introduce the α_1-AT gene into cultured cells *in vitro* (transfection) and these would produce the protein [78]. Furthermore, reintroduction of transfected cells into the peritoneal cavity of experimental animals resulted in release of α_1-AT into the plasma and the lung [78]. More recently attempts have been made to introduce the α_1-AT gene into epithelial cells lining the bronchial tree on the assumption that local gene expression would increase the anti-elastase screen at the site of lung damage.

Potential mechanisms of gene delivery include the transfer of plasmid DNA in liposomes and DNA attached to ligands which bind to specific receptors on the target cells. However, most work has been carried out with viral vectors.

(i) Retroviruses

Retroviruses are RNA viruses that contain sequences coding for their RNA and structural proteins in addition to the enzyme reverse transcriptase. Once the virus enters the cell the RNA is released and reverse transcriptase changes the RNA sequences into DNA and inserts them into the DNA of the infected cell. Thereafter the cell DNA insert makes further

RNA copies which are made into the virus and its structural proteins and new viruses are released.

Manipulation of the virus RNA can exclude the sequences that code for the structural proteins and include the gene to be replaced (in this case α_1-AT). The result is 'infection' of the target cell, introduction of some virus RNA and the replacement gene into the cell's DNA and finally 'normal' expression of the replacement gene without viral replication.

At present this approach has several drawbacks including:

1. Efficient transduction requires the target cell to be replicating.
2. The retroviral vectors can become contaminated with replication competent viruses leading to infection.
3. The viral RNA may become inserted into the cellular genome at a critical site activating oncogenes and resulting in malignant change.

Only extensive *in vivo* experimentation will determine the long-term safety of the retroviral approach.

(ii) Adenovirus vectors

An alternative and probably safer approach is the use of the DNA adenoviruses. These have several advantages over retroviruses. First, they can carry larger segments of DNA. Second, they can be obtained in very high titers and can 'infect' non-replicating cells, which makes them very attractive as a means of gene delivery to the airway epithelium. Finally, there are less concerns about safety as the vectors rarely undergo recombination and there are no known malignancies associated with adenovirus infection.

The vector is constructed by removal of the E3 region (which will allow encapsidation of the recombinant sequence containing the α_1-AT gene) and part of the E1a coding sequence to impair the viral replication. The α_1-AT gene expression cassette consists of the α_1-AT gene and the adenovirus major late promoter

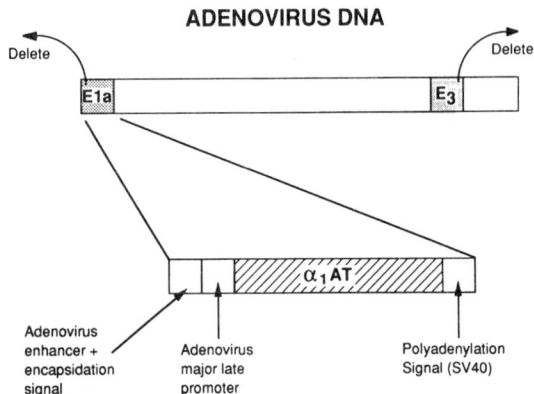

Fig. 6.7 Diagrammatic representation of the construction of the adenovirus vector for delivery of the α_1-AT gene to bronchial epithelium. See text for details. (Adapted from reference [79].)

as well as a polyadenylation sequence (Fig. 6.7). Using this vector, the α_1-AT gene has been delivered into the lungs of experimental animals. The viral DNA undergoes illegitimate recombination with the epithelial cell genome and the α_1-AT gene is expressed. The isolated epithelial cells secret the protein and it can be detected in bronchial lining fluid for up to a week [79].

Although these early experiments seem encouraging several problems remain. The major one is that the adenovirus structural proteins are antigenic and thus will induce a local immune response. Because the virus 'infects' non-replicating cells the treatment will have to be repeated on a regular basis as old cells die and are replaced. Activation of the immune system will render the vector ineffective due to prevention of cell infection by subsequent treatments. Furthermore even if gene delivery can be effectively repeated and remain efficiently transcribed, the success will depend upon subsequent delivery of the α_1-AT to the lung interstitium to prevent lung damage at this site.

(d) The Z defect

As mentioned earlier the Z α_1-AT accumulates at the rough endoplasmic reticulum because of polymerization [30]. Gene replacement will not prevent this process but if polymerization can be inhibited the protein should be transported normally. In this respect insertion of a blocking peptide into the A sheets may have therapeutic potential if delivery can be facilitated to the hepatocytes. Clearly further studies are indicated to assess this possibility.

(e) Transplantation

In severe α_1-AT deficiency transplantation of both liver and lung have been undertaken successfully. The former has been carried out in advanced liver disease and the plasma α_1-AT (which is made by the liver) changes phenotype in days [80]. Clearly in these patients intravenous or inhaled replacement therapy would no longer be necessary.

Single or double lung, as well as heart/lung, transplantation has also been carried out for patients with severe respiratory disease. There is uncertainty as to whether replacement therapy should follow transplantation. However, since the lung disease occurs gradually over a 30–40-year period and current survival after transplantation is considerably shorter, it is possibly unnecessary as a measure to prevent recurrence of emphysema. On the other hand episodes of acute rejection and atypical infection are inflammatory processes (albeit predominantly lymphocyte mediated) and it may be necessary to provide short courses of supplementation to cover these events.

Other potential therapies will be covered at the end of the next section on emphysema in non-α_1-AT deficient subjects.

6.4 EMPHYSEMA IN THE ABSENCE OF α_1-AT DEFICIENCY

Although the simple concept of emphysema relating to a disturbance in the elastase/anti-elastase balance is at least intellectually valid in the presence of severe α_1-AT deficiency, its relevance to the non-deficient

patient is less clear. Nevertheless the overall credibility of this hypothesis is so high that its principles have been applied to the pathogenesis of emphysema in subjects with normal plasma α_1-AT. However, the processes that lead to disturbance of the 'normal' proteinase/antiproteinase balance are less clear but a summary of potential mechanisms is outlined in Table 6.2.

In theory this could happen for one of three general reasons:

1. There may be a functional deficiency of the inhibitors due to excessive inactivation in the lung or failure to mount an appropriate acute phase response in the presence of inflammation thereby producing a persistent or intermittent *relative* deficiency.
2. The proteinase burden may be increased beyond the protective capacity of the antiproteinase in the lung.
3. A combination of both a relative inhibitor deficiency and an increased proteinase burden may be sufficient to tip the biochemical balance in favour of the enzymes.

Whichever mechanism applies, the assumption is that the enzymes predominate either continuously or intermittently, resulting in unchecked degradation of connective tissue leading to COPD. Because of the lessons and concepts that have derived from studies in α_1-AT deficiency, most of the research has again focused upon the balance between α_1-AT and NE and in particular factors which affect the function of α_1-AT.

Until the late 1970s extensive studies of plasma α_1-AT had failed to provide any further clues to the pathogenesis of emphysema other than identification of the rare deficiency states. However, animal models had shown that emphysema only occurred if the elastase was placed into the lungs directly. Furthermore Kimbel and colleagues [81] had shown that lung lavage prior to instillation of elastase resulted in the development of more severe emphysema. This suggested that the secretions contained a protective inhibitor

Table 6.2 Possible mechanisms of emphysema in subjects with normal α_1-AT

Functional deficiency of α_1-antitrypsin inactivation	– oxidation of active site – cleavage of active site – complexing with enzyme – peptide insertion into tertiary structure
inadequate acute phase response	– Taq 1 polymorphism?

Deficiency of other inhibitors	– metalloproteinase inhibitors – TIMP
	– cysteine proteinase inhibitors – cystatins
	– other serine proteinase inhibitors
	    – anti-leukoprotease
	    – elafin

Increased elastase burden	– raised cellular elastase content
	– increased recruitment
	    – excess chemotactic factors
	    – greater cell response
	– increased degranulation

Other enzymes	– metalloelastase (macrophage) – cathepsin B – collagenase

that had been removed by the lavage procedure. The likely candidate as a lung inhibitor appeared to be α_1-AT.

Studies showed that α_1-AT was present in secretions of patients with COPD and that it was partially complexed with NE [20]. Furthermore during clinical exacerbations the α_1-AT level rose but the degree of NE complex fell and free elastase activity was found suggesting the remaining α_1-AT was in some way inactivated [20].

Studies have shown that there are four ways in which α_1-At can be inactivated:

1. Oxidation of the critical methionine residue at the centre of the active site [82].
2. Cleavage of the reactive site loop releasing the carboxy terminus [83].
3. The formation of irreversible complexes with proteolytic enzymes [84].
4. More recent data have shown that insertion of small peptides into the tertiary structure between the A sheets can also inactivate α_1-AT [85].

6.4.1 LUNG LAVAGE α_1-AT

In 1979 Gadek and colleagues published a key paper on lung lavage α_1-AT. They studied the function of α_1-AT in lavage fluids from healthy smokers and non-smokers. The results shown that α_1-AT function was normal in healthy non-smokers but on average reduced by 40% in smokers [86]. This finding was not unexpected as previous studies had shown that oxidation of α_1-AT resulted in loss of inhibitory function [82] and that cigarette smoke was one agent capable of effecting this change [87]. In addition, studies *in vivo* using an animal model confirmed that smoke exposure reduced lung α_1-AT function [88] and oxidation of the methionine residues was confirmed biochemically in the lungs of healthy smokers [89].

Thus the mechanism resulting in emphysema appeared straightforward. Cigarette smoking (the major risk factor) resulted in significant inactivation of α_1-AT by oxidation of the active site of the protein. In addition to this direct effect of cigarette smoke, macrophages from the lungs of smokers spontaneously released more reactive oxygen species that could also inactivate α_1-AT *in vitro* [90]. The net effect of these two mechanisms would be to reduce lung α_1-AT function in smokers' lungs by oxidation of the active site resulting in a significant disturbance of the α_1-AT/elastase balance in the lung. It was suggested that the reason most of the lavage α_1-AT remained active, even in smokers, reflected the mixing of protein from wide areas of the lung – some with fully active α_1-AT and some with completely 'inactive' α_1-AT [91]. It was hypothesized that the areas where all the α_1-AT was fully oxidized, and hence non-functional, were the sites of tissue destruction by NE.

This concept has subsequently dominated the field of emphysema research and the potential for intervention with antioxidants and even oxidation-resistant α_1-AT has been suggested (Fig. 6.8). However, studies by other groups have failed to consolidate this hypothesis. With the exception of one study showing a very transient and minimal decrease in α_1-AT function following smoking [92], other investigators have failed to find any difference in α_1-AT function in lavage from healthy smokers and non-smokers [93,94]. Furthermore there is also disagreement concerning the inhibitory activity of lung α_1-AT with some groups finding it to be fully functional in lavage fluids [92,95] and others finding a degree of inactivation [93,94,96]. This disparity may reflect technical differences in the studies since concentration [97] and storage [96] of samples can both alter α_1-AT function. Furthermore the original observation of oxidized α_1-AT in smokers' lavage fluid has not been confirmed. The only direct study using a specific monoclonal antibody failed to detect significant amounts of oxidized α_1-AT in lavage fluids [98]. Indirect confirmation of this latter result was obtained by incubating lavage fluids with the enzyme methionine sulfoxide peptide reductase which restores the inhibitory

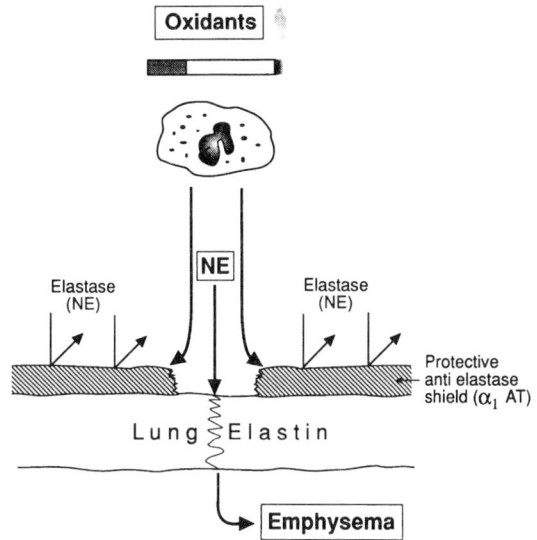

Fig. 6.8 Diagrammatic representation of the hypothesis implicating cigarette smoking in the pathogenesis of emphysema. Oxidants released from cigarette smoke and activated inflammatory cells inactivate the protective anti-elastase shield. NE can then penetrate the shield and destroy lung elastin resulting in the development of emphysema.

activity of oxidized α_1-AT [99] but failed to alter α_1-AT function in normal lavage fluids [96].

On balance no clear picture emerges, which makes it unlikely that oxidation of α_1-AT is the only explanation for the susceptibility to emphysema in smokers. There are other mechanisms that reduce the inhibitory activity of α_1-AT including cleavage of the active site and previous complex formation with enzyme. These two mechanisms result in a change in the molecular size of the α_1-AT making it smaller (49 000 KDa) or larger (approximately 80 000 KDa) respectively compared to native active α_1-AT (52 000–54 000 KDa). Studies have shown that α_1-AT of these molecular weights can be present in lavage fluids from emphysema patients [100] but not in healthy subjects [96]. Thus the inactivity of lung lavage α_1-AT in healthy subjects remains unexplained although it appears to be more positively charged [96]. Perhaps this may relate to the presence of a peptide insert into the native molecule [85] although the mechanism is currently unknown.

An alternative to inactivation is that the inhibitory characteristics of the α_1-AT is changed in a less dramatic way. Studies have shown that the α_1-AT in smokers' lavage has a slightly reduced association rate constant for NE [101]. This change is small but may affect the way α_1-AT, NE and lung elastin interact to favour elastin degradation. Certainly similar changes in association rate constant are found in the Z phenotype protein and this is less efficient than comparable amounts of the M protein in connective tissue from degradation by neutrophils [102]. Thus even if smoking does not reduce the absolute inhibitory capacity of α_1-AT *in vivo* it may alter it more subtly in a way which facilitates connective tissue degradation.

In general terms the lavage studies summarized above would suggest that changes in lung α_1-AT function are not central to pathogenesis of emphysema in non-deficient subjects. However, this may be a consequence of asking the wrong question and one of finding the wrong answer. The studies have been limited to differences between healthy smokers and non-smokers. Since most smokers do not develop significant emphysema one would not expect a major clue to emerge except in the 10–20% of subjects who are susceptible to the development of disease. Furthermore a difference would only be found easily in these subjects during the study if the development of emphysema is a continual rather than an intermittent process. Perhaps the evidence could emerge by studying patients with established disease who currently smoke and those who have stopped (when disease progression will have stopped and presumably the α_1-AT/NE balance will have been restored). Only one such study has been carried out [100] and although there was more evidence of cleaved α_1-AT in smokers'

lavage the inhibitory function was no different to that in the ex-smokers' lavage. It remains possible that the presence of established disease may have altered the results but the majority of the evidence to date does not implicate inactivation of α_1-AT in lung secretions as a major cause of an elastase/anti-elastase balance in emphysema.

The studies outlined above have been limited to lung lavage α_1-AT and it is believed that emphysema is the result of elastase activity near the lung interstitial elastin fibres. It may be that α_1-AT function at this site is more relevant to the pathogenesis of the disease. However, lung α_1-AT is thought to derive from the plasma by transudation through the lung interstitium and thus lavage α_1-AT should partly reflect the interstitial α_1-AT. Similarly if a direct effect of cigarette smoke on α_1-AT is difficult to demonstrate in lavage fluids it is even less likely to affect α_1-AT function in the interstitium. Nevertheless other local events in the interstitium may be of importance in determining the elastase anti-elastase balance (see later).

The final possibility is that α_1-AT function is not affected but the concentrations of protein do not increase appropriately during the acute phase response of inflammation. In support of this hypothesis genetic studies in patients with emphysema have shown an increased incidence of a polymorphism of the α_1-AT gene [103]. This polymorphism is related to a single change in the nucleotide sequence of an area beyond the end of the gene itself that alters a recognition sequence for the restriction enzyme *Taql*, resulting in a failure of the enzyme to cleave DNA at this site [104]. Recent analysis of this polymorphism shows that the area involved is an enhancer sequence [105] that can amplify gene expression. Thus the patients with the polymorphism may not be able to mount an appropriate acute phase response because of failure of the enhancer region to increase gene expression. If so the increase in elastase burden that would be predicted when the lung becomes inflamed would not be counteracted by an appropriate rise in the anti-elastase concentration provided by α_1-AT. As this polymorphism is the single most common genetic defect found in unrelated patients with emphysema (22%) further studies to determine its implications are clearly warranted.

6.4.2 INCREASE IN ELASTASE BURDEN

Although most research has concentrated on the anti-elastase side of the elastase/anti-elastase balance it is equally possible that the balance could be disturbed in favour of the enzymes if the enzyme load exceeded the capacity of the lung to inhibit it. Thus the pathogenesis of emphysema could be dependent upon the activity of the cells capable of damaging the connective tissue.

Normal lung lavage contains a small number of neutrophils recruited as part of the normal host defence to inhaled antigens. The number of neutrophils in the lungs of smokers is increased [53], perhaps due to the release of chemotactic factors such as LTB4 and IL8. If this process is not adequately controlled or the cells respond excessively the enzyme load could be increased sufficiently to exceed the capacity of the inhibitor screen. This may occur for several reasons:

1. There may, in some smokers, be excessive release or activity of chemotactic factors from the lung.
2. The neutrophils may respond excessively to the standard chemoattractant stimulus resulting in greater recruitment for a given signal.
3. The neutrophils from susceptible smokers may contain increased amounts of elastase compared to control subjects.
4. The neutrophils may degranulate excessively leading to more connective tissue damage.

(a) Chemotactic factors

Little is known about the true chemotactic gradient that exists across the lung tissues. Undoubtedly PMN migrate into the lung, nicotine itself is chemotactic [106]; and lung lavage fluids from smoke-exposed animals demonstrate increased chemotactic activity, possibly because of complement C3 activation [107]. Furthermore alveolar macrophages [108] and bronchial epithelium [109] release chemotactic factors. The control of these processes is poorly understood, although inactivators of chemotaxis also exist and may play a role in modulating the response in individual subjects.

For instance lung lavage in α_1-AT deficient subjects contains large numbers of neutrophils [47], and the alveolar macrophages release the chemoattractant leukotriene B4 [51]. However, in addition a deficiency of a chemotactic factor inactivator has been described in α_1-AT deficiency [110] and part of the excessive recruitment in these patients may result from the inability to control the magnitude of the response because of this factor deficiency. Whether similar mechanisms play a role in patients with normal α_1-AT remains unknown.

(b) Enhanced response to chemotactic agent

Since there is a 'normal' traffic of neutrophils to the lung and since the numbers are increased in smokers, it suggests that increased chemotactic response is a feature of smokers. Indeed circulating neutrophils seem to be sensitized to chemotactic signals even in passive smokers [111]. However, studies have again shown a wide degree of chemotactic response to a standard stimulus although patients with emphysema show increased response to a standard chemoattractant compared to age and smoking-matched controls (Fig. 6.9). The reasons for this increase have yet to be clarified although preliminary studies (Fig. 6.10) suggest that neutrophils

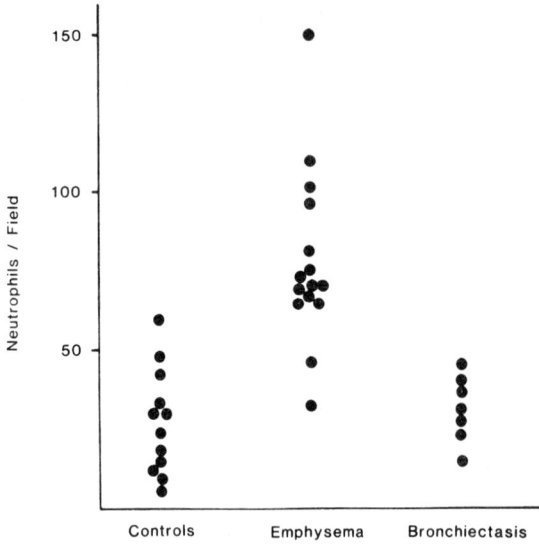

Fig. 6.9 The chemotactic response of isolated neutrophils to the chemoattractant FMLP (10^{-8} M). Individual results are shown for control subjects as well as those with emphysema and bronchiectasis (reproduced with permission from reference [115].)

from these patients show increased (P <0.02) receptors for formyl peptides (median = 495 × 10^3/cell; range 207–1080) compared to age and smoking-matched controls (median = 288; range 114–855). Again it is uncertain whether the increased chemotactic response

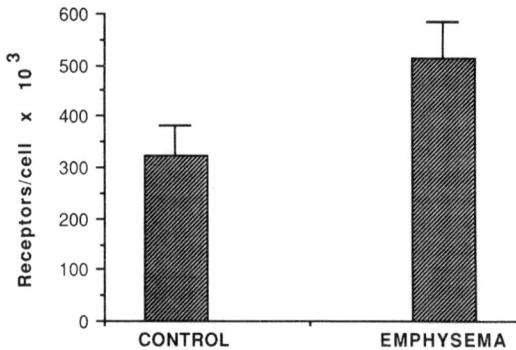

Fig. 6.10 The average number of formyl peptide receptors/cell is shown for 11 age matched healthy control subjects and 10 patients with emphysema. The bar lines are ± SE (P < 0.02).

represents cause or effect, although no increased response was found in patients with bronchiectasis (Fig. 6.9), suggesting it was a feature of emphysema rather than lung inflammation in general.

(c) Cell elastase content

There have been some studies of the elastase content of PMN in patients with established lung disease. Early studies suggested that the elastase from PMN in COPD patients was qualitatively different [112]. In addition Rodriguez and colleagues [113] and Kramps, Bakker and Dijkman [114] provided evidence that PMN elastase content was increased in COPD patients with the PiM phenotype whereas subjects with α_1-AT deficiency did not show such an increase [114]. However, it was uncertain whether this increase in PiM subjects was the cause or effect.

Elastase is preformed in the bone marrow during differentiation and stored in the azurophil granules and the gene is not expressed in mature circulating neutrophils [115]. Thus the enzyme load per cell has already been determined by the time the cell is released into the circulation. The elastase content of PMN shows a wide range in healthy subjects [116] and if those with high levels also smoked each cell recruited to the lung would deliver a greater amount of elastase. However, although early studies suggested that PMN elastase was increased in emphysema [114], subsequent studies have shown that it is not increased [116]. Thus the possibility of an increased elastase burden by this mechanism remains unproven, although a recent study has suggested that variations in elastase content may explain the variability in lung disease seen in subjects with PiZ α_1-AT deficiency [117].

(d) Excess degranulation

Neutrophil activation, adherence and phagocytosis results in release of elastase from the cell. If this response is excessive in emphysema patients each cell recruited to the lung would destroy more connective tissue than in a healthy smoker. Again evidence would support this possibility. Neutrophils isolated from patients with emphysema degrade more fibronectin *in vitro* than cells from control subjects matched for age and smoking [116]. Since this effect is almost solely mediated by NE [118], the results demonstrate the enhanced ability of cells from emphysema subjects to release this enzyme and thereby potentially lead to NE-induced lung damage.

At first sight, although potentially of importance, it may seem that the mechanisms outlined above may not be sufficient to disturb the elastase/anti-elastase balance. Lung lavage studies have shown that active α_1-AT is present in the lungs of smokers [96], emphysema patients [100] and even those with α_1-AT deficiency [47]. If an imbalance were to exist and thereby explain the disease one might expect no enzyme inhibitory capacity to remain in the susceptible subjects who have or are developing disease. However, this does not have to be the case. Firstly, as explained previously, the α_1-AT function in lavage represents an average from many areas and thus local absence of function could be hidden by mixing with samples from areas where function remains normal.

Secondly, and perhaps more importantly, studies have shown that PMN have the ability to degrade connective tissue matrices even in the presence of active enzyme inhibitors [119]. This relates to the ability of the cell to adhere tightly to connective tissue substrates and release enzyme in the interface between the two whilst effectively excluding the surrounding inhibitors [119]. It could be argued that this mechanism is so effective that emphysema would occur in all subjects with PMN recruitment to the lung, irrespective of α_1-AT status. However, α_1-AT does have some effect and will limit the degradation perhaps by limiting enzyme activity to the immediate vicinity of the cell. More widespread release and enzyme activity would be less easy to control in the presence of low concentrations of α_1-AT (as in α_1-AT deficiency).

This mechanism of a privileged microenvironment of connective tissue degradation remains to be fully elucidated although it may be a critical factor in patients with normal α_1-AT. Direct evidence would be difficult to obtain but indirect evidence suggests that NE is present in emphysematous lungs and is associated with elastin (its putative target in emphysema). Such close proximity suggests release of NE at this site [120, 121], although one study has suggested that this finding may be artefactual [122]. Nevertheless once released and attached to elastin, NE can degrade the connective tissue even in the presence of α_1-AT [123]. Thus the neutrophil has the potential to degrade elastin before, during and after migration, even in the presence of α_1-AT. This ability suggests a mechanism whereby emphysema can develop in subjects with normal α_1-AT if long-term recruitment and activation of PMN occurs.

(e) Other steps in cell recruitment

Once activated in the circulation the PMN has to adhere to the endothelial cells prior to migration into the tissues. This involves the interaction between cell surface adhesion molecules, primarily the CD11/CD18 family of neutrophil integrins, and the endothelial ligand ICAM1. It is possible that variations in this response may also affect susceptibility to the development of emphysema although studies have yet to be carried out. However, indirect studies have shown that neutrophil transit times are increased in the lungs of smokers [124] and this may be related to a decrease in cell deformability [125]. The exact mechanism and its implications are uncertain, a delay in transit could facilitate endothelial adherence and hence migration into the tissues. However, patients with emphysema show a more rapid neutrophil transit time [126], suggesting that reduced deformability is a less important mechanism in the presence of disease.

(f) Other cells

Although neutrophils are the richest source of NE, the enzyme is present in mast cells [127] and, perhaps more importantly, a subpopulation of monocytes [128]. The latter cell is the precursor of alveolar macrophages and also has to migrate from the blood into the lung. The process of adherence is therefore of major importance and recent studies have shown that the adherent monocytes contain small amounts of NE and release it during the adherence process [128]. Thus they may contribute to the lung elastase load, although the significance of this contribution needs to be determined.

6.4.3 OTHER ENZYMES

The importance of the mechanism discussed above still assumes that neutrophil elastase is the major mediator of tissue damage in emphysema. Although evidence points to a major role for NE, other enzymes have been implicated in elastin degradation in emphysema, either directly or indirectly.

Elastolytic enzymes

Enzymes other than NE could be implicated in emphysema either because of:

1. intrinsic elastolytic activity
2. their ability to interact with α_1-AT thereby reducing its inhibitory function
3. a combination of both mechanisms.

Several other elastolytic enzymes have been identified including two in the neutrophil (cathepsin G and proteinase 3). The elastinolytic activity of cathepsin G is rela-

tively weak compared to NE [129], but it has been shown to act synergistically with NE to degrade more elastin than either alone [130]. This may be of some importance since although both enzymes are stored within the azurophil granule in similar quantities [131], little cathepsin G is detected even in secretions rich in NE [132]. However, *in vivo* studies have shown that cathepsin G does not enhance the potential of NE to produce emphysema. Thus it is unlikely that cathepsin G has a major role in elastin degradation alone unless its activity around the site of PMN/substrate contact is in some way facilitated.

Proteinase 3 on the other hand is a more potent elastase than NE at pH 6.5, but less potent at neutral pH [133]. Although the pH around inflammatory cells in the lung is uncertain, proteinase 3 has been shown to produce emphysema in a hamster model [133]. The release of proteinase 3 *in vivo* and its relationship to emphysema have yet to be studied.

Macrophage 'elastase'

Alveolar macrophages posses the potential to degrade elastin although the nature of the elastase involved has been the subject of much research and some confusion. An early study did suggest that macrophage homogenates could produce mild emphysema although the enzyme responsible was not identified [134]. Further studies confirmed that macrophages had the capacity to release elastolytic enzymes [135] and in 1981 Banda and Werb characterized a macrophage elastase from murine cells [136], confirming that it was a metalloproteinase (dependent upon metal ions for activity). This resulted in a long search for a similar enzyme in human cells which was complicated by the ability of macrophages to internalize NE by receptor binding [137]. Subsequent studies confirmed that human macrophages produce a metallo-elastase but only in continued culture over 24 hours [138]. This was complicated by the ability of the cells under other circumstances to produce a natural inhibitor of metalloproteinases [139]. Meanwhile other studies have shown that macrophages also produce a cysteine proteinase (cathepsin L) which has the ability to degrade elastin at acidic pH [140]. This enzyme has yet to be shown to produce emphysema but is likely to be active in the acidic environment beneath adherent cells [141]. On the other hand, recent studies showed that a further enzyme (cathepsin B), known to be present in macrophages [142], has the potential to produce emphysema in experimental animals [143].

Thus there are several enzymes with a potential role in elastin degradation and possibly an association with emphysema. Studies in lavage fluids have not provided clear evidence to support the role of any of these potential candidates. 'Elastase'-like activity has been identified in lavage fluids from normal subjects. Two studies showed that some of the enzyme activity was abolished following the addition of an ion chelating agent (EDTA) suggesting it was a metallo-enzyme similar to that derived from the macrophage [144,145], although there was also evidence to suggest that some enzyme activity could also be attributed to NE [144]. Values for smokers were higher than non-smokers [144], and although this may be transient [146] the results supported an elastase/anti-elastase balance in these subjects. There has been only one study demonstrating significant amounts of NE-like activity in lavage although the heterogeneity of the patients makes interpretation of the data difficult [147]. However, these observations still failed to explain why only a minority of smokers develop emphysema. The study by McLeod *et al.* [148] partly addressed this problem by demonstrating that macrophages from smokers, but especially those from patients with disease, secrete greater quantities of 'elastase' (Fig. 6.11). Unfortunately little was done to characterize this enzyme.

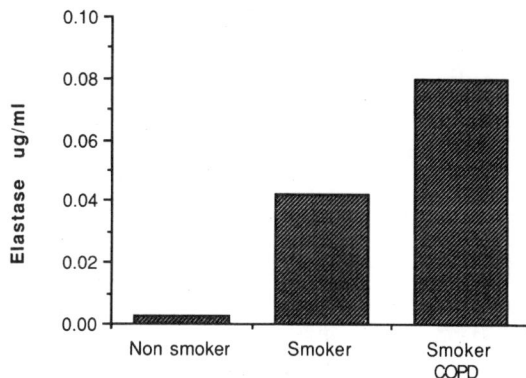

Fig. 6.11 Median 'elastase' activity is shown for macrophages obtained from healthy non-smokers, smokers and smokers with COPD. (Adapted from reference [148].)

Perhaps the most complete study was that by Burnett *et al.* [149] who demonstrated that a low level of true elastase activity was present in lung lavages and was a combination of serine and metallo-elastase possibly associated with lipids (such as cell membranes). This activity was increased in lavage from patients with emphysema. However, NE was not identified suggesting that the serine proteinase was proteinase 3 or cathepsin G [149]. Although cathepsin B has been identified in lung lavage fluids [150], the study by Burnett *et al.* [149] did not demonstrate any cysteine elastase activity, suggesting that there was no cathepsin L present and that cathepsin B may act via a non-elastolytic mechanism. Indeed the potential effect *in vivo* may be even more complex since neutrophil elastase can activate cathepsin B in the secretions by limited cleavage of a proenzyme [151]. Therefore it is possible that NE may have a direct effect on lung connective tissues *in vivo* but may also act indirectly by activation of cathepsin B, leading to an additive or synergistic effect.

Thus the nature and role of lung elastases needs to be clarified although data would suggest that neutrophil elastase has little role in healthy and stable lavage fluids. Whether these other elastases have a direct effect on lung elastin is uncertain, but they and others have the potential to affect the elastase/anti-elastase balance more indirectly by damage to the anti-elastases. Cathepsin L [152], the mouse metallo-elastase [153] and bacterial enzymes [154] can all inactivate α_1-AT as an anti-elastase. Thus the presence of any or all of these enzymes could reduce the protective anti-elastase screen thereby permitting lung destruction by enzymes normally inhibited by α_1-AT. Further studies of the role of these and other enzymes need to be undertaken.

6.5 OTHER ANTI-ELASTASES

The presence and significance of other elastase inhibitors in the lung remains a highly controversial issue. The problem has been approached in several ways including enzyme inhibition, immunological measurement and immunohistochemistry. Each approach has its own advantages and disadvantages and interpretation may be complicated by a variety of technical factors.

The simplest approach is to assess the ability of lung lavage fluids to inhibit the enzyme which has been implicated in lung damage (in this case NE). The results can then be compared with the concentration of known inhibitors, or those thought to be important, to determine their function and contribution to the anti-elastase screen. However, problems arise if several proteins inhibit the same enzyme and the function of each cannot be determined individually. For instance anti-leukoprotease (ALP) is present in the lung (see below) and is also an inhibitor of NE. Thus it can be difficult to determine the contribution of this inhibitor compared to α_1-AT if the function of neither is known.

However, α_1-AT also inhibits the enzyme porcine pancreatic elastase (PPE) whereas ALP does not. Thus in a mixture of α_1-AT and ALP it is possible to assess α_1-AT function with PPE and then α_1-AT and ALP function with NE. Subtraction of the two results would give the

contribution of ALP to the anti-elastase screen (Fig. 6.12). When these techniques have been applied workers have found that less than 50% of the NE inhibition in lavage can be attributed to α_1-AT [96,155]. Other workers have assessed samples in different ways with opposite results. For instance, Gadek and colleagues specifically removed α_1-AT from lavage fluids and demonstrated that only 10% of the inhibitory capacity remained [49]. Furthermore studies of lavage fluids from subjects with α_1-AT deficiency had little NE inhibitory capacity compared to subjects with normal α_1-AT [50]. However, this has not been confirmed by other workers where adequate NE inhibition was found in lavage fluids from α_1-AT deficient subjects [47].

These discrepancies would suggest that technical factors may be influencing the results. *In vitro* studies have shown that concentrating lavage samples (a technique used frequently in early studies) results in significant loss of protein and inactivation of inhibitors [97]. Furthermore storage of unconcentrated samples also inactivates the inhibitors [96] and would thus give a falsely low value for their inhibitor capacity. In ad-

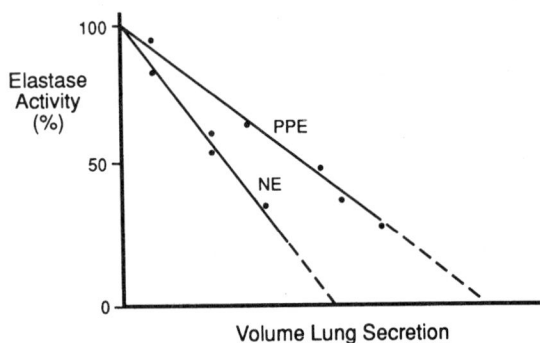

Fig. 6.12 The inhibition of NE and PPE is shown for increasing volumes of lung secretion. The inhibition lines differ indicating that the secretion is a more effective inhibitor of NE. These results would indicate the presence of anti-elastases in addition to α_1-AT (which accounts for most of the PPE inhibition). If α_1-AT were the only inhibitor present the two lines would be identical (see text for details).

dition the use of low enzyme concentration and high substrate concentration [156] in the assays used to assess inhibitory capacity also leads to an under-estimation of the true result. Finally, the substrate used to assess enzyme activity will also affect the results [157]. Thus many factors have to be considered to determine the validity of the final result using biological fluids containing several inhibitors.

An alternative approach is to purify the inhibitors and then assess their function. However, this approach assumes that all inhibitors are known and that purification procedures do not affect protein function. Recent studies have used this approach and indicated that although ALP is present in lavage fluids it is largely inactive and hence contributes little to the anti-elastase screen [158], although the reasons for inactivation were not addressed. It thus remains possible that the issue of elastase inhibitors and their contribution to the anti-elastase screen may never be resolved by current methods to assess their function. However, results from these studies confirm that α_1-AT and ALP are present in airways secretions. In addition an inhibitor distinct from, but functionally similar to, α_1-AT has been identified in lavage fluids [159] and a low affinity inhibitor of NE similar in size but distinct from ALP has also been demonstrated [48]. Further studies are clearly indicated to determine the role of these and other inhibitors in protection of the lung.

However, some studies have been carried out with other inhibitors, indicating a role in the protection of the lung.

6.5.1 ANTI-LEUKOPROTEASE (ALSO REFERRED TO AS SECRETORY LEUKOPROTEASE INHIBITOR (SLPI) OR BRONCHIAL MUCOUS PROTEINASE INHIBITOR (BMPI))

Anti-leukoprotease is an 11–12 KDa non-glycosylated protein present in a variety of body secretions including the lung secretions. The protein has been identified in serous glands [160] and is present in high concentrations in bronchial secretions where it exceeds the concentrations of α_1-AT [48]. However, it is also present in Clara cells and has been identified in peripheral airways [160]. Although there is some disagreement about its function in lavage fluids (see above), all groups have shown that it is present immunologically at lower concentrations than α_1-AT [158,161, 162]. Nevertheless its lower concentration does not mean that it is less important than α_1-AT in the pathogenesis of emphysema. The protein can be secreted from the basolateral aspect of airways cells [163] and is found immunologically in association with elastin [164], which is where NE has also been identified (see above). The protein is more effective than α_1-AT inhibiting NE that is already bound to elastin [123], and ALP is also very efficient at limiting connective tissue destruction by neutrophils that are closely adherent [165].

Thus the immunohistologic and *in vitro* studies would suggest that ALP may be an important inhibitor of NE activity in the lung interstitium where connective tissue destruction is believed to be central to the pathogenesis of emphysema. Quantitative and/or qualitative deficiency of ALP has not been verified in patients with emphysema although low concentrations were found in sputum from patients with α_1-AT deficiency and emphysema compared to patients with normal α_1-AT [48].

6.5.2 ALPHA$_1$-ANTICHYMOTRYPSIN (α_1-ACh)

This is a 68 KDa acute phase protein which can double its plasma concentration within 8 hours [166]. It is an inhibitor of cathepsin G and has a higher affinity for cathepsin G than α_1-AT [167]. Studies have shown that α_1-ACh is present in bronchial secretions [168] and lavage fluids (Stockley, unpublished observations). However, studies have suggested that lung α_1-ACh is not able to inhibit cathepsin G [169] although it is locally produced in the lung [169], probably by macrophages and epithelial cells [170]. These latter observations of local production of α_1-ACh suggest it has a major role in the lung, perhaps as an inhibitor of neutrophil chemotaxis [171]. Clearly this inhibitory effect on chemotaxis would influence the elastase/anti-elastase balance by reducing cell migration and hence elastase delivery to the lung.

6.5.3 METALLOPROTEINASE INHIBITORS

Although the presence and hence the role of metallo-elastases in the lung is uncertain it seems logical that as with any enzyme system, inhibitors also exist. Indeed studies have shown that the tissue inhibitor of metalloproteinases (TIMP) is present in lung lavage fluids [172]. This might be expected since macrophages possess the ability to produce this inhibitor *in vitro* [139]. Its role has yet to be studied although it is likely to play a role inhibiting macrophage metallo-elastase at sites where this enzyme may be destructive.

The only other metalloproteinase inhibitor identified in lung fluids is α_2-macroglobulin. This 725 KDa protein is present in very low concentration [173] even though macrophages also possess the ability to produce the protein [174]. The low concentrations are thought to reflect restriction of protein diffusion from plasma because of its large size [175]. Again its role is unknown but perhaps further studies will follow once a role for metalloproteinases in emphysema or other lung diseases has been established.

6.5.4 CYSTEINE PROTEINASE INHIBITORS (CYSTATINS)

Studies have shown that cystatins A, C and S are present in lung secretions [176]. However, the source and distribution of these inhibitors in the lung has yet to be assessed. Again studies will progress as the role of cysteine proteinases becomes clearer. The development of emphysema following cathepsin B administration [143] suggests that the relationship of this cysteine proteinase to its inhibitors may also influence the pathogenesis of disease in some patients.

6.5.5 OTHER INHIBITORS

Studies have shown that other elastase inhibitors also exist in the lung secretions [48,155,159] including cleavage products of the plasma inhibitor inter-α-trypsin inhibitor [177]. Their role particularly in the presence of other major anti-elastases (α_1-AT and ALP) may be relatively minor.

6.6 OTHER ASPECTS OF COPD

Although the majority of this chapter has focused on the pathogenesis of emphysema there are other factors often associated with the disease (bronchitis, epithelial damage, reduced mucociliary clearance and bacterial colonization) and other diseases encompassed by the term COPD (bronchiectasis and cystic fibrosis). Proteolytic enzymes and NE in particular have also been implicated in these features and diseases [178,179].

Animal models of elastase-induced emphysema also show features of airways disease with goblet cell hyperplasia [180]. In addition NE is a potent secretogogue for mucus glands and has been implicated in the excess mucus production of bronchitis [181]. Furthermore NE can damage bronchial epithelium [182] and reduce ciliary beat frequency [183] *in vitro*. Thus an elastase/anti-elastase imbalance within the airways can produce bronchial as well as interstitial lung disease.

Clinical studies have shown that elastase activity is a regular feature of the bronchial secretions in bronchiectasis [184] and cystic fibrosis [185,186] as well as occurring during exacerbations of chronic bronchitis [20]. Although the mechanisms involved have yet to be clarified the secretions contain neutrophil chemotactic activity [187] and this probably results in a constant or intermittent neutrophil traffic which, at least at times, delivers sufficient NE to overcome the anti-elastases.

In addition NE has been implicated in the cleavage of lung immunoglobulins [188] and the neutrophil C3bi receptors required for successful phagocytosis [189]. These effects may play a role in the persistence of bacterial colonization in many of the patients. Removal of elastase activity by inhalation of antiproteases improved the bactericidal function of neutrophils [190] suggesting that such an approach may have a major role in morbidity and mortality due to bronchial disease. In this respect antiprotease therapy is already under investigation in cystic fibrosis and may have a major role in the future management of bronchiectasis from other causes as well as acute exacerbations of bronchitis.

6.7 INTERVENTION THERAPY

The concept that an imbalance between proteinases and antiproteinases is central to the pathogenesis of emphysema is so widely supported that development of therapeutic regimens aimed at specifically altering this balance are being actively pursued. The approaches being investigated depend upon the pathways thought to be important and the specificity depends upon the interpretation of the evidence implicating specific mediators or the belief in more general principles.

6.7.1 ANTIPROTEINASES

At present most activity is directed at developing strategies for the protection or supplementation of the anti-elastase screen, although this is largely based upon the assumption that it is inadequate in subjects without α_1-AT deficiency who smoke or who are developing emphysema. In this respect anti-oxidants have been suggested to consume the presumed release of oxidants from activated cells in the lungs of smokers or those inhaled with the cigarette smoke. The theory is to protect the anti-elastases (and α_1-AT in particular) from

inactivation by oxidation of the enzyme inhibitory site. Preliminary studies have been carried out with inhaled glutathione and shown that this enhances anti-oxidant concentration in the lower airways [191]. However, smokers already have enhanced glutathione levels in their lung fluids [192] and thus this approach may prove superfluous. Furthermore, as mentioned previously, it remains contentious as to whether α_1-AT function is reduced in the lungs of smokers or even patients with emphysema (see above).

It would also be possible to prevent inhibitor inactivation by enzymes other than NE (such as complexing with other serine proteinases or cleavage of the active site by enzymes such as macrophage elastase). This would require firm evidence of the enzymes involved and the development of specific antagonist to be delivered to the lung tissues.

An alternative approach to the protection of the lung anti-elastases is to increase their concentrations. This may be achieved by agents such as danazol or tamoxifen and is more likely to be successful in subjects with normal α_1-AT than in α_1-AT deficiency since the secretory process is not impaired. However, direct supplementation by the inhaled or intravenous route would seem to be more appropriate. Undoubtedly both routes of administration enhance the anti-elastase screen in lung fluids (see under α_1-AT deficiency) but it still remains uncertain whether either route would lead to a rise in inhibitor level that would be protective particularly if the 'normal' levels are not. If this approach of supplementation is adopted it may be possible to use 'super inhibitors' such as genetically engineered forms of α_1-AT that are resistant to inactivation by oxidants. Replacement of the active site methionine by valine results in an elastase inhibitor that cannot be inactivated by oxidants [74]. Thus if oxidation of α_1-AT is a major pathogenic process in emphysema the problem could be circumvented by delivery of an oxidant-resistant form to the lung. Again uncertainty about the role of oxidative inactivation makes the validity of this approach uncertain. Furthermore the ability to inactivate α_1-AT by oxidation may in itself be of major importance at times when the release of active NE is a necessary process. Since the role of NE in health is unknown it is possible that excessive inhibition may also prove to be harmful. This concern is of major importance when considering the role of specific anti-NE chemical agents (see below). However, indirect evidence might suggest that this is unlikely to be a problem with α_1-AT supplementation since monthly augmentation in α_1-AT deficiency (which markedly raises the α_1-AT level above normal) is not associated with increased morbidity [73].

The same principles apply to the use of other proteinase inhibitors including recombinant antileukoprotease and chemical inhibitors. Certainly these agents have been shown to prevent experimental emphysema in animal models when administered with NE [193,194] with one major exception. In the studies described by Snider and colleagues a lower affinity boronic acid inhibitor actually enhanced the effect of NE [195]. This unexpected and potentially harmful outcome (if used in man) was thought to relate to delivery of the NE inhibitor complex into the lung interstitium and release of the enzyme to lung elastin. On the basis of these experiments and concepts it is possible to develop a series of guidelines to influence the development and choice of a protective therapy:

1. The inhibitor should be specific for the putative damaging enzyme.
2. The inhibitor should be administered by a route which ensures it is effective at the site where tissue damage is assumed to occur.
3. The effect of the inhibitor should not be excessive, thereby preventing 'normal' enzyme activity which presumably has a role in maintenance of health – indeed lack of lysosomal enzymes in Chediak–Higashi syndrome is associated with recurrent lung infections [196].

4. The inhibitor should bind the enzyme sufficiently to prevent its subsequent release to connective tissue.
5. The inhibitor should work in the presence of activated neutrophils to prevent or limit the connective tissue destruction. In this respect smaller molecular weight inhibitors may prove most effective (Fig. 6.13).

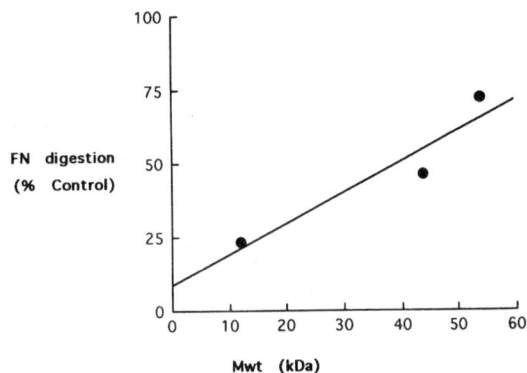

Fig. 6.13   The relationship between molecular size of the inhibitor and the ability to limit fibronectin degradation by neutrophils. The inhibitors studied were SLPI (approximately 11 kDa), recombinant α_1-AT which is not glycosylated (44 kDa) and native α_1-AT (54 kDa).

6.7.2 MODIFICATION OF NEUTROPHIL FUNCTION

If neutrophil enzymes in general and NE in particular cause emphysema, it may prove beneficial to modulate the destructive potential of the cell. Indeed this approach may be more realistic for two reasons. First, activation of the cell results in degradation of the connective tissue even in the presence of antielastases [119]. Second, clinical studies in emphysema suggest that although most patients have normal inhibitor concentrations their neutrophils show a greater destructive capacity [115].

The destructive effects of neutrophils could be modulated at several stages as indicated in Fig. 6.14. The cell could be modified during

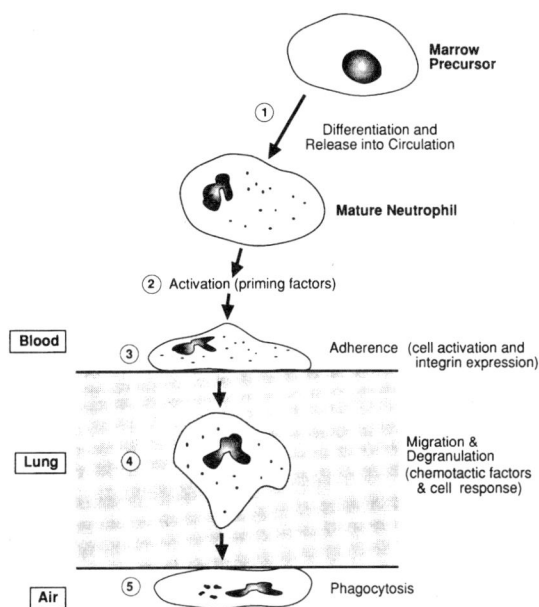

Fig. 6.14 Steps in neutrophil recruitment to the lung from differentiation to phagocytosis as part of the host defense. It is possible to modulate the process at several stages as indicated (1–5), see text for details.

differentiation to reduce its enzyme load [197]. Cell recruitment to the lung could be reduced by blocking the release of chemotactic factors, their binding to the cell, adherence to endothelial tissue and their chemotactic response. Finally therapies can be introduced that decrease neutrophil degranulation.

In vitro experiments have shown that is possible to modify all these processes although few studies have been performed *in vivo*. Corticosteroids reduce chemotactic response and this can occur rapidly *in vivo* [198]. Studies have shown that this is associated with a reduction in lung inflammation [199] and an increase in anti-elastase function in COPD [200]. This latter effect may result from reduced neutrophil recruitment to the lung, although steroids also reduce neutrophil degranulation [201] and hence elastase release. Clearly, long-term oral corticosteroid therapy is unlikely to be indicated but similar effects

may occur with inhaled steroids. Recent studies showed that such therapy reduced inflammation and bronchial cell count [202] although the neutrophil count did not alter. A further preliminary study showed that the chemotactic activity of lung secretions was also reduced by inhaled steroids [203], suggesting a further potentially protective mechanism of action. However, in a larger study colchicine (which alters neutrophil mobility) did not have a measurable effect on cell recruitment and the elastase/anti-elastase balance in lung lavage fluids [204].

Nevertheless, alternative approaches may still be proved to be practical. Non-steroidal anti-inflammatory agents can also influence neutrophil migration *in vitro* although the effect occurs over 1–2 weeks, suggesting it is modulating the cells' ability to respond to chemoattractants during cellular differentiation prior to release from the bone marrow [205]. In addition recent evidence has shown that the chemotactic response of mature neutrophils may be partially dependent upon a cell surface serine proteinase which is similar to cathepsin G [206]. Therefore proteinase inhibitors aimed at this enzyme may also have a role in reducing neutrophil recruitment and hence NE delivery to the lungs.

In summary, several agents that are currently available and other potential specific agents may have a major role in the future management of COPD based upon mechanisms that may alter lung proteinase/antiproteinase balance.

6.7.3 ASSESSMENT OF EFFICACY

Emphysema is a chronic progressive disease and it may take several years in order to be sure that intervention therapy has been effective by demonstrating a reduction in decline in lung function or CT appearance. This is of major importance especially because there are many potential mechanisms that could result in development of the disease (see above and other animal models below). Indeed clinical trials aimed at specific intervention in individual processes and specific inhibition of the enzymes implicated may be the only way to determine the pathogenesis of emphysema. In view of the large number of potential therapeutic approaches there have been extensive studies into the development of a biochemical marker that could be used to assess efficacy more rapidly. Whereas this will not replace the need for extensive long-term trials to assess the effect on clinical, physiologic and radiologic progression, a biochemical marker would help with the screening of realistic therapeutic approaches.

The current biochemical markers being investigated include those indicating elastase activity and those indicating lung elastin destruction.

6.7.4 ELASTASE ACTIVITY

Neutrophil elastase can be measured immunologically in the plasma as well as lung lavage fluids. With the exception of some lavage studies (see previously) the enzyme is usually inactive and complexed with inhibitors. The results therefore fail to indicate how active the enzyme has been and merely quantitate how much has been released. Thus alternative assays are required and two approaches have been adopted:

(a) Fibrinogen degradation products

Neutrophil elastase cleaves fibrinogen at the 21–22 amino terminal sequence of the $A\alpha$ chain. The generation of the $A\alpha$ 1–21 peptide should therefore be a specific indicator of elastase activity. Early studies using an indirect assay showed that this peptide was probably increased in smokers [207]. Levels were also increased in subjects with α_1-AT deficiency supporting the presence of increased NE activity in these subjects [208].

However, the development of more direct assays suggested that $A\alpha$ 1–21 was not a suitable marker [209]. The issue remains un-

resolved since the peptide is very labile and rapidly degrades to $A\alpha$ 1–19 [210]. Thus the validity of this marker still remains unproven.

(b) Elastin degradation products

Since emphysema is believed to be the result of excess elastin degradation, the ideal marker would be one that reflects this process. Studies have assessed the concentrations of desmosine (an elastin cross linking peptide) and elastin peptides themselves and shown that they are increased in experimental emphysema [211 and 212 respectively]. Desmosine values are also increased in smokers and COPD patients [213] as are elastin peptides [214] (Fig. 6.15).

However, there are concerns that these markers reflect generalized elastin degradation rather than that occurring only in the lung (Fig. 6.15). This is based upon the extreme longevity of lung elastin [215], suggesting that turnover in normal subjects is minimal and peptides and breakdown products related to the lung should not be detectable. The issue remains unresolved and preliminary studies with these markers continue since their validation will be critical to assess intervention therapy.

The exploration of potential intervention therapy still assumes that the elastase/antielastase balance is the key to the development of emphysema. However, although the best characterized animal model of emphysema involves elastase instillation other models also exist.

6.8 CADMIUM

Acute exposure to cadmium vapor has been reported to result in the development of lung fibrosis and emphysema in 2 subjects [216]. Animal experiments demonstrated that instillation of cadmium chloride into the airway resulted in the development of airspace enlargement [217] with some fibrosis. The distribution of the changes was predominantly

PLASMA

URINE

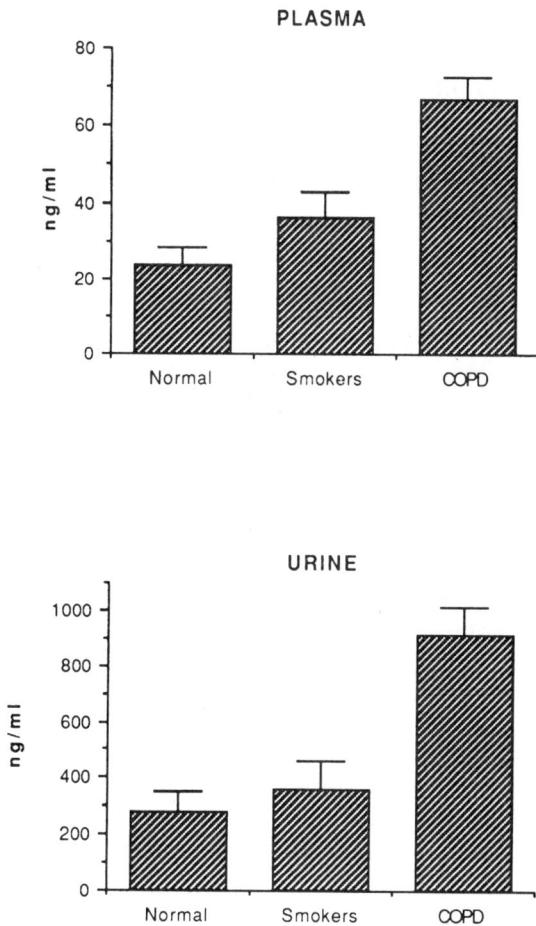

Fig. 6.15 The concentration of elastin degradation products (elastin peptides) in plasma and urine of healthy non-smokers (normal), healthy smokers and patients with COPD. The average data and SE bar lines are derived from reference [214].

centrilobular, although no loss of elastin was found. Nevertheless the addition of lathyrogens (agents which prevent the normal cross-linking of elastin) resulted in more severe change [218,219] possibly as the result of an additive effect of two independent mechanisms. In addition studies using neutrophil depleted animals suggested that proteolytic enzymes from these cells were not required in the development of this type of emphysema [219].

There is evidence that cadmium may be important in human disease other than the acute exposures described above. For instance it has been shown that fibrosis is often a feature of centrilobular emphysema in man [220] and cadmium is a constituent of cigarette smoke [221]. Furthermore the cadmium content of emphysematous lungs has been reported to be increased [222].

Thus the cadmium model may have some relevance to human disease, although the exact mechanism remains largely unknown.

6.9 HYPEROXIA AND NITROGEN DIOXIDE

Exposure of experimental animals to hyperoxia can result in airspace enlargement, possibly as a result of damage to collagen [223]. This process is not thought to be mediated via proteinases but provides some evidence that collagen plays a role in maintenance of lung architecture. However, few studies have been performed with this model.

On the other hand more studies have been carried out with emphysema produced by nitrogen dioxide. This pollutant causes emphysema-like changes in several animal species including rats [224], hamsters [225], rabbits [226] and dogs [227]. The process is associated with the loss of lung elastin [228] which may relate to degranulation of neutrophils during their migration into the lung [224]. Thus the NO_2 model may cause architectural changes indirectly as a result of neutrophil recruitment. In this respect it may be pathogenically similar to the elastase model.

6.10 STARVATION AND ELASTIN SYNTHESIS

Severe starvation has been associated with the development of airspace enlargement in experimental animals [229] with a reduction in lung elastin content. The changes may relate to disordered lung growth as a direct result of malnutrition. However, severe malnutrition in man has also been associated with emphysema

[230], although it is uncertain whether milder forms of malnutrition may be important in the majority of patients.

On the other hand disorders of lung elastin may play a role in some patients. Emphysema has been described in several connective tissue disorders, including Ehlers–Danlos syndrome [231] and cutis laxa [232]. In the latter condition elastin gene expression may be defective [233], although a defect of lysyl oxidase activity may also be present [234]. Lysyl oxidase is an enzyme required for cross-linking of elastin fibers, a process that is necessary for the formation of normal tissue elastin. The importance of this process is emphasized by the effect of lathyrogens (which prevent elastin cross-linking) in experimental emphysema [235]. Furthermore starvation and in particular copper deficiency [236], and zinc supplementation with copper deficiency [237] are thought to affect lysyl oxidase activity in animal emphysema models.

Finally there are animal models where emphysema develops spontaneously. In particular the tight skin mouse represents an autosomal dominant mutation characterized by multiple defects in connective tissue metabolism [238]. This genetic variant develops emphysema spontaneously [239] and this is associated with an increase in lung neutrophils [240]. Subsequent studies showed that the mice also had a deficiency of serum anti-elastases [241] and hence the condition was thought to be similar to the situation in α_1-AT deficiency where enzyme inhibitors were insufficient to protect the lung tissues from enzymes released from the neutrophils. However, a recent study involving cross-breeding of tight skin mice with beige mice (deficient in neutrophil elastase) has shown that emphysema still occurs and is likely to be related to defective connective tissue alone [242].

Nevertheless, these studies confirm that defects in elastin synthesis have the potential to cause emphysema-like lesions in both man and experimental animals. Recent data have shown that an enzyme with collagenolytic activity can also produce emphysema-like lesions in experimental animals [243]. This again questions the assumed central role of NE in the pathogenesis of emphysema and highlights another cell/enzyme/inhibitor/substrate pathway to be explored.

6.11 SUMMARY

There is extensive direct and indirect evidence to implicate proteolytic enzymes in the pathogenesis of COPD. However, the mechanisms are unclear in most patients with this clinical problem. This may reflect difficulties in dividing patients into clear pathologic groups or indicate that the common pathologic problem is the end result of diverse yet broadly similar pathologic processes. Perhaps our understanding of the critical steps in development of this disease or group of diseases will await the development and investigation of specific antagonists to the putative mediators involved.

Meanwhile, future studies should be directed at investigating factors which may alter proteinase/antiproteinase balance in subjects who already have COPD. Unlike healthy smokers these patients have already demonstrated their susceptibility to the development of disease. Differences between COPD patients whilst exposed to or removed from the known risk factors (such as smoking) may provide the best clues, especially when compared to healthy age and risk factor-matched control subjects. Further studies are clearly indicated but the wealth of information that has arisen has already influenced the management of many patients with severe COPD.

REFERENCES

1. Thurlbeck, W.M. (1976) *Chronic Airflow Obstruction in Lung Disease.* Saunders, Philadelphia.
2. Fletcher, C. and Peto, R. (1977) The natural history of chronic airflow obstruction. *Br. Med. J.*, **1**, 1645–8.

3. Jones, J.G., Minty, B.D., Lawler, P. *et al.* (1980) Increased alveolar epithelial permeability in cigarette smokers. *Lancet*, **1**, 66–8.

4. Laurell, C.-B. and Eriksson, S. (1963) The electrophoretical alpha-1-globulin pattern of serum in alpha-1-antitrypsin deficiency. *Scand. J. Clin. Lab. Invest.*, **15**, 132–40.

5. Gross, P., Pfitzer, E.A., Tolker, E. *et al.* (1964) Experimental emphysema. Its production with papain in normal and silicotic rats. *Arch. Environ. Health*, **11**, 50–8.

6. Eriksson S. (1964) Pulmonary emphysema and alpha$_1$-antitrypsin deficiency. *Acta Med. Scand.*, **175**, 197–205.

7. Janoff A. and Scherer J. (1968) Mediators of inflammation in leukocyte lysosomes. IX Elastinolytic activity in granules of human polymorphonuclear leukocytes. *J. Exp. Med.*, **128**, 1137–51.

8. Turino, G.M., Senior, R.M., Garg, B.B. *et al.* (1969) Serum elastase inhibitor deficiency and alpha-1-antitrypsin deficiency in patients with obstructive emphysema. *Science*, **165**, 709–11.

9. Ohlsson, K. (1971) Neutral leukocyte proteases and elastase inhibited by plasma alpha1-antitrypsin. *Scand. J. Clin. Lab. Invest.*, **28**, 251–3.

10. Lieberman, J. (1972) Digestion of antitrypsin deficient lung by leukoproteases. In: *Pulmonary Emphysema and Proteolysis*, (ed. C. Mittman), Academic Press, London, pp. 189–203.

11. Janoff, A., Sloan, B., Weinbaum, G. *et al.* (1977) Experimental emphysema induced with purified human neutrophil elastase: tissue localization of the instilled protease. *Am. Rev. Respir. Dis.*, **115**, 461–78.

12. Kuhn, C., Slodkowska, J., Smith, T. and Starcher, B. (1980) The tissue response to exogenous elastase. *Bull. Europ. Physiopath. Resp.*, **16** (suppl.), 127–37.

13. Wittels, E.H., Coalson, J.J., Welch, M.H. and Guenter, C.A. (1974) Pulmonary intravascular leukocyte sequestration: a potential mechanism of lung injury. *Am. Rev. Respir. Dis.*, **109**, 502–9.

14. Guenter, C.A., Coalson, J.J. and Jacques, J. (1981) Emphysema associated with intravascular leukocyte sequestration: comparison with papain-induced emphysema. *Am. Rev. Respir. Dis.*, **123**, 79–84.

15. Blackwood, R.A., Moret, J., Mandl, I. and Turino, G.M. (1984) Emphysema induced by intravenously administered endotoxin in an alpha1-antitrypsin-deficient rat model. *Am. Rev. Respir. Dis.*, **130**, 231–6.

16. Schwarzenberg, S.J., Sharp, H.L., Manthei, R.D. and Seelig, S. (1986) Hepatic α_1-antitrypsin mRNA content in cirrhosis with normal and abnormal protease inhibitor phenotypes. *Hepatology*, **6**, 1252–8.

17. Johannson, B.G., Kindmark, C-O., Trell, E.Y. and Wallheim, F.A. (1972) Sequential changes of plasma proteins after myocardial infarction. *Scand. J. Clin. Lab. Invest.*, **29** (suppl. 124); 117–26.

18. Stockley, R.A., Mistry, M., Bradwell, A.R. and Burnett, D. (1979) A study of plasma proteins in the sol phase of sputum from patients with chronic bronchitis. *Thorax*, **34**, 777–82.

19. Stockley, R.A. (1984) The measurement of soluble proteins in lung secretions. *Thorax*, **39**, 241–7.

20. Stockley, R.A. and Burnett, D. (1979) Alpha$_1$-antitrypsin and leukocyte elastase in infected and non-infected sputum. *Am. Rev. Respir. Dis.*, **120**, 1081–6.

21. Rabin, M., Watson, M., Kidd, V. *et al.* (1986) Regional location of α1-antichymotrypsin and α1-antitrypsin genes on human chromosome 14. *Som. Cell Mol. Genet.*, **12**, 209–14.

22. Perlino, E., Cortese, R. and Ciliberto, G. (1987) The human alpha-1-antitrypsin gene is transcribed from two different promoters in macrophages and hepatocytes. *EMBO J.*, **6**, 2767–72.

23. Eriksson, S. (1965) Studies in alpha1-antitrypsin deficiency. *Acta Med. Scand.*, **177**, (suppl. 432).

24. Mornex, J-F., Chytil-Weir, A., Martinet, Y. *et al.* (1986) Expression of the alpha-1-antitrypsin gene in mononuclear phagocytes of normal and alpha-1-antitrypsin deficient individuals. *J. Clin. Invest.*, **77**, 1952–61.

25. Verbanac, K.M. and Heath, E.C. (1986) Biosynthesis processing and secretion of M and Z variant human α_1-antitrypsin. *J. Biol. Chem.*, **261**, 9979–89.

26. Foreman, R.C., Judah, J.D. and Colman, A. (1984) *Xenopus* oocytes synthesise but do not secrete the Z variant of human α_1-antitrypsin. *FEBS Lett.*, **168**, 84–8.

27. Nukiwa, T., Satoh, K., Brantly, M.L. *et al.* (1986) Identification of a second mutation in the protein coding sequence of the Z-type alpha-1-antitrypsin gene. *J. Biol. Chem.*, **261**, 15989–94.

28. Brantly, M.L., Courtney, M. and Crystal, R.G. (1988) Repair of the secretion defect in the Z form of α1-antitrypsin by addition of a second mutation. *Science*, **242**, 1700–2.

29. Sifers, R.N., Hardick, C.P. and Woo, S.L.C. (1989) Disruption of the 290-342 salt bridge is not responsible for the secretory defect of the PiZ α1-antitrypsin variant. *J. Biol. Chem.*, **264**, 2997–3001.

30. Lomas, D.A., Evans, D.Ll., Finch, J.T. and Carrell, R.W. (1992) The mechanism of Z α1-antitrypsin accumulation in the liver. *Nature*, **357**, 605–7.

31. Curiel, D.T., Holmes, M.D., Okayama, H. *et al.* (1989) Molecular basis of the lung and liver disease associated with the α1-antitrypsin deficiency allele M_{malton}. *J. Biol. Chem.*, **264**, 13938–45.

32. Seyama, K., Nukiwa, T., Takake K. *et al.* (1991) S_{iiyama} (serine 53 [TCC] to phenylalanine 53 [TTC]). *J. Biol. Chem.*, **266**, 12627–32.

33. Crystal, R.G. (1989) The α1-antitrypsin gene and its deficiency states. *Trends Genet.*, **5**, 411–7.

34. Takahashi, H. and Crystal, R.G. (1990) $Null_{isola de procida}$: a novel sub-class of α1-antitrypsin deficiency alleles caused by a deletion of all α1-antitrypsin coding exons. *Am. J. Hum. Genet.*, **47**, 403–13.

35. Satoh, K., Nukiwa, T., Brantly, M. *et al.* (1988) Emphysema associated with complete absence of α1-antitrypsin in serum and the homozygous inheritance of a stop codon in an α1-antitrypsin-coding exon. *Am. J. Hum. Genet.*, **42**, 77–83.

36. Holmes, M., Curiel, D., Brantly, M. and Crystal, R.G. (1989) Characterization of the intracellular mechanism causing alpha-1-antitrypsin $Null_{Granite Falls}$ deficiency state. *Am. Rev. Respir. Dis.*, **140**, 1662–7.

37. Curiel, D.T., Chytil, A., Courtney, M. and Crystal, R.G. (1989) Serum α1-antitrypsin deficiency associated with the common S-type (Glu^{264}–Val) mutation results from exaggerated pre-glycosylation intracellular degradation of α1-antitrypsin prior to secretion. *J. Biol. Chem.*, **264**, 10477–85.

38. Holmes, M.D., Brantly, M.L. and Crystal, R.G. (1990) Molecular analysis of the heterogeneity among the P-family of alpha-1-antitrypsin alleles. *Am. Rev. Respir. Dis.*, **142**, 1185–92.

39. Curiel, D.T., Stier, L.E. and Crystal, R.G. (1990) Molecular basis of α1-antitrypsin deficiency and emphysema associated with the α1-antitrypsin $M_{mineral springs}$ allele. *Mol. Cell Biol.*, **10**, 47–56.

40. Cook, P.J.L. (1974) Genetic aspects of the Pi system. *Postgrad. Med. J.*, **50**, 362–4.

41. Larsson, C., Dirksen, H., Sundstrom, G. and Eriksson, S. (1976) Lung function studies in asymptomatic individuals with moderately (PiSZ) and severely (PiZ) reduced levels of α1-antitrypsin. *Scand. J. Respir. Dis.*, **57**, 267–80.

42. Tobin, M.J., Cook, P.J.L. and Hutchison, D.C.S. (1983) Alpha1-antitrypsin deficiency: the clinical and physiological features of pulmonary emphysema in subjects homozygous for Pi type Z. *Br. J. Dis. Chest*, **77**, 14–27.

43. Cox, D.W. and Levison, H. (1988) Emphysema of early onset associated with a complete deficiency of alpha-1-antitrypsin (null homozygotes). *Am. Rev. Respir. Dis.*, **137**, 371–5.

44. Morse, J.O., Lebowitz, M.D., Knudson, R.J. and Burrows, B. (1977) Relation of protease inhibitor phenotypes to obstructive lung diseases in a community. *N. Engl. J. Med.*, **296**, 1190–4.

45. Lieberman, J., Winter, B. and Sastre, A. (1986) Alpha-1-antitrypsin Pi types in 965 COPD patients. *Chest*, **89**, 370–3.

46. Stockley R.A., (1979) Alpha₁-antitryspin phenotypes in cor pulmonale due to chronic obstructive airways disease. *Q. J Med.*, **191**, 419-28.

47. Morrison, H.M., Kramps, J.A., Burnett, D. and Stockley, R.A. (1987) Lung lavage fluid from patients with alpha-1-proteinase inhibitor deficiency or chronic obstructive bronchitis: antielastase function and cell profile. *Clin. Sci.*, **72**, 373–81.

48. Morrison, H.M., Kramps, J.A., Afford, S.C. *et al.* (1987) Elastase inhibitors in sputum from bronchitis patients with and without $alpha_1$-proteinase inhibitor deficiency: partial characterization of a hitherto unquantified inhibitor of neutrophil elastase. *Clin. Sci.*, **73**, 19–28.

49. Gadek, J.E., Fells, G.A., Zimmerman, R.L. *et al.* (1981) Antielastases of the human alveolar structures. Implications for the protease-antiprotease theory of emphysema. *J. Clin. Invest.*, **68**, 889–98.

50. Wewers, M.D., Casolaro, M.A. and Crystal, R.G. (1987) Comparison of alpha1-antitrypsin

levels and antineutrophil elastase capacity of blood and lung in a patient with the alpha1-antitrypsin phenotype null-null before and during alpha1-antitrypsin augmentation therapy. *Am. Rev. Respir. Dis.*, **135**, 539–43.

51. Hubbard, R.C., Fells, G., Gadek, J. *et al.* (1991) Neutrophil accumulation in the lung in alpha-1-antitrypsin deficiency: spontaneous release of leukotriene B4 by alveolar macrophages. *J. Clin. Invest.*, **88**, 891–7.

52. Larsson, C (1978) Natural history and life expectancy in severe alpha-1-antitrypsin deficiency, PiZ. *Acta Med. Scand.*, **204**, 345–51.

53. Reynolds, H.Y. and Newball, H.H. (1974) Analysis of proteins and respiratory cells from human lungs by bronchial lavage. *J. Lab. Clin. Med.*, **84**, 559–73.

54. Janus, E.D., Phillips, N.T. and Carrell, R.W. (1985) Smoking, lung function and alpha-1-antitrypsin deficiency. *Lancet*, **1**, 152–4.

55. Cohen, B.H., Ball, W.C., Bias, W.B. *et al.* (1975) A genetic-epidemiologic study of chronic obstructive pulmonary disease. *Johns Hopkins Med. J.*, **137**, 95–104.

56. Cohen, B.H., Diamond, E.L., Graves, C.G. *et al.* (1977) A common familial component in lung cancer and chronic obstructive pulmonary disease. *Lancet*, **ii**, 523–6.

57. Silverman, E.K., Miletich, J.P., Pierce, J.A. *et al.* (1989) Alpha-1-antitrypsin deficiency. High prevalence in the St. Louis area determined by direct population screening. *Am. Rev. Respir. Dis.*, **140**, 961–6.

58. Sveger, T. (1976) Liver disease in alpha-1-antitrypsin deficiency detected by screening of 200,000 infants. *N. Engl. J. Med.*, **294**, 1316–21.

59. Fagerhol, M.K. (1972) The incidence of alpha1-antitrypsin variants in chronic obstructive pulmonary disease. In: *Pulmonary Emphysema and Proteolysis*. (ed. C. Mittman), Academic Press, New York, pp. 51–4.

60. Jones, M.C. and Thomas, G.O. (1971) Alpha1 antitrypsin deficiency and pulmonary emphysema. *Thorax*, **26**, 652–62.

61. Cox, D.W. and Mansfield, T. (1987) Prenatal diagnosis of α1 antitrypsin deficiency and estimates of fetal risk for disease. *J. Med. Genet.*, **24**, 52–9.

62. Sveger, T. (1984) Prospective study of children with α1-antitrypsin deficiency: eight-year-old follow up. *J. Paediatr*, **104**, 91–4.

63. McNeil, T.F., Thelin, T., Aspegren-Jansson, E. and Sveger, T. (1986) Identifying children at high somatic risk: possible long-term effects on the parent's attitudes and feelings associated with the child. *Acta Psychiatr. Scand.*, **74**, 341–6.

64. Sharp, H.L., Bridges, R.A., Krivit, W. and Freier, E.F. (1969) Cirrhosis associated with alpha1-antitrypsin deficiency: a previously unrecognised inherited disorder. *J. Lab. Clin. Med.*, **73**, 934–9.

65. Eriksson, S., Carlson, J. and Velvez, R. (1986) Risk of cirrhosis and primary liver cancer in α1-antitrypsin deficiency. *N. Engl. J. Med.*, **314**, 736–9.

66. Psacharopoulos, H.T., Mowat, A.P., Cook, P.J.L. *et al.* (1983) Outcome of liver disease associated with α1 antitrypsin deficiency (PiZ). *Arch. Dis. Child.*, **58**, 882–7.

67. Perlmutter, D.H., May, L.T. and Sehgal, P.B. (1989) Interferon β2/interleukin 6 modulates synthesis of α1-antitrypsin in human mononuclear phagocytes and in human hepatoma cells. *J. Clin. Invest.*, **84**, 138–44.

68. Gadek, J.E., Fulmer, J.D., Gelfand, J.A. *et al.* (1980) Danazol-induced augmentation of serum α1-antitrypsin levels in individuals with marked deficiency of this antiprotease. *J. Clin. Invest.*, **66**, 82–7.

69. Wewers, M.D., Brantly, M.L., Casolaro, M.A. and Crystal, R.G. (1987) Evaluation of tamoxifen as a therapy to augment alpha-1-antitrypsin concentrations in Z homozygous alpha-1-antitrypsin deficient subjects. *Am. Rev. Respir. Dis.*, **135,** 401–2.

70. Eriksson, S. (1983) The effect of tamoxifen in the intermediate alpha$_1$-antitrypsin deficiency associated with the phenotype PiSZ. *Ann. Clin. Res.*, **15**, 95–8.

71. Gadek, J.E., Klein, H., Holland, P.V. and Crystal, R.G. (1981) Replacement therapy of alpha1-antitrypsin deficiency: reversal of protease-anti-protease imbalance within the alveolar structures of PiZZ subjects. *J. Clin. Invest.*, **68**, 1158–65.

72. Wewers, M.D., Casolaro, M.A., Sellers, S.E. *et al.* (1987) Replacement therapy for alpha-1-antitrypsin deficiency associated with emphysema. *N. Engl. J. Med.*, **316**, 1055–62.

73. Hubbard, R., Sellers, S., Czerski, D. *et al.* (1988) Biochemical efficacy and safety of monthly augmentation therapy for α1-antitrypsin deficiency. *JAMA*, **260**, 1259–64.

74. Rosenberg, S., Barr, P.J., Najarian, R.C. and Hallewell, R.A. (1984) Synthesis in yeast of a

functional oxidation-resistant mutant of human α1-antitrypsin. *Nature*, **312**, 77–80.

75. Casolaro, M.A., Fells, G., Wewers, M. *et al.* (1987) Augmentation of lung anti neutrophil elastase capacity with recombinant human α-1-antitrypsin. *J. Appl. Physiol.*, **63**, 2015–23.

76. Hubbard, R.C., McElvaney, N.G., Sellers, S.E. *et al.* (1989) Recombinant DNA-produced α1-antitrypsin administered by aerosol augments lower respiratory tract anti neutrophil elastase defenses in individuals with α1-antitrypsin deficiency. *J. Clin. Invest.*, **84**, 1349–54.

77. Wewers, M.D., Casolaro, M.A. and Crystal, R.G. (1987) Comparison of alpha-1-antitrypsin levels and anti neutrophil elastase capacity of blood and lung in a patient with the alpha-1-antitrypsin phenotype Null-Null before and during alpha-1-antitrypsin augmentation therapy. *Am. Rev. Respir. Dis.*, **135**, 539–43.

78. Garver, R.I., Chytil, A., Courtney, M. and Crystal, R.G. (1987) Clonal gene therapy: transplanted mouse fibroblast clones express human alpha-1-antitrypsin gene *in vivo*. *Science*, **237**, 762–4.

79. Rosenfeld, M.A., Siegfried, W., Yoshimura, K. *et al.* (1991) Adenovirus mediated transfer of a recombinant α1 antitrypsin gene to the lung epithelium *in vivo*. *Science*, **252**, 431–4.

80. van Furth, R., Kramps, J.A., van der Putten, A.B.M.M. *et al.* (1968) Change in α1-antitrypsin phenotype after orthotopic liver transplant. *Clin. Exp. Immunol.*, **66**, 669–72.

81. Kimbel, P. and Weinbaum, G. (1975) Role of leucoproteases in the genesis of emphysema. In: *Lung Metabolism*, A.F Junod and R. de Haller (eds), Academic Press, New York, pp. 25–41.

82. Johnson, D. and Travis, J. (1979) The oxidative inactivation of human α1-proteinase inhibitor. Further evidence for methionine at the reactive center. *J. Biol. Chem.*, **254**, 4022–6.

83. Johnson, D. and Travis, J. (1977) Inactivation of human α1-proteinase inhibitor by thiol proteinases. *Biochem. J.*, **163**, 639–41.

84. Travis, J., Baugh, R., Giles, P.J. *et al.* (1978) Human leukocyte elastase and cathepsin G: isolation, characterization and interaction with plasma proteinase inhibitors. In: *Neutral Proteinases of Human Polymorphonuclear Leukocytes.* (eds. K. Havemann and A. Janoff), Urban and Schwarzenberg, Baltimore, pp. 118–28.

85. Carell, R.W., Evans, D. Ll. and P. E. Stein (1991) Mobile reactive centre of serpins and the control of thrombosis. *Nature*, **353**, 576–8.

86. Gadek, J., Fells, G.A. and Crystal R.G. (1979) Cigarette smoking induces functional antiprotease deficiency in the lower respiratory tract of humans. *Science*, **206**, 1315–6.

87. Carp, H. and Janoff, A. (1978) Possible mechanisms of emphysema in smokers: *in vitro* suppression of serum elastase-inhibitory capacity by fresh cigarette smoke and its prevention by anti-oxidants. *Am. Rev. Respir. Dis.*, **118**, 617–21.

88. Janoff, A., Carp, H., Lee, D.K. and Drew, R.T. (1979) Cigarette smoke inhalation decreases alpha-1-antitrypsin activity in rat lung. *Science*, **206**, 1313–4.

89. Carp, H., Miller, F., Hoidal, J.R. and Janoff, A. (1982) Potential mechanisms of emphysema: α1-proteinase inhibitor recovered from lungs of cigarette smokers contains oxidised methionine and has decreased elastase inhibitory capacity. *Proc. Natl Acad. Sci.*, **79**, 2041–5.

90. Hubbard, R.C., Ogushi, F., Fells, G.A. *et al.* (1987) Oxidants spontaneously released by alveolar macrophages of cigarette smokers can inactivate the active site of α1-antitrypsin rendering it ineffective as an inhibitor of neutrophil elastase. *J. Clin. Invest.*, **80**, 1289–95.

91. Janoff, A., Carp, H., Laurent, P. and Raju, L. (1983) The role of oxidative processes in emphysema. *Am. Rev. Respir. Dis.*, **127**, S31–S38.

92. Abboud, R.T., Fera, T., Richter, A. *et al.* (1985) Acute effect of smoking on the functional activity of alpha-1-protease inhibitor in bronchoalveolar lavage fluid. *Am. Rev. Respir. Dis.*, **131**, 79–85.

93. Stone, P., Calore, J.D., McGowan, S.E. *et al.* (1983) Functional alpha-1-protease inhibitor in the lower respiratory tract of smokers is not decreased. *Science*, **221**, 1187–9.

94. Boudier, C., Pelletier, A., Pauli, G. and Bieth, J.G. (1983) The functional activity of alpha$_1$-proteinase inhibitor in bronchoalveolar lavage fluids from healthy human smokers and non smokers. *Clin. Chim. Acta*, **132**, 309–15.

95. Gadek, J.E., Hunninghake, G.W., Fells, G.A. *et al.* (1980) Evaluation of the protease-antiprotease theory of human destructive lung disease. *Bull. Europ. Physiopath. Resp.*, **16** (suppl.), 27–40.

96. Afford, S.C., Burnett, D., Campbell, E.J. *et al.* (1988) The assessment of α1-proteinase inhibitor form and function in lung lavage fluid from healthy subjects. *Biol. Chem. Hoppe Seyler*, **369**, 1065–74.

97. Afford, S.C., Stockley, R.A., Kramps, J.A. *et al.* (1985) Concentration of bronchoalveolar lavage fluid by ultrafiltration: evidence of differential protein loss and functional inactivation of proteinase inhibitors. *Anal. Biochem.*, **151**, 125–30.

98. Campbell, E.J., Endicott, S.K. and Rios-Mollineda, R.A. (1987) Assessment of oxidation of alpha$_1$-proteinase inhibitor in bronchoalveolar lining fluid by monoclonal immunoassay. Comparison of smokers and non smokers. *Am. Rev. Respir. Dis.*, **135**, no. 4, part 2: A156.

99. Abrams, W.R., Weinbaum, G., Weissbach, L. *et al.* (1981) Enzymatic reduction of oxidised α-1-proteinase inhibitor restores biological activity. *Proc. Natl Acad. Sci.*, **78**, 7483–6.

100. Stockley, R.A. and Afford, S.C. (1984) Qualitative studies of lung lavage alpha$_1$-proteinase inhibitor. *Hoppe-Seyler's Z. Physiol. Chem.*, **365**, 503–10.

101. Ogushi, F., Hubbard, R.C., Vogelmeier, C. *et al.* (1991) Risk factors for emphysema. Cigarette smoking is associated with a reduction in the association rate constant of lung α1-antitrypsin for neutrophil elastase. *J. Clin. Invest.*, **87**, 1060–5.

102. Llewellyn-Jones, C., Lomas, D., Carrell, R.W. and Stockley, R.A. (1993) The effect of M and Z variants of α1-antitrypsin on connective tissue degradation. *Thorax*, **48**, 423.

103. Kalsheker, N.A., Hodgson, I., Watkins, G.L. *et al.* (1987) Deoxyribonucleic acid (DNA) polymorphism of the alpha$_1$-antitrypsin (AAT) gene in chronic lung disease. *Br. Med. J.*, **294**, 1511–4.

104. Stockley, R.A. and Burnett, D. (1992) Proteinases and proteinase inhibitors in the pathogenesis of pulmonary emphysema in humans. In: *Biochemistry of Pulmonary Emphysema.* (eds C. Grassi, J. Travis, L. Casali and M. Luisetti) Springer Verlag, London, pp. 47–69.

105. Morgan, K., Scobie, G. and Kalsheker, N. (1992) The characterization of a mutation of the 3' flanking sequence of the α1 antitrypsin gene commonly associated with chronic obstructive airways disease. *Eur. J. Clin. Invest.*, **22**, 134–7.

106. Totti, N., McCusker, R.T., Campbell, E.J. *et al.* (1984) Nicotine is chemotactic for neutrophils and enhances neutrophil responsiveness to chemotactic peptides. *Science*, **223**, 169–71.

107. Kew, R.R., Ghebrehiwet, B. and Janoff, A. (1986) The role of complement in cigarette smoke-induced chemotactic activity of lung fluids. *Am. Rev. Respir. Dis.*, **133**, 478–81.

108. Merrill, W.W., Naegel, G.P., Matthay, R. A. and Reynolds, H.Y. (1980) Alveolar macrophage-derived chemotactic factor. Kinetics of *in vitro* production and partial characterization. *J. Clin. Invest.*, **65**, 268–76.

109. Nakamura, H., Yoshimura, K., McElvaney, N.G and Crystal, R.G. (1992) Neutrophil elastase in respiratory epithelial lining fluid of individuals with cystic fibrosis induces interleukin-8 gene expression in a human bronchial epithelial cell line. *J. Clin. Invest.*, **89**, 1478–84.

110. Ward, P.A. and Talamo, R.C. (1973) Deficiency of the chemotactic factor inactivators in human serum with alpha-1-antitrypsin deficiency. *J. Clin. Invest.*, **52**, 512–9.

111. Anderson, R., Theron, A.J., Richards, G.A. *et al.* (1991) Passive smoking by humans sensitizes circulating neutrophils. *Am. Rev. Respir. Dis.*, **144**, 570–4.

112. Taylor, J.C. and Kueppers, F. (1977) Electrophoretic mobility of leukocyte elastase of normal subjects and patients with chronic obstructive pulmonary disease. *Am. Rev. Respir. Dis.*, **116**, 531–6.

113. Rodriguez, J.R., Seals, J.E., Radin, A. *et al.* (1979) Neutrophil lysozomal elastase activity in normal subjects and patients with chronic obstructive pulmonary disease. *Am. Rev. Respir. Dis.*, **119**, 409–17.

114. Kramps, J.A., Bakker, W. and Dijkman, J.H. (1980) A matched-pair study of the leukocyte elastase-like activity in normal persons and in emphysematous patients with and without alpha-1-antitrypsin deficiency. *Am. Rev. Respir. Dis.*, **121**, 253–61.

115. Takahashi, H., Nukiwa, T., Basset, P. and Crystal, R.G. (1988) Myelomonocytic cell lineage expression of the neutrophil elastase gene. *J. Biol. Chem.*, **263**, 2543–7.

116. Burnett, D., Chamba, A., Hill, S.L. and Stockley, R.A. (1987) Neutrophils from subjects with chronic obstructive lung disease show enhanced chemotaxis and extracellular proteolysis. *Lancet*, **ii**, 1043–6.

117. Hubbard, R., McElvaney, N. and Crystal, R.G. (1990) Amount of neutrophil elastase carried by neutrophils may modulate the extent of emphysema in α1-antitrypsin deficiency. *Am. Rev. Respir. Dis.*, **141**, A682.

118. Chamba, A., Afford, S.C. Stockley, R.A. and Burnett, D. (1991) Extracellular proteolysis of fibronectin by neutrophils: characterization and the effects of recombinant cytokines. *Am. J. Respir. Cell Mol. Biol.*, **4**, 330–7.

119. Campbell, E.J., Senior, R.M., McDonald, J.A. and Cox, D.W. (1982) Proteolysis by neutrophils. Relative importance of cell-substrate contact and oxidative inactivation of proteinase inhibitors *in vitro*. *J. Clin. Invest.*, **70**, 845–52.

120. Damiano, V.V., Tsang, A., Kucich, U. *et al.* (1986) Immunolocalization of elastase in human emphysematous lungs. *J. Clin. Invest.*, **78**, 482–93.

121. Yi-Min, G., Yuan-jeu, Z., Wei-ci, L. *et al.* (1990) Damaging role of neutrophil elastase in the elastic fiber basement membrane in human emphysematous lung. *Chin. Med. J.*, **103**, 588–94.

122. Fox, B., Bull, T.B., Guz, A. *et al.* (1988) Is neutrophil elastase associated with elastic tissue in emphysema? *J. Clin. Pathol.*, **41**, 435–40.

123. Morrison, H.M., Welgus, H.G., Stockley, R.A. *et al.* (1990) Inhibition of human leukocyte elastase bound to elastin: relative ineffectiveness and two mechanisms of inhibitory activity. *Am. J. Respir. Cell Mol. Biol.*, **2**, 263–9.

124. MacNee, W., Wiggs, B., Belzberg, A.S. and Hogg, J.C. (1989) The effect of cigarette smoking on neutrophil kinetics in human lungs. *N. Engl. J. Med.*, **321**, 924–8.

125. Drost, E.M., Selby, C., Lannan, S. *et al.* (1992) Changes in neutrophil deformability following *in vitro* smoke exposure mechanism and protection. *Am. J. Respir. Cell Mol. Biol.*, **6**, 287–95.

126. Selby, C., Drost, E., Lannan, S. *et al.* (1991) Neutrophil retention in the lungs of patients with chronic obstructive pulmonary disease. *Am. Rev. Respir. Dis.*, **143**, 1359–64.

127. Meier, H.L., Heck, L.W., Schulman, E.S. *et al.* (1985) Purified human mast cells and basophils release human elastase and cathepsin G by an IgE-mediated mechanism. *Int. Arch. Allergy Appl. Immunol.*, **77**, 179–83.

128. Campbell, E.J., Silverman, E.K. and Campbell, M.A. (1989) Elastase and cathepsin G of human monocytes. Quantification of cellular content, release in response to stimuli and heterogeneity in elastase-mediated proteolytic activity. *J. Immunol.*, **143**, 2961–8.

129. Reilly, C.F. and Travis, J. (1980) The degradation of human elastin by neutrophil proteinases. *Biochim. Biophys. Acta*, **621**, 147–57.

130. Boudier, C., Holle, C. and Bieth, J.G. (1981) Stimulation of the elastolytic activity of leukocyte elastase by leukocyte cathepsin G. *J. Biol. Chem.*, **256**, 10256–8.

131. Senior, R.M. and Campbell, E.J. (1983) Neutral proteinases from human inflammatory cells. *Clin. Lab. Med.*, **3**, 645–66.

132. Goldstein, W. and Doring, G. (1986) Lysosomal enzymes from polymorphonuclear leukocytes and proteinase inhibitors in patients with cystic fibrosis. *Am. Rev. Respir. Dis.*, **134**, 49–56.

133. Kao, R.C., Wehner, N.G., Skubitz, K.M. *et al.* (1988) Proteinase 3 – a distinct human polymorphonuclear leukocyte proteinase that produces emphysema in hamsters. *J. Clin. Invest.*, **82**, 1963–73.

134. Mass, B., Ikeda, T., Meranze, D.R. *et al.* (1972) Induction of experimental emphysema. Cellular and species specificity. *Am. Rev. Respir. Dis.*, **106**, 384–91.

135. Green, M.R., Lin, J.S., Berman, L.B. *et al.* (1979) Elastolytic activity of alveolar macrophages in normal dogs and human subjects. *J. Lab. Clin. Med.*, **94**, 549–62.

136. Banda, M.J. and Werb, Z. (1981) Mouse macrophage elastase. Purification and characterization as a metallo proteinase. *Biochem. J.*, **193**, 589–605.

137. Campbell, E.J., White, R.R., Senior, R.M. *et al.* (1979) Receptor mediated binding and internalization of leukocyte elastase by alveolar macrophages *in vitro*. *J. Clin. Invest.*, **64**, 824–33.

138. Senior, R.M., Connolly, N.L., Cury, J.D. *et al.* (1989) Elastin degradation by human alveolar macrophages. *Am. Rev. Respir. Dis.*, **139**, 1251–6.

139. Albin, R.J., Senior, R.M., Welgus, H.G. *et al.* (1987) Human alveolar macrophages secrete an inhibitor of metallo-proteinase elastase. *Am. Rev. Respir. Dis.*, **135**, 1281–5.

140. Reilly, J.J., Mason, R.W., Chen, P. *et al.* (1989) Synthesis and processing of cathepsin L, an elastase, by human alveolar macrophages. *Biochem. J.*, **257**, 493–8.

141. Silver, I.A., Murrills, R.J. and Etherington, D.J. (1988) Micro-electrode studies on the acid environment beneath adherent macrophages and osteoclasts. *Exp. Cell Res.*, **175**, 266–76.

142. Burnett, D., Crocker, J. and Stockley, R.A. (1983) Cathepsin B-like cysteine proteinase activity in sputum and immunohistologic identification of cathepsin B in alveolar macrophages. *Am. Rev. Respir. Dis.*, **128**, 915–9.

143. Lesser, M., Padilla, M.L. and Cardozo, C. (1992) Induction of emphysema in hamsters by intratracheal instillation of cathepsin B. *Am. Rev. Respir. Dis.*, **145**, 661–8.

144. Janoff, A., Raju, L. and Dearing, R. (1983) Levels of elastase activity in bronchoalveolar lavage fluids of healthy smokers and non smokers. *Am. Rev. Respir. Dis.*, **127**, 540–4.

145. Niederman, M.S., Fritts, L.I., Merrill, W.W. *et al.* (1984) Demonstration of a free elastolytic metalloenzyme in human lung lavage fluid and its relationship to alpha-1-antiprotease. *Am. Rev. Respir. Dis.*, **129**, 943–7.

146. Fera, T., Abboud, R.T., Richter, A. and Johal, S.S. (1986) Acute effect of smoking on elastase-like esterase activity and immunologic neutrophil elastase levels in bronchoalveolar lavage fluid. *Am. Rev. Respir. Dis.*, **133**, 568–73.

147. Smith, S.F., Guz, A., Cooke, N.T. *et al.* (1985) Extracellular elastolytic activity in human lung lavage: a comparative study between smokers and non-smokers. *Clin. Sci.*, **69**, 17–27.

148. McLeod, R., Mack, D.G., McLeod, E.G. *et al.* (1985) Alveolar macrophage function and inflammatory stimuli in smokers with and without obstructive lung disease. *Am. Rev. Respir. Dis.*, **131**, 377–84.

149. Burnett, D., Afford, S.C., Campbell, E.J. *et al.* (1988) Evidence for lipid-associated serine proteases and metalloproteases in human bronchoalveolar lavage fluid. *Clin. Sci.*, **75**, 601–7.

150. Burnett, D. and Stockley, R.A. (1985) Cathepsin B-like cysteine proteinase activity in sputum and bronchoalveolar lavage samples: relationship to inflammatory cells and effects of corticosteroid and antibiotic treatment. *Clin. Sci.*, **68**, 469–74.

151. Buttle, D.J., Abrahamson, M., Burnett, D. *et al.* (1991) Human sputum cathepsin B degrades proteoglycan, is inhibited by α_2-macroglobulin and is modulated by neutrophil elastase cleavage of cathepsin B precursor and cystatin C. *Biochem. J.*, **276**, 325–31.

152. Johnson, D.A., Barrett, A.J. and Mason, R.W. (1986) Cathepsin L inactivates α1-proteinase inhibitor by cleavage in the reactive site region. *J. Biol. Chem.*, **261**, 14748–51.

153. Banda, M.J., Clark, E.J. and Werb, Z. (1980) Limited proteolysis by macrophage elastase inactivates human α1 proteinase inhibitor. *J. Exp. Med.*, **152**, 1563–70.

154. Morihara, K., Tsuzuki, H. and Oda, K. (1979) Protease and elastase of *Pseudomonas aeruginosa*: inactivation of human plasma α1-proteinase inhibitor. *Inf. Immun.*, **24**, 188–93.

155. Boudier, C., Pelletier, A., Gast, A. *et al.* (1987) The elastase inhibitory capacity and the α1-proteinase inhibitor and bronchial inhibitor content of bronchoalveolar lavage fluids from healthy subjects. *Biol. Chem. Hoppe Seyler*, **368**, 981–90.

156. Morrison, H.M., Kramps, J.A., Afford, S.C. *et al.* (1987) The effect of assay conditions on the measurement of anti-elastase function in lung secretions. *Clin. Chim. Acta*, **162**, 165–74.

157. Kramps, J.A., Morrison, H.M., Burnett, D. *et al.* (1987) Determination of elastase inhibitory activity of alpha$_1$-proteinase inhibitor and bronchial antileukoprotease: different results using insoluble elastin or synthetic low molecular weight substrates. *Scand. J. Clin. Lab. Invest.*, **47**, 405–10.

158. Vogelmeier, C., Hubbard, R.C., Fells, G.A. *et al.* (1991) Anti-neutrophil elastase defence of the normal human respiratory epithelial surface provided by the secretory leukoprotease inhibitor. *J. Clin. Invest.*, **87**, 482–8.

159. Sallenave, J-M., Marsden, M.D. and Ryle, A.P. (1992) Isolation of elafin and elastase-specific inhibitor (ESI) from bronchial secretions. *Biol. Chem. Hoppe Seyler*, **373**, 27–33.

160. Mooren, H.W.D., Kramps, J.A., Franken, C. *et al.* (1983) Localisation of a low molecular weight bronchial protease inhibitor in the human peripheral lung. *Thorax*, **38**, 180–3.

161. Kramps, J.A., Franken, C. and Dijkman, J. (1988) Quantity of anti leucoprotease relative to α1-proteinase inhibitor in peripheral air spaces of the human lung. *Clin. Sci.*, **75**, 351–3.

162. Stockley, R.A. and Morrison, H.M. (1990) Elastase inhibitors of the respiratory tract. *Eur. Respir. J.*, **3** (suppl. 9), 9–15.

163. Dupuit, F., Jacquot, J., Spilmont, C. *et al.* (1993) Vectorial delivery of newly-synthe-

sised proteins by human tracheal gland cells in culture. *Epith. Cell Biol.*, **2**, 91–9.

164. Willems, L.N.A., Otto-Verberne, C.J.M., Kramps, J.A. *et al.* (1986) Detection of anti-leukoprotease in connective tissue of the lung. *Histochemistry*, **86**, 165–8.

165. Rice, W.G. and Weiss, S.J. (1990) Regulation of proteolysis at the neutrophil-substrate interface by secretory leukoprotease inhibitor. *Science*, **249**, 178–81.

166. Aronsen, K.F., Ekelund, G., Kindmark, C.O. and Laurell, C-B. (1972) Sequential changes of plasma proteins after surgical trauma. *Scand. J. Clin. Lab. Invest.*, **29** (suppl.), 127–36.

167. Beatty, K., Bieth, J. and Travis, J. (1980) Kinetics of association of serine proteinases with native and oxidised alpha-1-proteinase inhibitor and alpha-1-antichymotrypsin. *J. Biol. Chem.*, **255**, 3931–4.

168. Stockley, R.A. and Burnett, D. (1980) Alpha$_1$-antichymotrypsin in infected and non-infected sputum. *Am. Rev. Respir. Dis.*, **122**, 81–8.

169. Berman, G., Afford, S.C., Burnett, D. and Stockley, R.A. (1986) α-1-antichymotrypsin in lung secretions is *not* an effective proteinase inhibitor. *J. Biol. Chem.*, **261**, 14094–9.

170. Burnett, D., McGillivray, D.H. and Stockley, R.A. (1984) Evidence that alveolar macrophages can synthesise and secrete alpha$_1$-antichymotrypsin. *Am. Rev. Respir. Dis.*, **125**, 473–6.

171. Stockley, R.A., Shaw, J., Afford, S.C. *et al.* (1990) Effect of alpha-1-proteinase inhibitor on neutrophil chemotaxis. *Am. J. Respir. Cell Mol. Biol.*, **2**, 163–70.

172. Burnett, D., Reynolds, J.J., Ward, R.V. *et al.* (1986) Tissue inhibitor of metalloproteinase (TIMP) and collagenase inhibitory activity in sputum from patients with chronic obstructive bronchitis: the effect of corticosteroid therapy. *Thorax*, **41**, 740–5.

173. Stockley, R.A. (1987) Antielastases in lung lavage from patients with emphysema. In: *Pulmonary Emphysema and Proteolysis 1986*, (eds. J.C. Taylor and C. Mittman), Academic Press, Orlando, pp. 277–82.

174. White, R., Habicht, G.S., Godfrey, H.P. *et al.* (1981) Secretion of elastase and alpha-2-macroglobulin by cultured murine peritoneal macrophages: studies on their interaction. *J. Lab. Clin. Med.*, **97**, 718–28.

175. Burnett, D. and Stockley, R.A. (1981) Serum and sputum alpha$_2$-macroglobulin in patients with chronic obstructive airways disease. *Thorax*, **36**, 512–6.

176. Buttle, D.J., Burnett, D. and Abrahamson, M. (1990) Levels of neutrophil elastase and cathepsin B activities, and cystatins in human sputum: relationship to inflammation. *Scand. J. Clin. Lab. Invest.*, **50**, 509–16.

177. Hochstrasser, K., Albrecht, G.J., Schonberger, O.L. *et al.* (1981) An elastase-specific inhibitor from human bronchial mucus. Isolation and characterization. *Hoppe Seylers Z. Physiol. Chem.*, **362**, 1369–75.

178. Stockley, R.A. (1987) Bronchiectasis – new therapeutic approaches based on pathogenesis. In: *Clinics in Chest Medicine*. Saunders, Philadelphia, vol. 8, No. 3, pp. 481–94.

179. Stockley, R.A. (1988) Chronic bronchitis: the antiproteinase/proteinase balance and the effect of infection and corticosteroids. In: *Clinics in Chest Medicine*, Saunders, Philadelphia, vol. 9, pp. 643–56.

180. Lucey, E.C., Stone, P.J., Breuer, R. *et al.* (1985) Effect of combined human neutrophil cathepsin G and elastase on induction of secretory cell metaplasia and emphysema in hamsters with *in vitro* observations on elastolysis by these enzymes. *Am. Rev. Respir. Dis.*, **132**, 362–6.

181. Sommerhoff, C.P., Nadel, J.A., Basbaum, C.B. and Caughey, G.H. (1990) Neutrophil elastase and cathepsin G stimulate secretion from cultured bovine airway gland serous cells. *J. Clin. Invest.*, **85**, 682–9.

182. Amitani, R., Wilson, R., Rutman, A. *et al.* (1991) Effects of human neutrophil elastase and *Pseudomonas aeruginosa* proteinases on human respiratory epithelium. *Am. J. Respir. Cell Mol. Biol.*, **4**, 26–32.

183. Smallman, L.A., Hill, S.L. and Stockley, R.A. (1984) Reduction of ciliary beat frequency *in vitro* by sputum from patients with bronchiectasis: a serine proteinase effect. *Thorax*, **39**, 663–7.

184. Stockley, R.A., Hill, S.L., Morrison, H.M. and Starkie, C.M. (1984) Elastinolytic activity in sputum and its relation to purulence and lung function in patients with bronchiectasis. *Thorax*, **39**, 408–13.

185. Jackson, A.H., Hill, S.L., Afford, S.C. and Stockley, R.A. (1984) Sputum sol-phase proteins and elastase activity in patients with cystic fibrosis. *Eur. J. Respir. Dis.*, **65**, 114–24.

186. Suter, S., Schaad, U.B., Roux, L. *et al.* (1984) Granulocyte neutral proteases and *Pseudomonas* elastase as possible causes of airway damage in patients with cystic fibrosis., *J. Infect. Dis.*, **149**, 523–31.

187. Stockley, R.A., Shaw, J., Hill, S.L. and Burnett, D. (1988) Neutrophil chemotaxis in bronchiectasis: a study of peripheral cells and lung secretions. *Clin. Sci.*, **74**, 645–50.

188. Solomon, A. (1978) Possible role of PMN proteinases in immunoglobulin degradation and amyloid formation. In: *Neutral Proteinases of Human Polymorphonuclear Leukocytes* (eds K. Havemann and A. Janoff), Urban & Schwarzenberg, Baltimore, pp. 423–38.

189. Berger, M., Sorensen, R.U., Tosi, M.F. *et al.* (1989) Complement receptor expression on neutrophils at an inflammatory site, the *Pseudomonas*-infected lung in cystic fibrosis. *J. Clin. Invest.*, **84**, 1302–13.

190. McElvaney, N.G., Hubbard, R.C., Birrer, P. *et al.* (1991) Aerosol α1-antitrypsin treatment for cystic fibrosis. *Lancet*, **337**, 392–4.

191. Buhl, R., Vogelmeier, C., Critenden, M. *et al.* (1990) Augmentation of glutathione in the fluid lining the epithelium of the lower respiratory tract by directly administering glutathione aerosol. *Proc. Natl Acad. Sci.*, **87**, 4063–7.

192. Cantin, A., North, S.L., Hubbard, R.C. and Crystal, R.G. (1987) Normal alveolar epithelial lining fluid contains high levels of glutathione. *J. Appl. Physiol.*, **63**, 152–7.

193. Rudolphus, A., Kramps, J.A. and Dijkman, J.H. (1991) Inhibition of experimental emphysema by human antileukoprotease. *Eur. Respir. J.*, **4**, 31–9.

194. Janoff, A. and Dearing, R. (1980) Prevention of elastase-induced experimental emphysema by oral administration of a synthetic elastase inhibitor. *Am. Rev. Respir. Dis.*, **121**, 1025–9.

195. Stone, P.J., Lucey, E.C. and Snider, G.L. (1990) Induction and exacerbation of emphysema in hamsters with human neutrophil elastase inactivated reversibly by a peptide boronic acid. *Am. Rev. Respir. Dis.*, **141**, 47–52.

196. Chediak, M. (1952) Nouvelle anomalie leucocytaire de caractere constitutionnel et familial. *Rev. Haematol.*, **7**, 362–7.

197. Burnett, D., Crocker, J., Afford, S.C. *et al.* (1986) Cathepsin B synthesis by the HL60 promyelocytic cell line: effects of stimulating agents and anti-inflammatory compounds. *Biochim. Biophys. Acta*, **887**, 283–90.

198. Lomas, D.A., Ip, M., Chamba, A. and Stockley, R.A. (1991) The effect of *in vitro* and *in vivo* dexamethasone on human neutrophil function. *Agents Actions*, **33**, 279–85.

199. Wiggins, J., Elliot, J.A., Stevenson, R.D. and Stockley, R.A. (1982) Effect of corticosteroids on sputum sol phase protease inhibitors in chronic obstructive pulmonary disease. *Thorax*, **37**, 652–6.

200. Morrison, H.M., Afford, S.C. and Stockley, R.A. (1984) Inhibitory capacity of alpha$_1$-antitrypsin in lung secretions: variability and the effect of drugs. *Thorax*, **39**, 510–6.

201. Burnett, D., Chamba, A., Hill, S.L. and Stockley, R.A. (1989) Effects of plasma, tumour necrosis factor, endotoxin and dexamethasone on extracellular proteolysis by neutrophils from healthy subjects and patients with emphysema. *Clin. Sci.*, **77**, 35–41.

202. Thompson, A.B., Mueller, M.B., Heires, A.J. *et al.* (1992) Aerosolized beclomethasone in chronic bronchitis: improved pulmonary function and diminished airway inflammation. *Am. Rev. Respir. Dis.*, **146**, 389–95.

203. Weir, D., Jones, S., Chamba, A. *et al.* (1990) The effect of inhaled beclomethasone diprionate on peripheral neutrophil function in patients with chronic airflow obstruction. *Thorax*, **45**, 323p.

204. Cohen, A.B., Girard, W., McLarty, J. *et al.* (1990) A controlled trial of colchicine to reduce the elastase load in the lungs of cigarette smokers with chronic obstructive pulmonary disease. *Am. Rev. Respir. Dis.*, **142**, 63–72.

205. Ip, M., Lomas, D.A., Shaw, J. *et al.* (1990) Effect of non-steroidal anti-inflammatory drugs on neutrophil chemotaxis – an *in vitro* and *in vivo* study. *Br. J. Rheumatol.*, **29**, 363–7.

206. Lomas, D.A., Carrell, R.W. and Stockley, R.A. (1991) Inhibition of neutrophil chemotaxis by active mutants of α$_1$-antitrypsin. *Thorax*, **46**, 757p.

207. Weitz, J.I., Crowley, K.A., Landman, S.L. *et al.* (1987) Increased neutrophil elastase activity in cigarette smokers. *Ann. Intern. Med.*, **107**, 680–2.

208. Weitz, J.I., Landman, S.L., Crowley, K.A. *et al.* (1986) Development of an assay for *in vivo* human neutrophil elastase activity: increased elastase activity in patients with alpha-1-pro-

teinase inhibitor deficiency. *J. Clin. Invest.*, **78**, 155–62.

209. Mumford, R.A., Williams, H., Mao, J. *et al.* (1991) Direct assay of Aα (1–21), a PMN elastase-specific cleavage product of fibrinogen in the chimpanzee. *Ann. N.Y. Acad. Sci.*, **624**, 167–78.
210. Weitz, J.I. (1991) Development and application of assays for elastase-specific fibrinogen fragments. *Ann. N.Y. Acad. Sci.*, **624**, 154–66.
211. Janoff, A., Chanana, A.D., Joel, D.D. *et al.* (1983) Evaluation of the urinary desmosine radioimmune assay as a monitor of lung injury after endobronchial elastase instillation in sheep. *Am. Rev. Respir. Dis.*, **128**, 545–51.
212. Kucich. U., Christner, P., Weinbaum, G. and Rosenbloom, J. (1980) Immunologic identification of elastin-derived peptides in the serums of dogs with experimental emphysema. *Am. Rev. Respir. Dis.*, **122**, 461–5.
213. Harel, S., Janoff, A., Yu, S.Y. *et al.* (1980) Desmosine radioimmunoassay for measuring elastin degradation *in vivo. Am. Rev. Respir. Dis.*, **122**, 769–73.
214. Schriver, E.E., Davidson, J.M., Sutcliffe, M.C. *et al.* (1992) Comparison of elastin peptide concentrations in body fluids from healthy volunteers, smokers and patients with chronic obstructive pulmonary disease. *Am. Rev. Respir. Dis.*, **145**, 762–6.
215. Shapiro, S.D., Endicott, S.K., Province, M.A. *et al.* (1991) Marked longevity of human lung parenchymal elastic fibres deduced from prevalence of d-Aspartate and nuclear weapons-related radiocarbon. *J. Clin. Invest.*, **87**, 1828–34.
216. Lane, R.E. and Campbell, A.C.P. (1954) Fatal emphysema in two men making a copper cadmium alloy. *Br. J. Ind. Med.*, **11**, 118–22.
217. Thurlbeck, W.M. and Foley, F.D. (1963) Experimental pulmonary emphysema: the effect of intratracheal injection of cadmium chloride solution in the guinea pig. *Am. J. Pathol.*, **42**, 431–41.
218. Niewoehner, D.E. and Hoidal, J.R. (1982) Lung fibrosis and emphysema: divergent responses to a common injury. *Science*, **217**, 359–60.
219. Hoidal, J.R., Niewoehner, D.E., Rao, N.V. and Hibbs, M.S. (1985) The role of neutrophils in the development of cadmium-chloride-induced emphysema in lathyrogen-fed hamsters. *Am. J. Pathol.*, **120**, 22–9.

220. Leopold, J.G. and Gough, J. (1957) The centrilobular form of hypertrophic emphysema and its relation to chronic bronchitis. *Thorax*, **12**, 219–35.
221. Lewis, G.P., Jusko, W.J., Coughlin, L.L. and Hartz, S. (1972) Contribution of cigarette smoking to cadmium accumulation in man. *Lancet*, **i**, 291–2.
222. Hirst, R.N., Perry, H.M., Cruz, M.G. and Pierce, J.A. (1973) Elevated cadmium concentrations in emphysematous lungs. *Am. Rev. Respir. Dis.*, **108**, 30–9.
223. Riley, D.J., Berg, R.A., Edelman, N.H. and Prockap, D.J. (1980) Prevention of collagen deposition following pulmonary oxygen toxicity in the rat by cis-4-hydroxy-1-proline. *J. Clin. Invest.*, **65**, 643–51.
224. Glasgow, J.E., Pietra, G.G., Abrams, W.R. *et al.* (1987) Neutrophil recruitment and degranulation during induction of emphysema in the rat by nitrogen dioxide. *Am. Rev. Respir. Dis.*, **135**, 1129–36.
225. Lam, C., Kattan, M., Collins, A. and Kleinerman, J. (1983) Long term sequelae of bronchiolitis induced by nitrogen dioxide in hamster. *Am. Rev. Respir. Dis.*, **128**, 1020–3.
226. Haydon, G.B., Davidson, J.T. and Lillington, G.A. (1967) Nitrogen dioxide-induced emphysema in rabbits. *Am. Rev. Respir. Dis.*, **95**, 797–805.
227. Hyde, D., Orthoeffer, J., Dungworth, D. *et al.* (1978) Morphometric and morphologic evaluation of pulmonary lesions in beagle dogs chronically exposed to high ambient levels of air pollutants. *Lab. Invest.*, **38**, 455–69.
228. Kleinerman, J. and Ip, M.P.C. (1979) Effect of nitrogen dioxide on elastin and collagen contents of the lung. *Arch. Environ. Health*, **34**, 228–32.
229. Sahebjami, H. and Wirman, J.A. (1981) Emphysema-like changes in the lungs of starved rats. *Am. Rev. Respir. Dis.*, **124**, 619–24.
230. Wilson, D.O., Rogers, R.M. and Hoffman, R.M. (1985) Nutrition and chronic lung disease. *Am. Rev. Respir. Dis.*, **132**, 1347–65.
231. Cupo, L.N., Pyeritz, R.E., Olson, J.L. *et al.* (1981) Ehlers–Danlos syndrome with abnormal collagen fibrils, sinus of Valsalva aneurysms, myocardial infarction, panacinar emphysema and cerebral heterotopias. *Am. J. Med.*, **71**, 1051–8.
232. Harris, R.B., Heaphy, M.R. and Perry, H.O. (1978) Generalised elastolysis (cutis laxa). *Am. J. Med.*, **65**, 815–22.

233. Olsen, D.R., Fazio, M.J., Shambon, A.T. *et al.* (1988) Cutis laxa: reduced elastin gene expression in skin fibroblast cultures as determined by hybridization with a homologous cDNA and an exon1-specific oligonucleotide. *J. Biol. Chem.*, **263**, 6465–7.

234. Byers, P.H., Narayanan, A.S., Bornstein, P. *et al.* (1976) An x-linked form of cutis laxa due to deficiency of lysyloxidase. *Birth Defects*, **12**, 293–8.

235. Kuhn, C. and Starcher, B.C. (1980) The effect of lathyrogens on the evaluation of elastase-induced emphysema. *Am. Rev. Respir. Dis.*, **122**, 453–60.

236. O'Dell, B.L., Kilburn, K.H., McKenzie, W.N. and Thurston, R.J. (1978) The lung of the copper deficient rat. *Am. J. Pathol.*, **91**, 413–32.

237. Soskel, N.T., Watanabe, S., Hammond, E. *et al.* (1982) A copper deficient, zinc supplement diet produces emphysema in pigs. *Am. Rev. Respir. Dis.*, **126**, 316–25.

238. Green, M.C., Sweet, H.O. and Bunker, L.E. (1976) Tight-skin, a new mutation of the mouse causing excessive growth of connective tissue and skeleton. *Am. J. Pathol.*, **82**, 493–512.

239. Martorana, P.A., van Even, P.E., Gardi, C. and Lungarella, G. (1989) A 16-month study of the development of genetic emphysema in tight-skin mice. *Am. Rev. Respir. Dis.*, **139**, 226–32.

240. Giovanni, A., Rossi, A., Hunninghake, G.W. *et al.* (1984) Hereditary emphysema in the tight-skin mouse. *Am. Rev. Respir. Dis.*, **139**, 850–5.

241. Gardi, C., Martorana, P.A., van Even, P. *et al.* (1990) Serum anti-elastase deficiency in tight-skin mice with genetic emphysema. *Exp. Mol. Path.*, **52**, 46–53.

242. Starcher, B. and James, H. (1991) Evidence that genetic emphysema in tight-skin mice is not caused by neutrophil elastase. *Am. Rev. Respir. Dis.*, **143**, 1365–8.

243. D'Armiento, J., Dalal, S.S., Okaela, Y. *et al.* (1992) Collagenase expression in the lungs of transgenic mice causes pulmonary emphysema. *Cell*, **71**, 955–61.

N.B. Pride and J. Milic-Emili

Changes in the mechanical properties of the airways and airspaces are central to the disability in COPD. Increases in airway resistance, decreases in dynamic compliance and loss of lung recoil lead to hyperinflation of the lungs and chest wall and greatly increase the work of breathing. The unequal distribution of these changes leads to abnormal distribution of ventilation and is responsible for much of the inefficiency of the lungs as exchangers of O_2 and CO_2. In this chapter changes in lung mechanics will be considered at three stages: (1) mild disease as found in population studies of smokers, usually without symptoms; (2) established COPD with moderate to severe symptoms and airway obstruction studied in the stable state; (3) acute respiratory failure, defined as a significant deterioration of oxygenation from the chronic, stable state. A fuller account and bibliography of work on the first two stages up to 1985 is published elsewhere [1].

In clinical practice, lung mechanics almost always are assessed by simple measurements made during a forced expiratory maneuver. The major exception is acute respiratory failure in the intensive care unit, when resistance, compliance and work of breathing may be measured during tidal breathing. The relation between these two types of measurement is not intuitively obvious, although in fact forced expiratory volume in one second (FEV_1) provides a surprisingly good summary of the mechanical function of the lungs. The changes in lung distensibility and airway function which determine maximum expiratory flow will be described mainly in the section on established COPD, while measurements during tidal breathing will be described mainly in the section on acute respiratory failure.

7.1 MILD CHRONIC OBSTRUCTIVE PULMONARY DISEASE

The pathologic changes in smokers leading to airflow obstruction are thought to be predominantly in the small bronchi and bronchioles so investigations into mild COPD have concentrated on examining peripheral lung function [2]. In the early development of COPD considerable obstructive changes in the peripheral airways can be present without causing obvious reductions in total airways conductance or maximum expiratory flow, at least at volumes above functional residual capacity (FRC), as has been shown by wedging a bronchoscope in a subsegmental bronchus [3]. Consequently mild changes in lung mechanics in smokers can be detected best by tests which show non-uniform behavior of the lungs, such as enhanced airway closure or frequency-dependence of lung mechanics. Mild changes can also be detected by the shape of the maximum expiratory flow–volume curve and the response to helium–oxygen breathing.

Chronic Obstructive Pulmonary Disease. Edited by Dr P. Calverley and Professor N. Pride. Published in 1995 by Chapman & Hall, London. ISBN 0 412 46450 0

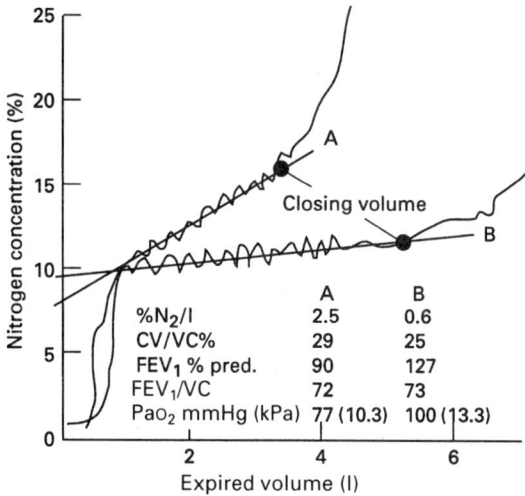

Fig. 7.1 Nitrogen concentration plotted against expired volume following a single vital capacity breath of 100% oxygen for two healthy middle-aged smokers. Greater slope (percentage N_2/l) in subject A indicates more uneven distribution of ventilation and asynchronous emptying. Abrupt change of slope at the closing volume (CV) indicates the volume at which some lung units in the most dependent lung zones stop emptying. Note arterial PO_2 (PaO_2) is lower in subject A suggesting ventilation–perfusion mismatching on basis of uneven distribution of ventilation.

7.1.1 ENHANCED AIRWAY CLOSURE

The size and patency of the airways are determined by the interaction between airway transmural pressure and the intrinsic properties of the airway wall. Transmural pressures are reduced as lung volume is reduced, but normal peripheral airways are stabilized against closure by the low surface tension of the airway lining liquid [4]; in healthy young subjects significant airway closure does not occur until lung volume is reduced below functional residual capacity (FRC) [5]. An early change in disease is enhanced airway closure at small lung volume. This has been assessed by determining the lung volume ('closing volume') at which a sudden increase

in expired gas concentration has been observed during a slow deflation from total lung capacity (TLC) (Fig. 7.1). In healthy non-smokers, closing volume in young adults is usually about 5–10% vital capacity (VC), rising to about 25–30% VC (and thus close to FRC) in old age. Increases in closing volume have been shown in asymptomatic young adult smokers with normal spirometry [6], but it is not certain that differences between smokers and non-smokers increase in middle age. Sometimes the closing volume has been assessed as an absolute volume (closing capacity (CC) which is closing volume plus residual volume (RV)), expressed as a ratio of TLC (CC/TLC). With more severe airway disease it becomes impossible to define a closing volume because expired N_2 rises continuously through the breath. The slope of expired N_2 versus volume has also been used as an indicator of disease.

7.1.2 FREQUENCY-DEPENDENT FALLS IN COMPLIANCE AND RESISTANCE

In contrast to most healthy non-smokers, many smokers show frequency dependence of lung compliance, values of dynamic compliance falling below the value of static inspiratory compliance as the breathing frequency increases [7]. This change has been observed consistently in smokers with few other abnormalities of lung function and with normal values for spirometry and total airway resistance. The implied increased inequality of time constants in the lung could be a result of changes in either the compliance or resistance of the various parallel lung compartments, of changes in the serial distribution of compliance between central airways and the periphery of the lung, or it might arise from the delay imposed on ventilation if some air spaces were only ventilated via collateral channels with long time constants. Measuring dynamic compliance is technically demanding; a more practical technique is to measure the fall in total respiratory resistance (lung and chest wall) with increasing frequency by using the forced oscillation technique applied at the mouth [8]. Because the resistance offered by the peripheral airways is normally less than one-third of the total airway resistance, this technique is probably less sensitive in detecting minor abnormalities than is frequency dependence of compliance.

7.1.3 REDUCTIONS IN MAXIMUM EXPIRATORY FLOW AND IN DENSITY DEPENDENCE OF MAXIMUM FLOW

Theory suggests that if narrowing first involves the peripheral airways, the earliest changes in maximum flow should occur in the termination of the maximum expiratory flow–volume (MEFV) curve toward residual volume (RV). Several studies have shown decreased flow confined to the lower 50% of VC in asymptomatic smokers, but this finding is not universal. Other investigators have found maximum flow at large volumes is also decreased in young smokers and even that abnormalities in maximum flow are more common at large volumes than at small volumes [2].

There is a wide variation in normal MEFV curves [9] so that a useful method for detecting mild abnormalities in an individual is to compare the differences in MEFV curves breathing air and after equilibration with a low density gas mixture of 80% He and 20% O_2. Density dependence of maximum flow (assessed by $\Delta \dot{V}max_{50}$, Fig. 7.2) is determined by the ratio of density-independent lateral pressure losses (due to laminar flow regimes) to density-dependent lateral pressure losses (due to turbulence and convective acceleration) between alveoli and the site of flow limitation. In some asymptomatic smokers there is a reduction in $\Delta \dot{V}max_{50}$, suggesting a greater contribution of density-independent flow regimes (presumably in peripheral airways) to the pressure drop between alveoli and flow-limiting airways. With increasing age $\Delta \dot{V}max_{50}$ on average does not change in

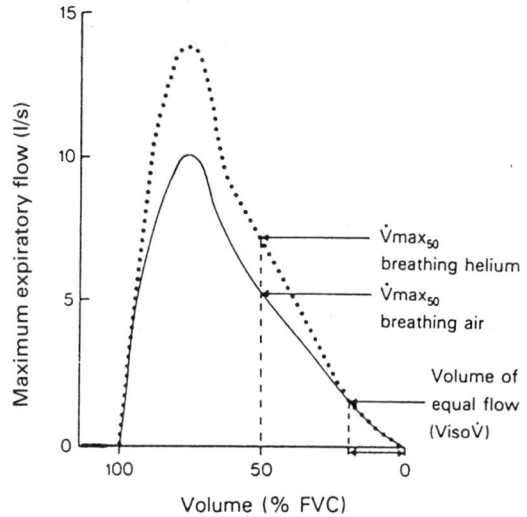

Fig. 7.2 Comparison of maximum expiratory flow–volume curves with the subject breathing air (solid line) and after equilibration with an 80% helium, 20% oxygen mixture (dotted line). Two measurements have been used: (1) the ratio $\dot{V}max_{50}$ helium/$\dot{V}max_{50}$ air ($\Delta \dot{V}max_{50}$); (2) the largest volume at which the two curves coincide (volume of equal flow, Viso$\dot{V}$) which is expressed as %FVC remaining to be expired.

non-smokers but decreases in smokers [10,11]. Unfortunately, reduction in $\Delta \dot{V}max_{50}$ has not been closely related to pathologic changes in peripheral airways in subjects who underwent lobectomy [12] or in lungs studied post-mortem [13]. Furthermore some patients with advanced COPD retain normal $\Delta \dot{V}max_{50}$ [14], possibly because the site of flow limitation remains in central airways; therefore measuring $\Delta \dot{V}max_{50}$ is unlikely to be a consistently reliable method for detecting mild COPD.

7.1.4 SIGNIFICANCE OF CHANGES IN PERIPHERAL LUNG FUNCTION

Prospective studies have shown that over a 10-year follow-up the great majority of smokers who developed a reduced FEV_1 had an initially abnormal single breath N_2 (SBN_2) test at a time FEV_1 was normal; but many other subjects with abnormal SBN_2 tests did not progress to an abnormal FEV_1 over that period [6,15,16]. With mild airway disease, certain smoking-related changes appear reversible in the first weeks after stopping smoking. Several studies have shown that frequency dependence of dynamic lung compliance was reduced within a few weeks of stopping smoking. Reductions in the slope of the SBN_2 test and in closing volume, small improvement in spirometry or indices from air–MEFV curves and an increased density dependence of maximum flow have all been described [17]. The tests used generally could not distinguish whether changes were in the peripheral airways or in the airspaces. In recent years interest in these 'sensitive' tests has waned; the proportion of total airflow resistance offered by airways less than 3 mm diameter in normal lungs is probably higher than originally estimated (section 7.2.3b) and changes in FEV_1 appear to provide an adequate index of progression of mild disease in smokers.

7.2 ESTABLISHED CHRONIC OBSTRUCTIVE PULMONARY DISEASE

When abnormal breathlessness on exertion develops in COPD, standard tests of overall lung mechanics, such as FEV_1 and airway resistance, are usually abnormal and there are increases in RV and FRC. In some patients there are also increases in TLC and in static lung compliance and loss of lung recoil pressure at a standard volume. The changes are distributed unevenly and frequency dependence of lung compliance and resistance persists. The increase in FRC potentially places the inspiratory muscles at a mechanical disadvantage due to their decreased resting length.

7.2.1 MAXIMUM FLOW–VOLUME CURVE

In clinical practice, changes in lung mechanics are usually assessed by measurements made during forced vital capacity maneuvers, with much more emphasis on expiratory than inspiratory maneuvers. The evolution of maximum flow–volume curves as COPD progresses is shown in Fig. 7.3. Characteristically the MEFV curve breathing air becomes increasingly convex toward the volume axis with the greatest proportionate reduction in maximum flow close to RV. Reductions in maximum inspiratory flow are less severe. Maximum flow–volume curves reflect a complex interaction between dynamic airway function, lung recoil and the forces applied to the lung surface by the respiratory muscles; all these aspects of respiratory mechanics are themselves strongly influenced by changes in lung volume. The usefulness of maximum flow–volume curves and derived measurements such as FEV_1, $FEV_1/FVC\%$ probably reflects their ability to integrate all these changes into a simple measurement which itself is related to the maximum breathing capacity.

7.2.2 CHANGES IN STATIC LUNG VOLUMES AND DISTENSIBILITY

Early studies with multibreath gas equilibration or washout methods established that RV and FRC were consistently increased in patients with COPD. With the introduction of the body plethysmograph technique for measuring thoracic gas volume, larger increases in FRC were found [18,19]. Originally these differences were explained on the basis that the standard gas-dilution methods only measured the gas that communicates with the airway, whereas plethysmography also measured trapped gas; however, it was shown subsequently that if gas dilution was prolonged sufficiently, the communicating gas volume in most patients with COPD was similar to that measured by plethysmography [20]. In the early 1980s various possible errors in the plethysmographic technique used in patients with increased airway resistance were identified. The major source of error appears to be that swings in mouth pressure

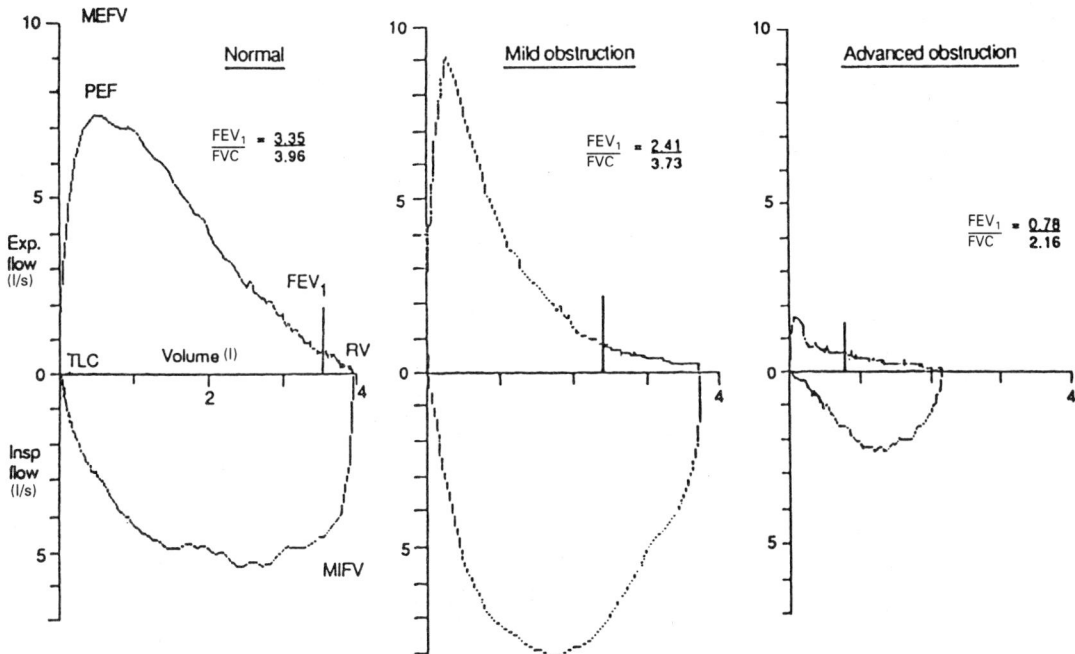

Fig. 7.3 Maximum expiratory and inspiratory flow–volume (MEFV, MIFV) curves in (left) a healthy subject, (middle) a subject with mild intrathoracic airways obstruction, (right) advanced intrathoracic airways obstruction. FEV_1 indicated on volume axis by vertical bar. TLC = total lung capacity, RV = residual volume, FVC = forced vital capacity. Note the development of convexity of flow to volume axis in mild obstruction which gives a diagnostic contour despite preservation of a large peak expiratory flow, FVC and only small reduction in FEV_1/FVC ratio. In advanced disease there is shrinkage on both volume and flow axes.

during panting can underestimate true swings in alveolar pressure, so that values of TLC derived from mouth pressure are higher than values based on swings in esophageal pressure. The tendency to overestimate TLC based on mouth pressure swings increases with increasing panting frequency and can probably be removed by panting at 1 Hz or less [21,22]. Despite the tendency to overestimate TLC with plethysmography, undoubtedly increases in TLC occur in some patients, particularly those with severe emphysema. This has been shown in emphysematous lungs studied post-mortem, and an acquired increase in TLC in life is suggested by chest radiographs taken at full inflation, which frequently show an abnormally low position of the diaphragm with loss of its normal curvature.

Changes in the static pressure–volume (PV) curve of the lungs are partly responsible for the changes in lung volumes. The characteristic changes are an increase in static compliance, reduction in static transpulmonary pressure (PL) at a standard volume, and decreased PL at TLC (Fig. 7.4). Such changes are not found in all patients with COPD and are generally regarded as indicating severe generalized emphysema. A few studies have compared various indices of lung distensibility with morphologic changes in lungs post-mortem or removed at surgery. In such comparisons, usually only one lung or even a single lobe is available; thus it is desirable to use measurements of distensibility that are independent of the volume, relative expansion, and maximum distending pressure of

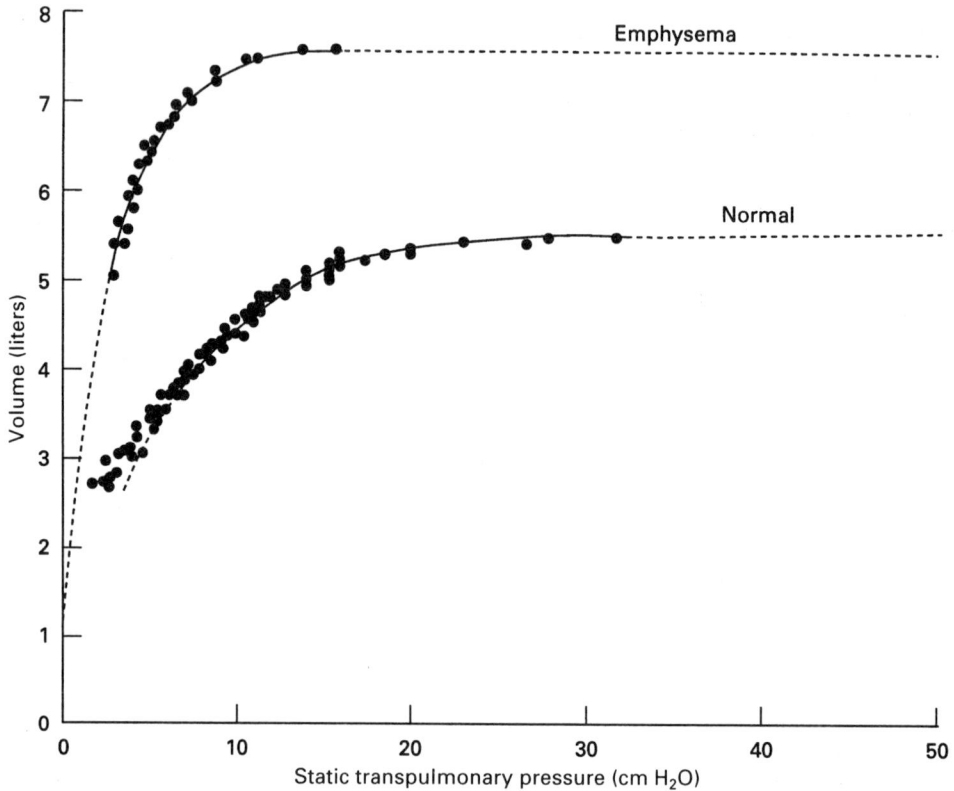

Fig. 7.4 Representative static expiratory pressure–volume curves of lungs in a subject with severe emphysema compared with a normal subject. Lung volume measured by body plethysmography. *Solid lines* through experimental points were derived by exponential curve-fitting procedure. *Broken lines*, extrapolation of curve to infinite pressure and to volume axis at zero pressure. Values of k (cmH$_2$O^{-1}): for emphysema, 0.325: normal, 0.143. (Adapted from Gibson *et al.* 1979 [24].)

the lung. This can be achieved either by measuring P$_L$ at a standard % of TLC or by modelling the volume–pressure curve as a single exponential and fitting the curve with the equation*

$$V = V_{max} - Ae^{-kP}$$

where Vmax represents the extrapolated volume at infinite pressure, *A* is a constant related to the intercept on the volume axis, and the parameter *k* is a shape factor, which when pressure (P$_L$) is measured in cmH$_2$O has the dimensions cmH$_2$O^{-1} (Fig. 7.4). The parameter *k* is particularly useful because it describes the shape of the curve independ-

ently of the absolute volume of the lung and the precise positioning of the PV curve on its axes. In human lungs *k* rises slightly with increasing age [23,24,25], reflecting increased concavity of the PV curve to the pressure axis; increases in *k* *in vivo* are also found in patients diagnosed as having severe emphysema by conventional clinical criteria, although the extent of increase observed has been variable. The value of *k* in normal human lungs examined post-mortem appears to be greater than *in vivo*, but allowing for this change, Greaves and Colebatch [26] found a good relation between an increase in *k* and the presence of relatively severe emphysema

*Despite different notation, this equation is identical with the equation used in Chapter 3 (p. 35–6).

in seven lungs studied post-mortem. Subsequent studies have shown a significant but loose relationship between k or P_L at 90% TLC and a macroscopic assessment of emphysema in surgical or post-mortem specimens [27,28] and also a relation between abnormalities in the volume–pressure curve and the mean number of alveolar attachments to small airways [29,30] (Chapter 2). That the relationships are not tighter is not surprising because the static PV curve represents the lumped characteristics of all lung units contributing to VC and would not be expected to bear a close relation to the gross morphologic changes that are characteristically distributed irregularly. Areas of lung affected by severe macroscopic emphysema, such as a bulla, may not change volume at all during a VC maneuver and contribute to the static PV curve only by displacing it to larger absolute volumes. Similarly, in centrilobular emphysema the affected spaces have a high RV and are less compliant than normal lung tissue and the surrounding lung, which is less severely affected by emphysema [31]. Despite the increase in static compliance, relative volume expansion (i.e., VC/RV ratio) between RV and TLC is reduced in emphysema because increase in RV outweighs any accompanying increase in TLC. Therefore as local emphysematous changes become more severe, the VC of these regions falls and their contribution to the overall PV curve of the lung declines. These considerations have led to the hypothesis ('the doughnut not the hole' [32]) that changes in the PV curve in emphysema are dominated not by the usually localized macroscopic changes but by a change in overall microscopic lung structure that accompanies (and possibly precedes) the macroscopic changes.

The evolution of changes in the PV curve in established COPD is not known. Because of the tendency to lose the volume contribution of the most emphysematous areas, a progressive loss of recoil pressure cannot be assumed. Studies of asymptomatic subjects with other known risk factors for emphysema, such as homozygous α_1-antitrypsin deficiency or recurrent pneumothorax, confirm that considerable changes in the PV curve can be found without accompanying severe airflow limitation and apparently at an early stage in the natural history of emphysema.

Changes in the static PV curve contribute to increases in FRC and RV in COPD and are probably essential for any true increase in TLC. Lung recoil pressure (P_L) at full inflation is reduced when TLC is increased, reflecting the reduced ability of the inspiratory muscles to lower pleural surface pressure at large volumes. Loss of lung recoil pressure increases the neutral position of the respiratory system (i.e. relaxation volume, Vr), and this may be enhanced by accompanying reductions in chest wall recoil pressure [33]. However, because of the slow expiratory flow rates caused by airway narrowing, FRC may be determined dynamically in patients with severe COPD; expiration is terminated by the initiation of the next inspiration before the respiratory system has sufficient time to reach its relaxation volume (Section 7.2.5). A combination of airway changes and loss of lung recoil probably also accounts for the increase in RV. Loss of lung recoil pressure results in airway closing pressures developing at larger lung volumes, but RV probably is also determined dynamically; in severe COPD the time to empty the lung is greatly prolonged with expiratory flow continuing at very low levels, presumably through dynamically narrowed airways, until RV is essentially limited by the breath-holding ability.

7.2.3 AIRWAY FUNCTION

(a) Determinants of maximum expiratory flow

Pressure–flow relations are highly dependent on lung volume and are best analyzed by constructing an iso-volume pressure–flow curve (IVPF) from many breaths made with varying efforts (Fig. 7.5) [34]. Ideally such curves are constructed at the same thoracic gas volume (as measured in a variable-volume body plethysmograph) rather than at a particular expired volume below TLC because the hyperinflation and reduced expiratory flow in patients with severe airflow limitation results in reduction in thoracic gas volume due to gas compression on forceful expiration being large in relation to the volume expired at the mouth [35]. IVPF curves based on thoracic gas volume usually show a plateau of flow in both normal subjects and patients with COPD at mid-VC. Compared with normal subjects, patients show a reduced maximum expiratory flow, the plateau of maximum expiratory flow is reached at lower driving pressure, and the $\Delta \dot{V}/\Delta P$ slope (conductance, G) is reduced at low flow (Fig. 7.5) [34,36]. This initial $\Delta \dot{V}/\Delta P$ slope is related to the overall static dimensions of the airways. Often there is also a reduced lung recoil pressure. A further difference from normal subjects is that plateaux of maximum expiratory flow develop at large lung volumes. Changes on the inspiratory limb of the IVPF

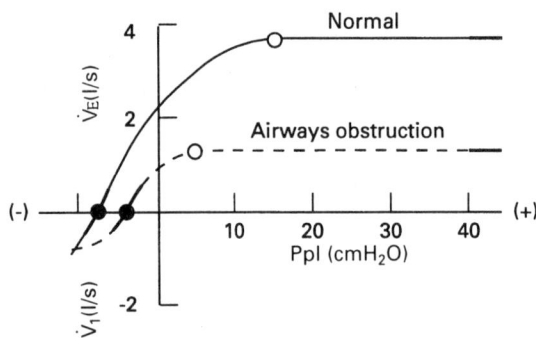

Fig. 7.5 Schematic isovolume pressure–flow (IVPF) curves at 50% VC for normal subject and patient with COPD. Compared with normal subject, in COPD airway conductance at low flow (-●-), the lowest pleural pressure (Ppl) at which maximum flow is achieved (○), maximum expiratory flow (–), and lung recoil pressure (indicated by distance from ● to zero Ppl) are all reduced. $\dot{V}E$ expiratory flow: $\dot{V}I$ inspiratory flow. There is no plateau of maximum inspiratory flow in either normal subject or COPD patients.

curve are less striking and both in normal subjects and patients with COPD maximum inspiratory flow does not show a plateau, the highest values being associated with the most negative pleural pressure.

As implied by such IVPF curves, the factors determining maximum flow are only indirectly related to the overall static dimensions of the airways. The airway narrowing found at low flow rates (or during breath holding) results from disease of the airway wall or lumen or from loss of the normal forces distending the airways. Additional dynamic narrowing of the airways develops on forced expiration. In normal subjects pressure losses down the airways on expiration reduce airway-distending pressures below the pressure present at the same lung volume during breath holding or inspiration. This leads to dynamic narrowing of all intrathoracic airways, which is most pronounced in the large intrathoracic airways. In COPD reduction in lung recoil pressure (reducing extra-airway distending pressure and effective driving pressure) and airway narrowing (increasing pressure losses down the airways for a given flow) both enhance dynamic narrowing of large intrathoracic airways on expiration. Hence the enhanced dynamic compression of central airways found in COPD does not necessarily indicate altered compliance of these airways (although atrophic changes and loss of cartilage have been described) but is commonly due to more peripheral airway or air space disease. The functional consequence of these dynamic effects is much greater reduction in maximum expiratory flow than in maximum inspiratory flow.

The role of loss of lung recoil in reducing maximum expiratory flow can be assessed by examining the relation between maximum expiratory flow and static transpulmonary pressure (syn. lung recoil pressure) curves (Fig. 7.6) [36,37,38]. In a few patients with mild or moderate airflow limitation, the relation between maximum expiratory flow ($\dot{V}max$)

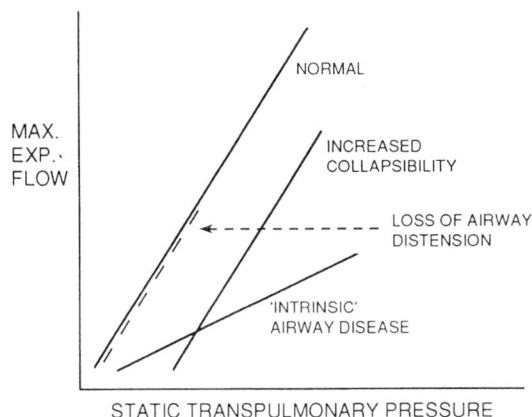

Fig. 7.6 Schematic changes in maximum expiratory flow versus lung recoil pressure curves. With loss of lung recoil pressure (----) the flow–pressure slope remains normal but is truncated at high pressures; with intrinsic airway obstruction the slope is reduced but points to the origin. With increased airway collapsibility the flow–pressure slope may be normal but displaced to higher pressures with an intercept on the pressure axis. Commonly in COPD the flow–pressure curve has both a positive pressure intercept and a reduced slope.

and lung recoil pressure (P_L) remains normal and the upstream conductance ($\dot{V}max/P_L$) remains normal. These patients usually have other evidence of emphysema (Chapter 3). When airflow limitation is more severe (FEV_1 <50% predicted value), maximum flow is almost always reduced at a standard lung recoil pressure (decrease in upstream conductance) [38]. This could be a result of any pathologic change that reduces the total cross-sectional area of the static lumen of the airways; in addition, an enhanced collapsibility of airways at or on the alveolar side of flow-limiting segments could have a similar effect even if resting dimensions are normal.

(i) Site of expiratory flow limitation

In normal subjects measurements of intrabronchial pressure suggest that equal pressure points (points in the tracheobronchial tree where lateral airway pressure equals pleural surface pressure) are in the central intrathoracic airways until ~ 75% of VC has been expired; at smaller lung volumes, equal pressure points move toward the periphery of the lung beyond the large bronchi·in which luminal pressure measurements are possible [39]. Probably there is a similar change in the sites of flow limitation. In patients with COPD, Macklem *et al.* [40] found variable results with some subjects in whom equal pressure points were in central airways over much of the VC, whereas in others equal pressure points were in airways peripheral to the bronchial catheter even at volumes >50% VC.

As discussed above, there is an analogous variability in the density dependence of maximum expiratory flow in COPD [14]. Overall, preservation of density dependence becomes increasingly uncommon as expiratory airflow limitation becomes more severe; nevertheless density dependence is preserved in a minority of patients, possibly because central airways are flow-limiting.

(b) Determinants of conductance at low flow

The relation between flow rate ($\dot{V}$) and driving pressure (alveolar pressure Palv) at low flow, shown in Fig. 7.5, corresponds to the airway conductance measured by shallow panting in a body plethysmograph. Reduced conductance, as found in COPD, indicates a reduction in overall airway dimensions under near-static conditions, which may be due to intrinsic disease of the airway wall or lumen or to loss of the normal forces distending the airways. The latter forces are closely related to lung recoil pressure. In theory, it is possible to dissect out the roles of intrinsic airway abnormality and loss of recoil by determining the conductance/lung recoil ratio at FRC. In practice a much better resolution can be obtained by studying the relation between conductance and lung recoil pressure over a range of lung volumes, because the increase

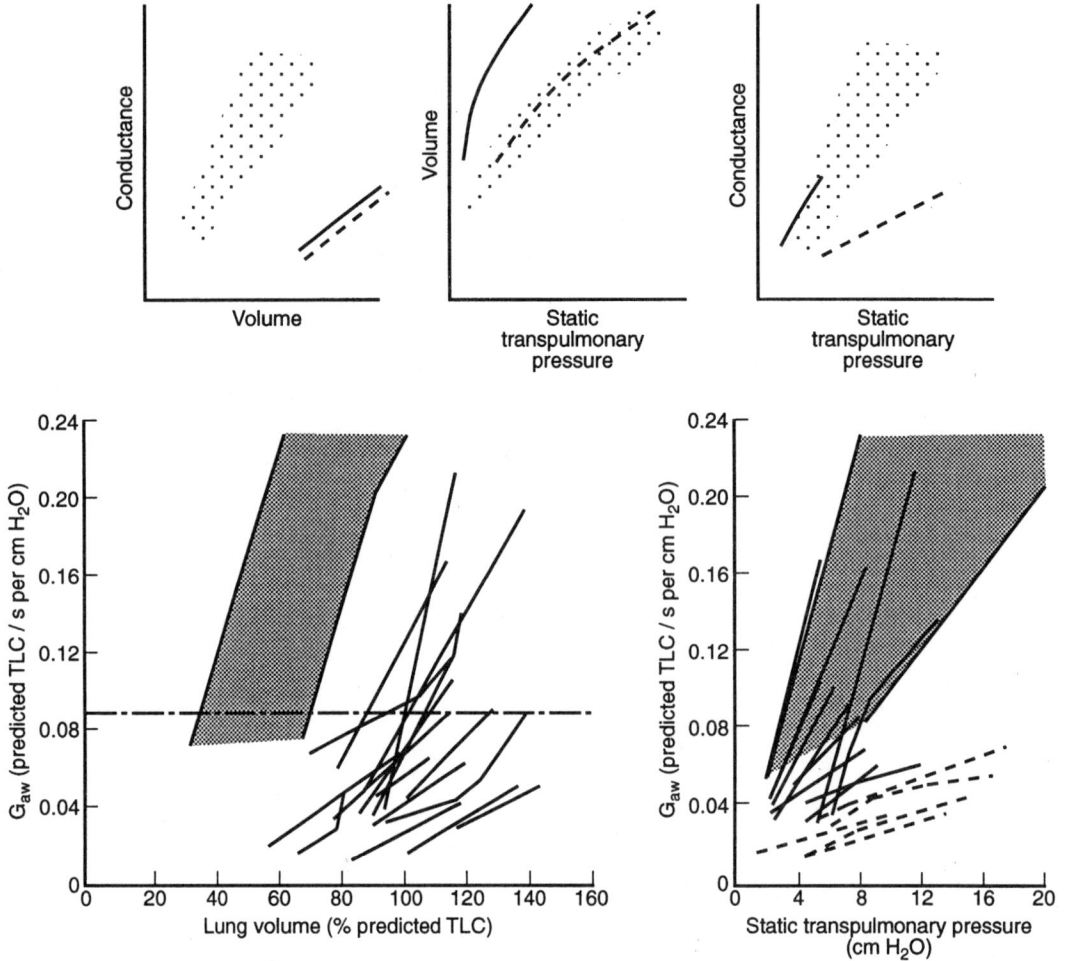

Fig. 7.7 Different mechanisms of reduction in airway conductance in chronic obstructive pulmonary disease (COPD). *Top*: Schematic diagram: At a given lung volume, conductance is reduced both with loss of lung recoil pressure (*solid lines*) and with intrinsic airway disease (*broken lines*), but when loss of lung recoil pressure is the only abnormality the conductance-static transpulmonary pressure curve may lie in normal range (*stippled area*). *Bottom* (*left*): conductance (Gaw) vs lung volume plots, horizontal interrupted line indicates a normal value of Gaw at FRC), (*right*) conductance vs static transpulmonary pressure in 17 patients with COPD. Shaded area represents normal range. Both Gaw and lung volume are corrected for height and gender by expressing as predicted TLC. (Data slightly redrawn from Leaver *et al.* [38].)

in lung recoil pressure as lung volume is increased is a major determinant of the normal increase in conductance as the lung is inflated (Fig. 7.7) [19,38,41]. The characteristic change in COPD is a reduced conductance/volume slope; however, in some patients, the relation between conductance and lung recoil pressure is normal, the abnormality in conductance being explained by loss of lung recoil (Fig. 7.7) [38,41]. Such patients usually show radiologic and functional evidence of emphysema. But in most patients with severe COPD, conductance is reduced at a standard lung recoil pressure and abnormality of the airways is present. The precise airway abnormality cannot be deduced; a reduced conductance/lung recoil slope could be caused by loss of parallel airways, smaller dimensions of the airways at low distending pressure, or reduced airway compliance.

Because of the linear relation between conductance and lung recoil, conductance ($\Delta\dot{V}/\Delta PL$) is the most appropriate measurement for this analysis. In clinical use, however, PL is usually not measured and allowance is made for the effect of lung volume. Specific airways conductance (SGaw) is usually measured; SGaw does not completely correct for the effect of lung volume because the conductance/volume slope usually intercepts at RV on the volume axis (Fig. 7.7). There are practical problems in measuring pressure–flow relations during panting in patients with COPD because of looping of these plots, particularly on expiration; in experimental studies pressure–flow relations are usually assessed at 0–0.5 1/s on inspiration. Another problem is that frequency dependence of pressure–flow relations – usually shown by a decline in resistance as breathing frequency – is increased in COPD [43]; even at the usual panting frequency of 1–2 Hz, differences in resistance between normal subjects and patients with COPD are less than during tidal breathing. Hence the measurement of resistance or conductance in practice does not provide a simple summary of airway function in established COPD.

(i)Site of increased airways resistance

Because resistance of the different serial generations of airways can be added to give the total airway resistance the important sites of airway narrowing can be assessed more easily in terms of resistance ($\Delta P/\Delta\dot{V}$) than of conductance ($\Delta\dot{V}/\Delta P$). Hogg, Macklem and Thurlbeck [44] studied the site of static intrinsic narrowing of the airways in nine post-mortem lungs from patients who died of COPD. Total airway resistance was measured by forced oscillation at the airway opening and was partitioned with the retrograde-catheter technique into that due to airways with diameters either larger or smaller than 2–3 mm. At low flows and at a lung recoil pressure of $5\,cmH_2O$, most of the increase in resistance lay in the peripheral airways of <2–3 mm diameter. The increase in resistance was present on inspiration as well as expiration, indicating that it was due to morphologic changes in the peripheral airways and not due to a 'check-valve' phenomenon.

Central airways resistance was only increased in three of the lungs and in each case there was also a proportionately greater increase in peripheral airway resistance. The proportion of the total airflow resistance accounted for by peripheral airways was very high at all lung volumes and averaged 75% at a lung recoil pressure of $5\,cmH_2O$. Subsequent studies of excised human lungs at post-mortem [45,46,47] have confirmed the conclusion of Hogg and colleagues that at low flows the predominant increase in resistance in lungs from patients dying from COPD was in the peripheral airways. Recent *in vivo* studies with an intrabronchial catheter have confirmed these results, resistance of airways smaller than 3 mm diameter contributing more than 50% of total pulmonary resistance in patients with COPD compared with about 25% in normal subjects [48].

These studies have important implications for the interpretation of changes in resistance (measured at low flow) in COPD. In life there is also a labile component to resistance, presumably due to bronchial muscle contraction or mucosal edema as shown by response to bronchodilator drugs or increased inspired O_2. This change probably involves more central airways. Nevertheless available evidence suggests that when total airway resistance is increased it is mainly due to a very large increase in peripheral airway resistance, implying that the hypertrophy of mucous glands in the central airways usually found in COPD does not lead to significant luminal narrowing.

(ii) Collateral ventilation

In advanced COPD many airways can be completely occluded. This would be expected to lead to the development of atelectasis or non-ventilated airspaces acting as effective right-to-left shunt. Yet neither atelectasis nor increase in shunt are features of advanced COPD except in patients in acute respiratory failure (Chapter 8); this is probably due to a reduction in the resistance to collateral ventilation related to the increase in FRC and destruction of alveolar walls in emphysema [49,50].

(c) Summary

The usual major site of fixed airway narrowing in COPD appears to be the peripheral airways of <2–3 mm diameter. There may be individual patients in whom obstructive changes in the central airways are of greater importance. Loss of lung recoil plays a role in many patients (particularly those with emphysema) by reducing the distending force on all intrathoracic airways, but is rarely the sole cause of severe airflow limitation. Static airway narrowing due to intrinsic disease of the airways and loss of lung recoil both enhance expiratory dynamic compression so that flow limitation develops at lower driving pressures and flows. In addition, atrophic changes in the airways and loss of support from surrounding lung may alter airway compliance, enhancing dynamic compression and the development of flow limitation. The site of flow limitation in the upper part of the VC may be more peripheral in many patients with COPD than in normal subjects. The large differences between maximum inspiratory and maximum expiratory flow at the same lung volume (far in excess of the expected hysteresis of airway dimensions and lung recoil pressure) emphasize the large role of dynamic factors in determining expiratory airflow limitation.

Tests of overall airway function such as airways conductance or FEV_1 reflect the predominant serial site of airway narrowing. Because of the low resistance of peripheral airways in normal lungs, for the past 20 years such tests have been correctly regarded as mainly reflecting large airway function in *normal* subjects even though more recent estimates of serial distribution of airway resistance in normal lungs also suggest that the peripheral airways are not quite so 'silent' as originally suggested. But when the predominant site of airway narrowing is in peripheral airways, as in COPD, this is reflected in reduced values of conductance and FEV_1. This is clearly indicated by the original studies of the lungs studied at necropsy by Hogg *et al.* and characterized by increased peripheral airway resistance; the patients in life had had severe reductions in FEV_1.

Reductions in tests of overall airway function in COPD breathing air do not provide any evidence on whether large or small airways are the site of increased resistance. Indeed the value of the FEV_1 in assessing the abnormality of lung mechanics is that it 'integrates' information on dynamic dimensions of *all* generations of airways and changes in lung recoil, providing a summary of lung size and the maximum rate of lung emptying. In practice, FEV_1 is the most consistent and important indicator of disability and prognosis.

7.2.4 CONTRIBUTIONS OF EMPHYSEMA AND INTRINSIC DISEASE OF THE AIRWAYS TO ALTERATIONS IN LUNG MECHANICS

Many studies of lung mechanics in COPD have attempted to distinguish changes due to primary disease of the airways from those due to emphysematous changes in the terminal bronchioles and air spaces. The most characteristic change in lung mechanics associated with severe emphysema is marked loss of recoil pressure but patients with

COPD thought to be due to primary bronchial disease also show some loss of lung recoil and increase in TLC [42]. It is not clear whether this is because of a direct effect of airway obstruction alone or whether it reflects the presence of lesser degrees of emphysema among patients thought on clinical and functional grounds to have primary airway disease. In general, emphysema becomes increasingly common and severe as airways obstruction worsens in COPD. As discussed above, some patients thought to have emphysema have shown preservation of a normal relation between total lung conductance and lung recoil pressure (Fig. 7.7) [38,41] and, less commonly, between maximum expiratory flow and lung recoil pressure [38,42]. Usually, however, emphysema and intrinsic disease of the airways coexist and both relations are abnormal. Thus only the minority of patients with predominant emphysema and little intrinsic

disease of the airways would be expected to show a normal relation between lung recoil and conductance or maximum flow.

Characteristically patients with severe airflow limitation who develop chronic hypercapnia show low values of dynamic lung compliance, have an increased inspiratory flow resistance, and a small tidal volume during resting breathing. These changes have been claimed to be characteristic of intrinsic disease of the airways rather than emphysema.

7.2.5 FLOW, VOLUME, AND PRESSURE DURING TIDAL BREATHING AT REST

(a) Pattern of breathing

Although minute ventilation at rest in patients with severe airflow limitation is usually normal or slightly increased, this requires considerable adjustments in respiratory muscle

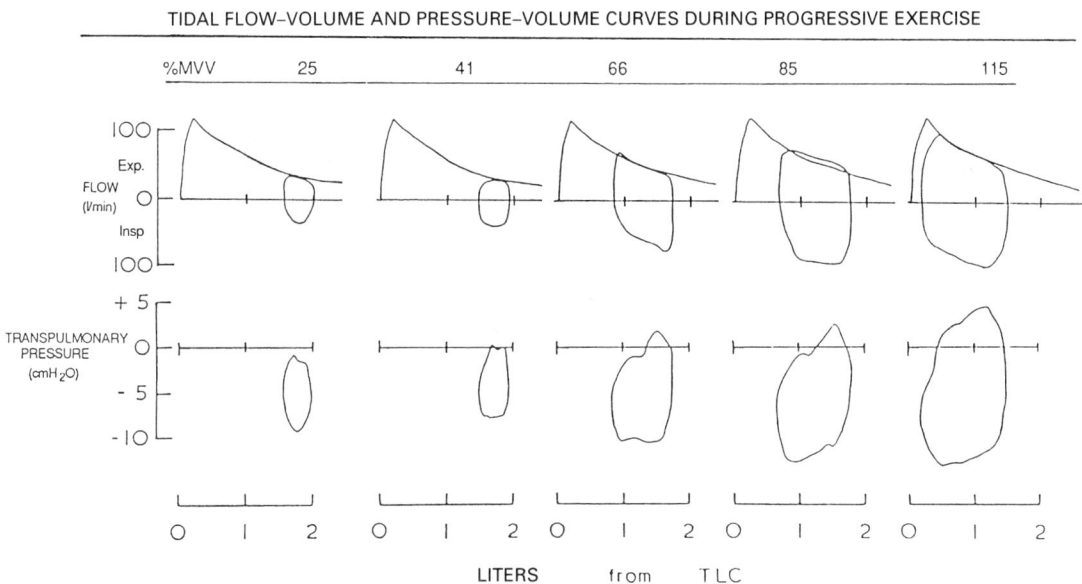

Fig. 7.8 Evolution of tidal flow–volume loops (*top series*) and tidal pleural pressure–volume loops (*bottom series*) as exercise increases in intensity. Tidal flow–volume loops are shown in relation to the subject's complete maximum expiratory flow–volume curve. The numbers show the associated minute ventilation (expressed as a percentage of the predicted maximum breathing capacity) and indicate the intensity of exercise load.

activation. The most obvious requirement is increased swings in pleural pressure to overcome increased airflow resistance and reduced dynamic compliance. However, there are also alterations in breathing pattern so that any increase in ventilation tends to be produced by increase in frequency rather than tidal volume (VT) [51], whereas inspiratory time (TI) in some patients is a lower proportion of total breath duration (TTOT) [52]. Furthermore, inspiration is initiated from an increased FRC, which may partly be determined by dynamic factors. These altered patterns of breathing ultimately depend on neurologic control mechanisms but are clearly constrained by the alterations in lung mechanics, particularly expiratory flow limitation. When maximum expiratory flow is severely reduced, expiratory flow during tidal breathing reaches maximum levels (Fig. 7.8). The effects of expiratory flow limitation may be slightly reduced both by decreasing TI/TTOT (thus allowing more time for expiration) and (more importantly) by breathing tidally at larger lung volumes, where airway size, and consequently maximum expiratory flow, is greater. However, both these adaptations increase the work of the inspiratory muscles – the former by increasing the mean inspiratory flow needed to sustain a given total ventilation, the latter by increasing the elastic work required to inflate the lungs and chest wall.

Thus, although airflow limitation is predominantly expiratory, compensation is achieved by increased work by the inspiratory muscles; most of the increased tidal swings in pleural (esophageal) pressures in these patients are inspiratory.

Some patients with severe COPD reduce their tidal volume and hypoventilate. This results in chronic hypercapnia. The rapid shallow breathing pattern observed in the hypercapnic COPD patients has in the past been regarded as an adaptive strategy used to prevent inspiratory muscle fatigue [53]. Recent studies do not support this contention [54].

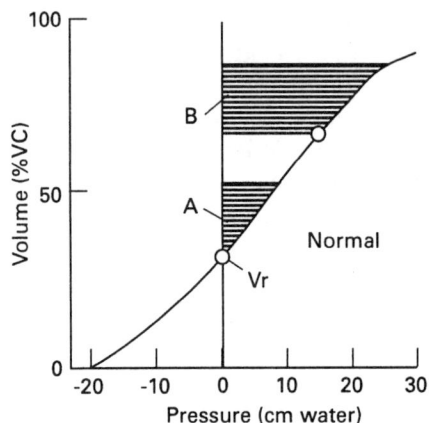

Fig. 7.9 Volume–pressure diagram of the relaxed respiratory system showing the increase in static elastic work caused by dynamic hyperinflation. VC, vital capacity; Vr, relaxation volume of the respiratory system. *Hatched area A*, elastic work for a breath that starts from relaxation volume. *Hatched area B*, elastic work for a similar breath that starts from a volume 29% VC higher than Vr. In case B, the intrinsic PEEP is 15 cmH$_2$O, as indicated by the upper circle, and WPEEPi is given by PEEPi × tidal volume.

(b) Dynamic hyperinflation

In normal subjects at rest, the end-expiratory lung volume (functional residual capacity, FRC) corresponds to the relaxation volume (Vr) of the respiratory system, i.e. the lung volume at which the elastic recoil pressure of the total respiratory system is zero (Fig. 7.9). Pulmonary hyperinflation is defined as an increase of FRC above predicted normal. This may be due to increased Vr due to loss of elastic recoil of the lung (e.g. emphysema) or to dynamic pulmonary hyperinflation which is said to be present when the FRC exceeds Vr. Dynamic hyperinflation exists whenever the duration of expiration is insufficient to allow the lungs to deflate to Vr prior to the next inspiration. This tends to occur under conditions in which expiratory flow is impeded (e.g. increased airway resistance) or when the expiratory time is shortened (e.g. increased breathing frequency). Expiratory flow may also be retarded by other mechanisms such as persistent contraction of the inspiratory muscles during expiration and expiratory narrowing of the glottic aperture. Most commonly, however, dynamic pulmonary hyperinflation is observed in patients who exhibit expiratory flow limitation during resting breathing

(c) Intrinsic Positive End-expired Pressure (PEEPi)

Under normal conditions, when end-expired volume equals Vr, the end-expiratory elastic recoil pressure of the total respiratory system (lungs and chest wall) is zero (case A in Fig. 7.9). In this instance, as soon as the inspiratory muscles contract, the alveolar pressure becomes subatmospheric and gas flows into the lungs. When breathing takes place at lung volumes higher than Vr, the end-expiratory elastic recoil pressure is positive (15 cmH$_2$O in case B of Fig. 7.9). The elastic recoil pressure present at end-expiration has been termed occult PEEP, auto PEEP, or intrinsic PEEP (PEEPi). When PEEPi is present, the onset of inspiratory muscle activity and inspiratory flow are not synchronous; inspiratory flow starts only when the pressure developed by the inspiratory muscles exceeds PEEPi because only then does alveolar pressure become subatmospheric. In this respect, PEEPi acts as an inspiratory threshold load which increases the static elastic work of breathing. This places a significant extra burden on the inspiratory muscles, which are operating under disadvantageous force-length conditions and abnormal thoracic geometry.

Patients with severe COPD may contract their abdominal muscles in the second half of expiration raising end-expired abdominal and pleural pressures, which fall rapidly with relaxation of abdominal muscles after the start of inspiration [55]. In spontaneously breathing patients who are *not* increasing pleural pressure at the end of tidal expiration by contracting abdominal muscles PEEPi can be estimated as the negative deflection in esophageal pressure from the start of inspiratory effort to the onset of inspiratory flow. This pressure is termed dynamic PEEPi. Values of dynamic PEEPi are usually lower than those of static PEEPi obtained by the end-expiratory occlusion technique used during mechanical ventilation [56].

(d) Effects of dynamic hyperinflation on work of breathing and mechanical performance of the inspiratory muscles

In 1954 McIlroy and Christie [57] observed that the mechanical work of breathing was increased in stable COPD patients which they attributed to increased airway and 'viscous' resistance of the lung. In later studies it was suggested that in COPD patients there is an increase of work of breathing also as a result of time constant inequality within the lung which causes an increase of effective dynamic pulmonary elastance and flow resistance [58], and PEEPi [59].

If PEEPi is absent and static elastance of the respiratory system (Est,rs) is linear over the volume change considered (ΔV), the static inspiratory work per breath is given by

$$WIst,rs = 0.5 \, Est,rs \, \Delta V \qquad (1)$$

If PEEPi is present, Eq. (1) becomes

$$WIst,rs = 0.5 \, Est,rs \, \Delta V + PEEPi \, \Delta V \qquad (2)$$

Fig. 7.9 illustrates the static elastic work required from the inspiratory muscles for the same tidal volume inhaled from Vr and from a higher lung volume. As shown by the hatched areas, WIst,rs increases markedly when the breath is taken at a higher lung volume. In this example, the increase in WIst,rs is due mainly to PEEPi, though an increase in Est,rs (as reflected by the decreased slope of the static PV curve at the higher lung volume) also plays a role. Clearly, during spontaneous breathing dynamic hyperinflation implies an increase of static inspiratory work, and hence in inspiratory muscle effort. Furthermore, as lung volume increases there is a concomitant decrease in effectiveness of the inspiratory muscles as pressure generators, because the inspiratory muscle fibers become shorter and their geometrical arrangement changes. Thus, in COPD patients there is a vicious cycle: in addition to these increases in static elastic work, resistive work on inspiration is invariably increased due to airway obstruction which in turn promotes dynamic hyperinflation with a concomitant increase in elastic work and impaired mechanical performance of the inspiratory muscles. With increasing severity of airway obstruction, a critical point is eventually reached at which the inspiratory muscles become fatigued.

7.2.6 ROLE OF ABNORMAL VENTILATORY MECHANICS IN LIMITING EXERCISE CAPACITY

Abnormalities in ventilatory mechanics predominate in limiting exercise tolerance in patients with severe COPD. This conclusion is based on studies that show that, whereas exercise is terminated when O_2 consumption and heart rate are below predicted maximum values, maximum exercise ventilation frequently attains the maximum breathing capacity (MBC) as predicted from the resting value of FEV_1 [51]. However, this prediction is rather imprecise and the formula commonly used in normal subjects (MBC [litres/min] = $35 \times FEV_1$ (litres)) considerably underestimates the maximum exercise ventilation achieved by patients with the most severe expiratory airflow limitation. Maximum exercise ventilation can be predicted better by measuring the maximum voluntary ventilation that can be sustained for 4 min [60], while maintaining isocapnia. Indirect methods using maximum inspiratory pressure or flow have also been proposed [61]. Detailed comparison of tidal and maximum flow–volume curves during exercise supports the role of ventilatory mechanics in limiting performance [62–64]. In the patients with most severe airflow limitation, tidal expiratory flow reaches the MEFV curve even at rest (Fig. 7.8); in those with less severe disease, flow limitation is reached on expiration once ventilation is increased to meet the metabolic needs of exercise. Increases in ventilation are achieved at first by increases in both V_T and frequency, but V_T becomes fixed at ~50% of VC and further increases in ventilation are then achieved by increasing frequency [51,65]. Because of expiratory flow limitation, to increase expiratory flow, tidal breathing has to take place closer to TLC and end-expiratory volume rises. However, this increase is achieved exclusively by an increase in rib cage volume [66]; as in normal subjects, there is a small decrease in end-expired abdominal volume. This change in chest cage configuration assists diaphragm function by minimizing the decrease in its length that would otherwise occur with increase in end-expired volume. At the breaking point of exercise, tidal inspiratory flow also approaches maximum levels.

These changes in breathing pattern are achieved by increased tidal swings in pleural pressure, which are predominantly due to more negative inspiratory pressures, at least until approaching the breaking point of exercise when more positive pleural pressures in the range 15–20 cmH_2O are generated. Some studies have suggested that the sensation of dyspnea during exercise is related to the generation of more negative inspiratory pressures.

These observations raise the possibility that the ability to sustain respiratory muscle force may ultimately limit exercise [65]. During strenuous exercise in patients with COPD the predicted O_2 requirements of the respiratory muscles have been estimated to be as much as 40% of the observed O_2 consumption [67]; thus, in contrast to normal subjects, there is significant competition between limb and respiratory muscles for the available O_2 (see Chapter 9 for further discussion).

7.3 ACUTE RESPIRATORY FAILURE (ARF)

Overall, surprisingly few studies have been made of the changes in lung mechanics in exacerbations of disease in COPD and it is only in the last few years that adequate studies of changes during the most severe episodes, requiring assisted ventilation, have been made. For the purposes of this section we define acute *respiratory* failure as worsening arterial oxygenation and acute *ventilatory* failure as an increase in arterial P_{CO_2}; implicitly these exacerbations will have occurred on the background of considerable and persistent underlying abnormalities in lung mechanics.

7.3.1 ORIGINS OF INCREASED WORK OF BREATHING

Acute ventilatory failure in COPD patients is most commonly triggered by airway infection. As a result, there is an acute increase in airway resistance which causes increased resistive work of breathing, and promotes dynamic hyperinflation. The latter is further exacerbated by the tachypnea which is invariably present in COPD patients with ARF. Expiratory flow limitation is present during tidal breathing. Dynamic hyperinflation promotes an increase in the static elastic work of breathing which can be due both to PEEPi and decreased lung compliance (Fig. 7.9). The highest values of PEEPi observed in stable COPD patients are in the order of 7–9 cmH$_2$O [68] but with ARF values up to 13 cmH$_2$O during spontaneous breathing [59] and 22 cmH$_2$O during mechanical ventilation [69] have been reported. As a result the work of breathing is markedly increased. This increase in work of breathing, in association with the impaired inspiratory muscle performance, promotes inspiratory muscle fatigue (Fig. 7.10). As a result, the patient may need to be mechanically ventilated.

The average inspiratory work of the respiratory system (WI,rs) and its components in 10 mechanically ventilated sedated paralyzed COPD patients with ARF are shown in Fig.

Acute Ventilatory Failure in COPD

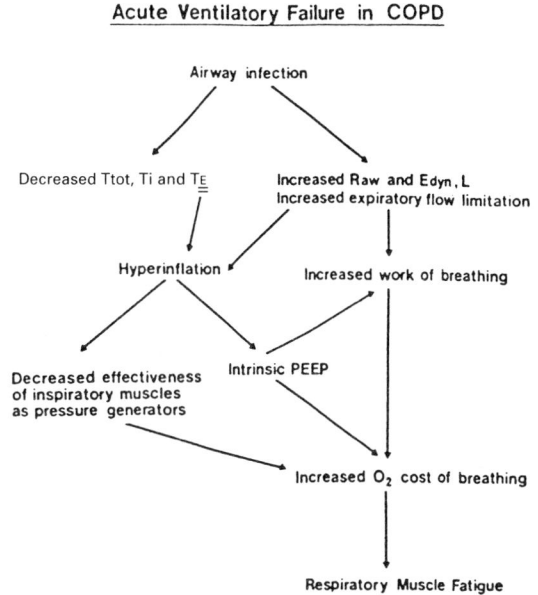

Fig. 7.10 Scheme of the pathophysiology causing acute ventilatory failure in COPD patients. T$_{TOT}$, total breathing cycle duration; T$_I$ and T$_E$, inspiratory and expiratory ti mes: Raw, airway resistance; Edyn,L, dynamic lung elastance (reciprocal of lung compliance).

7.11 together with the corresponding values obtained in 18 anesthetized paralyzed normal subjects [54]. The measurements were obtained during constant-flow inflation with tidal volume of 0.73 l, frequency of 12.5 breaths per minute and inspiratory duration of 0.92 s. WI,rs was two-fold greater in COPD patients than in normal subjects, the difference reflecting an increase of both static (WIst,rs) and dynamic (WIdyn,rs) work.

The increase in WIst,rs in these COPD patients was due entirely to the work due to PEEPi (WI,PEEPi) which represented 57% of the overall increase in WI,rs exhibited by the COPD patients relative to normal subjects. These studies agree with those of Guérin *et al.* [70] and Tantucci *et al.* [71] in finding normal values of Est,rs in COPD patients with ARF. By contrast, Broseghini *et al.* [69], who studied COPD patients during the first day of

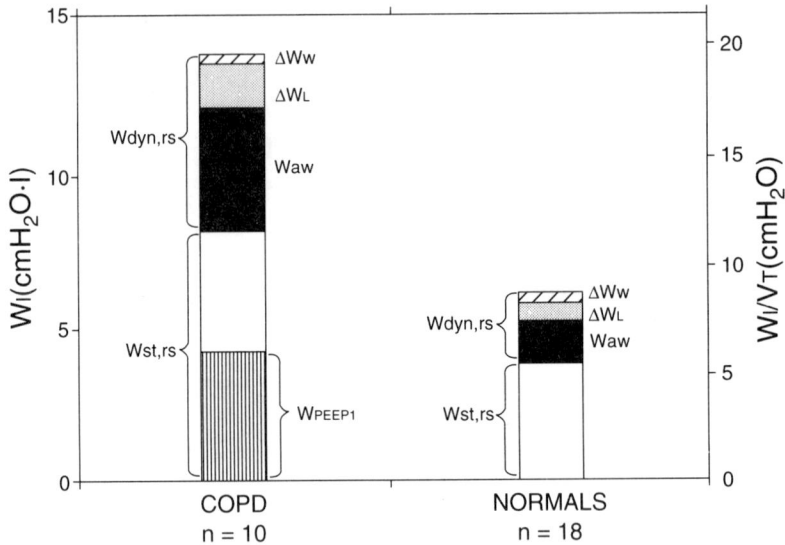

Fig. 7.11 Average values of inspiratory work (W_I) done on the respiratory system and its components in 10 COPD patients and 18 normal anesthetized paralyzed subjects with inflation flow of 0.8 l/s and tidal volume of 0.73 l. Wst,rs, total static work of respiratory system; W_{PEEPi} static work due to intrinsic PEEP; Wdyn,rs, total dynamic work of respiratory system; Waw, airway resistive work; ΔWw, viscoelastic work of chest wall; ΔW_L, work of lung due to time constant inequality and/or visoelastic pressure dissipations. Work per liter of inspired volume (W_I/V_T) is shown on right ordinate. (From Coussa *et al.* [54].)

mechanical ventilation found increased values of Est,rs (Table 7.1). This was due in part to the fact that these patients had a more marked degree of dynamic pulmonary hyperinflation, and hence their ΔV during mechanical ventilation impinged into the flat part of their static volume–pressure (V–P) curves (Fig. 7.9). Even in these patients, however, most of the increase of static work was due to PEEPi.

In the COPD patients in Fig. 7.11, increase in W_{Idyn},rs accounted for 43% of the overall increase in inspiratory work. Airway resistive work ($W_{I,aw}$) was, on average, 3.3 times higher than in the normal subjects, and contributed 34% of the overall increase in $W_{I,rs}$. The increase in $W_{I,aw}$ in the COPD patients reflects increased airway resistance (Raw). According to Guérin *et al.* [70] and Tantucci *et al.* [71] at similar inflation volume and flow, Raw in COPD patients with ARF was about 3.5 times higher than in normal subjects (Table

7.1). Higher values of Raw were found by Broseghini *et al.* [69], presumably because their patients were studied on the first day of ARF. The results in Fig. 7.11 do not include the resistive work done on the endotracheal tubes which is relatively high. With an endotracheal tube size 7 this work amounted to 4.8 $cmH_2O \times l$ and even with tube size 9 was 2.0 $cmH_2O \times l$ compared to a value of 3.8 $cmH_2O \times l$, for W_I, aw due to the lungs themselves.

The remainder of the increase in W_{Idyn},rs was accounted for by an increase in the additional work done on the lung (ΔW_{IL}); the dynamic work due to the tissues of the chest wall (ΔW_{IW}) was similar in COPD patients to that of normal subjects. ΔW_{IL} is the additional work done on the lung as a result of pressure dissipations caused by viscoelastic behavior of pulmonary tissue and/or time constant inequality [54,58,71]. As originally proposed by Mount [72] in 1955 to explain a decline in dynamic pulmonary compliance with increas-

Table 7.1 Mean values ($\pm$ SE) of baseline ventilatory settings and respiratory mechanics in mechanically ventilated COPD patients with ARF

Authors [Reference]	n	Time (days)	ΔV (l)	$\dot{V}$ (l/s)	T_I (s)	T_E (s)	PEEPi (cmH_2O)	ΔFRC (l)	Est,rs (cmH_2O/l)	Raw ($cmH_2O/l/s$)	ΔRrs ($cmH_2O/l/s$)	Rrs ($cmH_2O/l/s$)
Broseghini *et al.* [69]	8	1	0.69 $\pm$ 0.03	0.62 $\pm$ 0.01	1.20 $\pm$ 0.05	2.14 $\pm$ 0.05	13.6 $\pm$ 0.8	0.66 $\pm$ 0.10	17.9 $\pm$ 0.01	15.6 $\pm$ 3.1	10.8 $\pm$ 2.0	26.4 $\pm$ 4.7
Tantucci *et al.* [71]	6	1–4	0.80 $\pm$ 0.04	1.01 $\pm$ .03	0.93 $\pm$ 0.04	3.35 $\pm$ 0.04	4.6 $\pm$ 0.9	0.42 $\pm$ 0.18	11.1 $\pm$ 0.01	8.0 $\pm$ 1.8	5.5 $\pm$ 1.0	13.5 $\pm$ 1.0
Guérin *et al.* [70]	10	1–16	0.73 $\pm$ 0.02	0.80 $\pm$ 0.03	0.92 $\pm$ 0.01	3.98 $\pm$ 0.20	5.7 $\pm$ 0.9	0.34 $\pm$ 0.06	12.6 $\pm$ 0.7	7.2 $\pm$ 0.6	5.6 $\pm$ 0.5	12.8 $\pm$ 1.1

n, number of patients studied; time, days from onset of ARF; ΔV, tidal volume; $\dot{V}$ inspiratory flow; T_I, inspiratory time; T_E, expiratory time; PEEPi, intrinsic end-expiratory positive pressure; ΔFRC, difference between the end-expiratory lung volume during mechanical ventilation and the relaxation volume; Est,rs, static elastance of respiratory system; Raw, airway resistance; ΔRrs, additional resistance due to time constant inequality and/or viscoelastic behavior; Rrs, total resistance of respiratory system.

ing frequency of breathing, ΔW$_{IL}$ in normal subjects predominantly reflects viscoelastic behavior of the lungs which 'confers time-dependency of the elastic properties' [73]. By contrast, in COPD patients ΔW$_{IL}$ should include a substantial component due to time constant inequality [54,58]. This probably explains the higher values of ΔW$_{IL}$ found in the COPD patients with ARF in whom ΔW$_{IL}$ was, on average, 2.3 times higher than in normal subjects. This increase of ΔW$_{IL}$, however, represented only 9% of the overall increase in W$_I$,rs observed in the COPD patients.

Predictably, the increase of ΔW$_{IL}$ in COPD patients is associated with more marked time-dependency of pulmonary elastance than in normal subjects, as shown in Fig. 7.12, which depicts the relationship of static and dynamic elastance of the lung (Edyn,L =1/Cdyn,L) to inspiratory flow obtained at a fixed inflation volume (ΔV= 0.73 l) in 10 COPD patients with ARF [70] and 18 normal subjects [73]. Because inflation volume was fixed, an increase in inspiratory flow ($\dot{V}$I) implies a shorter duration in inspiration (TI), since $\dot{V}$I is proportional to 1/TI, the data in Fig. 7.12 actually depict TI dependence of elastic properties. While Est,L was independent of TI and $\dot{V}$I in both COPD patients and normal subjects, Edyn,L increased progressively with increasing $\dot{V}$, or, more appropriately, with decreasing duration of inspiration (TI). In COPD patients the

increase in Edyn,L with increasing $\dot{V}$ was greater than in normal subjects because of time constant inequality [7,58]. In normal lungs the time-dependency of pulmonary elastance is due almost entirely to viscoelastic behavior [72,73].

Table 7.1 depicts the 'effective' additional resistance (ΔRrs) due to time constant inequality within the lung and viscoelastic behavior of pulmonary and chest wall tissue in COPD patients with ARF. In this instance, ΔRrs represented about 40% of the total resistance of the respiratory system (Rrs) and was substantially higher than normal [69–71]. It should be noted, however, that ΔRrs exhibits marked time-dependency, i.e. it decreases progressively with decreasing TI [70,73]. The values of ΔRrs in Table 7.1 pertain to experimental TI ranging from 0.9 to 1.2 s.

Fig. 7.13 depicts the average relationships between Rrs and inspiratory flow obtained at fixed inflation volume (ΔV = 0.5 l) in 6 COPD patients with ARF [71] and 16 normal subjects [74]. At all comparable flow rates, Rrs was about three-fold higher in the COPD patients. In both normals and COPD patients Rrs (= Raw + ΔRrs) was highest at the lowest flow and decreased progressively with $\dot{V}$ up to 1 l/s. At this $\dot{V}$, Rrs had a minimal value. This phenomenon is due to the fact that as $\dot{V}$ decreased there was a greater decrease of ΔRrs as compared to the concomitant increase of Raw.

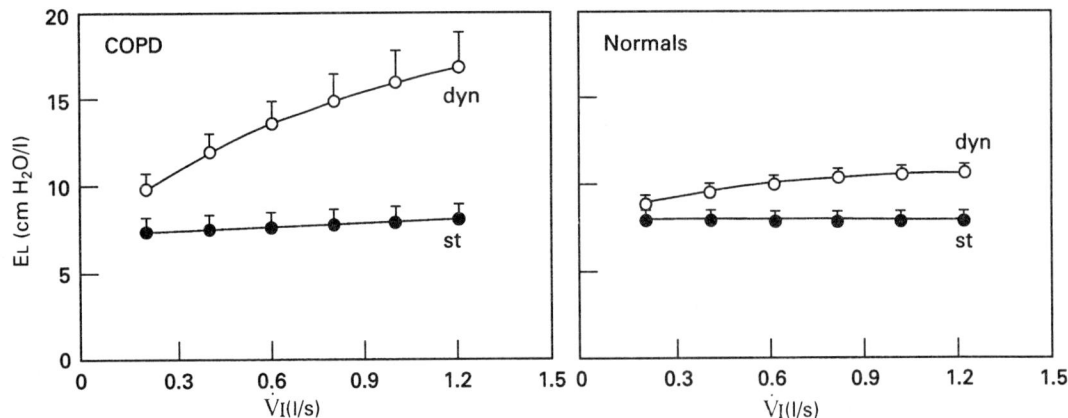

Fig. 7.12 Change in average values of static (st) and dynamic (dyn) elastance (EL) of the lungs at constant inflation volume (ΔVol of 0.73 l) delivered at varying inspiratory flow (V̇I) in 10 COPD patients with ARF [70] *left* and 18 normal subjects [73] *right*. Because ΔV was constant, increasing V̇I corresponds to shortening TI. Bars = SE.

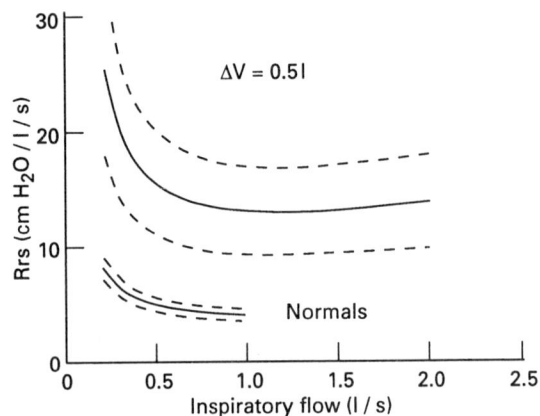

Fig. 7.13 Average relationship between total respiratory system resistance (Rrs) and inspiratory flow at constant inflation volume of 0.5 l in 6 sedated paralyzed COPD patients with ARF [71] and 16 normal anesthetized and paralyzed subjects [74].

At V̇ >1 l/s, Rrs tended to increase slightly in the COPD patients, reflecting the fact that over this range of V̇ the increase of Raw becomes predominant. The initial decrease in Rrs with increasing flow represents a clinically important aspect because it occurs in the inflation

flow range commonly used in the ICU setting (0.5 to 1 l/ s). Fuller accounts of ΔWI,L and ΔWI,w can be found elsewhere [54,73].

7.3.2 IMPLICATIONS OF PEEPi DURING MECHANICAL VENTILATION

The putative role of mechanical ventilation is to reduce the activity of the inspiratory muscles to tolerable levels during patient-triggered mechanical ventilation (e.g. assisted mechanical ventilation). This end is not always achieved because the pressure which has to be generated by the patient to trigger the ventilator necessarily includes PEEPi. If this is high, the inspiratory effort required by the patient may be excessive [75]. In contrast, during controlled mechanical ventilation all of the work of breathing is done by the ventilator. Nevertheless, PEEPi must be taken into account for correct measurement of respiratory compliance [76] and, more importantly, in terms of its adverse effects on cardiac output. In fact, PEEPi may severely decrease venous return and cardiac output [77], depending upon intravascular volume status, myocardial function, and other factors [78].

Patients with high levels of PEEPi are difficult to wean from mechanical ventilation and may become ventilator-dependent [79].

7.3.3 MONITORING PEEPi

Fundamental in the management of the mechanically-ventilated COPD patients is to monitor PEEPi. Indeed, measurement of PEEPi should become a part of routine monitoring in mechanically-ventilated patients, particularly those with airway obstruction. This will allow for reliable measurement and interpretation of other frequently determined cardiopulmonary variables, such as respiratory system compliance, pulmonary capillary wedge pressure, etc. The potential adverse effects of PEEPi require that, in addition, management should be specifically directed towards those factors contributing to the de-

velopment of PEEPi. This includes medical therapy aimed at reducing the severity of airflow obstruction as well as excessive minute ventilation (due to fever, metabolic acidosis, inadequate pain relief, etc.). The inspiratory flow settings should be adjusted to maximize the time available for passive expiration.

A simple way to detect the presence of dynamic hyperinflation, and hence of PEEPi, is to monitor the expiratory flow–time profile. When PEEPi is absent, there is a period of zero flow prior to the next spontaneous or mechanical lung inflation. By contrast, when PEEPi is present there is flow throughout expiration, which is abruptly terminated by the next spontaneous breath or by mechanical lung inflation (Fig. 7.14 left).

In mechanically-ventilated patients, PEEPi will not normally register on the ventilator

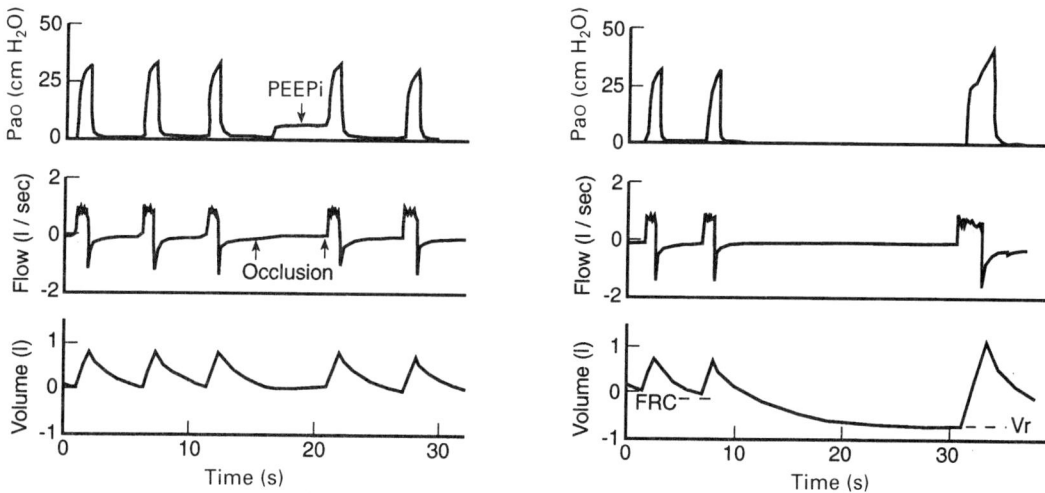

Fig. 7.14 *Left*: Records of pressure at the airway opening (Pao), flow, and changes in lung volume during mechanical ventilation in a sedated paralyzed COPD patient. Note that flow continues throughout expiration and is abruptly terminated by the onset of the next breath indicating the presence of dynamic hyperinflation and PEEPi. PEEPi is measured by end-expiratory airway occlusion indicated by the first arrow. Upon occlusion, the airway pressure rises and reaches a plateau that corresponds to the static end-expiratory elastic recoil pressure of the respiratory system (=PEEPi). In this patient PEEPi amounted to 5.5 cmH$_2$O. *Right*: Records as in left panel, illustrating the measurement of ΔFRC which is the difference between end-expiratory lung volume during steady state mechanical ventilation (FRC) and the relaxation volume of the respiratory system (Vr) in the same patient. A prolonged expiratory time was inserted during steady state mechanical ventilation that allowed the patient to exhale to Vr. ΔFRC in this patient amounted to 0.67 l. From Eissa and Milic-Emili [80].

manometer. During exhalation, the ventilator manometer is exposed to ambient pressure as the exhalation valve is open. Only the expiratory pressure dissipations due to the valve resistance or the applied PEEP will register on the ventilator manometer. Despite the fact that the alveolar pressure may be positive throughout exhalation, the manometer will not reflect the increased pressure unless the expiratory port is occluded. If the expiratory port is occluded at end-expiration, alveolar pressure and circuit pressure equilibrate, and PEEPi is seen on the ventilator manometer [77]. Fig. 7.14 (*left*) illustrates this method to determine PEEPi in a COPD patient during controlled mechanical ventilation. End-expiratory occlusion was done using the end-expiratory hold button on a Siemens 900C Servo ventilator. Following occlusion, the airway pressure rises until it reaches a plateau which corresponds to PEEPi. It should be noted, however, that most ventilators are not equipped with an end-expiratory hold button.

During controlled mechanical ventilation the magnitude of dynamic hyperinflation can be determined by inserting a prolonged expiratory time during steady state mechanical ventilation [69,80] (Fig. 7.14 *left*). In this way ΔFRC (i.e., the difference between the end-expiratory lung volume during steady state mechanical ventilation and Vr) is obtained.

7.3.4 STRATEGIES TO REDUCE THE INSPIRATORY LOAD CAUSED BY PEEPi

As implied in Fig. 7.10, treatment of COPD patients with respiratory failure should be aimed toward increasing the expiratory duration as well as decreasing respiratory flow-resistance. To the extent that tachypnea is due to fever and/or airway infection, resolution of these by conventional treatment should be beneficial. Similarly, effective bronchodilator administration may be useful in reducing both flow-resistance and PEEPi [81]. A less conventional but promising approach to deal with PEEPi is the use of continuous positive airway pressure

(CPAP). Indeed, CPAP has been found to reduce the magnitude of inspiratory muscle effort and the work of breathing in stable patients with severe COPD [75]. Furthermore, CPAP has also been found to reduce the work of breathing and dyspnea in patients with severe COPD during weaning from mechanical ventilation [56]. This is related to a reduction in the inspiratory workload imposed by PEEPi. CPAP administered through a face or nasal mask [82] may also be of therapeutic benefit during an acute exacerbation of severe COPD in the non-intubated patient. Conceivably, the early use of CPAP in this setting could preclude the need for intubation and mechanical ventilation in some COPD patients. Finally, it should also be noted that application of external PEEP during patient-triggered mechanical ventilation can counterbalance and reduce the inspiratory load imposed by PEEPi [75].

7.3.5 DETECTION OF EXPIRATORY FLOW LIMITATION DURING RESTING BREATHING

Patients with severe airway obstruction commonly exhibit expiratory flow limitation during resting breathing, particularly during acute exacerbations of their disease [1]. Such patients in general exhibit pronounced pulmonary hyperinflation with markedly increased work of breathing and markedly impaired inspiratory muscle function. Patients who are flow limited during mechanical ventilation are difficult to wean [79,83]. Accordingly, detection of airflow limitation in COPD patients with ARF appears to be crucial.

Several methods have been proposed to detect expiratory flow limitation in mechanically ventilated patients: (1) removal of external PEEP, if present [84]; (2) addition of a resistance to the expiratory circuit [84], and (3) application of a negative pressure of 5 cmH₂O at the airway opening during a single expiration [85]. The latter method can also be applied during spontaneous breathing [86].

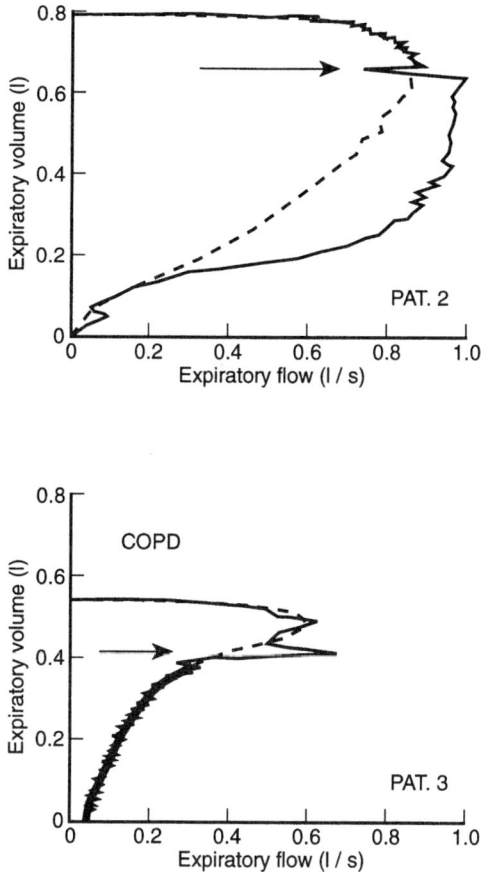

Fig. 7.15 Expiratory flow–volume relationships during passive expiration in a mechanically ventilated patient with COPD (*bottom*) and in a patient without airway obstruction (*top*). *Broken line*: baseline expiration; *solid line*: subsequent expiration during which a negative pressure of –5 cmH₂O was applied at points indicated by arrows and maintained throughout the rest of expiration. For further information see text. From Valta *et al.* [85].

Fig. 7.15 depicts expiratory flow–volume curves obtained during passive expiration in a mechanically ventilated COPD patient with ARF (patient #3) and in a subject without airways obstruction (patient #2). In patient #2 application of negative pressure during expiration resulted in a sustained increase of expiratory flow indicating absence of expiratory flow limitation during tidal breathing. By con-

trast, in patient #3 application of the negative pressure resulted in no change of expiratory flow, except for a transient change immediately after application of the negative pressure which reflects displacement of gas from the expiratory line due to rapid decompression [85, 87]. This lack of response to negative pressure (apart from the transient) occurs when expiratory flow limitation is present. Thus, expiratory flow limitation can be readily detected by analysis of expiratory flow–volume or flow–time relationships before and after application of negative pressure.

REFERENCES

1. Pride, N.B. and Macklem, P.T. (1986) Lung mechanics in disease, in *Handbook of Physiology, Mechanics of Breathing*, sect. 3, vol. 3, ch. 37, (eds P.T. Macklem and J. Mead), American Physiological Society, Bethesda, pp. 659–92.
2. Macklem, P.T. and Permutt, S. (eds) (1979) *Lung Biology in Health and Disease. The Lung in Transition between Health and Disease*. vol. 12 Dekker, New York.
3. Wagner, E.M., Bleecker, E.R., Permutt S. and Liu, M.C. (1992) Peripheral airways resistance in smokers. *Am. Rev. Respir. Dis.*, **146**, 92–5.
4. Macklem, P.T., Proctor, D.F., and Hogg, J.C. (1970) The stability of peripheral airways. *Respir. Physiol.*, **8**, 191–203.
5. Leblanc, P., Ruff, F. and Milic-Emili, J. (1970) Effects of age and body position on 'airway closure' in man. *J. Appl. Physiol.*, **28**, 448–51.
6. Buist, A.S., Vollmer, W.M., Johnson, L.R. and McCamant, L.E. (1988) Does the single-breath N₂ test identify the smoker who will develop chronic airflow limitation? *Am. Rev. Respir. Dis.*, **137**, 293–301.
7. Woolcock, A.J., Vincent, N.J. and Macklem, P.T. (1969) Frequency dependence of compliance as a test for obstruction in the small airways. *J. Clin. Invest.*, **48**, 1097–106.
8. Coe, C.I., Watson, A., Joyce H. and Pride, N.B. (1989) Effects of smoking on changes in respiratory resistance with increasing age. *Clin. Sci.*, **76**, 487–94.
9. Black, L.F., Offord, K. and Hyatt, R.E. (1974) Variability in the maximal expiratory flow volume curve in asymptomatic smokers and in non-smokers. *Am. Rev. Respir. Dis.*, **110**, 282–92.

10. Dosman, J., Bode, F., Urbanetti, J. *et al.* (1975) The use of a helium–oxygen mixture during maximum expiratory flow to demonstrate obstruction in small airways in smokers. *J. Clin. Invest.*, **55**, 1090–9.

11. Hutcheon, M., Griffin, P., Levison, H. and Zamel, N. (1974) Volume of isoflow. A new test in detection of mild abnormalities of lung mechanics. *Am. Rev. Respir. Dis.*, **110**, 458–465.

12. Cosio, M., Ghezzo, H., Hogg, J.C. *et al.* (1978) The relations between structural changes in small airways and pulmonary function tests. *N. Engl. J. Med.*, **298**, 1277–81.

13. Berend, N. and Thurlbeck, W.M. (1982) Correlations of maximum expiratory flow with small airway dimensions and pathology. *J. Appl. Physiol., Respirat. Environ. Exercise Physiol.*, **52**, 346–51.

14. Meadows, J.A. III, Rodarte, J.R. and Hyatt, R.E. (1980) Density dependence of maximal expiratory flow in chronic obstructive pulmonary disease. *Am. Rev. Respir. Dis.*, **121**, 47–54.

15. Oloffson, J., Bake, B., Svardsudd, K. and Skoogh, B.E. (1986) The single breath N_2-test predicts the rate of decline in FEV_1. The study of men born in 1913 and 1923. *Eur. J. Respir. Dis.*, **69**, 46–56.

16. Stanescu, D.C., Rodenstein, D.O., Hoeven, C. and Robert A. (1987) 'Sensitive tests' are poor predictors of the decline in forced expiratory volume in one second in middle-aged smokers. *Am. Rev. Respir. Dis.*, **135**, 585–90.

17. Cherniack, R.M. and McCarthy, D.S. (1979) Reversibility of abnormalities of pulmonary function, in *Lung Biology in Health and Disease. The Lung in Transition between Health and Disease*, (eds P.T. Macklem and S. Permutt), vol. 12. ch. 15, Dekker, New York, pp. 329–42.

18. Bedell, G.N., Marshall, R., DuBois, A.B. and Comroe, J.H. Jr. (1956) Plethysmographic determination of the volume of gas trapped in the lungs. *J. Clin. Invest.* **35**, 664–70.

19. Butler, J., Caro, C.G., Alcala, R. and DuBois, A.B. (1960) Physiological factors affecting airway resistance in normal subjects and in patients with obstructive respiratory disease. *J. Clin. Invest.*, **39**, 584–91.

20. Tierney, D.F. and Nadel, J.A. (1962) Concurrent measurements of functional residual capacity by three methods. *J. Appl. Physiol.*, **17**, 871–3.

21. Rodenstein, D.O. and Stanescu, D.C. (1982) Reassessment of lung volume measurement by helium dilution and by body plethysmography in chronic airflow obstruction. *Am. Rev. Respir. Dis.*, **126**, 1040–4.

22. Shore, S.A., Huk, O., Mannix, S. and Martin, J.G. (1983) Effect of panting frequency on the plethysmographic determination of thoracic gas volume in chronic obstructive pulmonary disease. *Am. Rev. Respir. Dis.*, **128**, 54–9.

23. Colebatch, H.J.H., Greaves, I.A. and Ng, C.K.Y. (1979) Exponential analysis of elastic recoil and aging in healthy males and females. *J. Appl. Physiol. Respirat. Environ. Exercise Physiol.*, **47**, 683–91.

24. Gibson, G.J., Pride, N.B., Davis, J. and Schroter, R.C. (1979) Exponential description of the static pressure-volume curve of normal and diseased lung. *Am. Rev. Resp. Dis.*, **120**, 799–811.

25. Knudson, R.J. and Kaltenhorn, W.T. (1981) Evaluation of lung elastic recoil by exponential curve analysis. *Respir. Physiol.*, **46**, 29–42.

26. Greaves, I.A. and Colebatch, H.J.H. (1980) Elastic behaviour and structure of normal and emphysematous lungs post-mortem. *Am. Rev. Resp. Dis.*, **121**, 127–36.

27. Pare, P.D., Brooks, L.A., Bates, J. *et al.* (1982) Exponential analysis of the lung pressure-volume curve as a predictor of pulmonary emphysema. *Am. Rev. Respir. Dis.*, **126**, 54–61.

28. Nagai, A., Yamawaki, I., Thurlbeck, W.M. and Takizawa, T. (1989) Assessment of lung parenchymal destruction by using routine histological tissue sections. *Am. Rev. Respir. Dis.*, **139**, 313–9.

29. Saetta, M., Ghezzo, H., Won Dong, K. *et al.* (1985) Loss of alveolar attachments in smokers. *Am. Rev. Respir. Dis.*, **132**, 894–900.

30. Petty, T.L., Silvers, G.W. and Stanford, R.E. (1986) Radial traction and small airways disease in excised human lungs. *Am. Rev. Respir. Dis.*, **133**, 132–5.

31. Hogg, J.C., Macklem, P.T., Nepszy, S.J. *et al.* (1969) Elastic properties of the centrilobular emphysematous space. *J. Clin. Invest.*, **48**, 1306–12.

32. Nagai, A. and Thurlbeck, W.M. (1991) Scanning electron microscopic observations of emphysema in humans. *Am. Rev. Respir. Dis.*, **144**, 901–8.

33. Sharp, J.T., Van Lith, P., Vej Nuchprayoon, C. *et al.* (1968) The thorax in chronic obstructive lung disease. *Am. J. Med.*, **44**, 39–46.

34. Fry, D.L. and Hyatt, R.E. (1960) Pulmonary mechanics: a unified analysis of the relationship between pressure, volume, and gas flow in the lungs of normal and diseased subjects. *Am. J. Med.*, **29**, 672–89.

35. Ingram, R.H., Jr and Schilder, D.P. (1966) Effect of gas compression on pulmonary pressure, flow, and volume relationships. *J. Appl. Physiol.*, **21**, 1821–6.

36. Pride, N.B., Permutt, S., Riley, R.L. and Bromberger-Barnea, B. (1967) Determinants of maximal expiratory flow from the lungs. *J. Appl. Physiol.*, **23**, 646–62.

37. Mead, J., Turner, J.M., Macklem, P.T. and Little, J.B. (1967) Significance of the relationship between lung recoil and maximum expiratory flow. *J. Appl. Physiol.*, **22**, 95–108.

38. Leaver, D.G., Tattersfield, A.E. and Pride, N.B. (1973) Contributions of loss of lung recoil and of enhanced airways collapsibility to the airflow obstruction of chronic bronchitis and emphysema. *J. Clin. Invest.*, **52**, 2117–28.

39. Macklem, P.T. and Wilson, N.J. (1965) Measurement of intrabronchial pressure in man. *J. Appl. Physiol.*, 20, 653–63.

40. Macklem, P.T., Fraser, R.G. and Brown, W.G. (1965) Bronchial pressure measurements in emphysema and bronchitis. *J. Clin. Invest.*, **44**, 897–905.

41 Colebatch, H.J.H., Finucane, K.E. and Smith, M.M. (1973) Pulmonary conductance and elastic recoil relationships in asthma and emphysema. *J. Appl. Physiol.*, **34**, 143–53.

42. Leaver, D.G., Tattersfield, A.E. and Pride, N.B. (1974) Bronchial and extrabronchial factors in chronic airflow obstruction. *Thorax*, **29**, 394–400.

43. Grimby, G., Takishima, T., Graham, W. *et al.* (1968) Frequency dependence of flow resistance in patients with obstructive lung disease. *J. Clin. Invest.*, **47**, 1455–65.

44. Hogg, J.C., Macklem, P.T. and Thurlbeck, W.M. (1968) Site and nature of airway obstruction in chronic obstructive lung disease. *N. Engl. J. Med.*, **278**, 1355–60.

45. Silvers, G.W., Maisel, J.C., Petty, T.L. *et al.* (1974) Flow limitation during forced expiration in excised human lungs. *J. Appl. Physiol.*, **36**, 737–44.

46. Van Brabandt, H., Cauberghs, M, Verbeken, E. *et al.* (1983) Partitioning of pulmonary impedance in excised human and canine lungs. *J. Appl. Physiol., Respirat. Environ. Exercise Physiol.*, **55**, 1733–42.

47. Verbeken, E.K., Cauberghs, M., Mertens, I. *et al.* (1992) Tissue and airway impedance of excised normal, senile and emphysematous lungs. *J. Appl. Physiol.*, **72**, 2343–53.

48. Yanai, M., Sekizawa, K., Ohrui, T. *et al.* (1992). Site of airway obstruction in pulmonary disease: direct measurement of intrabronchial pressure. *J. Appl. Physiol.*, **72**, 1016–23.

49. Hogg, J.C., Macklem, P.T. and Thurlbeck, W.M. (1969) The resistance of collateral channels in excised human lungs. *J. Clin. Invest.*, **48**, 421–31.

50. Terry, P.B., Traystman, R.J., Newball, H.H. *et al.* (1978) Collateral ventilation in man. *N. Engl. J. Med.*, **298**, 10–15.

51. Spiro, S.G., Hahn, H.L., Edwards, R.H.T. and Pride, N.B. (1975) An analysis of the physiological strain of submaximal exercise in patients with chronic obstructive bronchitis. *Thorax*, **30**, 415–25.

52. Sorli, J., Grassino, A., Lorange, G. and Milic-Emili, J. (1978) Control of breathing in patients with chronic obstructive lung disease. *Clin. Sci. Mol. Med.*, **54**, 295–304.

53. Bellemare, F. and Grassino, A.E. (1983) Force reserve of the diaphragm in patients with chronic obstructive pulmonary disease. *J. Appl. Physiol.*, **55**, 8–15.

54. Coussa, M.L., Guerin, C., Eissa, N.T. *et al.* (1993) Partitioning of work of breathing in mechanically ventilated COPD patients. *J. Appl. Physiol.*, **75**, 1711–9.

55. Ninane, V., Yernault, J-C. and de Troyer, A. (1993) Intrinsic PEEP in patients with chronic obstructive pulmonary disease: role of expiratory muscles. *Am. Rev. Respir. Dis.*, **148**, 1037–42.

56. Petrof, B.J., Legare, M., Goldberg. P. *et al.* (1990) Continuous positive airway pressure reduces work of breathing and dyspnea during weaning from mechanical ventilation in severe chronic obstructive pulmonary disease. *Am. Rev. Respir. Dis.*, **141**, 281–9.

57. McIlroy, M.B. and Christie, R.V. (1954) The work of breathing in emphysema. *Clin. Sci.*, **13**, 147–54.

58. Otis, A.B., Mckerrow, C.B., Bartlett, R.A. *et al.* (1956) Mechanical factors in distribution of pulmonary ventilation. *J. Appl. Physiol.*, **8**, 427–43.

59. Fleury, B., Murciano, D., Talamo, C. *et al.* (1985) Work of breathing in patients with chronic obstructive pulmonary disease in acute respiratory failure. *Am. Rev. Respir. Dis.*, **131**, 822–7.

60. Freedman, S. (1970) Sustained maximum voluntary ventilation. *Respir. Physiol.*, **8**, 230–44.

61. Dillard, T.A., Hnatiuk, O.W. and McCumber, T.R. (1993) Maximum voluntary ventilation. Spirometric determinants in chronic obstructive pulmonary disease patients and normal subjects. *Am. Rev. Respir. Dis.*, **147**, 870–5.

62. Potter, W.A., Olafsson, S. and Hyatt, R.E. (1971) Ventilatory mechanics and expiratory flow limitation during exercise in patients with obstructive lung disease. *J. Clin. Invest.*, **50**, 910–9.

63. Leaver, D.G. and Pride, N.B. (1971) Flow-volume curves and expiratory pressures during exercise in patients with chronic airways obstruction. *Scand. J. Respir. Dis* , **77** Suppl., 23–7.

64. Stubbing, D.G., Pengelly, L.D., Morse, J.L.C. and Jones, N.L. (1980) Pulmonary mechanics during exercise in subjects with chronic airflow obstruction. *J. Appl. Physiol. Respirat. Environ. Exercise Physiol.*, **49**, 511–5.

65 Gallagher, C.G. (1990) Exercise and chronic obstructive pulmonary disease. *Med. Clin. North. Am.*, **74**, 619–41.

66. Grimby, G., Elgefors, B. and Oxhoj, H. (1973) Ventilatory levels and chest wall mechanics during exercise in obstructive lung disease. *Scand. J. Respir. Dis.*, **54**, 45–52.

67. Levison, H. and Cherniack, R.M. (1968) Ventilatory cost of exercise in chronic obstructive pulmonary disease. *J. Appl. Physiol.*, **25**, 21–27.

68. Haluszka, J., Chartrand, D.A., Grassino, A.E. *et al.* (1990) Intrinsic PEEP and arterial PCO_2 in stable patients with chronic obstructive pulmonary disease. *Am. Rev. Respir. Dis.*, **141**, 1194–7.

69. Broseghini, C., Brandolese, R., Poggi, R. *et al.* (1988) Respiratory mechanics during the first day of mechanical ventilation in patients with pulmonary edema and chronic airway obstruction. *Am. Rev. Respir. Dis.*, **138**, 355–61.

70. Guérin, C., Coussa, M-L., Eissa, N.T. *et al.* (1993) Lung and chest wall mechanics in mechanically ventilated COPD patients. *J. Appl. Physiol.*, **74**, 1570–80.

71. Tantucci, C., Corbeil, C., Chassé, M. *et al.* (1991) Flow resistance in patients with chronic obstructive pulmonary disease in acute respiratory failure. *Am. Rev. Respir. Dis.*, **144**, 384–9.

72. Mount, L.E. (1955). The ventilation flow-resistance and compliance of rat lungs. *J. Physiol. (London)*, **127**, 157–67.

73. D'Angelo, E., Robatto, F.M. and Calderini, E. *et al.* (1991) Pulmonary and chest wall mechanics in anaesthetized paralyzed humans. *J. Appl. Physiol.*, **70**, 2602–10.

74. D'Angelo, E., Calderini, E., Torri, G. *et al.* (1989) Respiratory mechanics in anesthetized paralyzed humans: effect of flow, volume and time. *J. Appl. Physiol.*, **67**, 2556–64.

75. Smith, T.C. and Marini, J.J. (1988) Impact of PEEP on lung mechanics and work of breathing in severe airflow obstruction. *J. Appl. Physiol.*, **65**, 1488–99.

76. Rossi, A., Gottfried, S.B., Zocchi, L. *et al.* (1985) Measurement of static compliance of the total respiratory system in patients with acute respiratory failure during mechanical ventilation. *Am. Rev. Respir. Dis.*, **131**, 672–7.

77. Pepe, P.E. and Marini, J.J. (1982) Occult positive end-expiratory pressure in mechanically ventilated patients with airflow obstruction. *Am. Rev. Respir. Dis.*, **126**, 166–70.

78. Johanson, W.G. and Peters, J.I. (1988) Respiratory failure: pathophysiology and treatment, in *Textbook of Respiratory Medicine* (eds J.F. Murray and J.A. Nadel), Saunders, Philadelphia, pp. 2017–34.

79. Kimball, W.R., Leith, D.E. and Robbins, A.G. (1982) Dynamic hyperinflation and ventilator dependence in chronic obstructive pulmonary disease. *Am. Rev. Respir. Dis.*, **126**, 991–5.

80. Eissa, N.T. and Milic-Emili, J. (1991) Modern concepts in monitoring and management of respiratory failure. *Anesthesiology Clin. North Am.*, **9**, 199–218.

81. Poggi, R., Brandolese, R., Bernasconi, M. *et al.* (1989) Doxofylline and respiratory mechanics: short term effects in mechanically ventilated patients with airflow obstruction and respiratory failure. *Chest*, **96**, 772–8.

82. Petrof, B.J., Kimoff, R.J., Cheong, T.H. *et al.* (1989) Nasal continuous positive airway pressure reduces inspiratory muscle effort during sleep in severe chronic obstructive pulmonary disease (abstract). *Am. Rev. Respir. Dis.*, **139**, A496.

83. Gottfried, S.B. (1991) The role of PEEP in the mechanically ventilated COPD patient, in *Ventilatory Failure* (eds J.J. Marini and C. Roussos), Springer-Verlag, Berlin, pp. 392–418.

84. Gottfried, S.B., Rossi, A., Higgs, B.D. *et al.* (1985) Noninvasive determination of respiratory system mechanics during mechanical ventilation for acute respiratory failure. *Am. Rev. Respir. Dis.*, **131**, 414–20.

85. Valta, P., Corbeil, C., Campodonico, R. *et al.* (1994) Detection of expiratory flow limitation during mechanical ventilation. *Am. J. Respir. Crit. Care Med.*, in press.

86. Koulouris, N., Valta, P., Lavoie, A. *et al.* (1993) A simple method to detect expiratory flow limitation during spontaneous breathing. *Am. Rev. Respir. Dis.*, **147**, A781.

87. Knudson, R.J., Mead, J. and Knudson, D.E. (1974) Contribution of airway collapse to supramaximal expiratory flows. *J. Appl. Physiol.*, **36**, 653–67.

PULMONARY GAS EXCHANGE

8

R. Rodriguez-Roisin and J. Roca

8.1 INTRODUCTION

The ultimate goal of the respiratory system is to exchange oxygen (O_2) and carbon dioxide (CO_2), to meet the metabolic needs of the body. In order to properly transfer both gases, ventilation and blood flow must be adequately apportioned and matched within the lungs. Of the four classic mechanisms determining abnormal arterial blood respiratory gases – alveolar hypoventilation, impaired alveolar–endcapillary diffusion to O_2, increased shunt, and ventilation–perfusion ($\dot{V}A/\dot{Q}$) mismatching – the last is by far the most common cause of impaired pulmonary gas exchange in respiratory disease. All the abnormalities alluded to above except alveolar hypoventilation may be viewed as intrapulmonary determinants of pulmonary gas exchange. Other key extrapulmonary determinants of respiratory blood gases include the fractional concentration of O_2 in the inspired gas, the hemodynamic status (cardiac output), and the metabolic demands (O_2 consumption) of the body.

The underlying structural abnormalities in chronic obstructive pulmonary disease (COPD), which include widespread airway narrowing with varying degrees of parenchymal destruction, together with rarefaction, distortion and/or obliteration of pulmonary vessels are at the origin of the maldistribution of alveolar ventilation and pulmonary blood

flow which leads to abnormal respiratory arterial blood gases and, ultimately, to respiratory insufficiency. Ventilation–perfusion mismatching is the principal determinant of pulmonary gas exchange under both acute and chronic conditions even though alveolar hypoventilation often emerges as a key mechanism producing hypercapnia [1,2]. By contrast, mild to moderate shunt is only present in acute respiratory insufficiency, or during its recovery, and the role of diffusion limitation to O_2 is negligible.

The present chapter reviews pulmonary gas exchange in COPD patients predominantly using the results obtained with the multiple inert gas elimination technique (MIGET) over the past two decades. This technique provided a quantum leap forward in the assessment of gas exchange abnormalities. We will first review the different clinical presentations of COPD to gain insight into the correlations between structure and function. Subsequently, the response to exercise and the effects of the breathing of O_2 and those induced by drugs on pulmonary gas exchange will be discussed.

8.2 MULTIPLE INERT GAS ELIMINATION TECHNIQUE (MIGET)

The potential and limitations of MIGET have been explored extensively [3,4]. It has three major advantages. First, it gives both

Chronic Obstructive Pulmonary Disease. Edited by Dr P. Calverley and Professor N. Pride. Published in 1995 by Chapman & Hall, London. ISBN 0 412 46450 0

quantitative and qualitative estimates of the distributions of $\dot{V}A/\dot{Q}$ ratios. Second, it does so without itself changing the airway caliber or pulmonary vascular tone, because there is no need to alter inspired O_2 concentrations during measurements. Third, it facilitates the interpretation of the complex interplay between intrapulmonary (abnormal $\dot{V}A/\dot{Q}$ relationships, shunt, and diffusion limitation to O_2) and extrapulmonary (inspired O_2 concentration, total ventilation, cardiac output, and O_2 consumption) factors influencing pulmonary gas exchange.

Furthermore, the extent of $\dot{V}A/\dot{Q}$ inequality detected by MIGET exceeds that derived from topographical measurements such as radioactive tracer gas scans, computed tomograms, or positron emission tomography (PET), in particular when used in patients with chronic, generalized lung disease, such as COPD [5–7]. The latter techniques all have a limited spatial resolution which grossly underestimates the intra-regional $\dot{V}A/\dot{Q}$ abnormalities.

Full technical details of MIGET have been reported [8]. In summary, the arterial, mixed venous and mixed expired concentrations of six infused inert gases, measured with gas chromatography, are used to calculate the ratio of arterial (Pa) to mixed venous pressures (P$\bar{v}$) (retention) and the ratio of mixed expired or alveolar (PA) to mixed venous pressure (excretion). Retention and excretion are then used to compute a multicompartment $\dot{V}A/\dot{Q}$ distribution. These six gases include a wide spectrum of solubilities (from the relatively insoluble gas, sulfur hexafluoride, to the most soluble, acetone, through those of intermediate solubility, i.e. ethane, cyclopropane, enflurane or halothane, and ether). The use of inert gases has two major advantages: first, the limitations due to a non-linear dissociation curve on gas exchange, as found for O_2 and CO_2, are not present; second, a large range of solubilities is used. It is known that the gas exchange behavior of any gas in the face of $\dot{V}A/\dot{Q}$ abnormalities is a function of its solubility [8].

The principle modulating inert gas elimination within the lung established by Kety in the early 1950s [9], and then further extended by Fahri and co-workers in the middle 1960s [10], is based on the simple concept that the uptake (retention) and the elimination (excretion) of an inert gas in any ideal homogeneous region of the lung under the assumption of steady state conditions is regulated by the following expression,

$$Pa/P\bar{v} = PA/P\bar{v} = \lambda / (\lambda + \dot{V}A/\dot{Q})$$

where λ corresponds to solubility. Notice that for a $\dot{V}A/\dot{Q}$ ratio of zero (shunt), the retention (Pa/P$\bar{v}$) is 1.0 for all gases, whereas for a $\dot{V}A/\dot{Q}$ ratio of infinity (dead space), the excretion (PA/P$\bar{v}$) is 0 for all gases.

Figure 8.1 depicts a typical distribution of $\dot{V}A/\dot{Q}$ ratios in a young, healthy non-smoker at rest, in a semi-recumbent position, breathing room air. The amounts (distributions) of alveolar ventilation and of pulmonary perfusion (Y axis) are plotted against a wide range of 50 $\dot{V}A/\dot{Q}$ ratios (from 0 to infinity) on a log scale (X axis). Each data point represents a particular amount of alveolar ventilation or pulmonary blood flow, the lines having been drawn to facilitate visual interpretation. Total blood flow or total alveolar ventilation correspond to the sum of all data points of their respective distributions. The logarithmic rather than linear axis of $\dot{V}A/\dot{Q}$ ratios is based on established practice in the field of pulmonary gas exchange. A logarithmic normal distribution of ventilation and blood flow is one of the simplest distributions and allows the spread to be defined by a simple variable, that is the standard deviation on a log scale (see below).

Both distributions are unimodal with three major common findings: symmetry, location around a mean $\dot{V}A/\dot{Q}$ ratio of 1.0, and a narrow dispersion ($\dot{V}A$ and $\dot{Q}$ to $\dot{V}A/\dot{Q}$ ratio between 0.1 and 10.0). Thus, in young healthy subjects there is no blood flow diverted to the left to a zone of low $\dot{V}A/\dot{Q}$ ratios (poorly ventilated lung units) nor ventilation distributed to the right to a zone of high $\dot{V}A/\dot{Q}$ ratios (in-

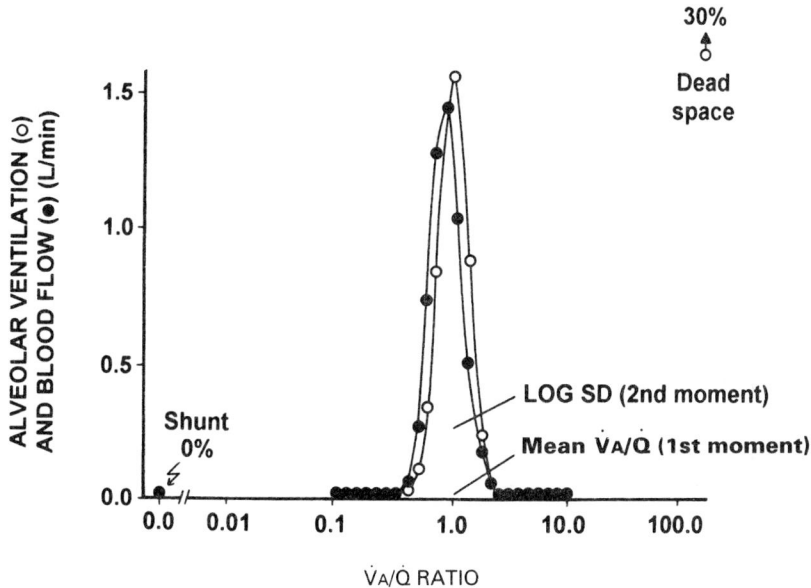

Fig. 8.1 Distributions of alveolar ventilation (*open symbols*) and pulmonary blood flow (*closed symbols*) (Y-axis) plotted against V̇A/Q̇ ratio on a log scale (X-axis) from a healthy, young individual at rest, breathing room air. The first moment of each distribution corresponds to its mean V̇A/Q̇ ratio (blood flow, Q̄, or ventilation, V̄) and the dispersion (second moment) of each distribution, expressed as the standard deviation on a log scale, is known as log SD Q (blood flow) or log SD V (ventilation). These indices are two of the most common markers used to assess V̇A/Q̇ mismatch.

completely perfused, but still finite, lung units). Shunt as detected by MIGET is defined as areas with zero V̇A/Q̇ ratio (in practice less than 0.005). Postpulmonary shunt (which corresponds to bronchial and Thebesian circulations) is not detected by MIGET. Consequently shunt measured by MIGET is lower than the conventional venous admixture ratio (Q̇s/Q̇t) (1–2 % of cardiac output) breathing room air which includes perfusion through very low V̇A/Q̇ units as well as the postpulmonary shunt [11]. When breathing 100% O$_2$ the influence of poorly ventilated units with low V̇A/Q̇ ratios is considerably decreased by wash out of nitrogen and so the difference between shunt measured by MIGET and 100% O$_2$ is greatly reduced. The normal value of inert physiologic dead space (infinite V̇A/Q̇ ratio, in practice above 100) (approximately 30% of overall alveolar venti-

lation) is also slightly less than that computed with the traditional Bohr's formula (VD/VT). While the Bohr's formula includes the dead space-like effects of all lung units whose alveolar PCO$_2$ values are less than the arterial PCO$_2$, the inert gas measurement represents only the dead space-like effects of those alveoli whose V̇A/Q̇ ratios are greater than 100.

The first moment of each distribution, i.e. the mean V̇A/Q̇ ratio of each distribution, and the second moment (or dispersion), log SD, are commonly used to quantitate the degree of V̇A/Q̇ mismatch. The second moment (square root) of the pulmonary blood flow (log SD Q) and of alveolar ventilation (log SD V) distributions reflects the variance (standard deviation) of V̇A/Q̇ ratios about the mean. In a perfectly homogeneous lung, log SD Q and log SD V should be zero. In practice, in a normal healthy individual they range between 0.3 and 0.6 [12]. By computing a multicompartmental lung model with a log normal distribution of pulmonary perfusion or alveolar ventilation, or both, West [13] earlier demonstrated that log SD Q or log SD V values of 1.0 and 1.5 imply moderate and severe degrees of $\dot{V}A/\dot{Q}$ mismatch, respectively. The degree of $\dot{V}A/\dot{Q}$ inequality can also be expressed as the total percentage of ventilation and perfusion in defined regions of the $\dot{V}A/\dot{Q}$ spectrum. Thus, the percentage of blood flow distributed in areas of $\dot{V}A/\dot{Q}$ ratios below 0.1 and above 0.005 (and, therefore, excluding shunt) is conventionally named 'low $\dot{V}A/\dot{Q}$ mode' and the amount of ventilation distributed to the region of $\dot{V}A/\dot{Q}$ ratios located between 10.0 and 100 (and, therefore, excluding dead space) is regarded as 'high $\dot{V}A/\dot{Q}$ mode' [8]. Using this technique no more than three modes of a distribution can be recovered and only smooth distributions can be obtained. Arterial–alveolar difference averaged for the group of inert gas indices also can be calculated and used to give indirect estimates of the degree of $\dot{V}A/\dot{Q}$ abnormalities [14]. Other approaches, equally valid, have plotted the retention minus excretion data of inert gases versus their partition blood:gas coefficient and interpolated various points for intermediate coefficients, giving thus a qualitative assessment of $\dot{V}A/\dot{Q}$ mismatch [15]. Finally, the amount of $\dot{V}A/\dot{Q}$ inequality can be assessed qualitatively by describing the morphologic pattern of each distribution, which can be narrowly or broadly unimodal, or clearly bimodal.

MIGET can also assist in addressing the potential presence of diffusion limitation for O_2 because equilibration of inert gases is in practice not diffusion limited [8,9]. Accordingly, the technique can be used to compute the PaO_2 predicted from the degree of both $\dot{V}A/\dot{Q}$ mismatch and shunting compared to the measured actual PaO_2. If the measured PaO_2 is not similar to the estimated values, this indicates that other potential mechanisms

of hypoxemia, such as diffusion limitation to O_2, increased intrapulmonary parenchymal O_2 consumption or increased postpulmonary shunt, are occurring [8]. Ventilation–perfusion mismatch has been shown to explain the measured PaO_2 in patients with COPD [16]. In contrast, limitation of diffusion of O_2 has been shown to explain at rest 20% and during exercise 40% of the increased alveolar–arterial PO_2 difference found in patients with cryptogenic fibrosing alveolitis (idiopathic pulmonary fibrosis) [17] (Fig. 8.2).

8.3 MECHANISMS OF ABNORMAL GAS EXCHANGE

With the use of MIGET, different degrees of $\dot{V}A/\dot{Q}$ inequality have been documented which by and large are consistent with the clinical severity of COPD. Increased intrapulmonary shunt is absent in stable chronic conditions, and during acute exacerbations rarely exceeds 10% of total pulmonary blood flow even in the presence of abundant, viscous bronchial secretions [17]. Moreover, in spite of the well-known finding of a reduced gas transfer factor (TLCO) in the most severe advanced cases of pulmonary emphysema, all of the studies using MIGET have consistently excluded the presence of alveolar–end capillary diffusion limitation for O_2 at rest or during exercise, as an additional intrapulmonary mechanism causing hypoxemia.

8.3.1 SEVERE, ADVANCED COPD

Combining measurements of arterial blood respiratory gases and routine pulmonary function tests and certain clinical features, Burrows *et al.* [18] in the middle 1960s were able to subdivide COPD patients into two distinct presentations. Type B patients, or 'blue bloaters', presented with marked cough and sputum production, fluid retention, recurrent cor pulmonale, polycythemia, and were more likely to be hypoxemic and hypercapnic. By

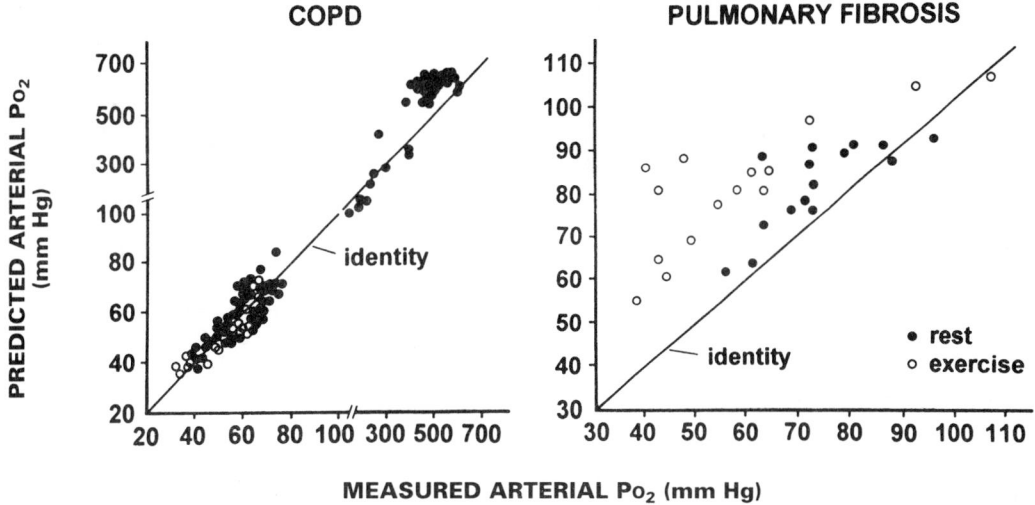

Fig. 8.2 Plots of individual predicted (estimated) PaO_2 (Y-axes) (reflecting $\dot{V}A/\dot{Q}$ mismatch as assessed by MIGET) versus actual PaO_2 (X-axes) at rest (*closed symbols*) and during exercise (*open symbols*) in patients with COPD (*left-hand panel*) (upon breathing room air or 100% O_2) and with cryptogenic fibrosing alveolitis (*right-hand panel*). Note that whilst in the former there were no differences between PaO_2, in the latter predicted PaO_2 was always significantly higher than measured PaO_2. This suggests the coexistence of limitation of alveolar to endcapillary O_2 diffusion as an additional cause of hypoxemia in patients with lung fibrosis. (Taken from reference [17] and reference [20] with permission.)

contrast, the gas exchange of Type A patients, or 'pink puffers' who complained of severe shortness of breath and were found at autopsy to have significant pulmonary emphysema, was characterized by a normal or low $PaCO_2$, only a mild decrease of the PaO_2 at rest, and a low carbon monoxide diffusing capacity (transfer factor) (TLCO) and Krogh coefficient (KCO or TLCO divided by alveolar volume).

Wagner *et al.* [20] in the late 1970s, in choosing 23 stable patients with advanced COPD for study (FEV$_1$ range 19–58% predicted), with mild to severe gas exchange disturbances (PaO_2 range 38–71 mmHg; $PaCO_2$ range 25–64 mmHg; TLCO range 17–157% predicted) aimed to find stable patients who reflected as closely as possible the two classic clinical types suggested by Burrows and colleagues ten years earlier. In these patients $\dot{V}A/\dot{Q}$ ratio distributions were remarkably abnormal and displayed three distinct $\dot{V}A/\dot{Q}$

patterns (Figure 8.3). The first $\dot{V}A/\dot{Q}$ profile showed the presence of lung units with very high $\dot{V}A/\dot{Q}$ ratios or a 'high $\dot{V}A/\dot{Q}$ mode' (type H). With this pattern most of the ventilation was located in the zone of higher $\dot{V}A/\dot{Q}$ ratios. The second pattern was characterized by a mode including a large proportion of blood flow perfusing lung units with very low $\dot{V}A/\dot{Q}$ units or a 'low $\dot{V}A/\dot{Q}$ mode' (type L), most of the blood flow being into areas of lower $\dot{V}A/\dot{Q}$ ratios. Finally, the third pattern was a mixed 'high-low $\dot{V}A/\dot{Q}$ mode' (type H-L), including additional modes both above and below the main body. Overall, the dispersions of blood flow or ventilation, or both, were moderately to severely increased (each above 1.0). Specific amounts of distributions of blood flow to low $\dot{V}A/\dot{Q}$ ratios and of ventilation distributed to high $\dot{V}A/\dot{Q}$ areas were not reported. Interestingly, whereas 7 of the 8 patients classified as Burrows' type A showed a $\dot{V}A/\dot{Q}$ distribution of pattern H, only one

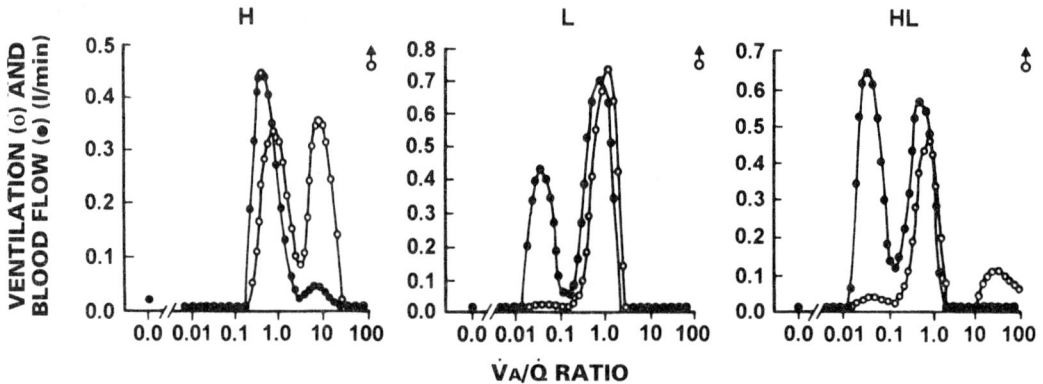

Fig. 8.3 Typical $\dot{V}A/\dot{Q}$ distributions in patients with advanced COPD (from left to right and from top to bottom): Type H (high $\dot{V}A/\dot{Q}$ mode) represents a $\dot{V}A/\dot{Q}$ pattern characterized by a substantial amount of ventilation distributed to high $\dot{V}A/\dot{Q}$ regions; type L (low $\dot{V}A/\dot{Q}$ mode) depicts a $\dot{V}A/\dot{Q}$ profile in which a marked amount of blood flow is diverted to low $\dot{V}A/\dot{Q}$ areas; and, type HL illustrates both former abnormal $\dot{V}A/\dot{Q}$ patterns. Whilst shunt (left closed symbol) is trivial, dead space (right open symbol with arrow) space is always moderately increased in all three patterns. (Taken from reference [20] with permission.)

had pattern L. By contrast, in the 12 patients characterized as Burrows' Type B, the three $\dot{V}A/\dot{Q}$ patterns (H, L, and H-L) were equally present (one-third each). Among the remaining 3 patients with clinical features of mixed Types A and B COPD, 2 had a pattern H-L and the third the pattern H.

These results suggested that patients with Type A COPD were very likely to have high $\dot{V}A/\dot{Q}$ areas, and were unlikely to have distinct low $\dot{V}A/\dot{Q}$ areas unless they had clinical evidence of Type B COPD as well. It was postulated that pattern H was likely produced by continued ventilation of regions with reduced blood flow. Conceivably, these regions might represent emphysematous regions where destruction of the alveolar walls results in the loss of the pulmonary vasculature. In contrast, patients of the Burrows' Type B variety commonly have distinct low or high $\dot{V}A/\dot{Q}$ areas, or both, although there is clearly much more variability within this group. Thus, pattern L was likely to represent regions subtended by airways partially blocked by mucus secretions and plugging, smooth muscle hypertrophy, wall edema, bron-

chospasm, distortion, or some combination of all these abnormalities. Other findings of interest were the essential absence of intrapulmonary shunt and the presence of a mild to moderate increase in dead space (range 30–42% of alveolar ventilation) in most of the patients. The absence of shunt suggests that the efficiency of collateral ventilation is very active or that complete airways occlusion does not occur.

Of further interest was the lack of correlation between spirometry (FEV_1) and respiratory blood gases. Similarly, the three patterns of $\dot{V}A/\dot{Q}$ ratio distributions did not correlate with spirometry (Fig. 8.4), airways resistance, arterial blood gases or transfer factor. There was, however, some correlation between the loss of elastic recoil (or increased static compliance) and the presence of the type H pattern.

Subsequently, more than a dozen studies [20–35] including approximately 200 patients with severe or very severe airflow obstruction (mean FEV_1 equal to or below 36% predicted), many of them with hypoxemia (with or without chronic hypercapnia) and some with

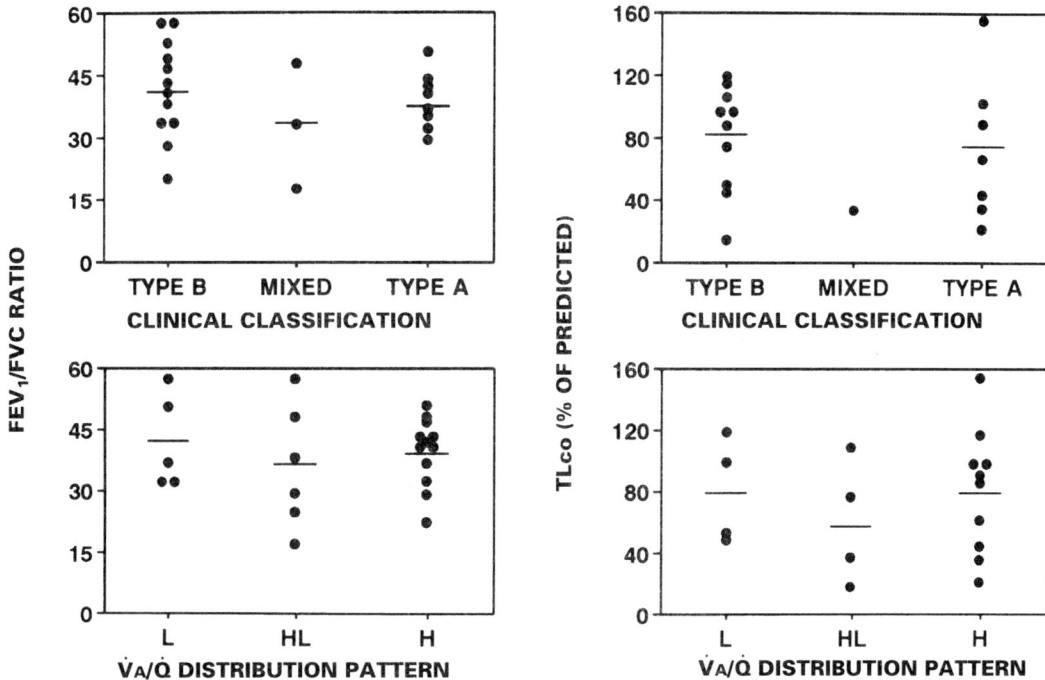

Fig. 8.4 Plots of spirometry and transfer factor (TLco) (Y-axes)versus Burrows' clinical classification *(top)* and $\dot{V}_A/\dot{Q}$ patterns *(bottom)* (X-axes). No correlation was found between routine lung function tests and clinical data or inert gas measurements. (Taken from reference [20] with permission.)

pulmonary hypertension, have been reported. All but 2 studies [25,28] were carried out in patients with stable disease, spontaneously breathing room air. Most of them documented $\dot{V}_A/\dot{Q}$ patterns similar to those reported originally by Wagner *et al.* [20], although the relationship established with the clinical COPD types of Burrows *et al.* could not be established as clearly as in the study of Wagner *et al.* The amounts of blood flow or ventilation distributed to regions with low or high $\dot{V}_A/\dot{Q}$ ratios, respectively, were modest (range equal to or below 10% of cardiac output) in all but a few of the reports. As in the original study of Wagner *et al.* [20], the correlation between spirometric and gas exchange indices was very poor. In one study [27], however, despite the same amount of airflow obstruction the $\dot{V}_A/\dot{Q}$ mismatching was less severe with broadly unimodal pat-

terns of ventilation and blood flow, clearly at variance with the bimodal or trimodal shapes shown previously [20]. Different clinical circumstances may explain such differences. We have shown that the severity of $\dot{V}_A/\dot{Q}$ abnormalities and their patterns during episodes of acute exacerbation of COPD may improve over a period of few weeks of adequate treatment [31]. In this sequential study of patients with acute hypercapnic respiratory failure not needing mechanical ventilation (Fig. 8.5), one month after the onset of study all spirometric and gas exchange indices had improved. Arterial Po_2 increased and $Paco_2$ decreased and some distributions of $\dot{V}_A/\dot{Q}$ inequalities became unimodal. These data suggest that part of the $\dot{V}_A/\dot{Q}$ abnormalities during exacerbations are related to partially reversible pathophysiologic abnormalities of airway narrowing, such as mucus plugging,

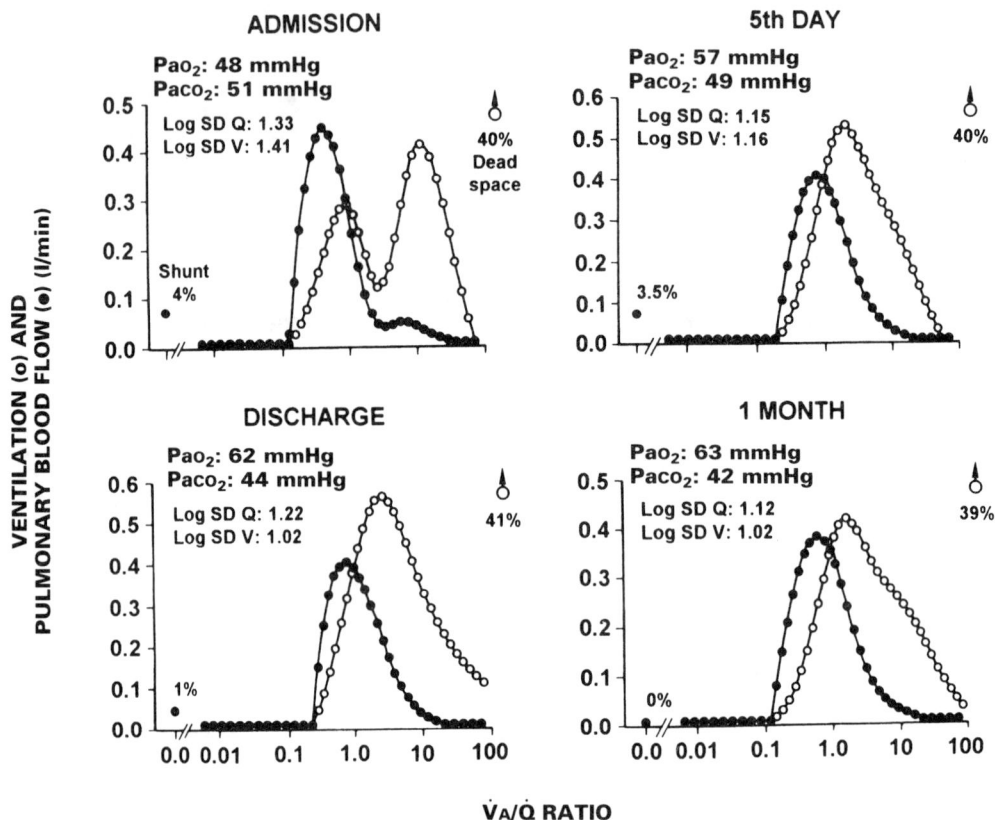

Fig. 8.5 Evaluation of $\dot{V}A/\dot{Q}$ distributions in a representative patient with COPD and acute respiratory failure breathing spontaneously ($FIO_2 = 0.24$) (from left to right and from top to bottom):On admission inequalities $\dot{V}A/\dot{Q}$ (log SD Q and log SD V ranges 1.0–1.5) were moderately to severely abnormal. With appropriate medical care there was a progressive, although partial, amelioration both in $\dot{V}A/\dot{Q}$ distributions and arterial blood respiratory gases. A modest shunt (less than 5% of cardiac output) is observed during the first days of the acute exacerbation; note also that the bimodal blood flow distribution is present on admission only. (Taken from reference [31] with permission).

bronchial wall edema, bronchoconstriction, and/or air trapping.

Two studies of COPD patients needing mechanical support for acute exacerbation of the disease have shown qualitatively similar $\dot{V}A/\dot{Q}$ patterns, although quantitatively more severe than those documented in patients breathing spontaneously [25,28]. The main difference was the presence of intrapulmonary shunt, which was always slightly increased (range 4–10% of cardiac output). This suggests that some airways were completely occluded, possibly by

inspissated bronchial secretions. However, if a patient with COPD shows a shunt of 20% or more of cardiac output despite a normal chest radiograph, which excludes extensive atelectasis, pneumonia, lung collapse or pulmonary edema, then the possibility of a reopening of the foramen ovale due to increase in right atrial pressure should be considered [36]. Contrast enhanced echocardiogram or angiocardiography may help to differentiate between intrapulmonary and intracardiac shunt [37]. In the presence of a true shunt, breathing 100% O_2 for

30 minutes or more fails to increase PaO_2 to more than 300–350 mmHg [38].

A further finding was the crucial role of both cardiac output and ventilatory pattern in influencing gas exchange when patients were discontinued from mechanical ventilation [28]. During weaning, while cardiac output increased considerably due to the abrupt increase in venous return (following the reduction of intrathoracic pressure) and total ventilation was maintained, tidal volume was reduced and respiratory frequency increased and became less efficient (Fig. 8.6). As a result, both the dispersion of alveolar ventilation and the overall $\dot{V}A/\dot{Q}$ heterogeneity increased resulting in further $\dot{V}A/\dot{Q}$ mismatch. A striking observation was that there was only a small and non-significant increase in shunt from mechanical ventilation to spontaneous breathing (from 3 to 9% of cardiac output) despite the substantial increases in cardiac output and mixed venous PO_2. This is at variance with the well-known, although poorly understood, strong linear relationship between increase in pulmonary blood flow and shunt fraction, commonly observed in patients with acute lung injury [39,40]. In an experimental model of shunt plus low $\dot{V}A/\dot{Q}$ mode, Wagner et al [41] showed that the relationship between pulmonary blood flow and shunt fraction was heavily dependent on inspired O_2 concentration (the higher the FIO_2, the more the increase in the former relationship). They suggested that the increase in shunt fraction with cardiac output depended more on vascular tone of non-injured areas of the lungs than on tone of the low $\dot{V}A/\dot{Q}$ areas which remain hypoxic at all values of inspired O_2.

Another striking finding in the study of Torres *et al.* [28] was that respiratory blood

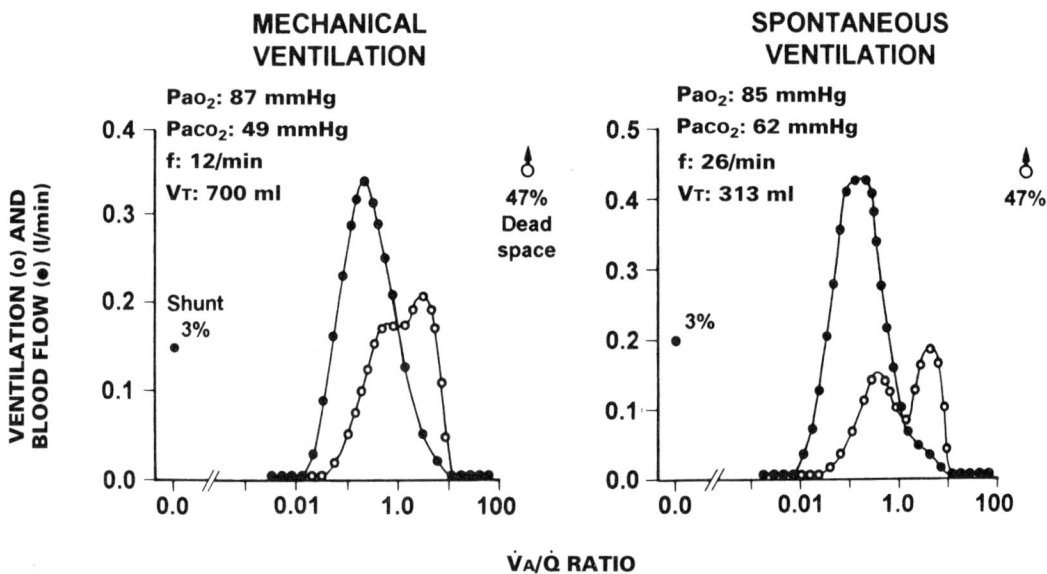

Fig. 8.6 $\dot{V}A/\dot{Q}$ distributions during weaning (FIO_2 = 0.36) in a representative patient with COPD, after 9 days of mechanical ventilation (left-hand panel) During spontaneous ventilation (right-hand panel) there was more hypercapnia secondary to an abnormal ventilatory pattern dysfunction (rapid and shallow breathing), which further deteriorated $\dot{V}A/\dot{Q}$ relationships. Cardiac output increased abruptly (*not shown*) resulting in increased mixed venous PO_2 and, consequently, in less hypoxemia. (Taken from reference [28] with permission).

gases remained unaltered despite increases in mixed venous P_{O_2} and O_2 delivery (arterial O_2 content times cardiac output). In other words, the potentially beneficial effect of the increased cardiac output on Pa_{O_2} was offset by the deleterious influence of the change in ventilatory pattern on Pa_{O_2}. Despite these problems, weaning in these patients was successful. When patients were removed from the ventilator in this study [28], O_2 consumption (calculated according to the Fick principle) did not change. Lemaire and co-workers [42] also stressed the importance of cardiac output variations and other hemodynamic changes together with an increase in O_2 consumption as causes of unsuccessful weaning, in a similar group of patients with severe COPD in the face of myocardial infarction and left ventricular dysfunction. These data [28,42] have been complemented with another study using both inert gas and lung isotopic scanning measurements whilst discontinuing mechanical ventilation in patients with COPD after more than 5 days of attempted weaning from the ventilator [43]. During spontaneous breathing, the isotopic craniocaudal difference of $\dot{V}_A/\dot{Q}$ ratios was closely correlated to the dispersion of pulmonary blood flow. Further, the patients with the smallest tidal volume whilst breathing spontaneously showed the largest amount of blood flow to areas of low $\dot{V}_A/\dot{Q}$ units, the lowest isotopic $\dot{V}_A/\dot{Q}$ ratio at the bases, and the largest isotopic craniocaudal difference in $\dot{V}_A/\dot{Q}$ ratios. These results suggested that the abnormal ventilatory pattern induced during spontaneous breathing was the major determinant of the $\dot{V}_A/\dot{Q}$ inequalities, probably preferentially located at the bases of the lungs. Interestingly, this $\dot{V}_A/\dot{Q}$ worsening was not influenced by inspiratory pressure support, a ventilatory approach that exerts an adjustable level of positive pressure to the airways during inspiration. In these and other studies [42,44], however, it has been shown that O_2 consumption usually increases during weaning which could tend to induce a

decrease in Pa_{O_2}. By computing a lung model of $\dot{V}_A/\dot{Q}$ mismatch alone, Wagner showed that Pa_{O_2} can fall by 10 mmHg when there is a 10% rise in O_2 consumption [45]. The behaviour of Pa_{O_2} in this $\dot{V}_A/\dot{Q}$ model is more sensitive than in the shunt model because here the Pa_{O_2} is located on the upper flat part of the oxyhemoglobin curve, and this allows larger variations.

We have also to be aware of the potential influence of an increased CO_2 production on Pa_{CO_2}. Malnutrition is an important clinical and therapeutic problem in COPD patients which is receiving increasing attention [46]. Normally, the amount of CO_2 produced per minute is a function of the metabolic rate and the substrate used for fuel. In healthy individuals, the absorption and metabolism of carbohydrate loads causes an increase in CO_2 output (from about 70 to 100 % of the O_2 consumed), as the whole body fuel utilization is shifted from predominantly fat to essentially carbohydrate and also from the thermogenic effect of food *per se*. In hospitalized patients receiving excessive hypernutrition, basal CO_2 production can increase by approximately 50% [47]. With such an increase in CO_2 production, presumably minute ventilation has to be doubled to avoid arterial CO_2 retention. In patients who receive high glucose loads in association with total parenteral nutrition, the respiratory quotient can increase to 1.0 (resting normal value, 0.8), such that CO_2 output increases markedly. Patients without primary respiratory problems increase ventilation proportionately and accommodate to the increased CO_2 production without major problems. In contrast, patients with COPD prone to hypercapnic respiratory failure are less able to excrete this load by increasing ventilation, and hypercapnia may worsen. Failure to wean from mechanical ventilation in patients with COPD may occur due to this increased CO_2 load [48]. It has been suggested that these patients should receive alimentation of fat emulsions, because these induce a lower production of CO_2 than isocaloric amounts of glucose [49]. The consequences of these nutritional problems on $\dot{V}A/\dot{Q}$ distributions have never been studied.

Although the role of sleep in patients with COPD is addressed extensively elsewhere (Chapter 12), it is worth noting that as well as alveolar hypoventilation, other potential mechanisms for worsening hypoxemia during sleep include a reduced functional residual capacity and worsening $\dot{V}A/\dot{Q}$ mismatch [50]. Unfortunately because steady state conditions cannot be assumed, specific data on $\dot{V}A/\dot{Q}$ distributions during sleep are not available.

8.3.2 MILD, EARLY COPD

Barberà *et al.* [32] studied 23 patients with a mild obstructive ventilatory pattern (mean FEV_1, 76% predicted). All but 2 patients had normal TLCO and total lung capacity was within the normal range. Mean PaO_2 and $PaCO_2$ were normal, but mean $AaPO_2$ was moderately increased (>15 mmHg). Overall, the dispersions of ventilation and blood flow were mildly abnormal (each log SD below 1.0), shunt was absent and dead space was normal. Blood flow distributions were broadly unimodal in two-thirds of the patients and modestly bimodal in the remaining one-third. By contrast, the ventilation distributions were never bimodal and were devoid of regions of very high $\dot{V}A/\dot{Q}$ ratios.

8.3.3 SMALL AIRWAYS DISEASE

In the only available study to date, Barberà *et al.* [51] studied 7 patients with functional criteria compatible with small airways disease (mean FEV_1 above 80% predicted but abnormalities of maximum mid-expiratory flow and single breath N_2 test). The results were compared to 6 individuals with normal lung function and also to 22 others with FEV_1 below 80% predicted. Patients with small airways dysfunction, but with normal PaO_2, showed a small but significant increase in alveolar–arterial PO_2 difference and milder $\dot{V}A/\dot{Q}$ mismatch, as expressed by modest increases in the dispersions of both blood flow and ventilation (each log SD below 1.0), compared to controls. No differences in these parameters were shown, however, between patients with mild airway dysfunction and those with early COPD and greater airflow obstruction. Although the interpretation of these data remains speculative, they are akin with the concept, at least theoretically, that functional abnormalities in peripheral airways can produce maldistribution of ventilation and $\dot{V}A/\dot{Q}$ mismatching in the face of a normal PaO_2.

8.4 OTHER CHRONIC DISORDERS WITH AIRFLOW OBSTRUCTION

8.4.1 BRONCHIAL ASTHMA

A wide spectrum of $\dot{V}A/\dot{Q}$ inequalities occurs in adult patients with asthma, from the nearly normal distributions in patients with episodic asthma in remission to very abnormal distributions found in patients with acute severe asthma needing mechanical ventilation [40,52]. In moderate to severe asthma the most common $\dot{V}A/\dot{Q}$ pattern is the presence of a bimodal or broadly unimodal blood flow distribution. A considerable percentage of pulmonary perfusion is diverted to alveolar units with low $\dot{V}A/\dot{Q}$ ratios, the amount being broadly proportional to the clinical severity of the disease. This is the principal component of hypoxemia. Shunt is conspicuously absent, even in the most life-threatening conditions, the distribution of alveolar ventilation is never bimodal, and dead space is normal or slightly increased only. Conceivably, the lack of shunt may be related to the efficiency of collateral ventilation which prevents collapse of alveoli beyond the occluded airways and also to the fact that airways obstruction is never totally complete; alternatively, it may reflect the efficiency of hypoxic pulmonary vasoconstriction. A consistent dissociation between spirometric data and gas exchange indices has been shown not only under baseline conditions, but also after the administration of some bronchodilators [52] or following various bronchial challenges [53]. This suggests that while the reduction of airflow rates is more related to the presence of narrowing of conducting airways, gas exchange abnormalities largely reflect the status of peripheral airways. In patients with asthma, especially in acute severe attacks, both cardiac output and minute ventilation tend to be increased, thus optimizing the baseline values of PaO_2 that otherwise would be much lower due to the deleterious effects of $\dot{V}A/\dot{Q}$ mismatch by itself.

8.4.2 CYSTIC FIBROSIS

Dantzker and co-workers [54] studied the $\dot{V}A/\dot{Q}$ inequalities in 6 adult patients with stable cystic fibrosis. Two were normoxemic and 4 hypoxemic, 2 with $PaO_2 < 60$ mmHg. While all patients had mild to moderate amounts of shunt, 3 patients showed additionally minor $\dot{V}A/\dot{Q}$ abnormalities, namely a broadening of the distribution of pulmonary blood flow; the distributions of ventilation were always unimodal and dead space was normal or increased. Unlike patients with asthma, gas exchange disturbances in cystic fibrosis were essentially characterized by the presence of shunt as the predominant mechanism of the underlying degree of hypoxemia. This is compatible with unventilated alveoli whose airways are completely occluded by abundant, inspissated secretions, and mucoid impaction; the coexistence of regions with low $\dot{V}A/\dot{Q}$ ratios may be related to the presence of poorly ventilated alveolar units.

Neither bronchial asthma nor cystic fibrosis showed a significant difference between predicted PaO_2 (according to inert gases) and measured PaO_2 (respiratory gases) (see above), thereby excluding the coexistence of diffusion impairment to O_2 transfer as a complementary mechanism of hypoxemia.

8.5 STRUCTURE AND FUNCTION

Only one study [32] has investigated the influence of the morphologic changes of both pulmonary emphysema and small airway abnormalities on $\dot{V}A/\dot{Q}$ mismatching. In this study with mild COPD, emphysema was the morphologic variable that correlated best with the respiratory gas indices. The emphysema severity correlated positively with the alveolar–arterial PO_2 difference ($AaPO_2$), negatively with PaO_2 and was significantly positively related to the dispersion of blood flow and that of alveolar ventilation (Fig. 8.7). The more severe the degree of emphysema, the more abnormal the $\dot{V}A/\dot{Q}$ mismatch. The degree of abnormality in the dispersion of pulmonary perfusion suggests the development of areas of lower than normal $\dot{V}A/\dot{Q}$ ratios, Likewise, these findings suggest that poorly ventilated areas associated with emphysema may be one of the structural determinants of hypoxemia in these patients. Thus, it can be hypothesized that the loss of alveolar attachments of bronchiolar walls observed in emphysema may result in both distortion and narrowing of the lumen of bronchioles. The latter may cause reduced alveolar ventilation in the dependent alveolar units, and hence low $\dot{V}A/\dot{Q}$ ratios. Likewise, it has been shown that centrilobular emphysema areas have a greater residual volume and a lower compliance leading therefore to a decreased ventilation-to-volume ratio [55]. This is an additional mechanism to account for a reduction in effective ventilation in peripheral alveoli. Reduction in ventilation of some areas produces lung units with continued blood flow and thus low $\dot{V}A/\dot{Q}$ areas. Accordingly, this abnormality in $\dot{V}A/\dot{Q}$ relationships becomes evident in the dispersion of blood flow.

The correlation between emphysema and abnormalities in the dispersion of alveolar ventilation (Fig. 8.7) may be, at least in part, related to the loss of pulmonary capillary network of emphysematous spaces (wasted ventilation). This would lead to the develop-

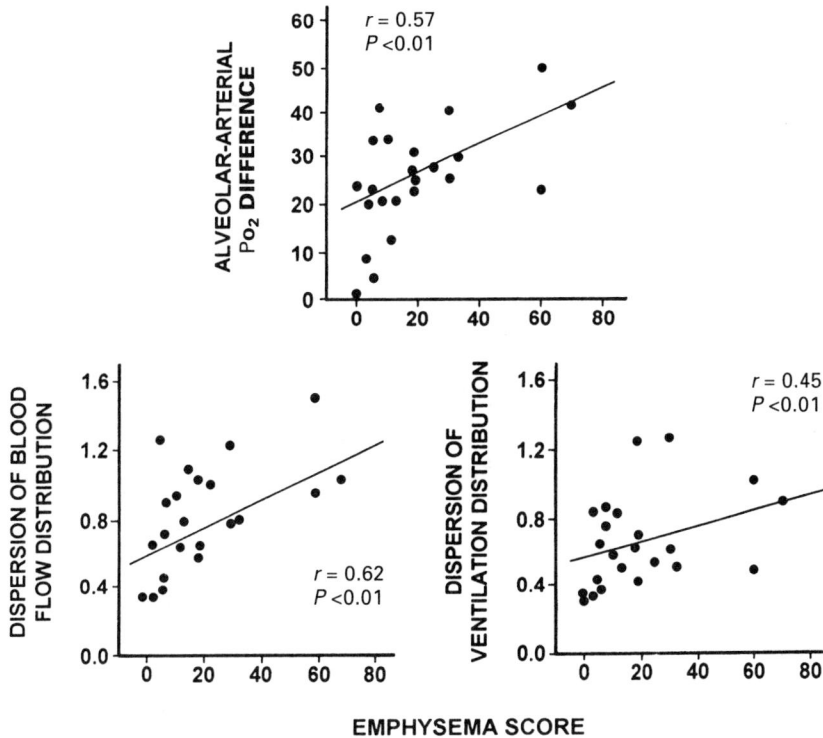

Fig. 8.7 Positive correlations between alveolar–arterial Po_2 difference (mmHg) and blood flow and alveolar ventilation dispersions (Y-axes) and emphysema score (X-axes) in patients with mild COPD. (Taken from reference [32] with permission.)

ment of lung units with high $\dot{V}A/\dot{Q}$ ratios, hence increasing dispersion of ventilation. Accordingly, the bimodal pattern of the ventilation distribution, with a large amount of ventilation diverted to high $\dot{V}A/\dot{Q}$ ratios (type H) alluded to above in patients with advanced Type A COPD, would be an extension of this phenomenon likely reflecting large areas of destroyed parenchyma.

Despite the lack of relationships between chronic abnormalities in small airways and the respiratory gas indices, which is consistent with the absence of correlation between these structural changes and the dispersion of blood flow, bronchiolar lesions were associated with $\dot{V}A/\dot{Q}$ mismatching as shown by the significant correlation found between the airway inflammation score and

the dispersion of ventilation (Fig. 8.8). A potential explanation for this correlation might be that a non-homogeneous distribution of inspired air, as a result of the airway narrowing caused by the bronchiolar impairment, accounted for the increased dispersion of ventilation, particularly evident when the latter is broadly unimodal and devoid of very high $\dot{V}A/\dot{Q}$ ratios as in this case.

The absence of correlation between small airways abnormalities and both the dispersion of blood flow and the percentage of perfusion to low $\dot{V}A/\dot{Q}$ ratios cannot be extrapolated to the common $\dot{V}A/\dot{Q}$ findings shown in patients with more advanced COPD during recovery from acute exacerbations [20,28,31]; in these patients a bimodal blood

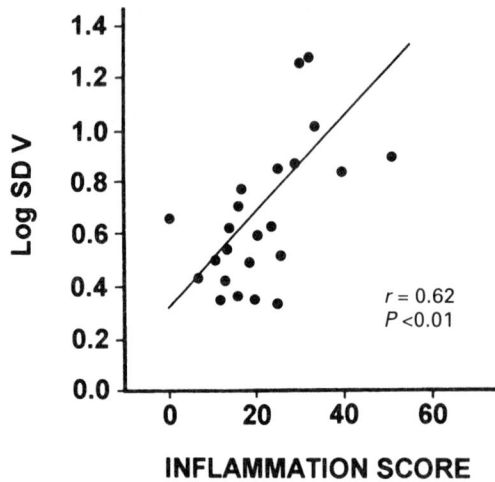

Fig. 8.8 Positive correlation between the dispersion of alveolar ventilation (Y-axis) and inflammatory bronchial changes (X-axis) in patients with mild COPD. (Taken from reference [32] with permission.)

flow pattern distribution is common and may be attributed to the superimposition of acute and potentially reversible airway changes, such as bronchial wall edema or mucus plugging, on the chronic airway abnormalities.

More recently, the same group of investigators have assessed the potential correlation between the pulmonary vascular abnormalities and the $\dot{V}A/\dot{Q}$ relationships in the same COPD patients prior to lobectomy for small neoplasms [56]. It was shown that the lower the degree of pulmonary vascular reactivity to the breathing of 100% O_2, the greater the thickness of the intimal layer of the pulmonary vascular arteries. Further, the thickness of the intimal layer was related to gas exchange indices and also to the degree of bronchiolar inflammation. Obviously, this is crucial to the development of further $\dot{V}A/\dot{Q}$ worsening. Moreover, thickening in small pulmonary arteries can interfere with the adaptability of these vessels to various O_2 concentrations and the maintenance of $\dot{V}A/\dot{Q}$ matching.

SUMMARY

According to these data, it can be postulated that there may be a spectrum of $\dot{V}A/\dot{Q}$ abnormalities in patients with COPD. At one end of the spectrum, there would be those patients with mild to moderate airflow obstruction and little or no abnormality in arterial blood gases, whose $\dot{V}A/\dot{Q}$ mismatch is mild, being essentially characterized by broadly unimodal profiles of the dispersions of blood flow and alveolar ventilation. At the other end, there would be those patients with severe advanced disease and marked gas exchange abnormalities. These individuals will show dramatic $\dot{V}A/\dot{Q}$ inequalities, with bimodal profiles of blood flow or alveolar ventilation distributions, or both, according to clinical conditions, reflecting thus different degrees of progression of disease. Conceivably, Type B Burrows's patients with high $\dot{V}A/\dot{Q}$ areas have lesions of emphysema as well as of chronic airway changes, but Type A COPD patients with areas of low $\dot{V}A/\dot{Q}$ units are rarely observed. These patients with severe COPD show always increased dead space and occasionally modest shunts, particularly during exacerbations. In between these extremes would be many patients, with different degrees of $\dot{V}A/\dot{Q}$ mismatch, depending on evolution, clinical condition and therapeutic regimen.

8.6 GAS EXCHANGE DURING EXERCISE

In the normal human at maximum exercise, O_2 transport can increase as much as 15 to 20 times compared to resting conditions [57]. By contrast, in patients with severe COPD O_2 consumption at maximum symptom-limited exercise only increases 3–4 times resting levels to approximately one liter per minute. Such a limitation is basically due to the inability of the lungs to match pulmonary O_2 uptake and elimination of CO_2 to higher levels of whole body metabolic O_2 consumption and CO_2 production. Physical decondi-

FACTORS DETERMINING ARTERIAL OXYGENATION DURING EXERCISE IN COPD

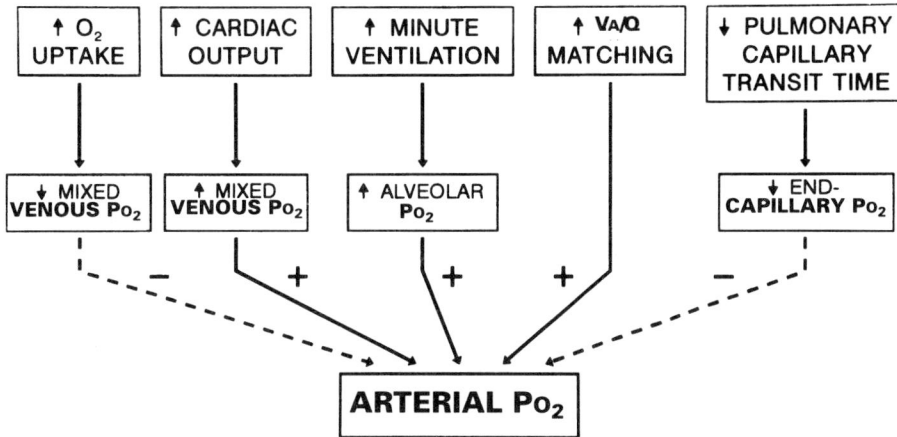

| ↑ O_2 UPTAKE | ↑ CARDIAC OUTPUT | ↑ MINUTE VENTILATION | ↑ $\dot{V}A/\dot{Q}$ MATCHING | ↓ PULMONARY CAPILLARY TRANSIT TIME |

| ↓ MIXED VENOUS Po_2 | ↑ MIXED VENOUS Po_2 | ↑ ALVEOLAR Po_2 | | ↓ END-CAPILLARY Po_2 |

−   +   +   +   −

ARTERIAL Po_2

Fig. 8.9 Arterial Po_2 increases because either cardiac output and/or minute ventilation (extrapulmonary determinants) increase or $\dot{V}A/\dot{Q}$ mismatching (intrapulmonary determinant) improves; other extrapulmonary factors, such as increased O_2 uptake (consumption) and decreased of pulmonary capillary blood transit time (due to increased cardiac output in the absence of pulmonary capillary recruitment/distensibility), may tend to reduce Pao_2. Arterial Po_2 is thus the end-point variable of the complex interaction between all these elements. Similar interplay is observed in other situations, such as discontinuing from mechanical ventilation or after the administration of vasoactive drugs.

tioning also plays a role limiting exercise performance in these patients. The behavior of both Pao_2 and $Paco_2$ during exercise in these patients rely on complex interactions between intrapulmonary (essentially $\dot{V}A/\dot{Q}$ mismatching) and extrapulmonary factors (i.e. cardiac output, total ventilation and O_2 consumption) modulating respiratory gases (Fig. 8.9). As during weaning, during exercise Pao_2 and $Paco_2$ do not necessarily reflect parallel variations in $\dot{V}A/\dot{Q}$ inequality because of the influential role of these extrapulmonary factors.

The original MIGET study of Wagner *et al.* [20], performed in patients with severe COPD during exercise, showed a complete absence of systematic changes in the measured respiratory gases and in $\dot{V}A/\dot{Q}$ distributions; likewise, there was no evidence of a diffusion defect for O_2. A later study [26], in a smaller series of patients with similarly advanced COPD, showed the same results for intrapul-

monary determinants of respiratory gases ($\dot{V}A/\dot{Q}$ relationships and diffusion limitation) but falls in Pao_2 and mixed venous Po_2 and a rise in $Paco_2$ occurred during exercise.

Two further studies [30,58] have assessed the effects of submaximal exercise (approximately at 60% of maximal O_2 consumption) in patients with COPD, with severe airflow obstruction, mild to moderate impairment of gas exchange and no pulmonary hypertension. In the first study [30], it was shown that, unlike patients with more advanced disease, exercise had a beneficial effect on $\dot{V}A/\dot{Q}$ distributions with a reduced dispersion of ventilation and a more homogeneous distribution of pulmonary blood flow (Fig. 8.10); as expected, inert dead space fell significantly. It was hypothesized that these improvements were related to less severe structural abnormalities.

In the second study Barberà *et al.* [58] showed, in patients with even milder COPD,

	REST		EXERCISE
$\bar{Q}$	0.79 ± 0.06		1.18 ± 0.12 *
Log SD Q	0.90 ± 0.06	* $P <0.05$	0.78 ± 0.07 *
$\bar{V}$	2.14 ± 0.27		2.23 ± 0.27
Log SD V	1.03 ± 0.11		0.83 ± 0.09 *

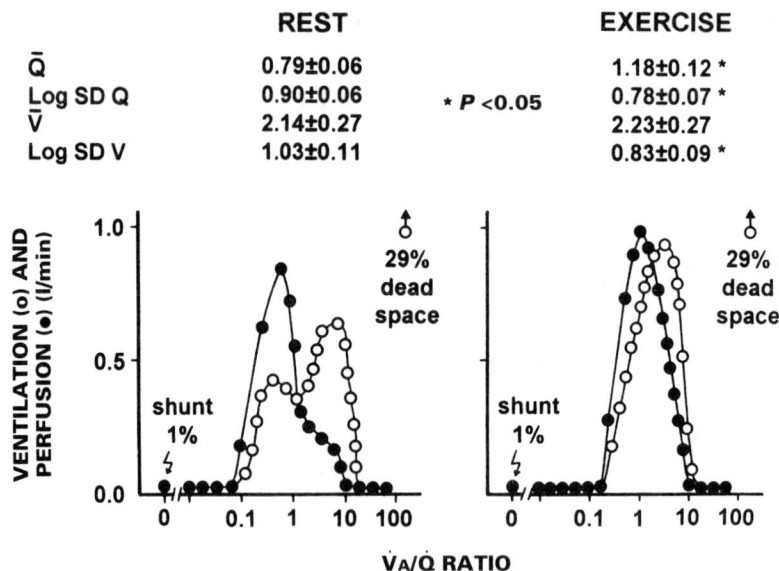

Fig. 8.10 Overall improvement of $\dot{V}A/\dot{Q}$ distributions during submaximal exercise (right-hand panel) in patients with severe airway obstruction and mild gas exchange impairment. Qualitatively, compared to resting conditions (left-hand panel) the profiles of both blood flow and alveolar ventilation dispersions ameliorated: they became unimodal, without low or high $\dot{V}A/\dot{Q}$ regions, and narrower. Quantitatively, both the mean $\dot{V}A/\dot{Q}$ ratios of blood flow ($\bar{Q}$) and ventilation ($\bar{V}$) distributions increased whereas their respective dispersions (log SD Q and log SD V) decreased. These changes tend to optimize pulmonary gas exchange along the same direction. Shunt and dead space remain unaltered. (Data correspond to the mean for 8 patients, whilst $\dot{V}A/\dot{Q}$ distributions represent one single patient.) (Taken from reference [30] with permission.)

that, as a group, both PaO_2 and $AaPO_2$ improved during exercise with no significant changes in $PaCO_2$. The main mechanism of adaptation of gas exchange was a relatively greater increase in minute ventilation than in cardiac output. This accounted for a shift of blood flow distribution to higher $\dot{V}A/\dot{Q}$ ratios, optimizing the efficiency of the lung as a gas exchanger. Furthermore, the greater the structural derangement of the airways, as assessed by the total pathologic score of the membranous bronchioles, the more the improvement in the dispersion of alveolar ventilation from resting to maximum symptom-limited exercise conditions. This reduction in the dispersion of ventilation post-exercise suggests a preferential diversion of ventilation to alveolar units with normal $\dot{V}A/\dot{Q}$ ratios. Conceivably, normal areas with an adequate $\dot{V}A/\dot{Q}$ matching are more sensitive to ventilation or blood flow changes, or both, than are alveolar units with abnormal $\dot{V}A/\dot{Q}$ ratios. A complementary explanation for the improvement in the distribution of ventilation could be related to pulmonary mechanical changes during exercise. It can be speculated that lung volume increases due to a decreased internal diameter of the membranous bronchioles, hence leading to an increased functional residual capacity, thereby enhancing a more homogeneous distribution of ventilation. In other words, there is an increase in and a more efficient distribution of ventilation which results in an overall improvement in pulmonary gas exchange in these patients.

8.7 GAS EXCHANGE RESPONSE TO OXYGEN

The response to high O_2 concentrations in patients with COPD is broadly similar irrespective of the clinical severity of the disease. With little $\dot{V}A/\dot{Q}$ mismatch, PaO_2 rises almost linearly as the inspired O_2 is increased. As the severity of $\dot{V}A/\dot{Q}$ inequality worsens, the rate of rise of PaO_2 is reduced and becomes more curvilinear [59]. We have shown in patients with COPD and acute respiratory failure needing mechanical ventilation that full nitrogen wash out of alveolar units, even in patients with poorly ventilated alveolar units with low or very low $\dot{V}A/\dot{Q}$ ratios, is rapid and that steady state conditions are easily reached by about 30 min [60]. The coexistence of a modest shunt, however, further decreases the elevation of PaO_2. In clinical practice, however, physicians administer low inspired O_2 concentrations (0.24 or 0.28) delivered through high flow masks to patients with COPD and acute respiratory failure, to provide modest but effective increases in PaO_2 (of the order of 10–15 mmHg) without inducing detrimental CO_2 retention, to optimize O_2 delivery to peripheral tissues.

Although $\dot{V}A/\dot{Q}$ inequality is no longer a barrier to O_2 exchange when 100% O_2 is breathed, 100% O_2 always worsens $\dot{V}A/\dot{Q}$ mismatch, as assessed by a significant increase in the dispersion of blood flow, without changes in shunt or in the dispersion of alveolar ventilation (Fig. 8.11) [28,60]; in contrast, pulmonary arterial pressure and pulmonary vascular resistance remain essentially unchanged. The impairment in $\dot{V}A/\dot{Q}$ relationships implies release or abolition of hypoxic pulmonary vasoconstriction. The total absence of further increases in shunt suggests that reabsorption atelectasis does not take place, either because collateral ventilation is

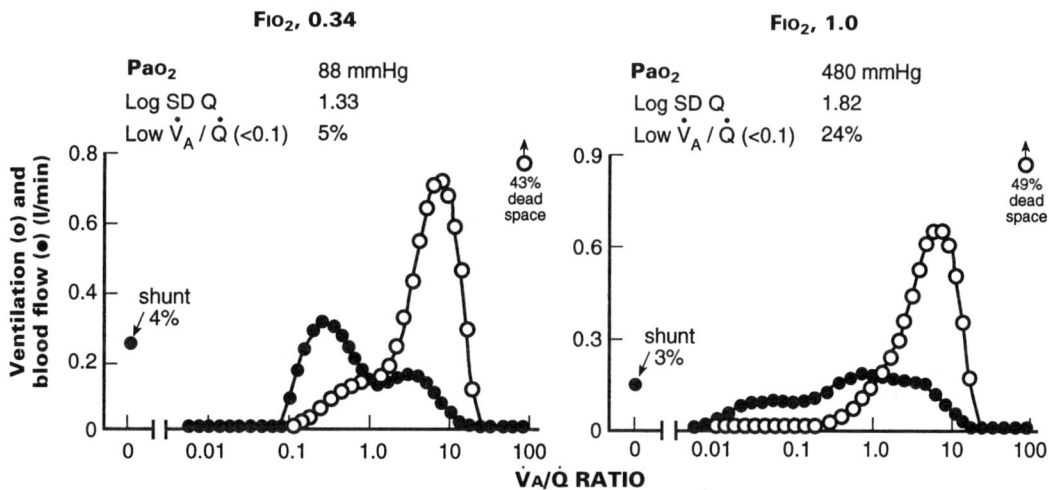

Fig. 8.11 Effect of 100% O_2 breathing on $\dot{V}A/\dot{Q}$ distributions in a representative patient with COPD and acute respiratory failure needing mechanical ventilation (right-hand panel) [59]. Compared to low inspired O_2 concentrations (left-hand panel), the most striking finding was the increase in the dispersion of pulmonary blood flow (log SD Q), suggesting that hypoxic pulmonary vasoconstriction was mitigated. Note that PaO_2 increased to considerable levels indicating full nitrogen wash out, whilst shunt remained constant and dead space increased minimally only. (Data correspond to the mean for 4 patients, whilst $\dot{V}A/\dot{Q}$ distributions are representative of one single patient).

very efficient or regional airway obstruction is never complete.

In our experience, a similar $\dot{V}A/\dot{Q}$ pattern of response to the breathing of O_2 is shown in most patients breathing spontaneously with severe asthma, of acute [61] or chronic forms [62], or in those with cryptogenic fibrosing alveolitis [17]. Only patients with life-threatening status asthmaticus requiring mechanical support increase shunt during 100% O_2 breathing, together with release of hypoxic vasoconstriction [63]; this suggests either the development of atelectasis or, more likely, vascular recruitment of small and not detectable pre-existing shunts. In patients with acute 'wet lung' diseases requiring mechanical ventilation, the breathing of O_2 induces a less uniform gas exchange pattern depending on the underlying type of acute respiratory failure. For example, in severe bacterial pneumonia breathing 100% O_2 abolishes hypoxic vasoconstriction while shunt remains unaltered [64], a pattern similar to that shown in patients with chronic respiratory disorders [17,28]. By contrast, in patients with adult respiratory distress syndrome (ARDS) a mild to moderate increase in shunt without release of hypoxic pulmonary vasoconstriction results [60]. This response suggests the presence of critical alveolar units (with low inspired $\dot{V}A/\dot{Q}$ ratios) unstable and vulnerable to high O_2 concentrations over time. These units tend to collapse easily, so leading to the development of reabsorption atelectasis [65]. When there is no release of hypoxic vasoconstriction, the amount of shunt is always greater, irrespective of the FIO_2,[65]. In contrast, in patients with COPD, breathing high inspired O_2 concentrations reduces airways resistance [66]. This should tend to improve the distribution of ventilation, and reduce the amount of areas with low $\dot{V}A/\dot{Q}$ ratios and, consequently, the dispersion of pulmonary blood flow.

An intriguing finding was that, irrespective of the FIO_2, inert shunt was always less than venous admixture ratio; there were no differences, however, between venous admixture ratio and the sum of inert shunt plus the percentage of blood flow diverted to low $\dot{V}A/\dot{Q}$ ratios. At low levels of FIO_2, this is explained because the inert shunt and the low $\dot{V}A/\dot{Q}$ areas are incorporated into the measurement of venous admixture ratio. In contrast, when breathing 100% O_2 shunt and venous admixture ratio should be equal because the wash out of nitrogen abolishes all alveolar units with poorly ventilated $\dot{V}A/\dot{Q}$ ratios. Although the reasons for this difference remain to be elucidated, release of hypoxic vasoconstriction in the bronchial and pulmonary circulations whilst breathing 100% O_2 could be an alternative explanation.

Using traditional gas exchange variables, such as the Bohr dead space, Aubier *et al.* [67] concluded that, in patients with COPD and acute-on-chronic respiratory insufficiency, the administration of 100% O_2 resulted in a remarkable increase in $PaCO_2$. Since the respiratory muscles maintained ventilation at nearly the same level as when breathing room air, they suggested that the increase in $PaCO_2$ was mainly attributed to an increased dead space; additional mechanisms included a small reduction in both tidal volume and the Haldane effect. This conclusion has been disputed by Stradling [68] who advocated that the increase in $PaCO_2$ could be explained entirely by the latter two mechanisms together with that from flattening the slope of the CO_2 pressure/content relationship with a rise in $PaCO_2$. Unfortunately, no information is available with MIGET to assess the effects of high O_2 concentrations on $\dot{V}A/\dot{Q}$ distributions in acute respiratory failure.

8.8 THE EFFECTS OF DRUGS

8.8.1 BRONCHODILATORS

Ringstedt *et al.* [29], by studying a small group of patients with advanced COPD and mild respiratory failure, before and after a continuous intravenous infusion of terbutaline (β_2-agonist bronchodilator), explored the role of the pulmonary vascular tone in modulating gas exchange in these patients. Following terbutaline, cardiac output increased and systemic blood pressure and pulmonary vascular resistance decreased. In addition, while PaO_2 decreased and mixed venous PO_2 and O_2 delivery increased, $PaCO_2$ remained unchanged. There was further $\dot{V}A/\dot{Q}$ worsening, as assessed by increases both in the perfusion to low $\dot{V}A/\dot{Q}$ ratios and in the dispersion of blood flow. Although FEV_1 and minute ventilation increased, these increments were not significant. Thus, the $\dot{V}A/\dot{Q}$ worsening could have resulted from an increased dispersion of pulmonary blood flow and/or a decrease in the overall $\dot{V}A/\dot{Q}$ ratio, due to the increased cardiac output, not efficiently counterbalanced by the simultaneous increased minute ventilation. The concomitant significant increase in mixed venous PO_2 may have also contributed to further worsening of $\dot{V}A/\dot{Q}$ mismatch by releasing hypoxic pulmonary vasoconstriction. However, it was not possible to differentiate between these mechanisms from the data provided. In the same study [29], it was shown, in another small group of patients with COPD with more airflow obstruction, more hypoxemia, more hypercapnia, and also more pulmonary hypertension, that cardiac output increased without changes in pulmonary artery pressure or in pulmonary vascular resistance. Minute ventilation increased modestly but without improvement in the indices of airflow obstruction. Respiratory arterial blood gases did not change, neither did the underlying $\dot{V}A/\dot{Q}$ abnormalities. In summary, although terbutaline caused an increase in cardiac output and consequently in mixed venous PO_2 similar to the former group of patients, this subpopulation of patients with more severe airways obstruction, higher pulmonary hypertension, and worse pulmonary gas exchange, did not modify their gas exchange pattern following terbutaline. Conceivably, the hypoxic vascular response could

have played a pivotal role in modulating pulmonary gas exchange before and after the administration of the drug. Thus, these patients with more severe COPD could have weaker or even absent hypoxic vascular response. This lack of hypoxic vascular response in advanced severe COPD could be related to either severe chronically established alveolar hypoxia or to structural changes in the pulmonary circulation coupled with areas of parenchymal destruction due to emphysema, or both. This is in keeping with the concept that the progressive increase of pulmonary vascular resistance seen in advanced COPD not only is due to irreversible structural vascular lesions but also includes a reversible vasoconstrictive component. This interpretation would be consistent with the work of Barberà *et al.* [55], investigating the influence of the structure of pulmonary arteries and the contribution of the hypoxic vascular response in preserving an adequate matching of ventilation and blood flow in patients with mild COPD.

In a double-blind, crossover, placebo-controlled study we have shown, in patients with advanced COPD during recovery from exacerbations, that intravenous administration of aminophylline during one hour produced no change in ventilation, hemodynamics or the $\dot{V}A/\dot{Q}$ distribution in the face of a modest increase in FEV_1; in comparison, breathing 100% O_2 increased the dispersion of pulmonary blood flow [35].

More recently, we have compared the short-term effect on gas exchange of fenoterol, a selective β_2-agonist, against that of ipratropium bromide, an anticholinergic agent, both given by inhalation, in a double-blind, placebo-controlled study in a series of patients with severe COPD and mild to moderate hypoxemia [69]. While fenoterol slightly decreased mean PaO_2 (by 7 mmHg) due to further worsening in the dispersion of pulmonary blood flow, gas exchange remained unaltered after ipratropium bromide. Although pulmonary hemodynamics were not measured, it was suggested that the pulmonary vascular tone was probably decreased by fenoterol, hence inducing further $\dot{V}A/\dot{Q}$ mismatch. This is at variance with the effects of intravenous salbutamol given to patients with acute severe asthma [61], in whom PaO_2 remained unchanged despite marked increases in cardiac output and similar changes in $\dot{V}A/\dot{Q}$ inequalities. This suggests that fenoterol may have a greater direct effect in reducing pulmonary vascular tone. It has been shown that at doses based on those used in clinical practice, fenoterol causes more adverse effects (cardiac, metabolic and systemic) than salbutamol or terbutaline in patients with mild asthma [70]. The most likely explanation is that fenoterol has been marketed at a higher dose than the other two β_2-agonists, despite having *in vitro* the same potency as isoprenaline; furthermore, it is suggested that fenoterol may be less selective for β_2 receptors.

8.8.2 VASODILATORS

Another good example of the influence of pulmonary vascular tone on gas exchange is given by the administration of oral nifedipine in patients with COPD and chronic respiratory failure [22]. After nifedipine there was a reduction in mean systemic arterial pressure and also in systemic vascular resistance. While cardiac output increased, pulmonary vascular resistance decreased without accompanying changes in pulmonary artery pressure. Similarly, PaO_2 decreased and there was further deterioration of $\dot{V}A/\dot{Q}$ relationships: blood flow was redistributed to areas with low $\dot{V}A/\dot{Q}$ units such that the dispersion of pulmonary perfusion increased. These changes suggest partial release of hypoxic pulmonary vasoconstriction and raise a real concern regarding the use of vasodilating drugs for the therapy of pulmonary vasoconstriction due to COPD. Similar results were shown by our group [30] in patients with

COPD with mild hypoxemia and less severe disease.

In another study [33], felodipine, a calcium antagonist vasodilator, was administered to patients with advanced COPD and chronic respiratory failure as an adjuvant to long-term oxygen therapy. Short-term infusion of the drug produced similar pulmonary gas exchange alterations to the two previous studies using nifedipine [22,30], explained also by a reduction of hypoxic vasoconstriction. Interestingly, while long-term oral administration of felodipine over a period of several weeks induced systemic and pulmonary hemodynamic changes similar to those produced during short-term therapy, $\dot{V}A/\dot{Q}$ relationships improved [33]. Although the mechanism remains to be elucidated, it was postulated that a redistribution of ventilation to areas with low $\dot{V}A/\dot{Q}$ ratios receiving simultaneously an increased amount of blood flow could be the most likely explanation. Similar deleterious effects on gas exchange have been shown following the use of vasoactive agents, such as dopamine and dobutamine, in patients with COPD and acute respiratory failure needing artificial ventilation [71].

A preliminary report [72] using inhaled nitric oxide (NO) in patients with severe COPD and chronic respiratory failure has shown a selective vasodilator effect but without gas exchange impairment. Similarly, inhalation of NO has been proven, in patients with adult respiratory distress syndrome (ARDS), to reduce pulmonary hypertension and optimize arterial oxygenation, without associated side effects [73]. Because of its unique properties [74], NO was designated the molecule of the year 1992 [75]. Thus, inhaled NO could be contemplated in the future as an agent of therapeutic benefit in patients with COPD and pulmonary hypertension, without inducing the well-known deleterious effects on gas exchange shown by more conventional vasoactive drugs.

8.8.3 ALMITRINE

There have been three studies [21,25,76] in patients with COPD and different degrees of ventilatory failure investigating the effects of oral almitrine bismesylate, a peripheral chemoreceptor stimulant, on pulmonary vascular tone and pulmonary gas exchange. In the first report [21], it was observed in a few patients, some with hypercapnic respiratory failure, that respiratory arterial blood gases improved significantly due to $\dot{V}_A/\dot{Q}$ amelioration. The only associated hemodynamic change was a modest increase in pulmonary vascular resistance without increase in pulmonary artery pressure. In another study [25], in patients requiring mechanical ventilation because of severe respiratory failure, conventional and inert gas exchange indices improved significantly together with a small but significant decrease in cardiac output and a mild increase in pulmonary vascular resistance. In all three studies [21,25,76], there was essentially a redistribution of pulmonary blood flow from regions of low $\dot{V}_A/\dot{Q}$ units to areas with normal $\dot{V}_A/\dot{Q}$ ratios. An even more dramatic improvement in pulmonary gas exchange, brought about by markedly reducing the amount of shunt (by an order of magnitude greater than that induced by NO [73]), has been shown in patients with ARDS following intravenous almitrine [77]. In both COPD and ARDS, it was suggested that enhancement of hypoxic pulmonary vasoconstriction was responsible for the overall improvement in pulmonary gas exchange. However, this beneficial effect on gas exchange in patients with COPD needs to be balanced against the unwanted side effects of almitrine, such as peripheral neuropathy and body weight loss, particularly if long-term administration is considered.

REFERENCES

1. Roussos, C. and Macklem, P.T. (1982) The respiratory muscles. *N. Engl. J. Med.*, **307**, 785–97.

2. Bégin, P. and Grassino, A. (1992) Inspiratory muscle dysfunction and chronic hypercapnia in chronic obstructive pulmonary disease. *Am. Rev. Respir. Dis.*, **143**, 905–12.

3. Wagner, P.D., Saltzman, H.A. and West, J.B. (1974) Measurements of continuous distributions of ventilation-perfusion ratios: Theory. *J. Appl. Physiol.*, **36**, 588–99.

4. Evans, J.W. and Wagner, P.D. (1977) Limits on $\dot{V}_A/\dot{Q}$ distributions from analysis of experimental inert gas elimination. *J. Appl. Physiol.*, **42**, 889–98.

5. Bergin, C., Müller, N., Nichols, D.M. *et al.* (1986) The diagnosis of emphysema: a computed tomography-pathologic correlation. *Am. Rev. Respir. Dis.*, **133**, 541–6.

6. Gould, G.A., MacNee, W., Maclean, A. *et al.* (1988) CT measurements of lung density in life can quantitate distal airspace enlargement – an essential defining feature of human emphysema. *Am. Rev. Respir. Dis.*, **137**, 380–92.

7. Brudin, L.H., Rhodes, C.G., Valind, S.O. *et al.* (1992) Regional structure-function correlations in chronic obstructive lung disease measured with positron emission tomography. *Thorax*, **47**, 914–21.

8. Roca, J. and Wagner, P.D. (1994) Principles and information content of the multiple inert gas elimination technique. *Thorax*, (in press).

9. Ketty, S. (1951) The theory and applications of the exchange of inert gas at the lungs and tissues. *Pharmacol. Rev.*, **3**, 1–41.

10. Fahri, L.E. (1967) Elimination of inert gas by the lung. *Respir. Physiol.* **3**, 1–11.

11. Wagner, P.D., Laravuso, R.B., Uhl, R.R. and West, J.B. (1974) Continuous distributions of ventilation-perfusion ratios in normal subjects breathing air and 100% O_2. *J. Clin. Invest.*, **54**, 54–68.

12. Wagner, P.D., Hedenstierna, G. and Bylin, G. (1987) Ventilation-perfusion inequality in chronic asthma. *Am. Rev. Respir. Dis.*, **136**, 605–12.

13. West, J.B. (1969) Ventilation-perfusion inequality and overall gas exchange in computer lung models of the lung. *Respir. Physiol.*, **7**, 88–110.

14. Gale, G.E., Torre-Bueno, J., Moon, R.E. *et al.* (1985) Ventilation-perfusion inequality in normal humans during exercise. *J. Appl. Physiol.*, **58**, 978–88.

15. Hlastala, M.P. and Robertson, H.T. (1978) Inert gas elimination characteristics of the normal and abnormal lung. *J. Appl. Physiol.*, **44**, 258–66.

16. Agustí, A.G.N. and Barberà, J.A. (1994) Chronic pulmonary diseases. *Thorax*, (in press).

17. Agustí, A.G.N., Roca, J., Gea, J. *et al.* (1991) Mechanisms of gas-exchange impairment in idiopathic pulmonary fibrosis. *Am. Rev. Respir. Dis.*, **143**, 219–25.

18. Burrows, B.E., Fletcher, C.M., Heard, B.E. *et al.* (1966) The emphysematous and bronchial types of chronic airways obstruction. A clinico-pathological study of patients in London and Chicago. *Lancet*, **i**, 830–5.

19. Wagner, P.D., Dantzker, D.R., Dueck, R. *et al.* (1977) Ventilation-perfusion inequality in chronic obstructive pulmonary disease. *J. Clin. Invest.*, **59**, 203–16.

20. Dantzker, D.R. (1984) Gas exchange, in *Chronic obstructive pulmonary disease* (ed. H.D. Montenegro), Churchill Livingstone, Edinburgh, pp. 141–60.

21. Mélot, C., Naeije, R., Rothschild, T. Mertens Ph. *et al.* (1983) Improvement in ventilation-perfusion matching by almitrine in COPD. *Chest*, **83**, 528–33.

22. Mélot, C., Hallemans, R., Naeije, R. *et al.* (1984) Deleterious effect of nifedipine on pulmonary gas exchange in chronic obstructive pulmonary disease. *Am. Rev. Respir. Dis.*, **130**, 612–6.

23. Marthan, R., Castaing, Y., Manier, G. and Guénard, H. (1985) Gas exchange alterations in patients with chronic obstructive lung disease. *Chest*, **87**, 470–5.

24. Castaing, Y., Manier, G. and Guénard, H. (1985) Effect of 26% oxygen breathing on ventilation and perfusion distribution in patients with COLD. *Bull. Eur. Physiopathol. Respir.*, **21**, 17–23.

25. Castaing, Y., Manier, G. and Guénard, H. (1986) Improvement in ventilation-perfusion relationships by almitrine in patients with chronic obstructive pulmonary disease during mechanical ventilation. *Am. Rev. Respir. Dis.*, **134**, 910–6.

26. Dantzker, D.R. and D'Alonzo, G.E. (1986) The effect of exercise on pulmonary gas exchange in patients with severe chronic obstructive pulmonary disease. *Am. Rev. Respir. Dis.*, **134**, 1135–9.

27. Roca, J., Montserrat, J.M., Rodriguez-Roisin, R. *et al.* (1987) Gas exchange response to naloxone in chronic obstructive pulmonary disease with hypercapnic respiratory failure. *Bull. Eur. Physiopathol. Respir.*, **23**, 249–54.

28. Torres, A., Reyes, A., Roca, J. *et al.* (1989) Ventilation-perfusion mismatching in chronic obstructive pulmonary disease during ventilator weaning. *Am. Rev. Respir. Dis.*, **140**, 1246–50.

29. Ringstedt, C.V., Eliasen, K., Andersen, J.B. *et al.* (1989) Ventilation-perfusion distributions and central hemodynamics in chronic obstructive pulmonary disease. *Chest*, **96**, 976–83.

30. Agustí, A.G.N., Barberà, J.A., Roca, J. *et al.* (1990) Hypoxic pulmonary vasoconstriction and gas exchange in chronic obstructive pulmonary disease. *Chest*, **97**, 268–75.

31. Rodriguez-Roisin, R., Roca, J. and Barberà, J.A. (1991) Extrapulmonary and intrapulmonary determinants of pulmonary gas exchange, in *Ventilatory Failure* (eds J.J. Marini and C. Roussos), Springer-Verlag, Berlin, pp. 18–36.

32. Barberà, J.A., Ramirez, J., Roca, J. *et al.* (1990) Lung structure and gas exchange in mild chronic obstructive pulmonary disease. *Am. Rev. Respir. Dis.*, **141**, 895–901.

33. Bratel, T., Hedenstierna, G., Nyquist, O. and Ripe, E. (1990) The use of a vasodilator, felodipine, as an adjuvant to long-term oxygen treatment in COLD patients. *Eur. Respir. J.*, **3**, 46–54.

34. Gunnarson, L., Tokics, L., Lundquist, H. *et al.* (1991) Chronic obstructive pulmonary disease and anaesthesia: formation of atelectasis and gas exchange impairment. *Eur. Respir. J.*, **4**, 1106–16.

35. Barberà, J.A., Reyes, A., Roca, J. *et al* (1992) Effect of intravenously administered amino-phylline on ventilation/perfusion inequality during recovery from exacerbations of chronic obstructive pulmonary disease. *Am. Rev. Respir. Dis.*, **145**, 1328–33.

36. Daly, J.J. (1968) Venoarterial shunting in obstructive pulmonary disease. *N. Engl. J. Med.*, **278**, 952–3.

37. Hervé, Ph., Petitpretz, P., Simonneau, G. *et al.* (1983) The mechanisms of abnormal gas exchange in acute massive pulmonary embolism. *Am. Rev. Respir. Dis.*, **128**, 1101.

38. Laver, M.B., Morgan, L., Bendixen, H.H. and Radford, E.P. Jr (1964) Lung volume, compliance and arterial oxygen tensions during controlled ventilation. *J. Appl. Physiol.*, **19**, 725–33.

39. Lynch, J.P., Mhyre, J.G. and Dantzker, D.R. (1979) Influence of cardiac output on intrapulmonary shunt. *J. Appl. Physiol.*, **46**, 315–21.

40. Wagner, P.D. and Rodriguez-Roisin, R. (1991) Clinical advances in pulmonary gas exchange. *Am. Rev. Respir. Dis.*, **143** , 883–8.

41. Wagner, P.D., Schaffartzik, W., Prediletto, R. and Knight, D.R. (1991) Relationships among cardiac output, shunt, and inspired O_2 concentration. *J. Appl. Physiol.*, **71**, 2191–7.

42. Lemaire, F., Teboul, J.L., Cinotti, L. *et al.* (1988) Acute left ventricular dysfunction during unsuccessful weaning from mechanical ventilation. *Anesthesiology*, **69**, 171–9.

43. Beydon, L., Cinotti, L., Rekik, N. *et al.* (1991) Changes in the distribution of ventilation and perfusion associated with separation from mechanical ventilation in patients with obstructive pulmonary disease. *Anesthesiology*, **75**, 730–8.

44. Hubmayr, R.D., Loosbrock, L.M., Gillespie, D.J. and Rodarte, J.R. (1988) Oxygen uptake during weaning from mechanical ventilation. *Chest*, **94**, 1148–55.

45. Wagner, P.D. (1982) Ventilation-perfusion inequality in catastrophic lung disease, in *Applied Physiology in Clinical Respiratory Care* (ed. O. Prakash), Martinus Nijhoff, The Hague, pp. 363–79.

46. Efthimiou, J., Fleming, J., Gomes, C. and Spiro, S.G. (1988) The effect of supplementary oral nutrition in poorly nourished patients with chronic obstructive pulmonary disease. *Am. Rev. Respir. Dis.*, **137**, 1075–82.

47. Azkanazi, J., Rosembaum, S.H., Hyman, A.I. *et al.* (1980) Respiratory changes induced by large glucose loads of total parenteral nutrition. *JAMA*, **243**, 1444–7.

48. Covelli, H.D., Black, J.W., Olsen, M.S. and Beckman, J.F. (1985) Respiratory failure precipitated by high carbohydrate loads. *Ann. Intern. Med.*, **132**, 579–85.

49. Efthimiou, J., Mounsey, P.J., Benson, D.N. *et al.* (1992). Effect of carbohydrate rich versus fat rich loads on gas exchange and walking performance in patients with chronic obstructive lung disease. *Thorax*, **47**, 451–6.

50. Douglas, N.J. and Flenley, D.C. (1990) Breathing during sleep in patients with obstructive lung disease. *Am. Rev. Respir. Dis.*, **141**, 1055–70.

51. Barberà, J.A., Roca, J., Rodriguez-Roisin, R. *et al.* (1988) Gas exchange in patients with small airways disease (abstract). *Eur. Respir. J.*, **1**, 27S.

52. Rodriguez-Roisin, R. and Roca, J. (1994) Bronchial asthma. *Thorax*, (in press).

53. Roca, J. and Rodriguez-Roisin, R. (1992) Asthma, allergen challenge and gas exchange. *Eur. Respir. J.*, **5**, 1171–2.

54. Dantzker, D.R., Patten, G.A. and Bower, J.S. (1982) Gas exchange at rest and during exercise in adults with cystic fibrosis. *Am. Rev. Respir. Dis.*, **125**, 400–5.

55. Hogg, J.C., Nepszy, S.J., Macklem, P.T. and Thurlbeck, W.M. (1969) Elastic properties of the centrilobular emphysematous space. *J. Clin. Invest.*, **48**, 1306–12.

56. Barberà, J.A., Riverola, A., Roca, J. *et al.* (1994) Pulmonary vascular abnormalities and ventilation-perfusion relationships in patients with mild chronic obstructive pulmonary disease. *Am. J. Respir. Crit. Care Med.*, **149**, 423–9.

57. Roca, J., Hogan, M.C., Story, D. *et al.* (1989) Evidence for tissue diffusion limitation of VO_{2max} in normal humans. *J. Appl. Physiol.*, **67**, 291–9.

58. Barberà, J.A., Roca, J., Ramirez, J. *et al.* (1991). Gas exchange during exercise in mild chronic obstructive pulmonary disease. Correlation with lung structure. *Am. Rev. Respir. Dis.*, **144**, 520–5.

59. Rodriguez-Roisin, R. (1993) Ventilation-perfusion relationships, in *Pathophysiologic Foundations of Critical Care* (eds M.R. Pinsky and J.F.A. Dhainaut), Williams & Wilkins, Baltimore, pp. 389–413.

60. Santos, C., Roca, J., Torres, A. *et al.* (1992) Patients with acute respiratory failure increase shunt during 100% O_2 breathing (abstract). *Eur. Respir. J.*, **5** (Suppl 5), 272S.

61. Ballester, E., Reyes, A., Roca, J. *et al.* (1989) Ventilation-perfusion mismatching in acute severe asthma: effects of salbutamol and 100% oxygen. *Thorax*, **44**, 258–67.

62. Ballester, E., Roca, J., Ramis, Ll *et al.* (1990) Pulmonary gas exchange in chronic asthma. Response to 100% O_2 oxygen and salbutamol. *Am. Rev. Respir. Dis.*, **141**, 558–62.

63. Rodriguez-Roisin, R., Ballester, E., Roca, J. *et al.* (1989) Mechanisms of hypoxemia in patients with status asthmaticus requiring mechanical ventilation. *Am. Rev. Respir. Dis.*, **139**, 732–39.

64. Gea, J., Roca, J., Torres, A. *et al.* (1991) Mechanisms of abnormal gas exchange in patients with pneumonia. *Anesthesiology*, **75**, 782–8.

65. Dantzker, D.R., Wagner, P.D. and West, J.B. (1975) Instability of lung units with low $\dot{V}A/\dot{Q}$ ratios during O_2 breathing. *J. Appl. Physiol.*, **38**, 886–95.

66. Astin, T.W. (1970) The relationships between arterial blood oxygen saturation, carbon

dioxide tension, and pH on airway resistance during 30 percent oxygen breathing in patients with chronic bronchitis with airway obstruction. *Am. Rev. Respir. Dis.,* **102**, 382–7.

67. Aubier, M., Murciano, D., Milic-Emili, *et al.* (1980) Effects of the administration of O_2 on ventilation and blood flow gases in patients with chronic obstructive pulmonary disease during acute respiratory failure. *Am. Rev. Respir. Dis.,* **122**, 747–54.

68. Stradling, J. (1987) Effects of the administration of O_2 on ventilation and blood gases in patients with chronic obstructive pulmonary disease during acute respiratory failure. *Am. Rev. Respir. Dis.,* **135**, 274.

69. Ferrer, A., Viegas, C., Montserrat, J.M. *et al.* (1991) Effects of fenoterol and ipratropium bromide on gas exchange in chronic obstructive pulmonary disease. *Eur. Respir. J.,* **4**, 224S.

70. Wong, C.S., Pavord, I.D., Williams, J. *et al.* (1990) Bronchodilator, cardiovascular, and hypokalaemic effects of fenoterol, salbutamol, and terbutaline in asthma. *Lancet,* **336**, 1396–9.

71. Rennotte, M.T., Reynaert, M., Clerbaux, Th. *et al.* (1989) Effects of two inotropic drugs, dopamine and dobutamine, on pulmonary gas exchange in artificially ventilated patients. *Intensive Care Med.,* **15**, 160–5.

72. Moinard, J., Manier, G., Pillet, O. *et al.* (1994) Effect of inhaled nitric oxide on hemodynamics and $\dot{V}_A / \dot{Q}$ inequality in patients with chronic destructive pulmonary disease. *Am. J. Respir. Crit. Care Med.,* **149**, 1482–7.

73. Rossaint, R., Falke, K.J., López, F.A. *et al.* (1993) Inhaled nitric oxide for the adult respiratory distress syndrome. *N. Engl. J. Med.,* **328**, 399–405.

74. Culotta, E. and Koshland, D.E. (1992) NO news is good news. *Science,* **258**, 1862–5.

75. Koshland, D.E. Jr. (1992) The molecule of the year. *Science,* **258**, 1861.

76. Castaing, Y., Manier, G., Varène, N. and Guénard, H. (1981) Effects of oral almitrine on the distribution of $\dot{V}_A / \dot{Q}$ ratio in chronic obstructive lung disease. *Bull Eur. Physiopath. Resp.,* **17**, 917–32.

77. Reyes, A., Roca, J., Rodriguez-Roisin, R. *et al.* (1988) Effect of almitrine on ventilation-perfusion distribution in adult respiratory distress syndrome. *Am. Rev. Respir. Dis.,* **137**, 1062–7.

RESPIRATORY MUSCLES

9

G.J. Gibson

The respiratory muscles are the only skeletal muscles whose regular contraction is necessary for the maintenance of life. In this respect their role is intermediate between that of other skeletal muscles and cardiac muscle. Their action may be altered profoundly in patients with COPD. In such individuals dysfunction of the respiratory muscles can have major effects on the maintenance of ventilation awake and asleep and during exercise, on the motion of the chest and abdomen, on pulmonary gas exchange and the symptom of dyspnea. The importance of abnormalities of muscle function in patients with COPD has been appreciated increasingly over the last 20 years as a result of many studies in all these areas.

9.1 ACTIONS OF THE RESPIRATORY MUSCLES

9.1.1 NORMAL ACTIONS

During quiet tidal breathing in normal subjects inspiration is achieved predominantly by contraction of the diaphragm and expiration is largely passive, dependent on the elastic recoil of the lungs and chest wall. The inspiratory action of the diaphragm is supported by other inspiratory muscles including the inspiratory intercostals, particularly the deepest parasternal layer of muscles and the scalene muscles [1]. Activation of these muscles has the effect of stabilizing the rib cage. The diaphragm has a complex action (Fig. 9.1): its contraction leads to shortening of the muscle fibers and caudal displacement with lowering of pleural pressure (Ppl) and increase in abdominal pressure (Pab). Due to the curvature of the diaphragmatic domes there is at lower lung volumes a circumferential 'zone of apposition' between the internal surface of the lower rib cage and the superior surface of the diaphragm. The increasing abdominal pressure produces forward motion of the abdominal contents and abdominal wall and also of the lower rib cage which is effectively exposed to abdominal pressure via this zone of apposition [2]. In addition the insertional action of the diaphragm via its attachments to the lower six ribs contributes to expansion of the rib cage. The upper part of the rib cage, however, is exposed to pleural pressure which becomes increasingly negative during inspiration; without the action of other inspiratory agonist muscles the upper ribs would tend to move inwards as the lower ribs and abdomen move outwards. The action of the rib cage and accessory muscles becomes increasingly important as ventilatory efforts increase, e.g. during exercise.

The importance of a further group of inspiratory muscles has been appreciated only in recent years as a result of studies on patients with sleep apnea and related conditions: these are the muscles which surround and

Chronic Obstructive Pulmonary Disease. Edited by Dr P. Calverley and Professor N. Pride. Published in 1995 by Chapman & Hall, London. ISBN 0 412 46450 0

Normal   COPD

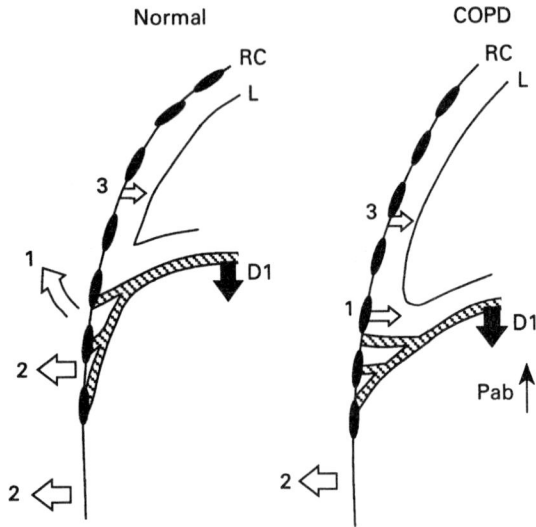

Fig. 9.1   Schematic diagram showing actions of the diaphragm on the chest wall in a normal subject (left) and patient with COPD (right). Normally the lower rib cage (RC) is expanded (1) by direct insertion and (2) by the effect of increasing abdominal pressure (Pab) via the zone of apposition; these effects are partly offset by (3) the deflating effect of pleural pressure (Ppl) as it becomes more negative. The net effect is inspiratory but mechanisms (1) and (2) become progressively less effective as lung volume increases. In the hyperinflated patient with COPD (right) the expanding effect of the diaphragm is compromised because (a) the zone of apposition is reduced and (b) the insertional effect (1) is now expiratory. Increased activity of other inspiratory muscles is necessary to compensate for these effects.

support the upper airway, particularly the pharynx and their phasic inspiratory contraction is necessary for maintenance of airway patency during inspiration [3]. Without their action during inspiration the upper airway would narrow and might close due to the subatmospheric pressure inside the airway. These muscles thus have a role in supporting the upper airway analogous to the action of the intercostal and scalene muscles maintaining the stability of the rib cage.

Expiration in normal subjects at rest is essentially passive: indeed, inspiratory muscle activity continues for a short period into expiration ('post-inspiratory braking') and this controls the rate of expiratory airflow. The major expiratory muscles are those of the abdominal wall; earlier studies using surface electromyographic (EMG) recordings or needle electrodes sampling the rectus abdominis and external oblique muscles showed that they were electrically silent during normal quiet expiration and activity became detectable only when ventilation was markedly increased. More recent study [4] of the deepest abdominal muscle, transversus abdominis, shows that when ventilation increases it is recruited more readily than the more superficial abdominal muscles. The transversus muscle is orientated circumferentially around the abdomen and is therefore likely to be more effective in raising abdominal pressure than either the rectus or external oblique muscles which run from the rib cage to the pelvis.

9.1.2 RESPIRATORY MUSCLE DYSFUNCTION IN COPD

The net effects of respiratory muscle contraction are related to the force of contraction and the mechanical load against which the muscles are required to act, or in simple terms to the ratio of load to power. In COPD both these factors are affected adversely, in that the mechanical load is increased (increased respiratory impedance) whilst the pressure generating capacity of the muscles over the tidal breathing range is impaired. The latter results from a combination of the effects of pulmonary hyperinflation affecting the mechanical advantage of the muscles, malnutrition resulting in muscle weakness and, possibly in some situations, respiratory muscle fatigue.

The hyperinflation associated with COPD leads to shortening and flattening of the diaphragm and impairs its capacity to generate pressure because of both length–tension and geometric factors (see below). In addition, the 'zone of the apposition' where the lower rib cage is exposed to Pab is less than in normal subjects while that exposed to Ppl is greater: these factors impair the ability of the diaphragm to expand the rib cage by both appositional and insertional effects (Fig. 9.1). In consequence patients with COPD show increased use of the rib cage muscles and the inspiratory accessory muscles, e.g. sterno-mastoid, may also be active even during quiet breathing. Inevitably this pattern becomes more pronounced as ventilation increases on exercise. The result is distorted and sometimes paradoxical motion of the rib cage. Although narrowing of the intrapulmonary airways in COPD is predominantly *expiratory*, the burden falls mainly on the *inspiratory* muscles. Earlier EMG studies using surface electrodes showed no activity in the superficial muscles of the abdominal wall during quiet breathing [5]. A recent study by Ninane *et al.* [6] using needle electrodes inserted into the different layers of abdominal muscles has, however, shown that expiratory phasic activity is present at rest in the deeper transversus abdominis muscle in many patients with COPD, especially those with more severe degrees of airway narrowing.

9.2 MORPHOLOGY AND ENERGETICS

Skeletal muscle comprises two main types of fiber, classified in terms of histochemical appearances and corresponding to important differences in metabolic activity. Type I or red fibers are relatively slowly contracting and resistant to fatigue. They are well endowed with mitochondria and metabolize predominantly by oxidative pathways. Type II fibers are fast contracting, may be either fatigue-resistant (Type IIA) or fatiguable (Type IIB); they metabolize by either oxidative or glycolytic pathways (IIA) or predominantly by glycolysis alone (IIB). Both in normal subjects and patients with COPD the proportion of Type I fibers in intercostal and diaphragmatic muscle is greater than that found in a pos-

tural muscle such as latissimus dorsi [7]. This is consistent with the general finding that muscles in regular use tend to have a relatively high proportion of fatigue-resistant Type I fibers. Although the proportions of Type I and Type II fibers are similar in COPD patients and normal subjects, patients show reduced diameter of individual fibers and greater variations in fiber size with abnormalities such as splitting of fibers. The reduced diameter of individual fibers correlates with body weight [7], an observation which may underlie the important effects of weight on mechanical function of the respiratory muscles. It is likely that all the respiratory muscles share in the muscle wasting seen in many patients with advanced COPD. Most attention has been paid to the diaphragm, for the obvious reasons that it is the main inspiratory muscle, and it is relatively easy to 'isolate' mechanically and to measure morphometrically. Autopsy studies show that diaphragmatic mass and thickness are broadly proportional to body weight. It does, however appear that in more advanced COPD the reduction in diaphragmatic weight is relatively greater than the associated reduction in body weight [8,9]. Rochester and Braun [10], using radiographic measurements *in vivo*, found that estimated diaphragmatic length at RV in patients with COPD was appreciably less than that in normal subjects at RV but, as the authors pointed out, this comparison is potentially misleading because the absolute lung volumes represented are very different. Arora and Rochester [9] argued that if comparisons were made at similar lung volume the differences in diaphragmatic length were very small. They therefore concluded that in relation to *absolute lung volume*, COPD has only a small effect on diaphragmatic length *in vivo*. At similar *relative* volumes, however (e.g. RV or FRC), patients with hyperinflation inevitably have a markedly reduced muscle length.

The normal respiratory muscles, particularly the diaphragm, are highly active metabolically, in comparison with a postural muscle such as latissimus dorsi; there is a greater activity of various enzymes involved in both glycolysis and oxidative metabolism, to a degree comparable to the activity found in highly trained limb muscles in athletes [11]. Although still greater than that found in latissimus dorsi, enzymatic activity in the diaphragm of patients with COPD is less than in normal subjects, suggesting relative 'detraining' of the diaphragm; this might be a consequence of relatively less use of the diaphragm associated with the greater use of other inspiratory muscles in these patients [11]. The respiratory muscles of patients with COPD show reductions in high energy metabolic fuels such as ATP and phosphocreatine [12]. Similar findings have been reported in non-respiratory muscles in these patients [13] and may contribute to generalized weakness. In addition to the reduction in muscle bulk in many patients with COPD, there is evidence that the contractile force per unit area of the diaphragm is reduced out of proportion to any reduction in muscle mass [14]. Possible factors which may be involved include electrolyte and mineral deficiencies, impaired muscle membrane function, reduction of critical energy metabolite concentrations and the effects of hypoxemia, hypercapnia and infection.

The increased mechanical impedance to breathing in patients with COPD implies an inevitable increase in the work of breathing and consequently in the rate of oxygen consumption ($\dot{V}O_2$) by the respiratory muscles. This results in a disproportionate increase in $\dot{V}O_2$ as ventilation increases on exercise [15]. Otis [16] introduced the concept of 'critical gain', the point on exercise when the increase in $\dot{V}O_2$ is more than used up by the increased requirements for oxygen of the respiratory muscles themselves. This appears to be a factor limiting exercise in some healthy elderly subjects [17] and may be relatively more important in patients with COPD. The oxygen cost of breathing is particularly in-creased in malnourished individuals and also is higher in those with more severe hyperinflation [18] (where the inspiratory muscles are required to operate at an increasingly worse mechanical advantage).

Several studies have consistently shown that patients with COPD have abnormally high resting energy expenditure (REE). This reflects increases in both the basal metabolic rate (BMR) and the thermic response to food [19]. The increased BMR may result from increased oxidation of either glucose [20] or fat [19]. It has been attributed to increased energy requirements of the respiratory muscles resulting from the increased work of breathing but this is unlikely to be the whole explanation. The REE expressed as a ratio of body weight or fat free mass is relatively greater in subjects who have sustained significant weight loss and increases as airway obstruction and maximum inspiratory pressure decline [21]. The weight loss which is a common feature of patients with advanced COPD occurs despite a normal or increased dietary intake. The increased thermic response to food of these patients reflects inefficient metabolism and adds to the burden which the respiratory muscles are required to sustain. This is particularly relevant to metabolism of carbohydrate which has a respiratory quotient (RQ) of 1.0, i.e. a relatively greater CO_2 output in relation to oxygen consumption than is seen with fat metabolism (RQ 0.7); carbohydrate metabolism therefore results in greater ventilatory demands and this may adversely affect exercise performance [22] or worsen the resting gas exchange of patients in a critical state. A further aspect of inefficient metabolism is an abnormally high oxidation of protein after food [19], associated with an overall reduction in protein synthesis in muscles generally [23]; this probably contributes to wasting and weakness of the respiratory and other muscles. Although the excretion of nitrogen is increased, this is proportional to the increase in REE so that, unlike patients with sepsis, those with COPD are not truly hypercatabolic [20].

The observations discussed above have important implications for attempts to improve the nutrition and hence respiratory muscle function of patients with COPD. The potential disadvantage of carbohydrate feeding has been mentioned and also it is likely that the caloric gain from nutrients, particularly in undernourished patients may be less than anticipated because of the greater oxygen cost of diet-induced thermogenesis.

9.3 MECHANICAL PROPERTIES OF RESPIRATORY MUSCLES

9.3.1 STATICS IN NORMAL SUBJECTS

The static tension developed by a skeletal muscle is determined by the length of the muscle with, in general, the greatest tension developed when the muscle is close to its resting, unstressed length. Neither length nor tension of the respiratory muscles is readily measurable *in vivo* but volume and pressure can be used as indirect indices of their respective magnitudes. In normal subjects the resting length of the diaphragm (and probably of the other inspiratory muscles) is at a volume close to FRC. Consequently the maximum pressure developed statically by the inspiratory muscles is seen at lung volumes close to FRC or RV and it declines as volume increases above FRC. Conversely, maximum expiratory pressures are greater at high lung volumes close to full inflation. Maximum static respiratory pressure measured at the mouth, with glottis open, is equal to alveolar pressure. Such measurements include a contribution (minor in normal subjects) from the passive recoil of the respiratory system, but mainly reflect the net pressure resulting from contraction of the respiratory muscles – agonists and antagonists combined. Figure 9.2 shows the relationships of maximum inspiratory (PI max) and expiratory (PE max) pressures to lung volume.

The contribution to inspiratory efforts of the diaphragm alone can be assessed by direct measurement of transdiaphragmatic pressure (Pdi) using balloon-tipped catheters or small transducers in the esophagus and stomach. Measurements during various maneuvers in normal subjects show that the diaphragm is often not contracting maximally during forceful voluntary inspiratory efforts [25,26]. The diaphragm has a unique dual role as a thoracic and abdominal muscle acting agonistically with the rib cage muscles in generation of negative intrathoracic pressures and with the abdominal wall muscles in the generation of positive abdominal pressures (e.g. during defecation or parturition). The largest values of Pdi (Pdi max) are obtained at volumes close to FRC during maximum efforts which combine both an inspiratory effort (reducing Ppl) and an expulsive effort (increasing Pab). Although such

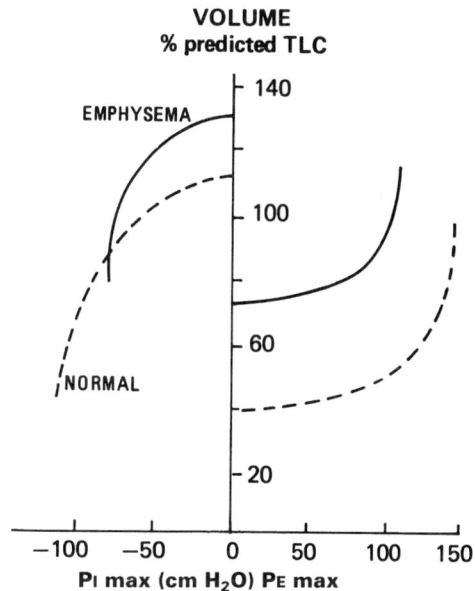

Fig. 9.2 Average values of maximum inspiratory (PI max) and expiratory (PE max) mouth pressures in groups of normal subjects and patients with emphysema plotted between RV and TLC, based on data of Decramer *et al.* [24].

'gymnastic' maneuvers can produce greater Pdi, they usually result in less negative pleural (inspiratory) pressures than do more natural efforts [25,26]. At volumes greater than FRC the value of Pdi max declines because of the length–tension relationship of the muscle. A further possible contributor to the reduced pressure is an increase in the radius of curvature of the diaphragm which, according to the law of Laplace, would result in a reduced pressure for a given linear tension. Most data on the diaphragm in normal subjects, however, suggest that the effect of length is quantitively much more important than the effect of curvature in determining the value of Pdi [27].

A similar shaped Pdi–volume relationship is seen if the diaphragmatic contraction is produced by electrical stimulation of the phrenic nerves. In the study of Smith and Bellemare [28] the diaphragm of normal subjects during phrenic stimulation at full inflation was still capable of generating an appreciable Pdi but this Pdi was not associated with an inspiratory *pleural* pressure, i.e. the Pdi resulted from an increase in Pab without any fall in Ppl. The distribution of Pdi in this and other situations depends critically on the relative compliances (stiffness) of the rib cage and abdomen and these, in turn, in more natural situations are influenced by contraction of other muscles. Clearly, however, the diaphragm at very large lung volumes might, in theory, become an expiratory rather than an inspiratory muscle.

In clinical testing of diaphragmatic function a commonly applied measurement is Pdi during a forceful 'sniff' which patients perform more easily and reproducibly than static efforts [29]. The effort is usually initiated at FRC and the values recorded are dependent on lung volume in a similar fashion to static measurements [30].

Measurements of static mouth pressures during maximum inspiratory and expiratory efforts assess global function of the respiratory muscles and suffice for clinical assessment in most cases. They are, however, inevitably effort-dependent and several attempts are likely to be required before reproducible values are obtained. The values obtained are very dependent on the type of mouthpiece used and there is a wide normal range. In normal subjects measurement of pressure in the nasopharynx during a forceful sniff is a useful alternative but such measurements are inaccurate in patients with COPD and increased airway resistance [31].

9.3.2 STATICS IN COPD

Many studies of maximum respiratory pressures in patients with COPD have shown impaired values of PI max [24,32] when these are measured at FRC or RV and more recent studies have confirmed similar findings for Pdi [25,26]. It is likely that geometric (length–tension) factors and weakness contribute in different proportions in different individuals. In relation to the absolute rather than relative lung volumes on the other hand, such pressures may appear normal or 'supernormal' [32]. This applies not only above the normal TLC (where the diaphragm and other inspiratory muscles of a healthy subject would not normally be capable of operating) but also sometimes at lower lung volumes. Recent data on maximum pressures across the diaphragm during forceful inspiratory efforts [25] or during phrenic nerve stimulation [33] have shown that diaphragmatic function is remarkably well preserved at least in well-nourished patients (Fig. 9.3). Despite the theoretical possibility that the diaphragm might become an expiratory muscle, in severe hyperinflation it retains an inspiratory action even at a markedly increased TLC [33]. These observations appear to imply that the respiratory muscles, and particularly the diaphragm, are capable of adapting to hyperinflation by an alteration in the length–tension characteristics of the muscle. The mechanism of any such adaptation is, however, uncertain: data from experimental animals have shown that

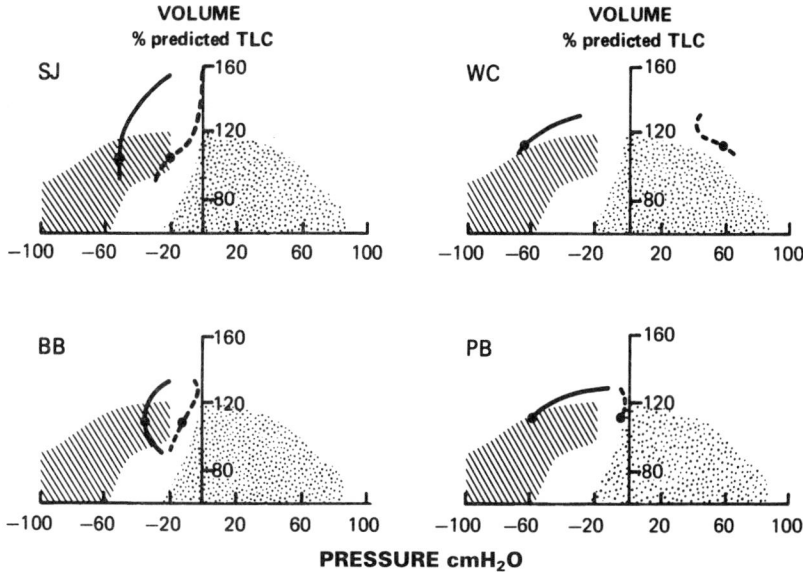

Fig. 9.3 Pleural (solid lines) and abdominal (broken lines) pressures during static maximal inspiratory efforts in four patients at various lung volumes with shaded and dotted areas representing the normal range of Ppl and Pab respectively. The horizontal distance between the two curves represents Pdi. (From Gibson *et al.* [25].)

chronic hyperinflation can be associated with a reduction in the number of sarcomeres in the diaphragmatic muscle, such that it retains its pressure-generating capacity at a shorter muscle length [34]. Evidence of such resorption of sarcomeres has not been demonstrated in man; the animal model in which it has been shown tends to produce relatively greater hyperinflation than occurs in most patients with COPD and the measurements of diphragmatic dimensions discussed above give little support to the concept of true shortening (i.e. a reduction in resting length of the muscle fibers). In subjects with mild–moderate degrees of hyperinflation it appears that reduction in diaphragmatic curvature is of little importance [10]. Increased radius of curvature and the consequent reduction in Pdi determined by the law of Laplace may become more important at high lung volumes in individuals with very severe hyperinflation or with acute increases in lung volume during exac-

erbations of disease, but little information is available in these groups.

Estimation of the length–tension properties of the respiratory muscles other than the diaphragm is more difficult but detailed radiographic measurements by Sharp and colleagues [35,36] have suggested that any changes in resting length associated with COPD are likely to be much less than those seen in the diaphragm and unlikely to impair the tension which these muscles are capable of generating.

The expiratory muscles are at no such mechanical disadvantage in the presence of an increased thoracic volume. Rochester and Braun [10] therefore argued that PE max could be used as an index of respiratory muscle strength in order to analyse the respective contributions of weakness and mechanical disadvantage to the impairment of PI max seen in many patients. On this basis they found that PE max (i.e. weakness) explained 46% and diaphragmatic length explained 35% of the variance in PI max. They therefore concluded that impairment of static inspiratory muscle function in COPD was due to a combination of mechanical disadvantage and general muscle weakness.

9.3.3 DYNAMICS

Under dynamic conditions, when airflow is occurring, the force of muscle contraction is dependent on the velocity of contraction in addition to any constraints which operate under static conditions. The greatest force is developed by a muscle when shortening during contraction is prevented (isometric contraction), but under dynamic conditions the force generated declines with increasing velocity of contraction. This corresponds to the situation which pertains during normal breathing with the airway open and lung volume increasing during inspiration and decreasing during expiration. The velocity of muscle shortening in turn depends upon the load placed upon the muscles; as this is increased in patients with COPD compared to normal the force–velocity characteristics of the respiratory muscles of patients with COPD should favor the generation of force (or pressure) compared with normal subjects, but the values obtained are always less than those which can be developed statically against an occluded airway. In patients, as in normal subjects, forced inspiratory flows are entirely dependent on the effort applied. During forceful expiration, however, maximum flow is much less dependent on effort at lower than at higher lung volumes, a feature which underlies the reproducibility of tests of forced expiration (Chapter 7). In patients with COPD this effect is increased, i.e. maximum expiratory flows are even less dependent on effort than in normal subjects.

Hyperinflation of the thorax and consequent flattening and shortening of the diaphragm in the tidal breathing range is associated with a change in the normal pattern of activation of the respiratory muscles, with relatively greater activity of the inspiratory intercostal and accessory muscles and consequently relatively more displacement of the rib cage and less of the abdomen [37,38]. The normal inspiratory positive swing of abdominal pressure during tidal breathing is attenuated and in some cases the net change becomes negative; in some individuals Pab follows Ppl with no significant contribution to pressure generation by the diaphragm (Fig. 9.4). The tidal swing in pleural pressure is inevitably greater than normal because of the greater impedance to breathing resulting from in-

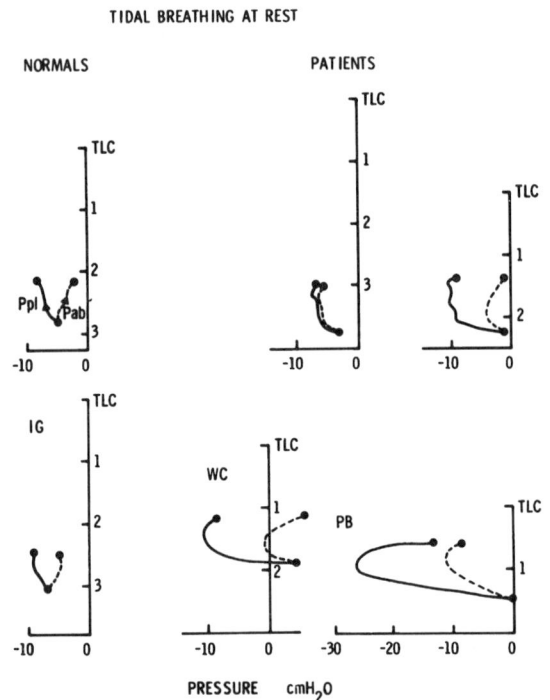

Fig. 9.4 Measurements of Ppl (solid line) and Pab (broken line) in four patients seated at rest and plotted against volume change during tidal breathing; two normal subjects are shown for comparison on the left. In the patients the swing in pleural pressure is greater because of increased impedance to breathing and Pab becomes more negative during part of inspiration. Pdi is given by the horizontal difference between the two pressure recordings.

creased airway resistance and sometimes also from reduced compliance associated with breathing at higher lung volumes. The most instructive way of examining the pressure relations during tidal breathing is by comparison with the pressure-generating capacity of the inspiratory muscles under static conditions when the severe constraints imposed by muscle function, especially when ventilation is required to increase, become apparent (Fig. 9.5).

Both EMG and pressure studies suggest that tidal expiration in patients with COPD is due mainly to passive recoil. Recent work [6] has, however, shown phasic expiratory activity in the transversus abdominis muscle, particularly in patients with more severe airway narrowing. Post-inspiratory 'braking' due to continuing *expiratory* contraction of *inspiratory* muscles occupies a much smaller proportion of the (prolonged) expiration of patients with COPD than is seen in normal subjects [40].

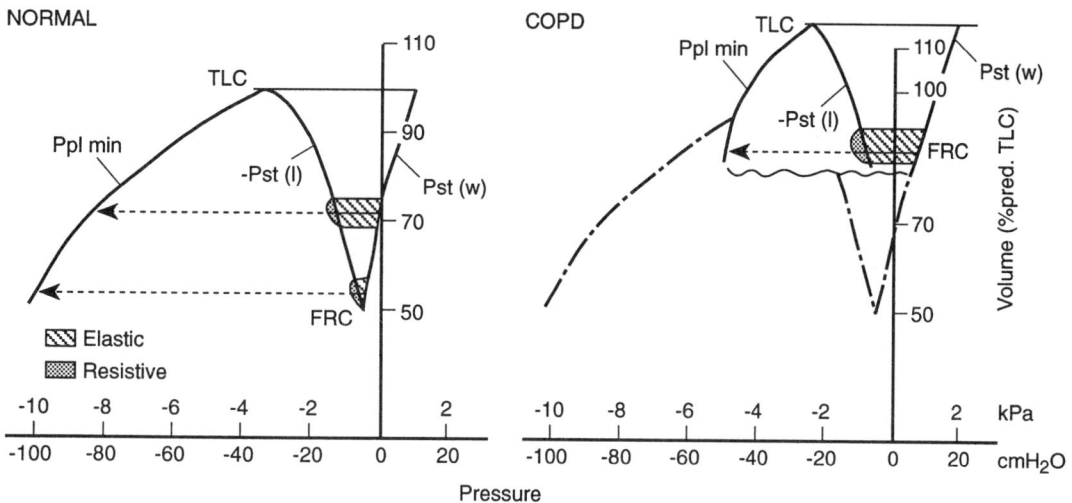

Fig. 9.5 Schematic relations of tidal and maximum inspiratory pressures in a normal subject (left) and a patient with COPD and hyperinflation (right) redrawn from Pride [39] with permission. Analysis is in terms of pleural pressure plotted against lung volume (% predicted TLC) (a) during maximum static inspiratory efforts (Ppl min), (b) when the respiratory muscles are relaxed (Pst(w) – which represents passive recoil of the chest wall) and (c) during breath holding (–Pst(l) – which represents the mirror image of the static recoil curve of the lungs). FRC in the normal subject represents the 'neutral' position of the respiratory system, i.e. Pst(w) = –Pst(l). The requirement for inspiratory muscle pressure during tidal breathing is indicated by the continuous horizontal line between Pst(w) and the dynamic Ppl (curved line) required to overcome elastic plus resistive forces; the pressure-generating capacity at the same lung volume is given by the horizontal line (continuous + broken) between Pst(w) and Ppl min. In the normal subject the lower hatched and stippled areas indicate work of breathing during an inspiration starting from FRC, while the upper hatched area indicates the greater elastic work of breathing necessary at a higher lung volume, where the pressure-generating capacity is less.

In the patient with COPD the end expired volume (FRC) is above the neutral position of the respiratory system and is associated with a positive relaxation pressure indicated by the horizontal distance between end tidal Pst(w) and Pst(l); this represents 'intrinsic PEEP' (see text) the presence of which increases the elastic work of inspiration. Adaptation of inspiratory muscle function allows a more negative Ppl min at high lung volumes than would be seen in a normal subject (whose equivalent curve is indicated by —.—.—.) but Ppl min at end expiration is less negative than at a normal FRC. The tidal requirement for inspiratory muscle pressure (Ppl) is a much higher proportion of the pressure-generating capacity than in a normal subject because of both an increase in load and a reduction in capacity.

Individuals with severe airway obstruction characteristically have expiratory flow limitation, even during tidal breathing, with a progressive reduction in tidal flow at low lung volumes (Chapter 7). This prolonged expiration results in termination of expiration at a lung volume (FRC) above the true neutral position of the respiratory system, a phenomenon recognized as 'dynamic hyperinflation', as inspiratory muscles start to contract and the next inspiration is initiated before expiratory flow ceases. This represents a mechanism of hyperinflation additional to that occurring as a result of loss of lung recoil pressure; it amounts to approximately half a litre or so at rest [41]. It places an additional burden on the inspiratory muscles because there is a greater elastic load associated with tidal breathing over a higher volume range (Fig. 9.5). The inspiratory muscles have to overcome an additional pressure ('intrinsic positive end expiratory pressure – PEEPi') before lung inflation can commence. PEEPi was first recognized in acutely ill patients during mechanical ventilation where it is easily identifiable as a positive pressure if the airway is occluded at end expiration. It is also seen as a consequence of dynamic hyperinflation in stable patients with severe COPD. Its magnitude is sometimes estimated from the fall in pleural (esophageal) pressure immediately preceding the onset of inspiratory flow [42,43]. Such a reduction in pleural pressure can be due also to relaxation of abdominal muscles, however; the recent demonstration of expiratory contraction of transversus abdominis in many patients with severe COPD implies that the assumption that this pre-inspiratory reduction in pleural pressure reflects 'intrinsic PEEP' may not necessarily be valid [6].

9.4 RESPIRATORY MUSCLE FATIGUE

The attractive concept of fatigue of the respiratory muscles as a cause of respiratory failure [44] has generated numerous studies over the past 15 years. The precise point at which fatigue develops and the most appropriate clinical test(s) for its detection have, however, remained elusive. Fatigue in the present context is defined [45] as a loss in the capacity for developing force and/or velocity of a muscle resulting from muscle activity under load and which is *reversible by rest*. The last point is important as it distinguishes fatigue from persistent weakness. Abnormalities of muscle function develop before the failure of a muscle as a generator of force; a clinical test of fatigue therefore needs to be sufficiently sensitive to detect this 'prodromal' phase so that, where possible, appropriate therapeutic steps can be taken to forestall power failure. Fatigue is not necessarily located peripherally in the neuromuscular apparatus. With 'central' fatigue the reduction in capacity results from an inability to maintain the necessary central motor drive. This may represent an important protective mechanism which avoids the adverse effects of prolonged forceful contraction. The possible mechanisms of fatigue arising peripherally in the neuromuscular apparatus include reduced substrate supply, depletion of muscle energy stores and local acid–base changes; these in turn are very dependent on local blood flow.

In limb muscles evidence of fatigue is detectable with continuous contractions of approximately 0.15 of the maximal tension that the muscle can develop. For intermittent contractions the fatigue threshold depends on the tension developed and the duration of each contraction. This principle has been applied to the diaphragm by calculation of the 'tension–time index' (TTdi), defined as the product of mean transdiaphragmatic pressure (as a fraction of Pdi max) and the 'duty cycle' which represents the proportion of each breathing cycle spent on inspiration, i.e. the time during which the diaphragm is contracting [46]. During ventilation at rest the critical TTdi beyond which fatigue is likely to become evident is approximately 0.15–0.20. In patients with COPD the mean Pdi during a breath is increased at the same time as Pdi max is decreased, hence the reserve is appreciably less than in normal subjects. Bellemare and Grassino [47] showed in patients with COPD that an increase in mean Pdi of only three-fold would be sufficient to produce evidence of fatigue whereas in normal subjects the corresponding increase had to be approximately eight-fold.

9.4.1 METHODS OF ASSESSMENT

Both EMG and mechanical indices have been proposed for the recognition of fatigue; the methods have been assessed mostly in normal subjects before and after breathing against a 'fatiguing' load such as a very high external resistance.

(a) Response to electrical stimulation

The standard method for limb muscles is measurement of the force of contraction in relation to stimulation at increasing frequency. This technique has been applied successfully to the sternomastoid muscle allowing construction of a frequency–force relationship [48]. The output of the diaphragm in terms of Pdi response to phrenic nerve stimulation can also be measured and a frequency–pressure curve constructed [49]. In fatigued healthy subjects the characteristic finding is of rapid recovery of the response to high frequency stimulation but markedly delayed recovery of the response to lower frequency stimulation – the phenomenon of 'low frequency fatigue' which is quantitated as a fall in the ratio of response to stimulation frequencies of 20 and 50 Hz (20:50 ratio).

(b) Spectral analysis of EMG

Fatigue is associated with a change in the frequency spectrum of the EMG during spontaneous muscle contraction [50]. There is an increase in amplitude of lower frequency components and a decrease in amplitude at higher frequencies. One way in which this can be quantitated is by calculating the ratio of the amplitudes of signals over arbitrary ranges of higher and lower frequencies (H/L ratio) [51]. Unlike low frequency fatigue (in response to stimulated contraction), the H/L ratio is rapidly restored to normal on recovery and may therefore be less sensitive [52]. Its arbitrary definition has been criticized and it has not been widely accepted as a specific index of fatigue [45].

(c) Maximum relaxation rate

Fatigued muscle relaxes abnormally slowly. Relaxation of the diaphragm can be quantitated from the decline in Pdi by calculating the maximum relaxation rate (MRR) or the time constant of relaxation, assuming a monoexponential decay [53]. In normal subjects the decline in pressure can be followed more simply by measurements with a balloon in the mouth or nasopharynx [54] but this is unreliable as a guide to changes in intrathoracic pressure in patients with abnormal pulmonary mechanics [31]. Although the MRR is a simple index of fatigue, its lengthening appears to parallel a decline in PImax [55] and consequently it lacks sensitivity as a predictor of *impending* fatigue.

9.4.2 RESPIRATORY MUSCLE FATIGUE IN COPD

Respiratory muscle fatigue has been demonstrated in experimental studies in patients with COPD using all the above indices but the relevance to normal breathing in these subjects remains unclear. The likely greater potential for the development of fatigue in patients with COPD compared with normal subjects was demonstrated by the study of Bellemare and Grassino [47], who emphasized the limited reserve available to these patients. Pardy and Roussos [56] showed that voluntary hyperventilation sufficient to reduce $PaCO_2$ by 10 mmHg was associated with a change in the H/L ratio compatible with the development of fatigue. Wilson *et al.* [57] showed the development of low frequency fatigue in the sternomastoid muscle after a 12-minute walk whereas this was not seen in normal subjects. The clinical significance of this finding is, however, uncertain as the performance of a second 12-minute walk shortly afterwards was not affected by its presence. Studies during acute exacerbations showed that the sternomastoid muscle was more easily fatiguable at the time of admission than during subsequent recovery but overt fatigue was identified in only a small proportion of patients admitted to hospital during an exacerbation [58]. Furthermore, although patients with COPD have a much higher TTdi than normal subjects, this does not generally lie in the fatiguing range unless they are made to breathe more slowly and deeply than they normally choose [47].The TTdi at rest is higher in hypercapnic than in eucapnic patients but a recent study by Begin and Grassino [59] showed that even in the severely hypercapnic it did not exceed the fatigue threshold.

An important adaptation to increased load in such patients is a reduction in tidal volume. Because of the irreducible dead space this breathing pattern predisposes to the development of hypercapnia but it may represent a mechanism for avoiding the development of fatigue [60].

9.5 CONSEQUENCES OF RESPIRATORY MUSCLE DYSFUNCTION IN COPD

9.5.1 TIDAL BREATHING AND EFFECT OF POSTURE

The characteristic tidal breathing pattern of patients with COPD with small tidal volume and rapid frequency results in part from abnormal respiratory muscle actions and may represent an adaptative mechanism which minimizes the risk of fatigue (see above). The increased lung volume associated with hyperinflation is accommodated mainly by a lower position of the diaphragm. An increase in anteroposterior (AP) diameter of the rib cage is a classic clinical sign of hyperinflation. Detailed radiographic measurements in subjects with COPD without kyphosis, however, have shown that the AP diameter and angulation of the ribs are similar at the same absolute lung volumes to those of normal subjects of similar age [61]. The 'clinical impression' is genuine but is simply a manifestation of the abnormally increased resting lung volume of such patients.

During quiet tidal breathing relative motion of the rib cage is increased and that of the abdomen decreased and this is related to the degree of hyperinflation [37]. Various other distortions have been reported, the most readily recognized is indrawing of the lateral rib cage margin on inspiration (so-called 'Hoover's sign'). Others include paradoxical inspiratory motion of the abdomen, inspiratory paradoxical motion of the lower sternum in the AP diameter and biphasic motion of the abdomen [37]. The development of Hoover's sign is related to reduction of the zone of apposition and consequent loss of the expanding effect of diaphragmatic contraction on the rib cage together with a change in orientation of diaphragmatic muscle fibres such that diaphragmatic contraction directly draws in the lower ribs [62]. Many patients with severe airway obstruction adopt a characteristic posture leaning forward with outstretched arms supported. This is associated with less shortness of breath and with improvements in PImax [63,64]. Sharp *et al.* [63] showed that patie nts with such postural relief of dyspnea tended to have paradoxical inspiratory motion of the abdomen in the upright posture associated with severe hyperinflation; it appears that in severely disabled individuals the leaning forward position aids diaphragmatic function by allowing the abdominal contents to stretch the diaphragm, improving the length–tension characteristics and allowing it to generate force more effectively. This is accompanied by a reduction in the activity of inspiratory accessory muscles [63].

9.5.2 BREATHING DURING SLEEP

The abnormalities of breathing during sleep in patients with COPD are discussed in detail elsewhere (Chapter 12). As in normal subjects, EMG activity of the respiratory muscles declines during sleep in comparison with the awake state and the changes are more marked in rapid eye movement (REM) sleep [65,66]. REM sleep in normal subjects is associated with marked inhibition of respiratory muscles other than the diaphragm, while in COPD activity of the other inspiratory muscles tends to be more variable [66]. Periods of hypopnea are seen in REM sleep, particularly during 'phasic' REM (pREM) sleep i.e. when eye movements are most marked. The pattern of such hypopneas varies with 'central' hypopnea resulting from pREM-related inhibition of the 'respiratory pump' muscles (i.e. diaphragm and/or inspiratory intercostals), while in some individuals 'obstructive' hypopneas are seen, associated with relatively greater inhibition of the upper airway stabilizing muscles such as genioglossus [67]. In addition to the direct effects of reduced respiratory muscle activity inducing hypoventilation, the end-expired volume in REM sleep falls in comparison with non-REM sleep due to a reduction in dynamic hyperinflation. This results from a lessening of the activity of inspiratory muscles (particularly scalenes and sternomastoid) during expiration. Dynamic hyperinflation persists in non-REM sleep; a recent preliminary report suggests that this can be counterbalanced by the application of nasal continuous positive airway pressure (CPAP) at night which reduces inspiratory muscle activity in non-REM sleep without any deterioration in gas exchange [68].

9.5.3 EXERCISE AND DYSPNEA

The increased requirements for ventilation during exercise are achieved by an increase in either frequency or tidal volume (or both); in addition the slowing of expiratory airflow implies a reduction in the relative duration of inspiration. Each of these factors adds to the burden placed on the inspiratory muscles; greater dynamic hyperinflation than at rest may further exacerbate the problem. Increasing end-expiratory and end-inspiratory lung volumes occur against a background of decreasing pressure-generating capacity of the inspiratory muscles due to the length–tension relationship. As a result the load/capacity ratio moves markedly in an adverse direction. The inspiratory change in abdominal pressure becomes more negative with recruitment of accessory muscles dominating the contribution of a severely compromised diaphragm [69]. At the same time expiratory abdominal muscle contraction becomes more evident with increasingly positive Pab during expiration. This tends to stretch the diaphragmatic fibers and hence potentially aids diaphragmatic contraction during the subsequent inspiration. Diaphragmatic descent may also be partially passive due to relaxation and the consequent fall in Pab at the start of inspiration. Strapping of the abdominal wall has been reported to give subjective relief to patients with COPD at rest, possibly by improving diaphragmatic function in a similar way and offloading other inspiratory muscles. It does not, however, improve exercise endurance, perhaps because it also impairs the ability of the abdominal muscles to aid inspiration by relaxation at its onset [70].

O'Connell and Campbell [71] compared patients with severe COPD with and without inspiratory dyspnea at rest; although they showed no significant differences in PI max values between these two groups, the dyspneic patients used a higher proportion of the maximum pressure available at that volume to generate inspiratory flow during quiet breathing. A study during exercise in patients with various cardiopulmonary diseases similarly showed a relation between dyspnea and the ratio of end-inspiratory pleural pressure to PI max [72], again emphasizing the need to interpret the load to breathing or the effort required to overcome this load in relation to the capacity available. In a recent study of a large number of patients with COPD Mahler and Harver [73] showed that dyspnea on exercise could be related to maximal respiratory pressures and this effect was independent of spirometric indices of lung function.

9.5.4 GAS EXCHANGE AND VENTILATORY CONTROL

Rochester and Braun [10] showed clearly the important relationship of inspiratory muscle function in COPD to the development of hypercapnia (Fig. 9.6). The general shape of the relationship was similar to that found in patients with neuromuscular disease but those with COPD have a greater load to breathing and consequently are likely to develop hypercapnia with a relatively better preserved value of PI max than patients with muscle weakness alone. The importance of inspiratory muscle dysfunction to the generation of chronic hypercapnia in these patients was emphasized in a recent large study by Begin and Grassino [59], who showed that $Paco_2$ was related best to an index of load (FEV_1 or respiratory resistance), to the dead space/tidal volume ratio and best of all to the relationship of load to capacity (expressed as either resistance/PI max or mean inspiratory pressure/PI max). One important contributor to the mean inspiratory pressure generated by the respiratory muscles during tidal breathing is intrinsic PEEP and this also has been shown to correlate with the severity of hypercapnia [42].

Inspiratory muscle function is relevant also to the assessment of ventilatory control in

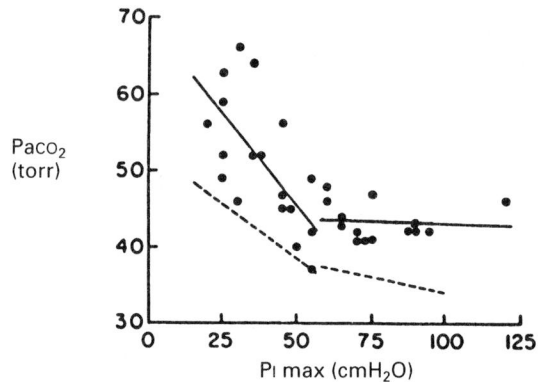

Fig. 9.6 Relationship between $Paco_2$ and PI max in patients with COPD (closed circles and solid lines). Also shown for comparison are the results of a similar analysis in patients with primary muscle disease and no significant airway obstruction (from Rochester and Braun [10].)

patients with COPD. The problems of interpretation of the ventilatory response to CO_2 in patients with adverse respiratory mechanics are well recognized. The mouth occlusion pressure was promoted as a more valid alternative in this situation but Gribbin *et al.* [74] showed that this also is open to criticism because of its dependence on respiratory muscle function, particularly as end-expiratory volume rises with CO_2 stimulation in these patients and consequently mouth occlusion pressure as a proportion of the maximum available inspiratory pressure rises markedly.

9.6 THERAPEUTIC POSSIBILITIES

9.6.1 REST AND VENTILATORY SUPPORT

The use in selected patients during exacerbations of assisted ventilation using intermittent positive pressure via an endotracheal tube has been standard practice for many years (Chapter 19). Of more recent interest is the use of long-term nocturnal ventilatory support by either negative pressure ventilation applied to the chest wall or by IPPV using a nasal mask. Some uncontrolled studies of negative pressure ventilation in hypercapnic patients suggested impressive results and were associated with apparent improvement in inspiratory muscle function. A recent large controlled study has, however, failed to show any benefit [76]. One potentially disadvantageous effect of such treatment is narrowing of the upper airway during inspiration due to more negative intra-airway pressures; this results in obstructive sleep apnoea in a few patients [77].

This type of ventilatory support for long-term use has largely been superseded by the development of nasal IPPV which is currently under evaluation. Again, uncontrolled studies have suggested benefit [78], even though reductions in daytime $PaCO_2$ could not be related to improved respiratory muscle strength [80] and further large studies are required.

The effects of continuous positive airway pressure (CPAP) have been studied during exercise and appear promising, allowing the maintenance of ventilation and exercise performance with a reduction in inspiratory muscle effort [81,82]. Whether this approach has a clinical role remains to be seen.

9.6.2 NUTRITIONAL TREATMENT

Several studies have examined the effect of dietary supplementation on respiratory muscle function in malnourished patients with COPD. Early uncontrolled studies reported benefit [83], while the results of controlled studies are variable with some showing no effect [84,85] and others reporting an improvement [86–88]. Positive results tend to be seen particularly in studies where weight gain is also achieved [87], but the improvements are generally modest and of doubtful cost effectiveness.

9.6.3 RESPIRATORY MUSCLE TRAINING

Several controlled and uncontrolled studies have examined the beneficial effects of specific training of the respiratory muscles. In general, training of muscles is task-specific, i.e. the benefits of training are seen in the task trained but not necessarily in other activities. Thus it is possible to improve respiratory muscle strength without necessarily any benefit on exercise performance. A recent meta-analysis of 17 randomized trials of respiratory muscle training in COPD [89] demonstrated how the effects of training depend upon method, duration, frequency and intensity of training used. When training by either resistive breathing or isocapnic hyperventilation was considered improvements in strength or endurance were demonstrable but overall there was no improvement in exercise performance.

9.6.4 PHARMACOLOGIC TREATMENT

The demonstration that methylxanthines such as theophylline potentiate the *in vitro* response of fresh and fatigued muscle strips to an electrical stimulus led to investigation of the value of such agents for this purpose *in vivo*. The concentrations used in *in vitro* studies, however, would be prohibitive *in vivo* in man. At more realistic therapeutic concentrations some [90], but not all [91], studies have shown a small increase in Pdi generated during maximal voluntary efforts, in the diaphragmatic response to a standard stimulus applied to the phrenic nerves or in the EMG power spectrum suggesting a reduction in fatigue. Minor improvements have been reported both in normal subjects and patients with COPD but it is difficult to dissociate direct effects on the contractile process from the indirect effects of increases in muscle blood flow or of bronchodilatation and associated reduction in lung volume. Such concomitant changes may well account for the modest improvements in muscle function reported. Other drugs which have been investigated include the β-sympathomimetic agents but the effects have generally been less than seen with methylxanthines.

9.7 CONCLUSIONS

The respiratory muscles of patients with COPD were largely neglected until the last 20 years. Over that time numerous studies have been performed, the constraints imposed on and by the muscles have become better understood and the importance of respiratory muscle function in determining breathlessness, exercise capacity, the development of respiratory failure, breathing during sleep and other manifestations has been clarified. The inspiratory muscles, in particular, are doubly compromised in patients with COPD and hyperinflation by an increase in load and a reduction in capacity. The latter results from the combination of distorted geometry and weakness due to impaired nutrition. Overall, however, the mechanical performance of the respiratory muscles, and particularly the diaphragm is generally better in practice than might have been predicted on theoretical grounds, although the adaptations which occur are still poorly understood.

REFERENCES

1. De Troyer, A. and Estenne, M. (1984) Co-ordination between rib cage muscles and diaphragm during quiet breathing in humans. *J. Appl. Physiol.*, **57**, 899–906.
2. Goldman, M.D. and Mead, J. (1973) Mechanical interaction between the diaphragm and rib cage. *J. Appl. Physiol.*, **35**, 197–204.
3. Van Lunteren, E. and Strohl, K.P. (1986). The muscles of the upper airways. *Clin. Chest Med.*, **7**, 171–85.
4. De Troyer, A., Estenne, M., Ninane, V. *et al.* (1990) Transversus abdominis muscle function in humans. *J. Appl. Physiol.*, **68**, 1010–6.
5. Campbell, E.J.M. and Friend, J. (1955) Action of breathing exercises in pulmonary emphysema. *Lancet*, **i**, 325–9.
6. Ninane, V., Rypens, F., Yernault, J-C. and De Troyer, A. (1992) Abdominal muscle use during breathing in patients with chronic airflow obstruction. *Am. Rev. Respir. Dis.*, **146**, 16–21.
7. Sanchez, J., Derenne, J.P., Debesse, B. *et al.* (1982) Typology of the respiratory muscles in normal men and in patients with moderate chronic respiratory diseases. *Clin. Respir. Physiol.*, **18**, 901–14.
8. Thurlbeck, W. (1978) Diaphragm and body weight in emphysema. *Thorax*, **33**, 483–7.
9. Arora, N.S. and Rochester, D.F. (1987) COPD and human diaphragm muscle dimensions. *Chest*, **91**, 719–24.
10. Rochester, D.F. and Braun, N.M.T. (1985) Determinants of maximal inspiratory pressure in chronic obstructive pulmonary disease. *Am. Rev. Respir. Dis.*, **132**, 42–7.
11. Sanchez, J., Bastien, C., Medrano, G. *et al.* (1984) Metabolic enzymatic activities in the diaphragm of normal men and patients with moderate chronic obstructive pulmonary disease. *Clin. Respir. Physiol.*, **20**, 535–40.
12. Campbell, J.A., Hughes, R.L., Sahgal, V. *et al.* (1980) Alterations in intercostal muscle morphology and biochemistry in patients with obstructive lung disease. *Am. Rev. Respir. Dis.*, **122**, 679–86.
13. Fiaccadori, E., Del Canale, S., Vitali, *et al.* (1977) Skeletal muscle energetics, acid-base equilibrium and lactate metabolism in patients with severe hypercapnia and hypoxaemia. *Chest*, **92**, 883–7.
14. Rochester, D.F. (1986) Body weight and respiratory muscle function in chronic obstructive pulmonary disease. *Am. Rev. Respir. Dis.*, **134**, 646–8.
15. Cherniack, R.M. (1959) The oxygen consumption and efficiency of the respiratory muscles in health and emphysema. *J. Clin. Invest.*, **38**, 494–8.
16. Otis, A.B. (1951) The work of breathing. *Physiol. Rev.*, **34**, 449–58.
17. Johnson, B.D., Reddan, W.G., Seow, K.C. and Dempsey, J.A. (1991) Mechanical constraints on exercise hyperpnea in a fit ageing population. *Am. Rev. Respir. Dis.*, **143**, 968–77.
18. Donahoe, M., Rogers, R.M., Wilson, D.O. and Pennock, B.E. (1989) Oxygen consumption of the respiratory muscles in normal and in malnourished patients with chronic obstructive pulmonary disease. *Am. Rev. Respir. Dis.*, **140**, 385–91.
19. Green, J.H. and Muers, M.F. (1991) The thermic effect of food in underweight patients with emphysematous chronic obstructive pulmonary disease. *Eur. Respir. J.*, **4**, 813–9.
20. Goldstein, S.A., Thomashow, B.M., Kvetan, V. *et al.* (1988) Nitrogen and energy relationship in malnourished patients with emphysema. *Am. Rev. Respir. Dis.*, **138**, 636–44.

21. Schols, A.M.W.J., Soeters, P.B., Mostert, R. *et al.* (1991) Energy balance in chronic obstructive pulmonary disease. *Am. Rev. Respir. Dis.*, **143**, 1248–52.

22. Efthimiou, J., Mounsey, P.J., Benson, D.N. *et al.* (1992) Effect of carbohydrate rich versus fat rich loads on gas exchange and walking performance in patients with chronic obstructive lung disease. *Thorax*, **47**, 451–6.

23. Morrison, W.L., Gibson, J.N.A., Scrimgeour, C. and Rennie, M.J. (1988) Muscle wasting in emphysema. *Clin. Sci.*, **75**, 415–20.

24. Decramer, M., Demedts, M., Rochette, F. and Billiet, L. (1980) Maximal transrespiratory pressures in obstructive lung disease. *Clin. Respir. Physiol.*, **16**, 479–90.

25. Gibson, G.J., Clark, E. and Pride, N.B. (1981) Static transdiaphragmatic pressures in normal subjects and in patients with chronic hyperinflation. *Am. Rev. Respir. Dis.*, **124**, 685–9.

26. Laporta, D. and Grassino, A. (1985) Assessment of transdiaphragmatic pressure in humans. *J. Appl. Physiol.*, **58**, 1469–76.

27. Braun, N.M.T., Arora, N.S. and Rochester, D.F. (1982) Force-length relation of the normal human diaphragm. *J. Appl. Physiol.*, **53**, 405–12.

28. Smith, J. and Bellemare, F. (1987) Effect of lung volume on *in vivo* contraction characteristics of human diaphragm. *J. Appl. Physiol.*, **62**, 1893–900.

29. Miller, J.M., Moxham, J. and Green, M. (1985) The maximal sniff in the assessment of diaphragmatic function in man. *Clin. Sci.*, **69**, 91–6.

30. Wanke, T., Schenz, G., Zwick, H. *et al.* (1990) Dependence of maximal sniff generated mouth and trans-diaphragmatic pressures on lung volumes. *Thorax*, **45**, 352–5.

31. Mulvey, D.A., Elliott, M.W., Coulouris, N.G. *et al.* (1991) Sniff, esophageal and nasopharyngeal pressures and maximal relaxation rates in patients with respiratory dysfunction. *Am. Rev. Respir. Dis.*, **143**, 950–3.

32. Byrd, R.B. and Hyatt, R.E. (1968) Maximal respiratory pressures in chronic obstructive lung disease. *Am. Rev. Respir. Dis.*, **98**, 848–56.

33. Similowski, T., Yan, S., Gauthier, A. *et al.* (1991) Contractile properties of the human diaphragm during chronic hyperinflation. *N. Engl. J. Med.*, **325**, 917–23.

34. Farkas, G.A., and Roussos, C. (1982) Adaptability of the hamster diaphragm to exercise and/or emphysema. *J. Appl. Physiol.*, **53**, 1263–72.

35. Sharp, J.T., Danon, J., Druz, W.S. *et al* (1974) Respiratory muscle function in patients with chronic obstructive pulmonary disease: its relationship to disability and to respiratory therapy. *Am. Rev. Respir. Dis.*, **110** no.6 suppl: 154–67.

36. Sharp, J.T., Beard, G.A., Sunga, M. *et al.* (1986) The rib cage in normal and emphysematous subjects: a roentgenographic approach. *J. Appl. Physiol.*, **61**, 2050–9.

37. Gilmartin, J.J. and Gibson, G.J. (1984) Abnormalities of chest wall motion in patients with chronic airflow obstruction. *Thorax*, **39**, 264–71.

38. Martinez, F.J., Couser, J.I. and Celli, B.R. (1990) Factors influencing ventilatory muscle recruitment in patients with chronic airflow obstruction. *Am. Rev. Respir. Dis.*, **142**, 276–82.

39. Pride, N.B. (1990) Chronic obstructive pulmonary disease (COPD): Pathophysiology, in *Respiratory Medicine* (eds R.A.L. Brewis, G.J. Gibson and D.M. Geddes), Bailliere-Tindall, London, pp. 507–20.

40. Citterio, G., Agostoni, E., Del Santo, A. and Marazzini, L. (1981) Decay of inspiratory muscle activity in chronic airway obstruction. *J. Appl. Physiol.*, **51**, 1388–97.

41. Morris, M.J., Madgwick, R.G., Frew, A.J., and Lane, D.J. (1990) Breathing muscle activity during expiration in patients with chronic airflow obstruction. *Eur. Respir. J.*, **3**, 901–9.

42. Haluszka, J., Chartrand, D.A., Grassino, A.E. and Milic-Emili, J. (1990) Intrinsic PEEP and arterial PCO_2 in stable patients with chronic obstructive pulmonary disease. *Am. Rev. Respir. Dis.*, **141**, 1194–7.

43. Dal Vecchio, L., Polese, G., Poggi, R. and Rossi, A. (1990) 'Intrinsic' positive end-expiratory pressure in stable patients with chronic obstructive pulmonary disease. *Eur. Respir. J.*, **3**, 74–80.

44. Macklem, P.T. and Roussos, C.S. (1977) Respiratory muscle fatigue: a cause of respiratory failure? *Clin. Sci.*, **53**, 419–22.

45. Respiratory Muscle Fatigue Workshop Group (1990) Respiratory muscle fatigue. *Am. Rev. Respir. Dis.*, **142**, 474–80.

46. Bellemare, F, and Grassino, A. (1982) Effect of pressure and timing of contraction on human diaphragm fatigue. *J. Appl. Physiol.*, **53**, 1190–5.

47. Bellemare, F. and Grassino, A. (1983) Force reserve of the diaphragm in patients with chronic obstructive pulmonary disease. *J. Appl. Physiol.*, **55**, 8–13.

48. Moxham, J., Wiles, C.M., Newham, D. and Edwards, R.H.T. (1980) Sternomastoid muscle function and fatigue in man. *Clin. Sci.,* **59**, 463–8.

49. Moxham, J., Morris, A.R.J., Spiro, S.G. *et al.* (1981) Contractile properties and fatigue of the diaphragm in man. *Thorax,* **36**, 164–8.

50. Haag, G.M. (1992) Interpretation of EMG spectral alterations and alteration indexes at sustained contraction. *J. Appl. Physiol.,* **73**, 1211–7.

51. Gross, D., Grassino, A., Ross, W.R.D. and Macklem, P.T. (1979) Electromyogram pattern of diaphragmatic fatigue. *J. Appl. Physiol.,* **46**, 1–7.

52. Moxham, J., Edwards, R.H.T., Aubier, M. *et al.* (1982) Changes in EMG power spectrum (high-to-low ratio) with force fatigue in humans. *J. Appl. Physiol.,* **53**, 1094–9.

53. Esau, S.A., Bye, P.T.B. and Pardy, R.L. (1983) Changes in rate of relaxation of sniffs with diaphragmatic fatigue in humans. *J. Appl. Physiol.,* **55**, 731–5.

54. Koulouris, N., Vianna, L.G., Mulvey, D.A. *et al.* (1989) Maximal relaxation rates of oesophageal, nose and mouth pressures during a sniff reflect inspiratory muscle fatigue. *Am. Rev. Respir. Dis.,* **139**, 1213–7.

55. Mulvey, D.A., Koulouris, N.G., Elliot, M.W. *et al.* (1991) Inspiratory muscle relaxation rate after voluntary isocapnic ventilation in humans. *J. Appl. Physiol.,* **70**, 2173–80.

56. Pardy, R.L. and Roussos, C. (1983) Endurance of hyperventilation in chronic airflow limitation. *Chest,* **83**, 744–50.

57. Wilson, S.H., Cooke, N.T., Moxham, J. and Spiro, S.G. (1984) Sternomastoid muscle function and fatigue in normal subjects and in patients with chronic obstructive pulmonary disease. *Am. Rev. Respir. Dis.,* **129**, 460–4.

58. Efthimiou, J., Fleming, J. and Spiro, S.G. (1987) Sternomastoid muscle function and fatigue in breathless patients with severe respiratory disease. *Am. Rev. Respir. Dis.,* **136**, 1099–105.

59. Begin, P. and Grassino, A. (1991) Inspiratory muscle dysfunction and chronic hypercapnia in chronic obstructive pulmonary disease. *Am. Rev. Respir. Dis.,* **143**, 905–12.

60. Rochester, D.F. (1991) Respiratory muscle weakness, pattern of breathing and CO_2 retention in chronic obstructive pulmonary disease. *Am. Rev. Respir. Dis.,* **143**, 901–3.

61. Walsh, J.M., Webber, C.L., Fahey, P.J. and Sharp, J.T. (1992) Structural change of the thorax in chronic obstructive pulmonary disease. *J. Appl. Physiol.,* **72**, 1270–8.

62. Gilmartin, J.J. and Gibson, G.J. (1986) Mechanisms of paradoxical rib cage motion in patients with chronic obstructive pulmonary disease. *Am. Rev. Respir. Dis.,* **134**, 683–7.

63. Sharp, J.T., Druz, W.S., Moisan, T. *et al.* (1980) Postural relief of dyspnoea in severe chronic obstructive pulmonary disease. *Am. Rev. Respir. Dis.,* **122**, 201–11.

64. O'Neill, S. and McCarthy, D.S. (1983) Postural relief of dyspnoea in severe chronic airflow limitation: relationship to respiratory muscle strength. *Thorax,* **38**, 595–600.

65. Hudgel, D.W., Martin, R.J., Capehart, M. *et al.* (1983) Contribution of hypoventilation to sleep oxygen desaturation in chronic obstructive pulmonary disease. *J. Appl. Physiol.,* **55**, 669–77.

66. Johnson, M.W. and Remmers, J.E. (1984) Accessory muscle activity during sleep in chronic obstructive pulmonary disease. *J. Appl. Physiol.,* **57**, 1011–7.

67. White, J.E.S., Drinnan, M., Smithson, A. *et al.* (1994) Respiratory muscle activity and oxygenation during sleep in chronic airflow obstruction. *Thorax* in press.

68. Petrof, B.J., Kimoff, R.J., Levy, R.D. *et al.* (1991) Nasal continuous positive airway pressure facilitates respiratory muscle function during sleep in severe chronic obstructive pulmonary disease. *Am. Rev. Respir. Dis.,* **143**, 928–35.

69. Dodd, D.S., Brancatisano, T. and Engel, L.A. (1984) Chest wall mechanics during exercise in patients with severe chronic airflow obstruction. *Am. Rev. Respir. Dis.,* **129**, 33–8.

70. Dodd, D.S., Brancatisano, T.P. and Engel. L.A. (1985) Effect of abdominal strapping on chest wall mechanics during exercise in patients with severe chronic airflow obstruction. *Am. Rev. Respir. Dis.,* **131**, 816–21.

71. O'Connell, J.M. and Campbell, A.H. (1976) Respiratory mechanics in airways obstruction with inspiratory dyspnoea. *Thorax,* **31**, 669–77.

72. Leblanc, P., Bowie, D.M., Summers, E. *et al.* (1986) Breathlessness and exercise in patients with cardiorespiratory disease. *Am. Rev. Respir. Dis.,* **133**, 21–5.

73. Mahler, D.A. and Harver, A. (1992) A factor analysis of dyspnoea ratings, respiratory muscle strength and lung function in patients with chronic obstructive pulmonary disease. *Am. Rev. Respir. Dis.,* **145**, 467–70.

74. Gribbin, H.R., Gardiner, I.T., Heinz, G.J. *et al.* (1983) Role of impaired inspiratory muscle function in limiting the ventilatory response to carbon dioxide in chronic airflow obstruction. *Clin. Sci.*, **64**, 487–95.

75. Braun, N.M.T. and Marino, W.D. (1984) Effect of daily intermittent rest of respiratory muscles in patients with severe chronic airflow limitation. *Chest*, **85**, 593–605.

76. Shapiro, S.H. Ernst, P., Gray-Donald, K. *et al.* (1992) Effect of negative pressure ventilation in severe chronic obstructive pulmonary disease. *Lancet*, **340**, 1425–9.

77. Levy, R.D., Cosio, M.G., Gibbons, L. *et al.* (1992) Induction of sleep apnoea with negative pressure ventilation in patients with chronic obstructive lung disease. *Thorax*, **47**, 612–5.

78. Elliott, M.W., Simonds, A.K., Carroll, M.P. *et al.* (1992) Domiciliary nocturnal nasal intermittent positive pressure ventilation in hypercapnic respiratory failure due to chronic obstructive lung disease. *Thorax*, **47**, 342–8.

79. Elliott, M.W., Mulvey, D.A., Moxham, J. *et al.* (1991) Domiciliary nocturnal nasal intermittent positive pressure ventilation in COPD: mechanisms underlying changes in arterial blood gas tensions. *Eur. J. Respir. Dis.*, **4**, 1044–52.

80. Strumpf, D.A., Millman, R.P., Carlisle, C.C. *et al.* (1991) Nocturnal positive-pressure ventilation via nasal mask in patients with severe chronic obstructive pulmonary disease. *Am. Rev. Respir. Dis.*, **144**, 1234–9.

81. O'Donnell, D.E, Sanii, R., Giesbrecht, G. and Younes, M. (1988) Effect of continuous positive airway pressure on respiratory sensation in patients with chronic obstructive pulmonary disease during submaximal exercise. *Am. Rev. Respir. Dis.*, **138**, 1185–91.

82. Petrof, B.J., Calderini, E. and Gottfried, S.B. (1990) Effect of CPAP on respiratory effort and dyspnoea during exercise in severe COPD. *J. Appl. Physiol.*, **69**, 179–88.

83. Wilson, D.O., Rogers, R.M., Sanders, M.H. *et al.* (1986) Nutritional intervention in malnourished patients with emphysema. *Am. Rev. Respir. Dis.*, **134**, 672–7.

84. Lewis, M.I., Belman, M.J. and Dorr-Uyemura, L. (1987) Nutritional supplementation in ambulatory patients with chronic obstructive pulmonary disease. *Am. Rev. Respir. Dis.*, **135**, 1062–8.

85. Knowles, J.B., Fairbarn, M.S., Wiggs, B.J. *et al.* (1988) Dietary supplementation and respiratory muscle performance in patients with COPD. *Chest*, **93**, 977–83.

86. Efthimiou, J., Fleming, J., Gomes, C. and Spiro, S.G. (1988) The effect of supplementary oral nutrition in poorly nourished patients with chronic obstructive pulmonary disease. *Am. Rev. Respir. Dis.*, **137**, 1075–82.

87. Whittaker, J.S., Ryan, C.F., Buckley, P.A. and Road, J.D. (1990) The effects of refeeding on peripheral and respiratory muscle function in malnourished chronic obstructive pulmonary disease patients. *Am. Rev. Respir. Dis.*, **142**, 283–8.

88. Rogers, R.M., Donahue, M. and Constantino, J. (1992) Physiologic effects of oral supplemental feeding in malnourished patients with chronic obstructive pulmonary disease: a randomised study. *Am. Rev. Respir. Dis.*, **146**, 1511–7.

89. Smith, K., Cook, D., Guyatt, G.H. *et al.* (1992) Respiratory muscle training in chronic airflow limitation: a meta-analysis. *Am. Rev. Respir. Dis.*, **145**, 533–9.

90. Murciano, D., Aubier, M., Lecocguic, Y. and Pariente, R. (1984) Effects of theophylline on diaphragmatic strength and fatigue in patients with chronic obstructive pulmonary disease. *N. Engl. J. Med.*, **311**, 349–53.

91. Moxham, J. and Green, M. (1985) Aminophylline and the respiratory muscles. *Bull. Eur. Physiopathol. Respir.*, **21**, 1–6.

VENTILATORY CONTROL AND DYSPNEA

10

P.M.A. Calverley

The progress of ideas in respiratory physiology has often been accelerated by the need for practical solutions. Thus the clinical problems of gas mask design in World War I led Haldane and co-workers to further study the stimulant effects of respiratory gases whilst the hypoxia of high altitude experienced by World War II fighter pilots generated new research about the chemical regulation of human breathing. The subsequent rise in the incidence of and mortality from chronic obstructive pulmonary disease gave a new clinical dimension to these problems. The dangers of high concentrations of oxygen during acute exacerbations of COPD were soon recognized [1] and led Campbell to apply new technologies to first identify the physiologic problem (hypercapnia), then hypothesize a mechanism for its production (reduced hypercapnic ventilatory drive) and finally suggest a practical solution (low flow oxgyen treatment by Venturi mask) [2].

About the same time Dornhorst's almost apocryphal (and certainly unreferenced) description of the two extremes of advanced COPD – 'pink and puffing' or 'blue and bloated' – launched a debate about whether these patients could not breathe or would not breathe when confronted with progressive lung disease, a controversy that continues in new forms to the present day. Meanwhile, Campbell and colleagues in a series of pioneering studies had begun the systematic investigation of respiratory sensation in general and breathlessness in particular. Their initial views were set out in a landmark symposium [3] whilst progress or lack of it has been reviewed more recently on a similar occasion [4].

This chapter will review some of the evidence underlying the ebb and flow of these ideas. More than most areas of respiratory medicine, studies of ventilatory control and dyspnea have been conditioned by the available technology and especially the problems of data handling. However, subtle and often unstated assumptions about the primary importance of blood gas tensions and the irrelevance of respiratory sensation and consciousness, have had a major effect on the hypotheses tested. These assumptions have now been challenged and hopefully the new approaches to these areas which have resulted will prove more useful to physiologists and clinicians alike.

10.1 ORGANIZATION OF VENTILATORY CONTROL

Conventional approaches envisage a hierarchy of command for ventilatory control [5,6] although there is considerably less agreement about whether the output of the control system is regulated to optimize ventilation or breathing pattern, however analyzed [7,8]. Inevitably most data about

Chronic Obstructive Pulmonary Disease. Edited by Dr P. Calverley and Professor N. Pride. Published in 1995 by Chapman & Hall, London. ISBN 0 412 46450 0

underlying mechanisms have involved animal studies where stimulation and ablation experiments are performed under anesthesia [5,9]. Whilst these establish that a neural connection exists, they do little to elucidate the integrated action of the system under conditions when mechanical and chemical homeostasis is disturbed as in COPD.

Respiration persists in these animals when the brain stem is sectioned at the pons or medulla [10]. The resulting metronomically regular breathing pattern is seldom seen in man except during deep general anesthesia [11] or stage 3/4 sleep [12]. It is believed to result from the interaction of three groups of tightly interconnected neurons [5,6]:

1. The dorsal respiratory group (DRG) which lies in the ventrolateral nucleus of the tractus solitarius and receives afferent impulses via the glossopharyngeal and vagus nerves from peripheral chemoreceptors and mechanoreceptors. The neurons here are mainly inspiratory but not all are influenced by stretch-receptor inputs. They project onto both the other neural groups and the phrenic nerve nucleus in the cervical cord.
2. The ventral respiratory group (VRG) extends throughout the medulla and includes neurons in the nucleus ambiguus, para-ambiguus and retrofacialis. The rostral neurones are thought to be inspiratory and the caudal ones expiratory. There are no direct connections with neural afferents from outside the CNS.
3. The pontine respiratory group corresponds to the neurones in the nucleus parabrachialis and the Kollicker–Fuse nucleus. These were thought to comprise the phase-spanning neurons that fire in late inspiration and early expiration. Recent data suggest they are a heterogeneous group of neurons rather than belonging to a specific type [13].

Neurons from the DRG and VRG synapse with phrenic and intercostal neurons in the spinal cord where neuronal firing can be further modified by multiple proprioceptive impulse principally from chest wall mechanoreceptors [14].

Respiratory rhythm is thought to rely on a central pattern generator [6,14] which acts as a rhythmic oscillator. The precise siting and nature of these respiratory pacemaker cells are still to be identified but extensive studies of the effects of lung inflation at different phases in the respiratory cycle in anesthetized animals have revealed characteristic patterns in neuronal firing in both inspiration and expiration. At the start of inspiration neurones from the DRG and VRG fire with increasing frequency to produce a ramp-like increase in respiratory muscle activation that seems to be limited by pulmonary stretch-receptor inputs, by pontine expiratory neuronal firing or by the inhibitory effects of the so-called post-inspiratory neurons [14]. After a brief pause the inspiratory neurons resume firing but at a lower frequency and their activity wanes as expiration proceeds. Since expiration is normally passive, activation of the expiratory muscles is not seen but when inspiratory drive increases there is a shortening of the duration of post-inspiratory neuronal firing with late expiratory neural activity.

Several mechanisms have been proposed to explain this activity. Inspiratory activity may continue to increase until it reaches some preset threshold or time when its specific 'off switch' inhibits it [5,9]. This begs the question of where such neurones lie and what determines the expiratory time. A more attractive option is based on the studies of Anderson and Sears [15] who suggested that the increase in neural activity during inspiration may be due to the withdrawal of tonic expiratory inhibition. A further alternative has been proposed by Richter and colleagues who believe in a reciprocal activation of inspiratory and expiratory neurones such that as the activity of one increases, so does the inhibitory effect of the other until finally inspiration or expiration is terminated [14].

These data have modified the way in which we analyze breathing patterns with an increased emphasis on the role of inspiratory time (TI) and total cycle duration (TTOT) as well as tidal volume. Minute ventilation, traditionally expressed as VT × f (respiratory frequency) can now be represented by VT/TI × TI/TTOT × 60 where VT/TI is the mean inspiratory flow which approximates to inspiratory neural drive assuming a linear increase in neural output and no mechanical restriction to VT whilst TI/TTOT is that proportion of each breath spent in inspiration (respiratory duty cycle). This approach has been helpful in analyzing the breathing pattern of COPD patients (see below).

Phasic respiratory motor output also controls the pharyngeal and laryngeal dimensions which has considerable importance for patients with COPD. Co-ordinated genioglossus activation before inspiration is essential if pharyngeal patency is to be maintained [16]. One group has reported that COPD patients with smaller upper airway dimensions are more likely to become hypercapnic, possibly because of an increase in pharyngeal resistance during sleep [17,18], although this is probably an unusual cause of hypercapnia [19]. Laryngeal braking of expiratory airflow appears to be an important mechanism for stabilizing expiratory lung volume which is a particular problem in COPD patients with hyperinflation [20]. The role of pursed-lip breathing and its neurologic basis as an adjunct to this remains uncertain [21].

10.2 FACTORS THAT MODULATE RESPIRATORY OUTPUT

Three major influences modify respiratory motor output namely chemoreceptor, mechanoreceptor and cortical factors. The relative importance of these will vary depending upon the situation.

10.2.1 CHEMORECEPTORS INPUTS

The peripheral chemoreceptors in man lie in the carotid body at the junction of the common and external carotid arteries, the aortic bodies having little demonstrable effect on human ventilation. Although only 15 mg in weight, they have a complex structure formed by Type 1a cells packed with neurotransmitters (mainly acetylcholine, substance P and dopamine) and Type 2 structural cells that surround a dense capillary network supplied directly from the carotid artery. With a blood flow equivalent to 2 1/100 g of tissue they are ideally sited to 'taste' the arterial gas tension of blood going to the brain. Local autonomic regulation of blood flow can further modify the chemoreceptor output [22]. Hypoxia produces a hyperbolic increase in carotid sinus nerve discharge [23] which may be signalled by intracellular changes in ADP or calcium. Carotid chemoreceptors are hypertrophied in some hypoxemic patients with COPD [24], but this does not seem to have functional significance.

Hypercapnia increases carotid sinus neural traffic linearly, probably due to local changes in pH [25]. The hypoxic and hypercapnic signals affect each other locally in a multiplicative way and travel in the glossopharyngeal nerves to the DRG where they are integrated with other inputs.

Peripheral chemoreceptor inputs contribute approximately 15% to resting ventilation and can be largely abolished by hyperoxia [26] which is thought to explain the beneficial role of supplementary oxgyen in normoxic COPD patients (Chapter 20). The relatively large falls in arterial P_{O_2} needed before chemoreceptor response occurs suggests that in most patients hypoxia is unimportant in eupneic ventilatory control. Chemoreceptor response to short-term hypoxemia is better related to oxygen saturation (Fig. 10.1), an important determinant of tissue oxygen delivery. Thus, chemoreceptor detection of hypoxemia is an important respiratory 'defence mechanism' which is very relevant at altitude

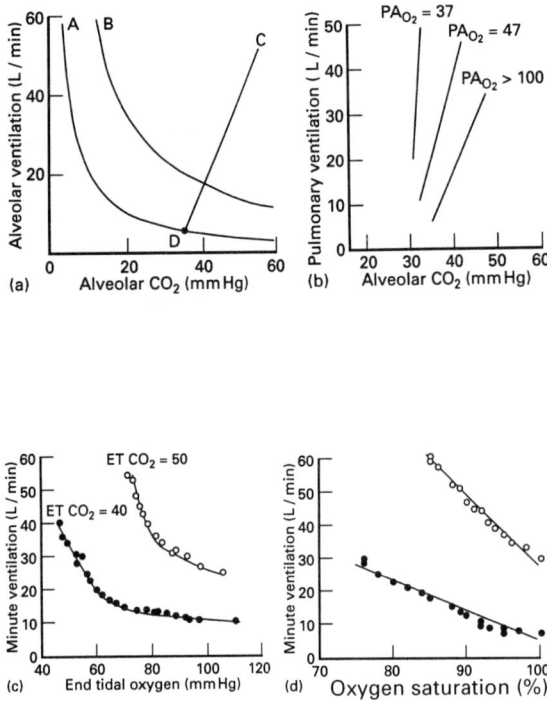

Fig. 10.1 Classical concepts of the chemical control of breathing in normal subjects. The relationship between alveolar ventilation and arterial CO_2 tensions are shown in the top left panel. The higher curve (B) represents a greater metabolic CO_2 production and the dotted line the effects of adding inspired CO_2. These apply to steady-state conditions only. The top right panel shows data obtained during CO_2 rebreathing at three different levels of arterial hypoxia. Note the critical dependence of the VE/PCO_2 slope on the oxygen tension. The converse is shown in the lower left panel which also illustrates the curvilinearity of the isocapnic hypoxic response. This can be corrected for by plotting arterial oxygen saturation SaO_2 on the absicissa as is now conventionally done when saturation is measured non-invasively.

when inspired oxygen tension falls and also enhances the effects of small changes in CO_2 tension at least when these occur acutely.

Changes in CO_2 tension produce a linear increase in ventilation, largely due to central chemoreceptor stimulation (Fig. 10.1). Unlike the anatomically discrete peripheral chemo-

receptors, the central chemoreceptors are disappointingly diffuse with continued disagreement about their exact site and nature. The classic studies of Pappenheimer [27] showed that perfusing the ventrolateral surface of the medulla with hydrogen ions increases ventilation. Changes in hydrogen ion rather than CO_2 are thought to be the major respiratory stimulus [28] although there is now some evidence that CO_2 has a more complex effect than that expected from changes in pH alone [29] and that other sites can respond to CO_2 [30]. Tonically discharging cells responding to limb flexion [31] or peripheral chemoreceptor stimulation [28] are found in this area intermingled with vasomotor neurones, as might be expected from the tight coupling of changes in ventilation and of circulation.

Traditionally hypoxia has been believed to act solely via its stimulant effects on peripheral chemoreceptors. However, when the chemoceptors are removed in animals, and more recently during extended periods of isocapnic hypoxemia in man, hypoxia has been shown to exhibit a central depressant effect [32]. This is probably mediated by the local production of adenosine, one of the range of neurotransmitters which can modify central ventilatory output [33]. Thus, studies in normal subjects before and after aminophylline, a specific adenosine antagonist, found that the fall in ventilation during sustained hypoxia was blocked [34]. Apart from the rather remote relevance of this to the clinical actions of theophylline, these observations may explain the occasional paradoxical falls in $PaCO_2$ seen after correction of hypoxemia during acute exacerbations of ventilatory failure as an increase in medullary PaO_2 may increase ventilation more than the simultaneous reduction of peripheral chemoreceptor hypoxic stimulation [35].

Interpretation of the effects of altered blood gas tensions on the ventilatory control system is now seen to be quite complex. Two further variables should also be considered. The factors determining the apneic threshold, ie the level of CO_2 below which respiration ceases, are poorly understood but do seem to depend on conscious and non-specific awareness [36]. Hypercapnia is a potent cerebral vasodilator and this will tend to reduce tissue CO_2 tensions for any given arterial CO_2 tension and hence reduce ventilatory output. Although direct data confirming this in COPD are lacking, there are elegant animal studies to suggest that this explains ventilatory depression in other circumstances such as sleep [37].

Finally, ventilation is closely related to metabolic CO_2 production in both normal subjects and COPD patients [38,39], but there is continuing uncertainty about how this comes about and whether the chemoreceptors are directly involved. The peripheral chemoreceptors can follow rapid changes in Pa_{CO_2} throughout the respiratory cycle, at least in normal subjects [40], but their removal in man does not abolish the ventilatory response to exercise [41]. Studies in sheep and men on hemodialysis have shown that ventilation falls as metabolic CO_2 is removed from the venous system even though Pa_{CO_2} is maintained constant [42,43]. This follows from the classic relationship between alveolar ventilation and Pa_{CO_2} shown in Fig. 10.1. Mechanisms to explain this include instability of the feedback mechanisms controlling ventilation, switching off the central chemoreceptors or an enhanced peripheral chemoreceptor activity.

10.2.2 MECHANORECEPTOR INPUTS

Afferent inputs from mechanoreceptors can augment or terminate inspiration in many animal models but their relevance to conscious man and particularly COPD patients, is much less clear. Three major groups have been identified, all travelling in the vagus nerve [44,45]:

1. Stretch-receptors: These slowly adapting receptors lie within the airways smooth muscle of the more distal airways and are stimulated by inflation and changes in gas tensions. They terminate inspiration, stimulate expiratory activity and are responsible for the Hering–Bruer reflex.

2. Rapidly-adapting receptors (RASR): These lie in the epithelium and submucosa of the larger airways and respond to stimulation by dust or ammonia by producing bronchoconstriction, cough and laryngeal narrowing. Increases in inspiratory airflow augment inspiratory neural activity via these receptors. Unlike the stretch-receptors which have a vasodepressor action, stimulation of RASR produces a vasopressor response.

3. Bronchial C and J receptors: These unmyelinated fibers are probably true irritant receptors and the bronchial ones are responsible for cough and the response to capsacin. Like the RASR, their stimulation promotes a rapid shallow breathing pattern. C fiber afferents are thought to be responsible for this pattern when these juxtacapillary receptors are stimulated during pulmonary edema.

Other reflex inputs include those from the rib cage and diaphragmatic muscle spindles which also project to the cortex [31,46] in addition to their well-recognized action at a spinal level. Spindle numbers are relatively low in the diaphragm which may be relevant to respiratory sensation (see below). Less well studied inputs include those from the rib cage joints and from the upper airways. Many of the latter appear to be state-dependent, and can only be elicited during sleep. However, pharyngeal stimulation with cold air can reduce the ventilatory response to CO_2 in normal subjects [47], whilst breathing chilled air during exercise can reduce minute ventilation for a given workload in COPD patients without change in spirometry [48] (Fig. 10.2).

The role of intrapulmonary receptors in respiratory regulation in conscious man is probably very small. Vagally mediated regulation of lung volumes which is present in the neonatal lung up to 8 weeks of age [16] can be detected during anesthesia [49,50]. The recent reports from patients undergoing heart/lung transplantations show that the ventilatory responses to hypoxia and hyper-

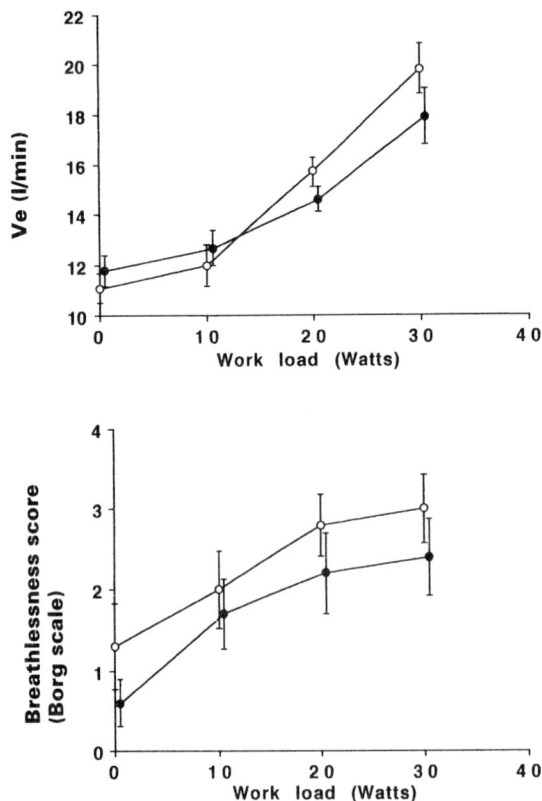

Fig. 10.2 The effect of breathing chilled air on exercise ventilation and breathlessness in stable COPD. Open circles are room air breathing, closed circles are chilled air breathing. These effects are most marked at the highest work levels in these severe patients. (Reproduced with permission from reference [48].)

capnia [51], exercise and the tidal volume response to added loads [52,53] are unaffected by total pulmonary denervation. One study has suggested some reduction in ventilatory response in patients after double lung transplantation [54] but this is probably explained by the postoperative mechanical limitations to breathing rather than the loss of reflex regulation.

10.2.3 CORTICAL INFLUENCES

The ability of the human respiratory system to modify automatic respiratory control so as to subserve the needs of speech or swallowing has long been recognized [55] but largely ignored because of the problems it creates in analyzing respiratory mechanisms. Studies by Newsom-Davis and Stagg were among the first to confirm the spontaneous breath to breath variations in normal human breathing [56]. This may be influenced by breathing route which appears to be selected largely for mechanical reasons [57] but the principal determinant is the level of consciousness. There is a progressive fall in breath to breath variability as sleep deepens from 12% during wakefulness to 4% during stage 4 sleep. When cortical activity increases once more in REM sleep, substantial variation to breathing returns especially in phasic REM, and tidal volume falls as well [58]. When automatic control of breathing is lost, profound nocturnal hypoventilation occurs as in Ondine's curse [59]. Even during wakefulness differences in the degree of concentration can affect breathing pattern. Thus Rigg *et al.* found that mental arithmetic did not influence the slope of the CO_2 response but the breathing pattern adopted during it, a finding similar to those of Mador and Tobin studying unstimulated breathing at rest [58,60]. These data support the view that cortical factors can regulate breathing pattern without the subject being aware of this.

10.2.4 VENTILATORY CONTROL – A UNIFYING HYPOTHESIS

This summary highlights the multiplicity of mechanisms which influence ventilation and which might be disturbed in diseases such as COPD. Conventionally such schemes have been integrated into a complex series of feedback loops which assume that the principal output variable is the maintenance of blood gas homeostasis as in the classic model of Grodins [61]. This is clearly not the case as the apparent redundancy of hypoxic drive at rest demonstrates. Changes in Pa_{CO_2} oscillations may influence chemoreceptors but seem un-

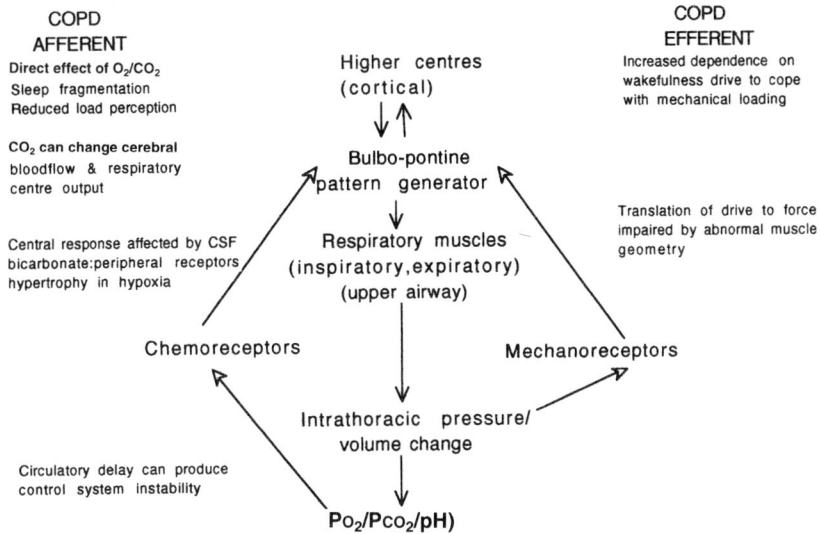

Fig. 10.3 Schematic summary of the components of the respiratory control system and their derangements in COPD patients.

likely to explain the immediate increase in ventilation that accompanies exercise [39] and, in any case, such changes are relatively well-buffered in normal subjects, let alone COPD patients, as short-term hypoventilation studies demonstrate [62].

One of the earliest attempts at explaining the integrated activity of the respiratory system came in 1965 when Priban and Fincham suggested that the system was regulated to minimize energy consumption [63]. There are now ample data to support this view. The most powerful model so far developed is that of Poon and colleagues [64,65].

Using conventional equations of steady-state gas exchange, lung mechanics and chemosensitivity together with a more recent analysis of inspiratory neural drive [66], this model has successfully predicted the pattern of breathing seen at rest, during exercise and with mechanical loading in normal subjects [66]. The key feature is the use of an optimizing function for medullary respiratory output such that the product of mechanical and chemical 'cost of breathing' is minimized. The model still has limitations as it makes no

allowance for active expiratory muscle activity or the visco-elastic mechanical behavior of the respiratory system. None the less, it fits well with developing ideas about the role of respiratory sensation in ventilatory control (see below).

10.3 SPECIFIC PROBLEMS OF VENTILATORY CONTROL IN COPD

Ventilatory control in COPD is only measurably deranged when respiratory impedance increases significantly although changes in breathing pattern and ventilation during maximal exercise have been reported in fit elderly people with a physiologic loss of lung elastic recoil [67]. Several factors affect ventilatory control in the COPD patient (Fig. 10.3):

1. Gas exchange is impaired in COPD with prolonged time-constants for gas mixing (Chapter 8). Differences in lung O_2 and blood CO_2 stores will blunt immediate changes in gas tensions as ventilatory stimulants. Conversely, end tidal gas ten-

sions are imperfect markers of blood gas status in tests of chemical control of breathlessness.

2. COPD is a complex mixture of internal resistive and elastic mechanical loads [68]. The resulting prolongation of mechanical time constants (the product of resistance and compliance, Chapter 7) is particularly sensitive to changes in respiratory frequency. Thus the total respiratory impedance is not constant but changes when ventilation increases, e.g. during exercise.

3. Pulmonary hyperinflation has a dynamic as well as a passive component and is associated with intrinsic PEEP (Chapters 7, 9). This acts as a threshold inspiratory load to breathe. The overinflated chest produces changes in chest wall configuration such that neither intercostals nor diaphragm muscle operate at their optimal length. Although sarcomere numbers may adapt to hyperinflation tending to restore optimum force generating capacity [69], the geometric disadvantages of hyperinflation persist (Chapter 9). Thus respiratory center output must be higher for an equivalent level of ventilation in the face of hyperinflation and airflow resistance.

4. The combination of arterial hypoxemia and increase in ventilatory demand during an acute exacerbation may precipitate respiratory muscle fatigue. The ability of the ventilatory control system to choose the breathing pattern which minimizes the risk of this is vital to the patient's survival.

10.4 ASSESSMENT OF VENTILATORY CONTROL IN COPD

A range of techniques have been used to study ventilatory control but each has significant disadvantages in the COPD patient (Table 10.1). The most widely used methods of inducing relatively rapid changes in blood gas tensions, often by rebreathing

techniques, may not yield physiologically relevant data. Use of ventilation as a measure of respiratory center output is limited by abnormal lung mechanics. Many of these problems can be overcome by using the mouth occlusion pressure ($P_{0.1}$) [70] but even this may not be representative of intrathoracic pressure swings in severe COPD [71]. Occlusion pressure is also influenced by posture [72] and by lung volume which may change during exercise or during rebreathing tests. The strengths and limitations of this approach have recently been reviewed [73]. In some studies of COPD patients, mouth occlusion pressure has been a particularly poor index of respiratory muscle activation [74], although these appear to be a minority. Despite these drawbacks, a large amount of data has accumulated about the results of such tests in COPD patients.

10.5 CHEMICAL CONTROL OF BREATHING IN COPD

Most studies of chemical control of breathing in COPD have tried to answer one or more of the following question:

1. Is the response to chemical stimuli abnormal?
2. Is this explicable solely by the increased mechanical load imposed on the respiratory system by the disease or does it reflect an inherent reduction in respiratory chemosensitivity?
3. Do patients who are 'blue and bloated' have different responses to hypoxia and/or CO_2 than those who are 'pink and puffing?'

While the answer to the first question is undoubtedly yes, the response to the other two is still confused reflecting the different methodologies employed in the patient groups studied.

It is over four decades since Donald and Christie noted that patients with severe obstructive lung disease had a reduced ventilatory response to CO_2 [75]. Many subsequent

Table 10.1 Methods of assessing ventilatory control – relevance to COPD

Test	Method	Result in COPD	Comment
Steady state CO_2 response	Ventilation measured at 2 stable CO_2 tensions; $\dot{V}/P_{CO_2}$ slope reflects CO_2 'sensitivity' or 'gain' of the system	Variable reduction	Time consuming 'classical' technique. Depends on adequate gas equilibration in blood and CSF – not easy in severe COPD. Chronic changes in blood buffering may affect this
Hyperoxic CO_2 rebreathing	Rebreathing from O_2-enriched closed system; rapid equilibration of blood/CSF CO_2 content. $\dot{V}/P_{CO_2}$ slope has 14-fold normal variability	Variable reduction	Quick, reproducible test. Ventilation may be limited mechanically, not by reduced drive. Ratio of free-breathing and loaded slope a measure of load compensation
Steady state of CO_2 at 2 levels of oxygen tension	Ratio of hypoxic: hyperoxic $\dot{V}/P_{CO_2}$ slopes gives an index of hypoxic drive	Normal or reduced	Demanding for patient and operator. Does allow for 'hypoxic depression' and CO_2 interaction. Seldom done
Progressive isocapnic hypoxia	Relatively rapid (4–10') test where ventilation is related to P_{O_2} (or Sa_{O_2}) with CO_2 held constant	Normal or reduced	Usually expressed as $\dot{V}/Sa_{O_2}$ as this is a linear plot. Useful for acute drug studies but hard to interpret when Pa_{O_2} already low; no allowance for hypoxic depression
Transient hypoxia/hyperoxic test	Rapid change in Pa_{O_2} will stimulate/supress peripheral chemoreceptors hence ventilation	No good data	Not applicable to COPD
Mouth occlusion pressure ($P_{0.1}$)	Pressure developed 100 msec after inspiration against a closed airway – should overcome problems of changing airflow/lung volume – relates to respiratory centre output	Variable increase at rest – $P_{0.1}/P_{CO_2}$ slope may be reduced, hypoxic response more so	Influenced by posture, lung volume and probably MIP. Mouth pressure may not reflect pleural $P_{0.1}$. Muscle shortening DOES occur after occlusion. Abdominal muscle activity increases $P_{0.1}$ for any given 'drive'. Still the best test in COPD
Integrated electromyogram (usually diaphragm)	Recorded from surface/esophageal electrodes. Expressed in arbitrary units; reflects activation of muscle recorded	Increased for any given Ppl in COPD. Increased by acute CO_2	Hard to interpret and technically very difficult. Surface electrodes influenced by diaphragm position/lung volume. Esophageal electrodes may move or other muscles may be activated. Not a routine test

studies have confirmed this, mainly using CO_2 rebreathing and with ventilation and/ or $P_{0.1}$ as their output variables [76–86]. Representative data from some of these are given in Table 10.2. There is a surprisingly good agreement in the severity of ventilatory depression between the groups, at least as compared with normals studied in the same fashion.

Early studies noted that normal subjects breathing against external inspiratory resist- ances showed similar falls in $\dot{V}E/P_{CO_2}$ to those seen in COPD [87]. This is associated with a compensatory increase in p0.1, although this is insufficient to maintain ventilation at the initial level (Fig. 10.4). These data show very similar $\dot{V}E/P_{CO_2}$ and $P_{0.1}/P_{CO_2}$ slopes to those seen at rest in patients with chronic mechani- cal loading due to COPD studied in the same laboratory (Fig. 10.4). One way of allowing for the effects of mechanical loading is to plot change in ventilation against change in $P_{0.1}$

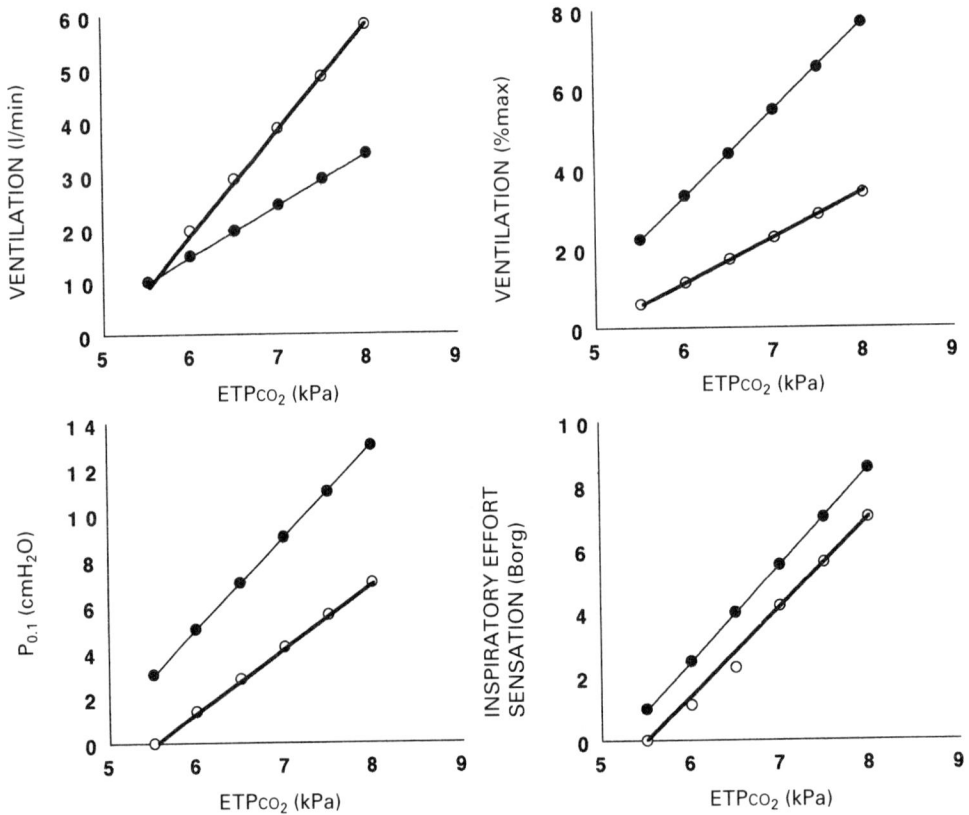

Fig. 10.4 Hypercapnic ventilatory responses in COPD. Data are derived from the mean values of each data point from a group of 12 normocapnic COPD patients studied when stable (mean FEV_1 0.92 l) (closed circles) and are compared to the matched group of control subjects (open circles). COPD patients have a reduced ventilatory response to increase in end tidal P_{CO_2} (ETP_{CO_2}) but a higher occlusion pres- sure response slope (left-hand panels). However, when ventilation is expressed as a percentage of the maximum voluntary ventilation, they are seen to use more of their ventilatory capacity in response to CO_2 (top right panel). The relationships between inspiratory effort sensation and CO_2 are similar in slope in both normal subjects and COPD patients but have a higher initial value in the COPD subjects and move in parallel with changes in $P_{0.1}$ (lower right panel).

Table 10.2 Ventilatory/neuromechanical response to altered gas tensions in COPD

Study	n	Method	Subjects	Results	Comments
[76]	42 COPD	Ventilation ($\dot{V}E$) inspiratory work (W) response to steady state CO_2	$PaCO_2$ 36–70 mmHg	$\dot{V}/PCO_2\downarrow$, $W/PCO_2\downarrow$ when $PaCO_2\uparrow$	An early study suggesting CO_2 retention related to reduced W response to CO_2
[77]	19 COPD	CO_2 rebreathing with measures as above	FEV 0.76 l $PaCO_2$ 36–65 mmHg	$\dot{V}/PCO_2$ generally $\downarrow$ W/PCO_2 0.3–0.45 kg/min/mmHg (normal = 0.4)	W/PCO_2 correlated with dyspnea; inversely related to $PaCO_2$, Hb, edema
[78]	7 control 8 COPD	Steady state CO_2 at 3 levels of O_2	COPD: RV/TLC↑, FEV 0.53	$\dot{V}/PCO_2\downarrow$ in COPD; hypoxic response normal in 2, reduced in 3	Changes in blood chemistry could not explain ↓ slopes – no mechanics data
[79]	7 control 8 COPD	Inspiratory work in steady state CO_2	COPD: RV↑, FEV 0.53	$\dot{W}/PCO_2\downarrow$	Suggests increased work alone cannot explain ↓ CO_2 slope – no CSF data here.
[80]	12 COPD	Steady state CO_2 at 2 levels of O_2 – CSF HCO_3 in 10	FEV 0.68 l $PaCO_2$ 40–66 mmHg	↓ $\dot{V}/PCO_2$ in 9 cases, $\dot{V}/PO_2$ normal in 6, absent in 2	CSF bicarbonate buffering could not explain reduce CO_2 slopes
[81]	26 control 14 COPD	$\dot{V}/PCO_2$, $P_{0.1}/PCO_2$ during rebreathing ± inspiratory resistance	COPD: FEV 38%p, FRC 134%p	$\dot{V}/PCO_2$ $P_{0.1}/PCO_2$ normal 2.4 0.6 eucapnic 0.7 0.6 hypercapnic 0.5 0.2	Loading ↑ $P_{0.1}$ response by 50% in control but not in COPD – FRC unchanged
[82]	15 control 17 COPD (9 high CO_2)	$\dot{V}/PCO_2$, $P_{0.1}/PCO_2$ during rebreathing	COPD normal CO_2 – FEV 82%p high CO_2 – FEV 26%p	$\dot{V}/PCO_2$ $P_{0.1}/PCO_2$ normal 2.95 0.52 eucapnic 1.37 0.41 hypercapnic 0.31 0.32	Data on 6 normal showed ↑ $P_{0.1}$ response with loading – not seen in COPD
[83]	17 control 20 COPD	CO_2 + hypoxic rebreathers	FEV 31%p FRC 175%p FEV 25%p FRC 190%p	eucapnic hypercapnic $\dot{V}/PCO_2$ 0.98 0.54 $P_{0.1}/PCO_2$ 0.55 0.37 $\dot{V}/SaO_2$ -0.3 -0.1 $P_{0.1}/SaO_2$ -0.21 -0.07	$P_{0.1}$ relatively preserved though $\dot{V}/PCO_2$ low – see problems of interpretation in text

Table 10.2 *Cont'd.*

[84]	14 COPD	CO_2 + hypoxic rebreathers	FEV 22%p	$\dot{V}/P_{CO_2}$ 0.49; $P_{0.1}/P_{CO_2}$ 0.4 V/S_{aO_2} −0.17; $P_{0.1}/S_{aO_2}$ −0.14	No correction of blunted hypoxic response after 6/12 O_2 therapy
[85]	20 COPD	CO_2 rebreath + lung mechanics (n=10)	FEV 27%p TLC 130%p	$\dot{V}/P_{CO_2}$ 0.92 $P_{0.1}/P_{CO_2}$ 0.3	Work done/min as % of CAPACITY doubled in COPD, though work/breath normal
[86]	15 COPD	$\dot{V}/P_{CO_2}$, $P_{0.1}/P_{CO_2}$ + cycle/walk exercise	FEV 37%p Pa_{CO_2} 37 mmHg	$\dot{V}/P_{CO_2}$ 0.94 $P_{0.1}/P_{CO_2}$ 0.59	No relationship between ventilatory control and exercise see also [175] $V_E/P_{0.1}$ highly correlated with VO_2 max and corridor walking distance
[111]	11 COPD	V/P_{CO_2}, $P_{0.1}/P_{CO_2}$ pre/post naloxone resistor	FEV 43%p Pa_{CO_2} 37 mmHg	$\dot{V}/P_{CO_2}$ 1.6 $P_{0.1}/P_{CO_2}$ 0.9	No effect from opioid block
[91]	8 COPD	CO_2 rebreathing with P_{di}/EMG_{di} and loading	FEV 38% Pa_{CO_2} 42 mmHg	Load ↓$\dot{V}/P_{CO_2}$ but variable effect on P_{di}/EMG slope	CO_2 'retainers' had higher FRC which limited ability to increase P_{di} when loaded
[90]	15 COPD (8 hypercapnic)	CO_2 rebreathing with $P_{0.1}$/EMG_{di} and EMG intercostal	FEV 29%	High CO_2 patients had rapid shallow breathing and lower $P_{0.1}$/EMG slopes	CO_2 'retainers' had lower MIP, suggesting weakness limited the ability to translate 'drive' into 'pressure'

Data are expressed in mmHg for gas tensions, $\dot{V}/P_{CO_2}$/P_{CO_2} as change in ventilation (litres) per mmHg rise in CO_2, $\dot{V}/S_{aO_2}$ as change in ventilation (litres) per % fall in oxygen saturation; $P_{0.1}$ is mouth occlusion pressure in cm H_2O with denominator as before. %p = % predicted. Note consistent reduction in $\dot{V}/P_{CO_2}$, that hypercapnia is associated with low $\dot{V}/S_{aO_2}$ and $P_{0.1}/S_{aO_2}$ but patients tend to have worse lung function. A large amount of the available ventilatory capacity is used during rebreathing and patients with the lowest ventilation/unit drive ($P_{0.1}$) have the worst exercise performance.

which can be derived as the ratio of $\dot{V}E/P_{CO_2}$ and $P_{0.1}/P_{CO_2}$ slopes. The values are remarkably consistent between studies and appear to be similar whether or not the patients are hypercapnic. If the data are expressed as a percentage of the maximum voluntary ventilation (derived from the FEV_1) with either P_{CO_2} or $P_{0.1}$ as the denominator, then most eucapnic COPD patients fall within the normal range of ventilation responses suggesting that the mechanical load explains the apparent reduction in chemosensitivity.

Similar results have been found when the effects of change in lung volume have been studied. Thus Gribbin *et al.* [85] found that Ppl min at a P_{CO_2} of 60 mmHg was only slightly less than normal in 10 COPD patients compared with 10 healthy controls but this represented 47% of the patient's static Ppl compared with 26% of the maximum pressure generation available to the controls.

Thus hyperinflation disguises some of the increased ventilatory drives seen in COPD and this emphasizes the relatively large amount of inspiratory muscle capacity these patients use. These observations are in keeping with earlier studies using inspiratory work on either the lungs or chest wall (W) as a measure of respiratory output independent of mechanical load [76,77]. Initial studies found that the relationship between W and $PaCO_2$ was displaced to the right and depressed slightly in hypercapnic COPD [76,79] whilst Lane and Howell reported several different patterns of response in similar patients with some failing to increase W as CO_2 rose [88]. All studies are agreed that there is an increase in resting work of breathing but the cause of the variable response to further stimulation is disputed.

The most popular explanation is that those individuals with a relatively flat response are those with a significant reduction in hypoxic drive to breathe. Thus, Flenley and Millar found that $W/PaCO_2$ lay in the normal range for eucapnic patients but was reduced in those with the greatest hypercapnia [79]. Lourenço and Miranda who used the grossly integrated electromyogram (EMG) output, also found reduced diaphragm activation in COPD patients who retained CO_2, although these studies had methodologic problems [89]. In an elegant study of both lung volume and hypercapnia in COPD, Altose *et al.* found that hypercapnic patients had lower $P_{0.1}/P_{CO_2}$ responses than did eucapnic patients although the latter group had surprisingly low $\dot{V}E/P_{CO_2}$ responses compared to other values in the literature [81].

These findings can be explained by the data of Gorini *et al.* [90] who studied $P_{0.1}$ and integrated diaphragm EMG in normocapnic and hypercapnic COPD patients and in normal subjects. The hypercapnic patients had lower $P_{0.1}$ and higher EMGdi values, suggesting that their central drive was high and the ability to develop pressure limited, a finding supported by their low MIP values compared with normocapnic patients. Similar findings have been reported in acute loading studies of normocapnic patients, in whom CO_2 retention was associated with a higher FRC and a lower Pdi for any level of diaphragm activation [91]. In a larger study of stable patients with COPD, Bradley, Fleetham and Anthonisen found no difference between the $P_{0.1}/P_{CO_2}$ slopes of normocapnic and hypercapnic patients but reported reduced $\dot{V}E/S_{aO_2}$ slopes in the latter [83]. This finding was extended in two further studies from the same group, the first showing that low flow oxygen throughout 12 or 24 hours per day did not change these blunted hypoxic responses [84] and the second that there was no relation between the O_2 and CO_2 responses and the underlying lung pathology [92]. This latter finding is somewhat at variance with the earlier data that relates to a much smaller number of patients.

However, there are problems in interpreting these data. The results of short-term tests of isocapnic hypoxia may not reflect those with longer periods of hypoxia (see above) and are vitally dependent on the initial $PaCO_2$ chosen. Unfortunately, this is not quoted in all of these reports. The lack of any reliable means of examining the interaction between changes in oxygen and CO_2 in these patients makes it hard to interpret the large number of patients in the hypercapnic group who appear to have no hypoxic response, although this is not a finding unique to such patients. Moreover, compensatory changes in CSF acid–base status in the face of chronic hypercapnia will mask acute changes which stimulate peripheral chemoreceptors and make interpretation of these data particularly difficult [93].

To overcome these difficulties, studies of family members unaffected by lung disease have been conducted [94,95]. These have shown reductions in both hypercapnic and hypoxic drives to breathing in individuals whose relatives subsequently develop hypercapnia but less frequently in those who do not. However, there must be some doubt about the method of subject selection and larger numbers of both cases and control subjects are needed to validate this approach.

In summary, the ventilatory response to changes in gas tensions is diminished in COPD patients but this appears to reflect mechanical loading rather than intrinsic chemoreceptor insensitivity in most cases. Some individuals with a high work of breathing do not increase this further when breathing CO_2 and this may be due to their inherently low chemoresponsiveness, shared by some family members. Such patients tend to have high arterial CO_2 tensions and correspondingly low oxygen tensions but not all hypercapnia is due to this mechanism. The failure to increase ventilation may reflect a choice between accepting an increased CO_2 tension which may have a modest stimulant effect in an already buffered CSF or using so much of the inspiratory force reserve that respiratory muscle fatigue occurs. Which patients follow which strategy is still unclear.

10.5.1 BREATHING PATTERN IN COPD

Studies on the impact of respiratory muscle loading on healthy individuals and revisions of the neurophysiology of normal breathing [5,9] have led to renewed interest in the pattern of breathing in COPD. The range of responses to any increase in respiratory impedance is limited and has been reviewed in detail [96,97]:

1. An increase in the stiffness of the chest wall by immediate respiratory muscle contraction. This will reduce the effect of subsequent changes in impedance and has been described as an operational length compensating mechanism [68].
2. Changes in inspiratory timing. These may involve either inspiratory duration (T_I), total cycle duration (T_{TOT}) or both. Lengthening T_I without changing T_{TOT} reduces mean inspiratory flow and may lead to hypoventilation and CO_2 retention. Optimum breathing patterns may be determined so as to minimize respiratory frequency, respiratory muscle oxygen consumption or 'the discomfort of breathing'.
3. An increase in inspiratory drive. This is the most widely adopted response to increases in impedance but is usually insufficient to completely off-set the effects of the added load unless it is a small one. It is conventionally represented by $P_{0.1}$ although this has its own limitations (Table 10.1).

Using the analysis of ventilation based on flow and timing and the simplified equation describing steady-state Pa_{CO_2} as used in the Poon model (Section 10.3), the breathing pattern in COPD can be interpreted in terms relevant to the response to ventilatory loading.

In normal subjects the response to increased respiratory resistance is to prolong T_I and reduce V_T. This occurs in COPD patients given a similar load to breathe but is not representative of their usual breathing patterns

Table 10.3 Breathing pattern, P0.1 and blood gases at rest in COPD

Study	n	Subject	V (l/min)	VT (l)	F (breath/min)	VT/TI (l/s/min)	TI/TTOT	P0.1 (cm H2O)	PaO2 (mmHg)	PaCO2 (mmHg)
[98]	8 COPD	FEV 38%p	15.4	0.93	16.9	0.66	0.39	2.48	77	36
	7 COPD	FEV 22%p	14.2	0.64	24.1	0.68	0.35	3.22	55	58
[99]	17	10 correctors[a]	9.4	0.55	17	0.52	0.38	3.4	52	51
	(14 COPD)	7 non-correctors	9.7	0.60	17	0.51	0.36	2.6	48	54
[100]	20 COPD	FEV 25%p air	11.4	0.37	31.6	0.56	0.33	8.3	38	61
	(acute	O2	9.8	0.37	28	0.50	0.33	4.9	120	68
	exacerbation)									
[101]	91 COPD	FEV 67%	9.2	0.50	18.6	–	–	–	–	39
	(wide range)									
[102]	15 COPD	FEV 27%p	10.9	0.64	17	0.50	0.37	–	74	40
	15 COPD	FEV 22%p	10.8	0.51	21.3	0.50	0.33	–	40	52
[83]	17 COPD	FEV 25%p	11.7	0.75	17.5	0.59	0.34	2.4	67	40
	20 COPD		11.4	0.58	21.6	0.56	0.34	3.0	57	45
[103][b]	8 normal	–	8.5	0.55	16.1	0.42	0.34	–	–	–
	12 COPD	FEV 15.49%p	11.2	0.55	21.7	0.53	0.36	–	75	<45
[90]	7 COPD	30%p	12.1	0.7	17.8	0.52	0.39	4.4	69	40
	8 COPD	28%p	10.1	0.48	21.1	0.49	0.34	3.6	59	55

Breathing pattern at rest in COPD. All studies except [b] use mouth piece and nose clip; [b] data derived from quantitative inductance plethysmography. [a] Study examined ability of medroxyprogesterone acetate, a ventilatory stimulant, to lower $PaCO_2$. All studies made while clinically stable unless otherwise stated. In general hypercapnic COPD patients have similar minute ventilation $V_E/P_{0.1}$ but slightly lower tidal volume (V_T) and higher breathing frequencies (f) than do normocapnic patients. Thus for a given dead space (V_D) the V_D/V_T ratio will be higher in the CO_2 group.

which are summarized in Table 10.3 [83, 98–103]. In general, minute ventilation is normal or even slightly higher than normal at rest whether instrumented with face mask or nose clip and mouth piece or whether free breathing where the minute ventilation and breathing pattern are recorded using inductive plethysmography [103]. The overall pattern is rapid and shallow but there are no differences in either minute ventilation or CO_2 production between those who develop CO_2 retention and those who do not. Central drive as reflected by $P_{0.1}$ is high but can be reduced by administration of relatively high flow oxygen (5 l/min) [100]. Patients retaining CO_2 have lower tidal volumes and shorter respiratory times together with a somewhat higher $P_{0.1}$ [83,98]. These changes in breathing pattern are load-dependent as is seen when acute inspiratory resistive loading is performed in stable COPD patients [104]. In this study there was a strong inverse correlation between changes in V_T and changes in T_I and the tendency to retain CO_2 ($r = -0.91$ and -0.87 respectively). Although it is an oversimplification of the complexities of gas exchange, falls in tidal volumes can be considered to encroach upon the fixed dead space of these patients and increase the V_D/V_T ratio and hence PCO_2 [98,101]. Chronic stimulation of ventilation with medroxyprogesterone acetate reduced PCO_2 in 11 of 15 hypercapnic patients by increasing V_T/T_I [99]. Conversely upper airway anesthesia has been reported increase PCO_2 in such patients although the changes in V_T and T_I were very modest [105]. None the less, this suggests that some tonic input from receptors in the pharynx or central airways occurs in COPD. Whether this is relevant to the normal regulation of ventilation is more questionable.

Studies in unanesthetized goats have shown that acute loading (50–80 $cmH_2O/$ l/sec) can double the levels of beta-endorphins in the CSF and that the corresponding fall in V_T parallels the rise in endorphins and can be reduced by naloxone infusion [106]. Since opiates can reduce the hypoxic and hypercapnic responses of normal individuals [107] and COPD is associated with both clinically increased respiratory impedance and reduced responses, it was reasonable to test whether these abnormalities resulted from increased elaboration of endogenous opioides. The results remain rather disappointing. The ventilatory responses to CO_2 and hypoxia in normal subjects and COPD are not influenced by naloxone infusion [108] nor are the hypoxic responses related to plasma levels of beta-endorphins [109]. However, the response to hypercapnic hypoxia is reduced by naloxone whilst the load compensating response as assessed by the increase in $P_{0.1}/P_{CO_2}$ slope with acute loading, was increased in 14 COPD patients given naloxone [110]. Interpretation of these data is affected by differences in the initial $P_{0.1}/P_{CO_2}$ between the responder and non-responder groups and others have not been able to replicate them [111]. None the less these studies merit extension to patients who have developed hypercapnia, preferably with accompanying data about the effects on respiratory sensation and resting breathing pattern.

10.6 HYPERCAPNIA, RESPIRATORY MUSCLE FATIGUE AND RESPIRATORY LOADING

The reduction in ventilatory response described above reflects a failure of the respiratory muscles to overcome the extra load upon them, a process subject to the usual arguments about cannot breathe and will not breathe. The function of the respiratory muscles in general and the role of respiratory muscle fatigue in stable COPD is reviewed elsewhere (Chapter 9). However, several types of fatiguing process have been thought relevant to ventilatory control. Although central muscle fatigue may occur in man, it has not been described in stable COPD [112].

High frequency fatigue whether defined electrically by a fall in the high/low EMG ratio [113] or prolongation of the maximum relaxation rate [114,115] is a relatively transient marker of excessive muscle loading. Low frequency fatigue which is characterized by sustained loss of force generation might explain the inability of the respiratory muscles to maintain the blood gas tensions. Several pieces of evidence would suggest this.

CO_2 retention in COPD is better related to the degree of hyperinflation than to the FEV_1 [101] (Fig. 10.5). When bronchoconstriction is induced in COPD patients by methacholine challenge, FRC rises and maximum inspiratory pressures fall [116]. Although the $\dot{V}_E/P_{CO_2}$ slope is reduced, $P_{0.1}/P_{CO_2}$ is unchanged, as in spontaneously hypercapnic patients (Table 10.2). Chronic and acute-on-chronic reductions in MIP reduce the denominator of the tension–time index (Chapter 9) and bring the patient nearer to the fatigue threshold. The force reserve in COPD is reduced at rest with a TTdi of the patient some tenfold greater than that in normal subjects [117]. Moreover, the conventional threshold for diaphragm fatigue of a TTdi of 0.15 was established in normal volunteers at low lung volumes and relatively modest flow rates. It is likely to be much lower in patients with a higher FRC who have to increase their flow rates during exercise thereby further reducing the inspiratory force reserve. Rapid shallow breathing occurs as fatigue develops in normal subjects [118] and is seen in hypercapnic patients. Finally, studies of acute high frequency fatigue in volunteers have reported reduced ventilatory responses to CO_2 [119].

However, it has proven very difficult to demonstrate respiratory muscle fatigue in patients and it was not a consistent finding even when weaning from assisted ventilation [120]. Contrary to previous belief, the diaphragm is fully activated in COPD and is at least as capable of generating pressure as in normal subjects once allowance is made for the altered chest wall geometry [112] (Fig. 10.6). The rapid

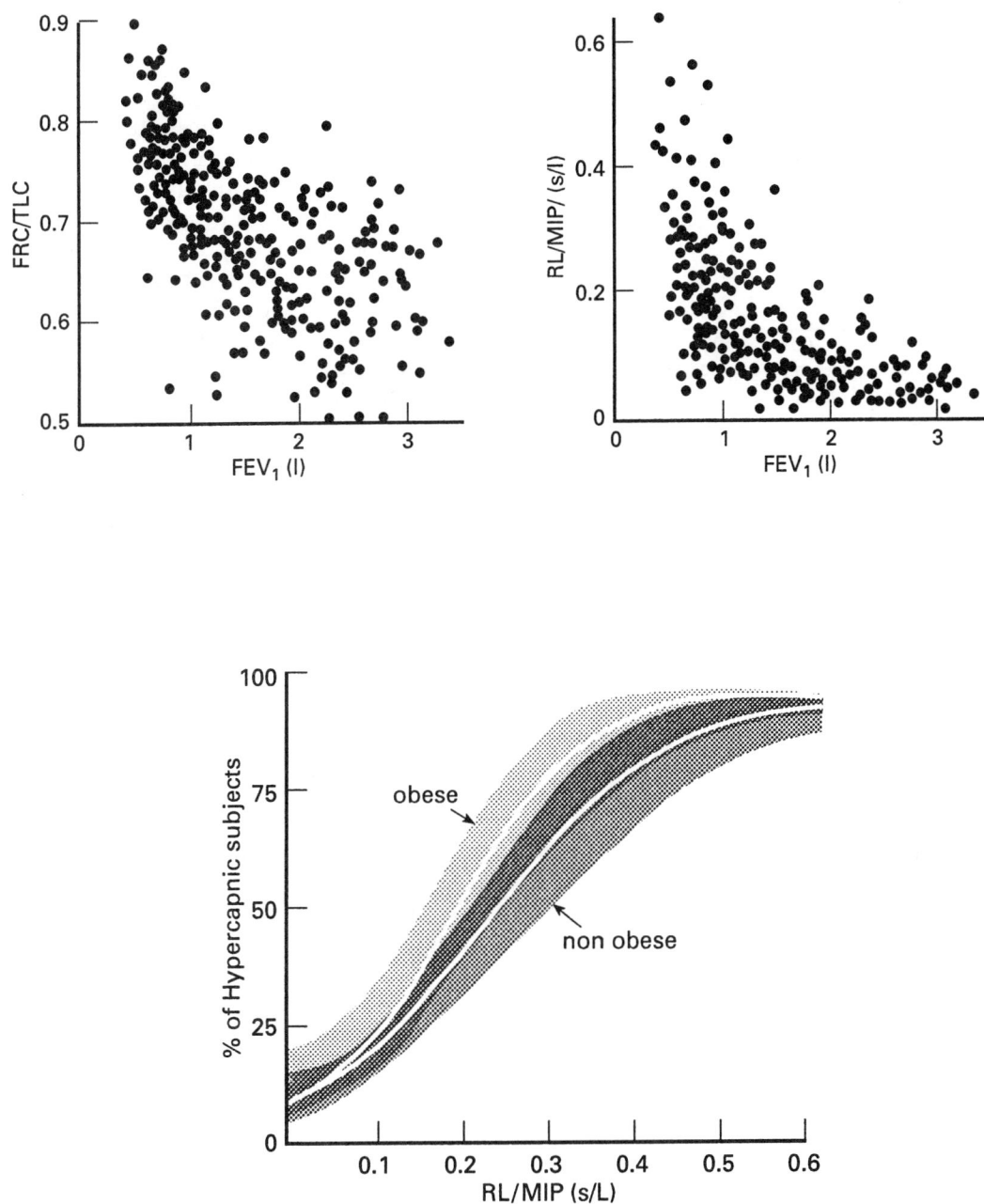

Fig. 10.5 The relationship between lung mechanics and carbon dioxide tension. The upper panel *(left)* shows that FEV_1 decreases in a curvilinear fashion with increasing lung volumes and gas trapping (FRC/TLC). *(right)* When CO_2 tensions are plotted against the pulmonary resistance divided by the maximum inspiratory pressure (RL/MIP), a surrogate measure of the burden on capacity of the respiratory muscles to meet ventilatory demands, then there is a closer relationship between CO_2 tension and this index suggesting that mechanical factors are the major determinants of hypercapnia in this study population, even when allowance is made for the effects of obesity (lower panel). (Modified from reference [124] with permission.)

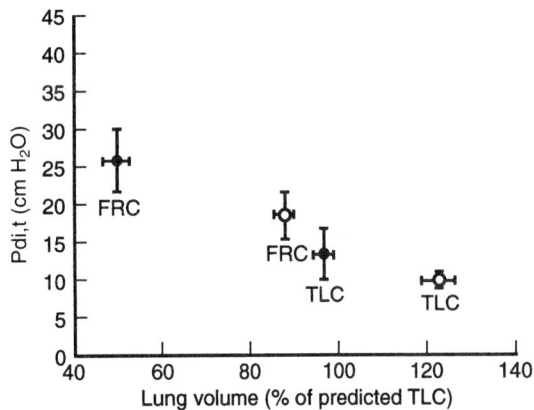

Fig. 10.6 Diaphragm twitch pressure at different lung volumes in normal subjects (closed circles) and COPD patients (open circles). These data show that COPD patients can activate their diaphragms just as well as normal subjects, if not better, once allowance is made for their altered geometry. (Modified from reference 112 with permission.)

shallow breathing pattern is a feature of any severe respiratory load [121] and does not imply even short-term respiratory muscle impairment, whilst indices such as maximum relaxation rate appear to be more load sensitive than fatigue sensitive [114] and cannot be used to infer the presence of respiratory muscle fatigue. Finally, when the inspiratory muscles are rested by negative pressure ventilation, there is no significant improvement in any fatigue-related index or in day-time performance [122]. It is possible that this may reflect a failure to use this treatment at night but this seems unlikely.

Recent attention has re-focused on the idea of the mechanical load due to hyperinflation (see above) and the importance of the threshold load provided by intrinsic PEEP. The severity of CO_2 retention can be related to the amount of PEEPi [123] or to the ratio of pulmonary resistance/maximum inspiratory pressure, an index of the imbalance between load and inspiratory capacity [124] (Fig. 10.5). Another study has shown that maximum voluntary ventilation, specific airways conductance and especially peak inspiratory flow

(PIF), are independent determinants of Pa_{CO_2} in stable COPD [125]. Thus, the load itself produces adjustments in the breathing pattern which are not associated with respiratory muscle fatigue but can produce hypercapnia. Factors like hyperinflation which worsen mechanical advantage appear to be especially important. All this seems to justify the original observation of one of the pioneers of respiratory physiology, Richard Riley, that 'hypercapnia is an adaptive mechanism by which the body tolerates an increase in work of breathing which would otherwise be intolerable' [126]. The mechanism by which this compromise is produced is the subject of the remainder of this chapter.

10.7 RESPIRATORY SENSATION AND DYSPNEA

Although breathlessness is the principal complaint of patients with COPD, its scientific study is relatively recent. This reflects the difficulties of applying a numerical dimension to a sensory term, a problem that has been reviewed in detail [127–129]. Before considering the limited amount of data directly relevant to patients with COPD, it is useful to establish what we mean by breathlessness, how we can measure it and what the underlying mechanisms producing this sensation might be.

10.7.1 WHAT IS BREATHLESSNESS?

The semantics of breathlessness have proven at least as difficult as those terms used to define COPD (Chapter 1). Medically, breathlessness is described as dyspnea – the sensation of difficulty in breathing. However, recent studies in normal subjects using cluster analysis statistical methods have shown that different stimuli are associated with different sensations [130]. These studies have been extended to a diverse group of patients including those with COPD, who were asked to relate their sensations to 45 different questions. COPD patients are more likely to describe their dyspnea as breathing discomfort and along with asthmatics, associate it with increased breathing effort and an inability to breathe deeply enough [131].

10.7.2 MEASUREMENT OF BREATHLESSNESS

Uncertainties about the quantitative nature of sensory responses led early investigators to assess sensation in terms of a sensory threshold. This was measured by the 'just noticeable difference' (JND) method [129] i.e. the intensity of stimulus which was detected on 50% of presentations. Here a sensation was either present or not but this method could not define the sensory intensity when the stimulus increased beyond this threshold value. These studies are examples of psychophysical techniques which quantitatively relate the characteristics or dimensions of a physical stimulus to the magnitude or attributes of the sensory response associated with it. Psychophysics has elucidated the sensory correlates of visual, auditory and kinesthetic responses [133] and has been central to the understanding of the mechanisms of breathlessness.

Scaling techniques, both nominal and ordinal, have been developed to assess suprathreshold sensory stimuli. Open magnitude scales relate sensory magnitude to stimulus intensity by assigning an arbitrary value to the magnitude which changes proportionately with the stimulus [129]. They are useful in defining variables that influence sensation but are time consuming to use, not suitable for repeated measures and involve log–log plotting of data to define the subjects perceptual sensitivity. More widely used is the visual analog scale (VAS), a form of cross-modality testing. The subject marks the sensory intensity along a 10 cm line with descriptors at each end, usually 'not breathless at all' to 'extreme or worst imaginable breathlessness'. It is relatively simple to use, reproducible, and does not need to be anchored at its upper extremes to an induced level of severe breathlessness. However, it does not have ratio properties.

Table 10.4 Borg Category Scale

0	Nothing at all
0.5	Very, very slight (just noticeable)
1	Very slight
2	Slight
3	Moderate
4	Somewhat severe
5	Severe
6	
7	Very severe
8	
9	Very, very severe (almost maximal)
10	Maximal

Modified from Borg [134], with permission.

The most widely used and versatile dyspnea scale is the category scale devised by Borg [134] (Table 10.4). The scale employs descriptors which in its modified form are spaced so that a doubling of numerical rating is associated with a doubling of sensory intensity. It is useful for use with a number of questions, e.g. How breathless are you? How much effort are you making to breathe?, and possibly some related variables, e.g. How tight does your chest feel? It allows easy comparison of absolute levels of sensation at a given intensity among a group of subjects and is amenable to parametric statistical analysis [135].

Comparisons between these scales show that VAS and Borg [136,137] are valid measures in normal subjects but the Borg scale tends to have a better reproducibility between days. Studies in COPD have confirmed the reproducibility of VAS [136] but there is concern about the between day reproducibility of Borg scaling [138].

These scales can be clinically useful in assessing the intensity of inspiratory effort or breathlessness at a particular time, e.g. before or after a corridor walk [139]. They are exquisitely dependent on the question asked and the degree to which the patient understands what is wanted of him and so require some explanation before use. They are sensitive to changes induced by physiologically relevant interventions, e.g. muscle training [140] or brochodilators [139] but do not give an overall impression of patient disability due to dyspnea.

This has been assessed using a different questionnaire-based approach. The earliest attempt was the British MRC Dyspnea Scale [141] where symptom severity was scored on a five point scale. This has been extremely useful epidemiologically but is not sensitive to small changes within an individual. Mahler and colleagues have developed two indices of breathlessness, the Baseline Dyspnea Index and the Transitional Dyspnea Index [142]. These questionnaires assessed three different attributes – functional impairment, magnitude of task and magnitude of effort. The BDI correlates well (r=0.6) with distance covered in a 12-minute walk test and with scores from the oxygen cost diagram, a type of VAS where the descriptors relate to every day activity. The TDI was designed to assess changes after some intervention over time and is related to the initial BDI assessment. These instruments take longer to administer than VAS or Borg scales and give a broader view of the impact of dyspnea on the patients life over time. They appear less suited to single dose pharmacologic testing but do not give such a comprehensive picture of disability as more formal quality of life scores (Chapter 21). Their use has shown that breathlessness is a separate defining characteristic of COPD patients in addition to other aspects of lung function such as spirometry and maximum inspiratory pressure generation [143]. Whether they will become a more useful clinical tool remains uncertain.

10.8 MECHANISMS OF DYSPNEA

Like the blind man describing an elephant, respiratory physiologists have groped for the mechanisms underlying dyspnea for the past 75 years. Certain findings are now widely accepted. There is no single stimulus which uniquely produces the sensation, neither are there specific dyspnea receptors in the muscles or the lung parenchyma. Conflicting results from reputable investigators are likely to reflect subtle differences in the protocol adopted or the questions asked rather than entirely different ·neurophysiologic mechanisms (for an example of this, see Killian *et al.*, *Breathlessness*, 1992, pp. 121–3, [4]). The early systematic reports of dyspnea related maximum exercise capacity to maximum voluntary ventilation to establish the measure of breathing reserve [144]. If the values exceeded 0.7–0.8, exercise would stop due to breathlessness. Inspection of the original data shows considerable variability in this index between individuals. Another approach was to relate the oxygen cost of breathing to exercise performance implying that limitations of muscle oxygen consumption might determine symptom onset [145]. Although long unfashionable, the relevance of these observations has increased recently. Several approaches have been used to study the mechanisms of dyspnea and these are largely complementary.

10.8.1 STUDIES OF MECHANICAL LOADING

The interaction between mechanical and chemical factors was explored during breath holding [146]. Fowler showed that breath-holding time could be increased by allowing the subjects to rebreathe their expired air at the end of the breath-hold, suggesting that mechanical rather than chemical factors were important in determining the break point. These data were extended during studies of partial curarization when subjects were able to breath-hold at a $PaCO_2$ of 60 mmHg for up to 4 minutes without reporting an increased sensation [147]. Subsequently Banzett and colleagues have challenged these views [148] which have been revised by the original workers in the light of further studies suggesting that a rise in PCO_2 does increase respiratory sensation in completely paralyzed individuals.

The detection of respiratory and elastic loads was first studied using just noticeable difference techniques. A 10–20% increase in elastic and 25–30% increase in resistive load was consistently detectable by normal subjects [132,149]. Taken together with the original breath-holding experiments, Campbell and Howell suggested that breathlessness arose when there was a mismatch between the pressure applied to the respiratory system and the resulting volume change. They translated these terms into ones relevant to the respiratory muscles, i.e. length and tension, and argued that length–tension inappropriateness was the principal mechanism underlying dyspnea [150]. Although no longer accepted as the most likely explanation, this theory produced an enormous stimulus to subsequent research.

10.8.2 STUDIES OF SENSORY PATHWAYS

Potential peripheral sensory mechanisms sensitive to changes in tension include vagally-mediated pulmonary stretch reflexes, tendon organs which are mainly in the diaphragm and sense force and muscle spindles which monitor muscle length. As in studies of ventilatory control, vagal blockade either by local anesthesia [151] or iatrogenically during lung transplantation does not affect respiratory sensation [53]. Tendon organs may register certain kinds of sensation, e.g. volume, and their stimulation can inhibit medullary inspiratory activity. Muscle spindles lie mainly in the intercostal muscles and provide an attractive mechanism of monitoring respiratory muscle shortening as extrafusal fibers will not shorten as much as intrafusal fibers when chest wall movement is restricted [152]. Chest wall vibration can either increase or reduce the sensation of breathlessness in asthmatic subjects or in normal subjects breathing against resistive loads although minute ventilation is maintained, and this is thought to be due to stimulation of muscle spindle afferents [46,153]. Stimulation of the intercostal

muscles can evoke cortical potentials [154] and so a pathway exists to signal information from the intercostals not only to the midbrain but to higher centers. Whether these are the only pathways is still debated as anesthesia up to T1 did not impair load detection. Others have shown that the upper airway is not sensitive to applied loads but suggested more recently that deformation of the trachea, a structure still innervated even after transplantation, may produce an alternative means of sensory detection.

10.8.3 STUDIES OF RESPIRATORY MUSCLES

The respiratory muscles are shortened and their pressure generation capacity reduced by hyperinflation. Studies at different lung volumes have confirmed that sensation increases at a given ventilation as FRC rises [155,156]. Moreover, these authors felt that the sense of inspiratory effort was the best correlate of breathlessness in these normal subjects rather than the sense of muscle tension [128,157]. When muscle function was compromised by sustaining a fatiguing contraction for a prolonged time, effort sensation rose and the ability to scale the load was impaired [158]. This led to the suggestion that inspiratory muscle fatigue may cause breathlessness and would be more likely to develop when hyperinflation was present as in COPD. This is only likely to be true if low frequency fatigue were common and this is not so. Bradley *et al.* showed that diaphragm fatigue and sensation are clearly dissociated [159] whilst more recently Clague *et al.* have shown in normal subjects that increases in effort sensation occur well before critical TTdi is reached at least during CO_2 rebreathing [160]. These latter studies show that inspiratory effort sensation was best related to TTrc and that rebreathing ceased when critical levels of TTrc were reached and respiratory sensation was maximum. High levels of inspiratory effort sensation may act

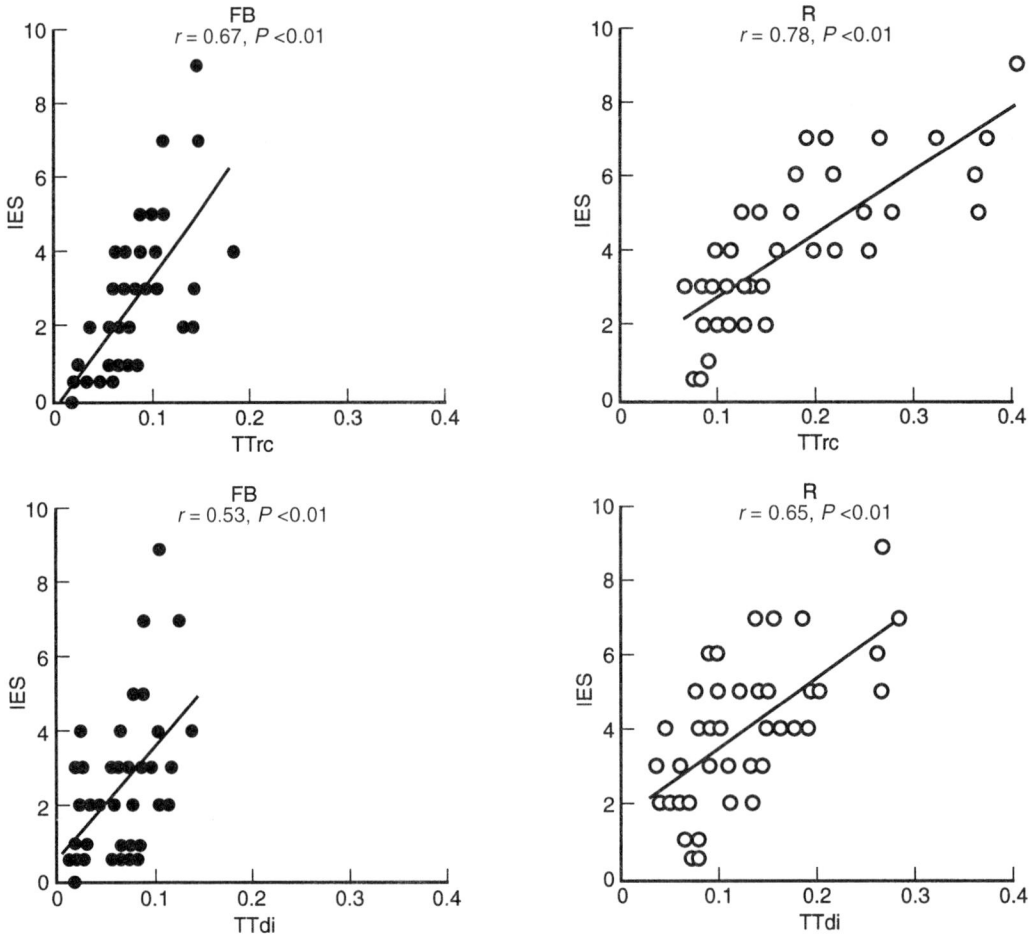

Fig. 10.7 The relationship between inspiratory effort sensation (IES), ribcage tension time index (TTrc) and diaphragmatic tension time index (TTdi) in normal subjects during free breathing (solid circles) and inspiratory resistive loading (open circles). Note the better correlation between sensation and ribcage tension time index, an indirect measure of respiratory muscle oxygen consumption. Although both tension time indices achieve levels which would be associated with inspiratory muscle fatigue if sustained long enough, these are only occurring at the end of the rebreathing test when the subject is asked to stop. Finally, acute loading changes the slope of the IES/tension time relationship because of the higher baselines values in keeping with Weber's law and this response occurs immediately with the onset of loading. Changes of this kind may be relevant to interpreting changes in ventilatory control reported in Table 10.2. (Reproduced from reference [159], with permission.)

as a physiologic monitor of impending muscle overload (Fig. 10.7).

Similarly, studies at lung volumes below FRC show that chest wall restriction may also increase the intensity of breathlessness [161]. Distortion of the chest wall can increase the activity of the inspiratory muscles and produce a more favorable chest wall configuration, e.g. leaning forward may reduce breathlessness [162]. The inability of some COPD patients to carry even light loads may reflect the loss of their pectoral muscles as accessory respiratory muscles which stabilize the chest wall [163].

Studies at rest and during exercise report consistent relationships between Ppl, a marker of inspiratory muscle contraction, and breathlessness. During loading the integrated electrical activity of the sternomastoid muscle appears to be as good or better an index than Ppl suggesting that total respiratory drive is important [164]. During exercise respiratory timing can modify the sense of breathlessness and in patients with a variety of lung diseases, the duration of inspiration and respiratory frequency appear to have a small but independent effect from Ppl on overall breathlessness intensity [165]. Comparisons of the sensation produced by elastic and resistive load suggest that breathing is regulated to minimize inspiratory pressure development [157]. Whether the other timing-related variables integrated together equate to TTrc is less clear at present although the limited studies available would support this [160]. If this is so, the original observations relating the oxygen cost of breathing to breathlessness will not have been too far from the truth.

10.8.4 STUDIES OF CENTRAL SENSORY PROCESSING

It is not clear where the intensity of these sensations is monitored. Research on the kinesthetic sensation of muscle suggests that there are corollary discharges to the cortex which indicate the intensity of any muscle contraction [133]. A similar mechanism has been proposed to explain how a subject can perceive increase in effort when voluntary muscle contractions are attempted during muscle paralysis. That sensory information from the integrated action of the respiratory system reaches the cortex is shown by the detection of cortical evoked responses after airway occlusions [166,167]. These appear maximal over the C4 EEG placement area which corresponds very approximately to the area of the sensory cortex thought to be innervated by

the diaphragm [168]. The adjacent motor cortex shows enhanced metabolic activity during increases in ventilation as assessed by PET scanning and also increases in intensity when ventilation rises during exercise (L. Adams, personal communication). Thus the motor and sensory cortex appear to be activated when ventilation increases and sensation is perceived. It is still unclear whether this activation occurs secondarily to some prior assessment of ventilatory stimulus in the mid-brain or whether the proposed comparatory function is itself cortical. Recent animal studies suggested that the peak intensity of the integrated diaphragm EMG during resistive loading was reduced after decerebration and favors the latter explanation [169].

10.8.5 THE ROLE OF THE BLOOD GAS TENSIONS

These explanations above have largely been developed from studies of resistive and elastic loading. Although chemosensitivity as currently assessed does not explain differences in the perception of breathlessness, there is now good evidence that increases in CO_2 can stimulate breathlessness independently of their effects on ventilation. Studies by Adams *et al.* have shown that oscillations in CO_2 tension did not relate to changes in breathlessness as closely as did those in ventilation [170] whilst Chonan *et al.* found that isocapnic voluntary and hypercapnic involuntary ventilation produced similar degrees of breathlessness [171]. Adams found that exercise and CO_2 were equivalent stimuli to increases in ventilation [170] but that low levels of both produced similar intensities of breathlessness to high levels of ventilation alone. When chest wall movement is restrained and ventilation maintained constant, increases in CO_2 will produce further increases in breathlessness [161]. These authors suggest that a loss of inhibitory mechanoreceptor feedback may explain this but Clague *et al.* found CO_2 to have a small independent effect in explaining effort sensation during loaded breathing even when pressure and timing factors were also measured [160]. Studies with hypoxia are harder to interpret as the response is very dependent on the preceding CO_2 tension and the oscillatory studies of Lane are technically more challenging [172]. None the less, it seems probable that neither hypoxia nor acidosis [173] causes breathlessness independent of their effects on ventilation.

There is considerable debate about the existence of a separate mechanism controlling voluntary ventilation. Although the studies of isocapnic voluntary ventilation do not support this [171], the Charing Cross group has found significant differences during exercise in the intensity of breathlessness compared with equivalent levels of ventilation where the subjects copy a preset breathing pattern [174]. Following their observations on cortical activation [168], they suggest that a separate voluntary pathway of corticospinal phrenic motor neurones exist which can override normal control mechanisms and modify the resulting sensation.

To summarize, it seems likely that respiratory effort can be sensed as an awareness of the outgoing motor discharge, the intensity of which may be modified by a number of afferent inputs which include mechanoreceptor and chemoreceptor derived information. Whether these latter further modify this sensation at a cortical level is not known but this is at least possible. Mechanical factors such as hyperinflation, muscle weakness, muscle fatigue or chest wall restriction contribute significantly to this afferent input as do changes in blood gas tensions. Voluntary controlled ventilation may be different in character but it is not known whether this is explained by different patterns of inspiratory muscle activation rather than separate neural pathways. Individuals vary in the intensity of sensation perceived for a given level of ventilation but the factors which determined this, whether genetic or acquired, have not yet been determined.

10.9 BREATHLESSNESS IN COPD

The study of dyspnea in COPD has been rather patchy following the development of ideas about mechanisms outlined above. Although many of the physiologic changes used to model dyspnea are applicable to COPD patients, most studies with altered lung volume and loaded breathing have been conducted in healthy volunteers. None the less one or more of these mechanisms is likely to operate in most patients. Experimental support for this comes from a number of observations.

As previously noted ventilatory and occlusion responses to CO_2 and hypoxia did not predict exercise performance or Borg scaled breathlessness intensity in COPD patients [86,175]. Swinburn, Wakefield and Jones found that supplementary oxygen reduced breathlessness in COPD but attributed this to changes in ventilation [176], whilst Lane *et al.* claimed that hypoxia had an independent effect but used a different protocol [88]. More recent studies during corridor walking have failed to find any relation to transient decreases in oxygen saturation and subsequent breathlessness intensity [177,178].

One problem in assessing the effect of changes in respiratory impedance in these patients is that they obey Weber's Law [179]. This was established for normal subjects using JND techniques and indicates that the ability to detect a stimulus depends upon the background level of that stimulus. Thus COPD patients with a high background impedance are less likely to detect additional changes in lung mechanics. Data from open magnitude scaling studies support this [180,181]. However, whether this applies to all forms of respiratory load is not clear. Our data in stable COPD patients suggest that resting levels of breathlessness are unrelated to FEV_1 but weakly correlate with FRC, so changes in FRC may be a more sensitive guide to changes in breathlessness. This agrees with data obtained during cycle exercise, where the change in breathlessness in COPD patients is independently related to that in dynamic FRC ($r = 0.63$, $p < 0.001$) [182]. Studies over a wider range of disease severity have reported considerable variations in the perceptual response to changes in lung volume in COPD [183].

The level of intrinsic PEEP is also related to the degree of breathlessness [184]. Reduction in the work of breathing in COPD by adding modest levels of CPAP or EPAP can diminish respiratory sensation [185]. As already noted, Ppl is a useful marker of the severity of breathlessness in COPD but is difficult to measure routinely. A reasonably surrogate is $P_{0.1}$ which reflects Ppl over a modest pressure range [135,160]. This may explain the relationship described by Burki that patients with a high $P_{0.1}$ and especially $P_{0.1}/\dot{V}E$ are more likely to complain of breathlessness [186].

Reduction in mechanical loads by bronchodilators can reduce breathlessness (Chapter 17). This can occur with even trivial changes in FEV_1 and may reflect more subtle adjustments in breathing pattern and the degree of hyperinflation. We have recently found that changes in PIF are a useful guide to the change in end of corridor walk breathlessness possibly because PIF makes an independent contribution to predicting maximum voluntary ventilation from that due to FEV_1 alone [187]. These data provide further support for the importance of respiratory muscle geometry in determining symptoms in COPD.

Finally, a major determinant of breathlessness in COPD is the attitude and mood of the patient [188]. This will determine exercise performance and symptom intensity, possibly for more physiologic reasons than previously envisaged.

10.10 VENTILATORY CONTROL AND DYSPNEA – A SYNTHESIS

It is increasingly clear that ventilatory control and respiratory sensations are intimately connected although perhaps not in the way initially envisaged. Mental activity can modify breathing pattern at rest and a loss of cortical input during sleep can produce an increase in tidal volume and a fall in frequency [189]. Breathing patterns during CO_2 rebreathing can change with mental activity and have been related to personality [190,191], whilst there seems to be an inverse relationship between the sensation during CO_2 rebreathing and the slope of the CO_2 response [192]. Moreover, those subjects with the greatest ability to perceive increases in ventilation show the smallest prolongation of inspiratory time when loaded with an external resistance adopting a rapid shallow breathing pattern [192]. Although initial data in COPD suggested that patients with the lowest sensory magnitude exponents were those most likely to retain CO_2 [180], more recent studies of external loading have shown much the same as in normal subjects, namely that those who perceive sensation most easily to loads compensate by developing rapid shallow breathing [193]. Thus breathing pattern is regulated by similar cortical mechanisms to those determining the intensity of respiratory sensation. Increasing the degree of alertness or cortical activity favors a rapid shallow breathing pattern which is the one associated with the lowest intensity of sensory discomfort. Respiratory sensation in general including dyspnea, appears to be well placed to act as the controller signal, the intensity of which must be minimized to optimize respiratory system function.

10.11 THERAPEUTIC IMPLICATIONS

Since ventilatory control is intimately connected to respiratory sensation, it is unlikely that changes in the one can be accomplished without affecting the other. There is abundant evidence that changes in intensity of breathlessness reflect changes in ventilation rather than changes in perceptual intensity. Thus, naloxone can reduce the intensity of sensation during acute inspiratory loads but does not alter the relationship between breathlessness and ventilation or mouth pressure [194]. The principal exception appears to be treatment which changes lung mechanics either by increasing respiratory muscle strength or reducing respiratory system loading. The main drugs which do this are the bronchodilators and their actions are reviewed elsewhere. Three other treatment approaches relevant to ventilatory control and breathlessness remain.

10.11.1 CHEMICAL STIMULATION OF BREATHING

Ventilatory stimulants act to increase minute ventilation, secondarily improving gas exchange by increasing the neural traffic from peripheral chemoreceptors, central chemoreceptors or both. The current therapies available have been reviewed [195]. Clinically their use is restricted to acute respiratory failure (see Chapter 19) where they can help maintain CO_2 tensions and avoid the use of intermittent positive pressure ventilation. Doxapram hydrochloride is the most widely used drug and is given intravenously in a dose titrated to the clinical response [196]. It acts on both central and peripheral chemoreceptors [197] contrary to earlier claims and has a generalized arousal effect which may help the narcotized patient to cope with physiotherapy.

Almitrine bismethylate is an investigational drug available in parts of Europe that is a highly specific peripheral chemoreceptor stimulant [198] which also modifies local ventilation and perfusion matching (Chapter 8). It improves hypoxemia by day and night in chronically hypoxic patients [199] but is associated with significant pulmonary hypertension during exercise which may limit exercise performance [200]. It has been given orally in multicenter studies of COPD to see if it affects morbidity and mortality [201,202] but its use has been limited by peripheral neuropathy which may be dose-dependent or simply unmasked by the drug.

Medroxyprogesterone acetate has been used as a central chemostimulant which produces modest changes in CO_2 tensions in COPD [203] but the estrogen-like side-effects have limited its practical use. The long-term use of oral ventilatory stimulants is less popular with increasing evidence of CO_2 retention determined by mechanical factors: any increase in overall ventilation is likely to increase symptoms. Whether a sub-set of relatively chemo-insensitive COPD patients with less severe mechanical problems exists, is unclear. If they do, then they will be the ones most likely to benefit from any new oral ventilatory stimulant therapy.

10.11.2 NON-PHARMACOLOGIC IMPROVEMENTS IN VENTILATORY CAPACITY

These are usually achieved by some form of exercise programme (Chapter 21). Increases in respiratory muscle strength and significant reductions in breathlessness have been reported with regular training [140]. However, overall the results of pulmonary rehabilitation have been disappointing [204,205]. An alternative strategy is that of 'respiratory muscle rest' using negative or positive pressure ventilation by day or night [206]. The theoretical problems of this approach have been reviewed [207,208] and typical results are summarized in Table 10.5 [122,209–218]. Data from the British NHLI Trial suggest that there are no changes in chemical ventilatory control or respiratory muscle strength in people treated with six months nasal IPPV (NIPPV) [218]. The high drop out rate and lack of control group makes these data of limited value. However, there does seem to be a role for acute intervention with NIPPV [219] to avoid intubation or aid extubation in patients during an acute exacerbation provided that they are able to cooperate and do not have excessive secretions. Empirical guidelines for the practical use of this treatment have been published [220].

Table 10.5 Intermittent ventilator therapy in stable COPD

Reference	Number started m (f)	Completed	Treatment allocation	Treatment	Period of treatment	FEV^a (l)	$PaCO_2$ (mmHg) Initial	$PaCO_2$ (mmHg) Final	MIP (cm H_2O) Initial	MIP (cm H_2O) Final	Comment
Braun and Marino [209]	18	18	Open	4–10 h daily	5 months	–	54	45	36%	58%	Hospitalization reduced
Cropp and Marco [210]	15(8)	15(8)	Randomized	3–6h daily	3 days	0.8	60	52	67	77	Sustainable ventilation increased
Gutierrez et al. [211]	5	5	Open	8h once weekly	4 months	27% p	59	51	45	62	Slower, deeper breathing pattern
Zibrak et al. [212]	20	9	Crossover	2–6h daily	6 months active	0.55	48	50	30	30	High dropout rate
Celli et al. [213]	16(9)	14(8)	Randomized	3–11h daily	3 weeks	0.6	45	42	–		Training improved exercise tolerance in both groups
Ambrosino et al. [214]	18(10)	18(10)	Randomized	6h daily	5 days	0.77	56	51	34	42	12-minute walk improved
Scano et al. [215]	11(6)	11(6)	Randomized	4h daily	7 days	28% p	60	51	41	45	Slower deeper breathing pattern

Table 10.5 Cont'd.

Reference	Number started m (f)	Completed	Treatment allocation	Treatment	Period of treatment	FEV[a] (l)	$PaCO_2$ (mmHg) Initial	Final	MIP (cm H_2O) Initial	Final	Comment
Shapiro et al. [122]	182(91)	111(57)	Randomized parallel group	205h total	12 weeks	30%	44	46	44	50	Data in treated group presented here – no different in sham treatment; no difference in walk time, cycle ergometry
Strumpf[b] et al. [216]	19	7	Randomized cross-over	3 month each limb	6 months	0.54	47	50	50	47	No difference between control/active treatment – no effect on dyspnea or sleep quality
Elliot et al.[b] [217,218]	12	8	Open	Overnight	12 months (7 cases)	0.6	58	51	34	42	More disabled, 7 already on home O_2. Improved sleep efficiency

[a] % figures refer to % predicted; [b] patients treated by nasal positive ventilation, all others by cuirass. In general only studies with substantially hypercapnic patients benefit. Significant placebo effects make reliance on uncontrolled studies unwise.

10.11.3 REDUCTIONS IN RESPIRATORY SENSATION

The idea of a specific 'anti-dyspnea' drug is attractive but most unlikely. Mitchell-Heggs reported 4 'pink puffers' who appeared to have reduced symptoms after taking 20 mg per day of diazepam [221]. These data have not been repeated with other benzodiazepines in COPD patients [222]. The similarities between dyspnea and pain, as well as the involvement of endogenous opioides in ventilatory control [223], have led to clinical trials of several opioid analgesics. Woodcock *et al.* [224] reported short-term improvement in breathlessness and exercise tolerance after 1 mg/kg dihydrocodeine together with reduced ventilation and resting oxygen consumption. Johnson, Woodcock and Geddes found that 15 mg dihydrocodeine t.d.s. increased treadmill walking distance by 16% and reduced breathlessness by 18% although these effects may not be sustained with regular treatment [225]. Oral morphine 0.8 mg/kg increased exercise capacity by 19% in 13 patients with COPD for a comparable level of breathlessness [226] and may alter the intensity of breathlessness for a given level of ventilation [227]. However, these results have not been found by all workers [228]. In all studies side-effects limited the regular use of these drugs, particularly constipation and sedation. For many patients these side-effects outweighed the benefits of the modest reductions in breathlessness.

Since mental state has a major effect on the perception of breathlessness, it is reasonable to consider antidepressant treatment in any breathless COPD patient with other factors to suggest even a reactive depressive illness and such treatment can achieve as much as more aggressive therapy with opiates. Likewise, good counselling and support can be very helpful in symptom control. Occasionally, for the patient *in extremis* with breathlessness during acute exacerbation, parenteral opiates for a short period can produce a dramatic improvement in both symptoms and breathing pattern which may allow time for other treatment to work. However, such a drastic step

can only be considered as a last resort of the experienced clinician.

Since oxygen reduces minute ventilation in normal subjects, it is not surprising that it improves breathlessness in COPD by similar mechanisms. Following initial studies of Woodcock, Gross and Geddes who found an increase in exercise tolerance after oxygen compared with compressed air [229], Davidson *et al.* showed a significant improvement in exercise tolerance and reduction in breathlessness in a controlled trial of oxygen treatment [230].

The greatest changes were seen with endurance exercise test but more recently the same group have shown a modest 'dose response' effect using self-paced walking tests where high flows of oxygen produced somewhat greater changes in exercise performance [230,231]. Whilst most of this effect is likely to follow from reduction in ventilation, stimulation of upper airway receptors by cold air may also diminish breathlessness [232] and improve exercise capacity [48]. Whether this explains the otherwise idiosyncratic benefits of nebulizer treatment in patients who show no spirometric or lung function improvement remains to be determined. Oxygen therapy is discussed further in Chapter 20.

At present, treatment options for breathlessness are limited. Careful assessment of the patient's potential response to bronchodilator drugs and corticosteroids, suitability for home oxygen and willingness to stop smoking are likely to lead to the greatest long-term benefit. For the more severely limited patient involvement in a rehabilitation programme that improves morale, explains how to cope with the physical limitations of the disease and occasionally deploys some of the treatments listed above, offers the best way of managing this difficult symptom.

REFERENCES

1. Donald, K.W. (1949) Neurological effects of oxygen. *Lancet*, ii, 1056–7.
2. Campbell, E.J.M. (1967) The management of acute respiratory failure in chronic bronchitis

and emphysema. *Am. Rev. Respir. Dis.*, **96**, 626–39.

3. Howell, J.B.L. and Campbell, E.J.M. (1966) *Breathlessness*. Blackwell Scientific, Oxford.

4. Jones, N.L. and Killian, K.J. (1992) *Breathlessness: The Campbell Symposium*. Boehringer Ingelheim (Canada), Hamilton.

5. von Euler, C. (1986) Brain stem mechanisms for generation and control of breathing pattern, in *Handbook of Physiology* (eds N.S. Cherniack and J.G. Widdicombe) Vol. 2, Part II, Section 3, Control of breathing. Am. Physiol. Soc. Bethesda, pp. 1–67.

6. Long, S. and Duffin, J. (1986) The neuronal determinants of respiratory rhythm. *Prog. Neurobiol.*, **27**, 101–82.

7. Mead, J. (1960) Control of respiratory frequency. *J. Appl. Physiol.*, **15**, 325–36.

8. Otis, A.B. (1954) The work of breathing. *Physiol. Rev.*, **34**, 449–58.

9. Clark, F.J. and von Euler, C. (1972) On the regulation of depth and rate of breathing. *J. Physiol. (Lond.)*, **222**, 267–95.

10. Berger, A.J., Mitchell, R.A. and Severinghaus, J.W. (1977) Regulation of respiration. *N. Engl. J. Med.*, **297**, 92–7.

11. Derenne, J-Ph., Couture, J., Iscoe, S. *et al.* (1976) Regulation of breathing in anaesthetized human subjects. *J. Appl. Physiol.*, **40**, 804–14.

12. Shea, S.A., Horner, R.L., Beuchetrit, G. and Guz, A. (1990) The persistence of a respiratory 'personality' into Stage IV sleep in man. *Respir. Physiol.*, **80**, 33–44.

13. Issa, F.G. and Remmers, J.E. (1992) Identification of a subsurface area in the ventral medulla sensitive to local changes in PCO_2. *J. Appl. Physiol.*, **72**, 439–46.

14. Richter, D.W. (1982) Generation and maintenance of the respiratory rhythm. *J. Exp. Biol.*, **100**, 93–107.

15. Anderson, P. and Sears, T.A. (1964) The role of inhibition in the phasing of spontaneous thalamo-cortical discharge. *J. Physiol. (Lond.)*, **173**, 459–80.

16. Rabette, P.S., Costelve, K.L. and Stocks, J. (1991) Persistence of the Hering–Breur reflex beyond the neonatal period. *J. Appl. Physiol.*, **71**, 474–80.

17. Chan, C.S., Grunstein, R.R., Bye, P.T.P., *et al.* (1989) Obstructive sleep apnea with severe chronic airflow limitation: comparisons of hypercapnic and eucapnic patients. *Am. Rev. Respir. Dis.*, **140**, 1274–8.

18. Chan, C.S., Bye, P.T.P., Woolcock, A.J. and Sullivan, C.E. (1990) Eucapnia and hypercap-

nia in patients with chronic airflow limitation. *Am. Rev. Respir. Dis.*, **141**, 861–5.

19. Jalleh, R., Fitzpatrick, M.F., Jan, M.A. *et al.* (1993) Alcohol and cor pulmonale in chronic bronchitis and emphysema. *Br. Med. J.*, **306**, 374.

20. Martin, J.G. and De Troyer, A. (1985) The thorax and control of functional residual capacity, in *The Thorax* (eds. C. Roussos and P.T. Macklem), Marcel Dekker, New York, pp. 899–922.

21. Ingram, R.H. and Schilder, D.P. (1967) Effect of pursed lips expiration on the pulmonary pressure-flow relationship in obstructive lung disease. *Am. Rev. Respir. Dis.*, **96**, 381–7.

22. Biscoe, T.J. and Purves, M.J. (1967) Factors affecting the cat carotid chemoreceptor and cervical sympathetic activity with special reference to passive hind limb movements. *J. Physiol. (Lond.)*, **190**, 425–41.

23. Biscoe, T.J., Bradley, G.W. and Purves, M.J. (1970) The relation between carotid body chemoreceptor discharge carotid sinus pressure and carotid body venous flow. *J. Physiol. (Lond.)*, **208**, 99–120.

24. Calverley, P.M.A., Howatson, R., Flenley, D.C. and Lamb, D. (1992) Clinicopathological correlations in cor pulmonate. *Thorax*, **47**, 494–8.

25. Pallot, D.J. (1987) The mammalian carotid body. *Adv. Anat. Embryol. Cell, Biol.*, **102**, 1–90.

26. Dejours, P. (1963) Control of respiration by arterial chemoreceptors. *Ann. N.Y. Acad. Sci.*, **109**, 682–95.

27. Pappenheimer, J.R., Fencl, V., Hersey, S.R. and Held, D. (1965) Role of cerebral fluids in control of respiration as studied in unanesthetized goats. *Am. J. Physiol.*, **208**, 436–50.

28. Bledsoe, S.W. and Hornbein, T.F. (1981) Central chemoreceptors and the regulation of their chemical environment, in *Regulation of Breathing* (ed. T.F. Hornbein), Marcel Dekker, New York, pp. 347–406.

29. Davidson, T.L., Sullivan, M.P., Swanson, K.E. and Adams, J.M. (1992) Cl-replacement alters the ventilatory response to central chemoreceptor stimulation. *J. Appl. Physiol.*, **74**, 280–5.

30. Bruce, E.N. and Cherniack, N.S. (1987) Central chemoreceptors. *J. Appl. Physiol.*, **62**, 389–402.

31. Shannon, R. (1986) Reflexes from respiratory muscles and costovertebral joints, in *Handbook of Physiology*, (eds. N.S. Cherniack and J.G. Widdicombe), Vol. 2, Part II, Section

3, Control of Breathing, Am. Physiol. Soc., Bethesda, pp. 431–448.

32. Easton, P.A., Slykerman, L.J. and Anthonisen, N.R. (1986) Ventilatory response to sustained hypoxia in normal adults. *J. Appl. Physiol.*, **61**, 906–11.

33. Parsons, S.T., Griffiths, T.L., Christie, J.M.L. and Holgate, S.T. (1991) Effect of theophylline and dipyridamole on the respiratory response to isocapnic hypoxia in normal human subjects. *Clin. Sci.*, **80**, 107–12.

34. Easton, P.A., Slykerman, L.J. and Anthonisen, N.R. (1988) Ventilatory response to sustained hypoxia after pretreatment with amino-phylline. *J. Appl. Physiol.*, **64**, 1445–50.

35. Rudolf, M., Banks, R.A. and Semple, S.J.G. (1977) Hypercapnia during oxygen therapy in acute exacerbations of chronic respiratory failure. *Lancet*, **2**, 483–6.

36. Prechter, G.C., Nelson, S.R. and Hubmayr, R.D. (1990) The ventilatory recruitment threshold for carbon dioxide. *Am. Rev. Respir. Dis.*, **141**, 758–64.

37. Parisi, R.A., Edelman, N.H. and Santiago, T.V. (1992) Central respiratory carbon dioxide chemosensitivity does not decrease during sleep. *Am. Rev. Respir. Dis.*, **145**, 832–6.

38. Wasserman, D.H. and Whipp, B.J. (1983) Coupling of ventilation to pulmonary gas exchange during non steady-state work in men. *J. Appl. Physiol.*, **54**, 587–93.

39. Wasserman, K.B., Whipp, B.J. and Casaburi, R. (1986) Respiratory control during exercise, in *Handbook of Physiology*, (eds. N.S. Cherniack and J.G. Widdicombe), Vol. 2, Part II, Section 3, Am. Physiol. Soc. Bethesda, pp. 595–619.

40. Band, D.M., Wolff, C.B., Ward, J. *et al.* (1980) Respiratory oscillations in arterial carbon dioxide tensions as a control signal in exercise. *Nature*, **283**, 84–5.

41. Wasserman, K., Whipp, B.J., Kogal, S.N. and Cleary, M.G. (1975) Effect of carotid body resection on ventilatory and acid-base control during exercise. *J. Appl. Physiol.*, **39**, 354–8.

42. Phillipson, E.A., Duffin, J. and Cooper, J.D. (1981) Critical dependence of respiratory rhythmicity on metabolic CO_2 load. *J. Appl. Physiol.*, **50**, 45–54.

43. De Backer, W.A., Heyrman, R.M., Wittesaele, W.M. *et al.* (1987) Ventilation and breathing patterns during hemodialysis-induced carbon dioxide unloading. *Am. Rev. Respir. Dis.*, **136**, 406–10.

44. Paintal, A.S. (1973) Vagal sensory receptors and their reflex effects. *Physiol. Rev.*, **53**, 159–227.

45. Coleridge, H.M. and Coleridge, J.C.G. (1986) Reflexes evoked from tracheobronchial tree and lungs, in *Handbook of Physiology*, (eds. N.S. Cherniack and J.G. Widdicombe), Vol. 2, Part II, Section 3, Control of Breathing. Am. Physiol. Soc., Bethesda, pp. 395–430.

46. Homma, I., Obata, T., Sibuya, M. and Uchida, M. (1984) Gate mechanisms in breathlessness caused by chest wall vibration in humans. *J. Appl. Physiol.*, **56**, 8–11.

47. Burgess, K.R. and Whitelaw, W.A. (1984) Reducing ventilatory response to carbon dioxide by breathing cold air. *Am. Rev. Respir. Dis.*, **129**, 687–90.

48. Spence, D.P.S., Graham, D.R., Ahmed, J. *et al.* (1993) Does cold air affect exercise capacity and dyspnea in stable chronic obstructive pulmonary disease? *Chest*, **103**, 693–6.

49. Gautier, H., Bonora, M. and Gaudy, J.H. (1981) Breuer–Hering inflation reflex and breathing in anesthetized humans and cats. *J. Appl. Physiol.*, **51**, 1162–8.

50. Zin, W.A., Behrakis, P.K., Luijoudijk, S.C.M. *et al.* (1986) Immediate response to resistive loading in anaesthetised humans. *J. Appl. Physiol.*, **60**, 506–12.

51. Sanders, M.H., Owens, G.R., Sciurba, F.C. *et al.* (1989) Ventilation and breathing pattern during progressive hypercapnia and hypoxia after human heart-lung transplantation. *Am. Rev. Respir. Dis.*, **140**, 38–40.

52. Kagawa, F.T., Duncan, S.R. and Theodore, J. (1991) Inspiratory timing of heart-lung transplant recipients during progressive hypercapnia. *J. Appl. Physiol.*, **71**, 945–50.

53. Tapper, D.P., Duncan, S.R., Kraft, S. *et al.* (1992) Detection of inspiratory resistive loads by heart-lung transplant recipients. *Am. Rev. Respir. Dis.*, **145**, 458–60.

54. Frost, A.E., Zamel, N., McClean, P. *et al.* (1992) Hypercapnic ventilatory response in recipients of double-lung transplants. *Am. Rev. Respir. Dis.*, **146**, 1610–2.

55. Hugelin, A. (1982) Suprapontine control of respiratory movement, in (eds. J.L. Feldman and A.J. Berger), *Proceedings of International Symposium: Central Neural Production of Periodic Respiratory Movements*. Lake Bluff, Illinois, pp. 60–63.

56. Newsom-Davis, J. and Stagg, D. (1975) Inter-relationships of the volume and time compo-

nents of individual breaths in normal man. *J. Physiol. (Lond.)*, **245**, 481–98.

57. Wheatley, J.R., Amis, T.C., and Engel, L.A. (1991) Oronasal partioning of ventilation during exercise in humans. *J. Appl. Physiol.*, **71**, 546–51.

58. Mador, M.J. and Tobin, M.J. (1991) Effect of alterations in mental activity on the breathing pattern in healthy subjects. *Am. Rev. Respir. Dis.*, **144**, 481–7.

59. Severinghaus, J.W. and Mitchell, R.A. (1962) Ondine's curse – failure of respiratory centre automaticity while awake. *Clin. Res.*, **10**, 122.

60. Rigg, J.R.A., Inman, E.M., Saunders, N.A. *et al.* (1977) Interaction of mental factors with hypercapnic ventilatory drive in man. *Clin. Sci.*, **52**, 264–75.

61. Grodins, F.S. (1950) Analysis of factors concerned in regulation of breathing in exercise. *Physiol. Rev.*, **30**, 220–39.

62. Catterall, J.R., Calverley, P.M.A. and MacNee, W. *et al.* (1985) Mechanisms of transient nocturnal hypoxaemia in hypoxic chronic bronchitis and emphysema. *J. Appl. Physiol.*, **59**, 1698–703.

63. Priban, I.P. and Fincham, W.F. (1965) Self-adaptive control and the respiratory system. *Nature*, **208**, 339–43.

64. Poon, C.S. (1987) Ventilatory control in hypercapnia and exercise: optimization hypothesis. *J. Appl. Physiol.*, **62**, 2447–59.

65. Poon, C.S. (1989) Effects of inspiratory resistive load on respiratory control in hypercapnia and exercise. *J. Appl. Physiol.*, **66**, 2391–9.

66. Poon, C.S., Lin, S-L. and Knudson, O.B. (1992) Optimization character of inspiratory neural drive. *J. Appl. Physiol.*, **72**, 2005–17.

67. Johnson, B.D., Saupe K.W. and Dempsey J.A. (1992) Mechanical constraints on exercise hyperpnea in endurance atheletes. *J. Appl. Physiol.*, **73**, 874–86.

68. Mead, J. (1979) Responses to loaded breathing. *Bull. Physiopathol. Respir.*, **15** (Suppl.), 61–71.

69. Farkas, G.A., and Roussos, C. (1983) Diaphragm in emphysematous hamsters: Sarcomere adaptability. *J. Appl. Physiol.*, **54**, 1635–40.

70. Whitelaw, W.A., Derenne, J-P. and Milic-Emili, J. (1975) Occlusion pressure as a measure of respiratory center output in conscious man. *Respir. Physiol.*, **23**, 181–99.

71. Murciano, D., Aubier, M., Bussi, S. *et al.* (1982) Comparison of esophageal, tracheal and mouth occlusion pressure in patients with chronic obstructive pulmonary disease during respiratory failure. *Am. Rev. Respir. Dis.*, **126**, 37–41.

72. Grassino, A.E., Derenne, J-P., Almirall, J. *et al.* (1981) Configuration of the chest wall and occlusion pressures in awake humans. *J. Appl. Physiol.*, **50**, 134–42.

73. Whitelaw, W.A., and Derenne, J-P. (1993) Airway occlusion pressure. *J. Appl. Physiol.*, **74**, 1475–83.

74. Elliot, M.W., Mulvey, D.A., Green, M. and Moxham, J. (1993) An evaluation of P0.1 measured in mouth and oesophagus, during carbon dioxide rebreathing in COPD. *Eur. Respir. J.*, **6**, 1055–9.

75. Donald, K.W. and Christie, R.V. (1949) The respiratory response to carbon dioxide and anoxia in emphysema. *Clin. Sci.*, **8**, 33–44.

76. Park, S.S. (1965) Factors responsible for carbon dioxide retention in chronic obstructive lung disease. *Am. Rev. Respir. Dis.*, **92**, 245–54.

77. Lane, D.J., and Howell, J.B.L. (1970) Relationship between sensitivity to carbon dioxide and clinical features in chronic airways obstruction. *Thorax*, **25**, 150–8.

78. Flenley, D.C. and Millar, J.S. (1967) Ventilatory response to oxygen and carbon dioxide in chronic respiratory failure. *Clin. Sci.*, **33**, 319–34.

79. Flenley, D.C. and Millar, J.S. (1968) The effects of carbon dioxide inhalation on the inspiratory work of breathing in chronic ventilatory failure. *Clin. Sci.*, **34**, 385–95.

80. Flenley, D.C., Franklin, D.H. and Millar, J.S. (1970) The hypoxic drive to breathing in chronic bronchitis and emphysema. *Clin. Sci.*, **38**, 503–18.

81. Altose, M.D., McCauley, W.C., Kelsen, S.G. and Cherniack, N.S. (1977) Effects of hypercapnia and flow resistive loading on respiratory activity in chronic airways obstruction. *J. Clin. Invest.*, **59**, 500–7.

82. Gelb, A.F., Klein, E., Schiffman, P. *et al.* (1977) Ventilatory response and drive in acute and chronic obstructive pulmonary disease. *Am. Rev. Respir. Dis.*, **116**, 9–16.

83. Bradley, C.A., Fleetham, J.A., and Anthonisen, N.R. (1979) Ventilatory control in patients with hypoxemia due to obstructive lung disease. *Am. Rev. Respir. Dis.*, **120**, 21–30.

84. Fleetham, J.A., Bradley, C.A., Kryger, M.H. and Anthonisen, N.R. (1980) The effect of low flow oxygen therapy on the chemical control

of ventilation in patients with hypoxemia COPD. *Am. Rev. Respir. Dis.*, **122**, 833–40.

85. Gribbin, H.R., Gardiner, I.T., Heinz, G.J. *et al.* (1983) Role of impaired inspiratory muscle function in limiting the ventilatory response to carbon dioxide in chronic airflow obstruction. *Clin. Sci.*, **64**, 487–95.

86. Chonan, T., Hida, W., Kikuchi, Y. *et al.* (1988) Role of CO_2 responsiveness and breathing efficiency in determining exercise capacity of patients with chronic airway obstruction. *Am. Rev. Respir. Dis.*, **138**, 1488–93.

87. Cherniack, R.M. and Snidal, D.P. (1956) The effect of obstruction to breathing on the ventilatory response to CO_2. *J. Clin. Invest.*, **35**, 1286–90.

88. Lane, R., Cockcroft, A., Adams, L. and Guz, A. (1987) Arterial oxygen saturation and breathlessness in patients with chronic obstructive airways disease. *Clin. Sci.*, **72**, 693–8.

89. Lourenco, R.V. and Miranda, J.M. (1968) Drive and performance of the ventilatory apparatus in chronic obstructive lung disease. *N. Engl. J. Med.*, **279**, 53–9.

90. Gorini, M.D., Spinelli, A., Duranti, R. *et al.* (1990) Neural respiratory drive and neuromuscular coupling in patients with chronic obstructive pulmonary disease (COPD). *Chest*, **98**, 1179–86.

91. Lopata, M., Onal, E. and Cromydas, G. (1985) Respiratory load compensation in chronic airway obstruction. *J. Appl. Physiol.*, **59**, 1947–54.

92. Jamal, K., Fleetham, J.A. and Thurlbeck, W.M. (1990) Cor pulmonale: correlation with central airway lesions, peripheral airway lesions, emphysema and control of breathing. *Am. Rev. Respir. Dis.*, **141**, 1172–7.

93. Dempsey, J.A. and Forster, H.V. (1982) Mediation of ventilatory adaptations. *Physiol. Rev.*, **62**, 262–346.

94. Mountain, R., Zwillich, C.W. and Weil, J. (1978) Hypoventilation in obstructive lung disease. The role of familial factors. *N. Engl. J. Med.*, **298**, 521–5.

95. Fleetham, J.A., Arnup, M.E. and Anthonisen, N.R. (1984) Familial aspects of ventilatory control in patients with chronic obstructive pulmonary disease. *Am. Rev. Respir. Dis.*, **129**, 3–7.

96. Cherniack, N.S. and Altose, M.D. (1981) Respiratory responses to loading, in *The Regulation of Breathing* (ed. T.K. Hornbein) Part II. Marcel Dekker, New York, pp. 905–64.

97. Cherniack, N.S. and Milic-Emili, J. (1985) Mechanical aspects of loaded breathing, in *Lung Biology in Health and Disease. The Thorax (part B)* (eds. Ch. Roussos and P.T. Macklem) Marcel Dekker, New York, pp. 905–64.

98. Sorli, J., Grassino, A., Lorange, G. and Milic-Emili, J. (1978) Control of breathing in patients with chronic obstructive lung disease. *Clin. Sci. Mol. Med.*, **54**, 295–304.

99. Skatrud, J.B., Dempsey, J.A., Bhansuli, P. and Irvin, C. (1980) Determinants of chronic carbon dioxide retention and its correction in humans. *J. Clin. Invest.*, **65**, 813–21.

100. Aubier, M., Murciano, D., Fournier, M. *et al.* (1980) Central respiratory drive in acute respiratory failure of patients with chronic obstructive pulmonary disease. *Am. Rev. Respir. Dis.*, **122**, 191–9.

101. Parot, S., Saunier, C., Gautier, H. *et al.* (1980) Breathing pattern and hypercapnia in patients with obstructive pulmonary disease. *Am. Rev. Respir. Dis.*, **121**, 985–91.

102. Javaheri, S., Blum, J. and Kazemi, H. (1981) Pattern of breathing and carbon dioxide retention in chronic obstructive pulmonary disease. *Am. J. Med.*, **71**, 228–34.

103. Loveridge, B., West, P., Anthonisen, N.R. and Kryger, M.H. (1984) Breathing pattern in patients with chronic obstructive pulmonary disease. *Am. Rev. Respir. Dis.*, **130**, 730–3.

104. Oliven, A., Kelsen, S.G., Deal, E.C. and Cherniack, N.S. (1983) Mechanisms underlying CO_2 retention during flow-resistive loading in patients with chronic obstructive pulmonary disease. *J. Clin. Invest.*, **71**, 1442–9.

105. Murciano, D., Aubier, M., Viau, F. *et al.* (1982) Effects of airway anesthesia on pattern of breathing and blood gases in patients with chronic obstructive pulmonary disease during acute respiratory failure. *Am. Rev. Respir. Dis.*, **126**, 113–7.

106. Scardella, A.T., Parisi, R.A., Phair, D.K. *et al.* (1986) The role of endogenous opioids in the ventilatory response to acute flow-resistive loads. *Am. Rev. Respir. Dis.*, **133**, 26–31.

107. Weil, J.V., McCullough, R.F., Kline, J.S. and Sodal, I.E. (1975) Diminished ventilatory response to hypoxia and hypercapnia after morphine in normal man. *N. Engl. J. Med.*, **292**, 1103–6.

108. Fleetham, J.A., Clarke, H., Dhringa, S. *et al.* (1980) Endogenous opiates and chemical control of breathing in humans. *Am. Rev. Respir. Dis.*, **121**, 1045–9.

109. Akiyama, Y., Nishimura, M., Suzuki, A. *et al.* (1990) Naloxone increases ventilatory response to hypercapnic hypoxia in healthy adult humans. *Am. Rev. Respir. Dis.*, **142**, 301–5.

110. Santiago, T.V., Remolina, C., Scoles, V. and Edelman, N.H. (1981) Endorphins and the control of breathing. Ability of naloxone to restore flow-resistive load compensation in chronic obstructive pulmonary disease. *N. Engl. J. Med.*, **304**, 1190–5.

111. Simon, P.M., Pope, A., Lahive, K. *et al.* (1989) Naloxone does not alter response to hypercapnia or resistive loading in chronic obstructive pulmonary disease. *Am. Rev. Respir. Dis.*, **139**, 134–8 (abstract).

112. Similowski, T., Yan, S., Gauthier, A.P. *et al.* (1991) Contractile properties of the human diaphragm during chronic hyperinflation. *N. Engl. J. Med.*, **325**, 917–23.

113. Moxham, J., Edwards, R.H.T., Aubier, M. *et al.* (1982) Changes in EMG power spectrum (high to low ratio) with force fatigue in humans. *J. Appl. Physiol.*, **53**, 1094–9.

114. Goldstone, J.C., Green, M. and Moxham, J. (1994) Maximum relaxation rate of the diaphragm during weaning from mechanical ventilation. *Thorax*, **49**, 54–60.

115. Levy, R.D., Esau, S.A., Bye, P.T.P. and Pardy, R.L. (1984) Relaxation rate of mouth pressure with sniffs at rest and with inspiratory muscle fatigue. *Am. Rev. Respir. Dis.*, **130**, 38–41.

116. Oliven, A., Cherniack, N.S., Deal, E.C. and Kelsen, S.G. (1985) The effects of acute bronchoconstriction on respiratory activity in patients with chronic obstructive pulmonary disease. *Am. Rev. Respir. Dis.*, **131**, 236–41.

117. Bellemare, F. and Grassino, A. (1983) Force reserve of the diaphragm in patients with chronic obstructive pulmonary disease. *J. Appl. Physiol.*, **55**, 8–15.

118. Roussos, C., Fixley, M., Gross, D. and Macklem, P.T. (1979) Fatigue of inspiratory muscles and their synergic behaviour. *J. Appl. Physiol.*, **46**, 897–904.

119. Mador, M.J., and Tobin, M.J. (1992) The effect of inspiratory muscle fatigue on breathing pattern and ventilatory response to CO_2. *J. Physiol. (Lond.)*, **455**, 17–32.

120. Cohen, C.A., Zagelbaum, G., Gross, D. *et al.* (1982) Clinical manifestations of respiratory muscle fatigue. *Am. J. Med.*, **73**, 308–16.

121. Tobin, M.J., Perez, W., Guenther, S.M. *et al.* (1987) Does ribcage abdominal paradox signify respiratory muscle fatigue? *J. Appl. Physiol.*, **63**, 851–60.

122. Shapiro, S.H., Ernst, P., Gray-Donald, K. *et al.* (1992) Effect of negative pressure ventilation in severe pulmonary disease. *Lancet*, **340**, 1425–9.

123. Haluszka, J., Chartrand, D.A., Grassino, A. and Milic-Emili, J. (1990) Intrinsic PEEP and arterial PCO_2 in stable patients with chronic obstructive pulmonary disease. *Am. Rev. Respir. Dis.*, **141**, 1194–7.

124. Begin, P. and Grassino, A.E. (1991) Inspiratory muscle dysfunction and chronic hypercapnia in chronic obstructive pulmonary disease. *Am. Rev. Respir. Dis.*, **143**, 905–12.

125. Molho, M., Shulimzon, T., Benzaray, S. and Katz, I. (1993) Importance of inspiratory load in the assessment of severity of airways obstruction and its correlation with CO_2 retention in chronic obstructive pulmonary disease. *Am. Rev. Respir. Dis.*, **147**, 45–9.

126. Riley, R.L. (1954) The work of breathing and its relation to respiratory acidosis. *Ann. Intern. Med.*, **41**, 172–6.

127. Katz-Salamon, M. (1988) Respiratory psychophysics: a methodological overview, in *Respiratory Psychophysiology* (eds. von Euler, C. and M. Katz-Salamon), Stockton Press, New York, pp. 65–78.

128. Stubbing, D.G., Ramsdale, E.H., Killian, K.J. and Campbell, E.J.M. (1983) Psychophysics of inspiratory muscle force. *J. Appl. Physiol.*, **54**, 1216–21.

129. Mahutte, C.K., Campbell, E.J.M. and Killian, K.J. (1983) Theory of resistive load detection. *Respir. Physiol.*, **51**, 131–9.

130. Simon, P.M., Schwartzstein, R.M., Weiss, J.W. *et al.* (1989) Distinguishable sensations of breathlessness induced in normal volunteers. *Am. Rev. Respir. Dis.*, **140**, 1021–9.

131. Elliot, M.W., Adams, L., Cockcroft, A. *et al.* (1991) The language of breathlessness: use of verbal descriptions by patients with cardiopulmonary disease. *Am. Rev. Respir. Dis.*, **144**, 826–32.

132. Campbell, E.J.M., Freedman, S., Smith, P.S. and Taylor, M.E. (1961) The ability to detect added elastic loads to breathing. *Clin. Sci.*, **20**, 222–31.

133. McCloskey, D.I., Ebeling, P. and Goodwin, G.M. (1974) Estimation of weights and tensions and apparent involvement of a sense of effort. *Exp. Neurol.*, **42**, 220–32.

134. Borg, G. (1982) Psychophysical basis of perceived exertion. *Med. Sci. Sports Exer.*, **14**, 377–81.

135. Clague, J.E., Carter, J., Pearson, M.G. and Calverley, P.M.A. (1990) Relationship between inspiratory drive and perceived inspiratory effort in normal man. *Clin. Sci.*, **78**, 493–6.

136. Muza, S.R., Silverman, M.T., Gilmore, C.G. *et al.* (1990) Comparisons of scales used to quantitate the sense of effort to breathe in patients with chronic obstructive pulmonary disease. *Am. Rev. Respir. Dis.*, **141**, 909–13.

137. Wilson, R.C. and Jones, P.W. (1989) A comparison of the visual analogue scale and modified Borg scale for the measurement of dyspnoea during exercise. *Clin. Sci.*, **76**, 277–82.

138. Mador, M.J. and Kufel, T.J. (1992) Reproducibility of visual analog scale measurements of dyspnea in patients with chronic obstructive pulmonary disease. *Am. Rev. Respir. Dis.*, **146**, 82–7.

139. Hay, J.G., Stone, P., Carter, J. *et al.* (1992) Bronchodilator reversibility, exercise performance and breathlessness in stable chronic obstructive pulmonary disease. *Eur. Respir. J.*, **5**, 659–64.

140. Larson, J.L., Kim, M.J., Sharp, J.T. *et al.* (1988) Inspiratory muscle training with a pressure threshold device in patients with chronic obstructive pulmonary disease. *Am. Rev. Respir. Dis.*, **138**, 689–96.

141. MRC Committee on Research into Chronic Bronchitis (1966) Instructions for use of the questionnaire on respiratory symptoms. W.J. Holman, Devon.

142. Mahler, D.A., Weinberg, D.H., Wells, C.K., and Feinstein, A.R. (1984) The measurement of dyspnea: contents, interobserver agreement and physiologic correlates of two new clinical indices. *Chest*, **85**, 751–8.

143. Mahler, D.A., and Harver, A. (1992) A factor analysis of dyspnea ratings, respiratory muscle strength and lung function in patients with chronic obstructive pulmonary disease. *Am. Rev. Respir. Dis.*, **145**, 467–70.

144. Cournand, A. and Richards, D.W. (1941) Pulmonary insufficiency. *Am. Rev. Tubercl.*, **44**, 26–41.

145. McIlroy, M.B., and Christie, R.V. (1954) The work of breathing in emphysema. *Clin. Sci.*, **13**, 147–54.

146. Fowler, W.S. (1954) Breaking point of breath-holding. *J. Appl. Physiol.*, **6**, 539–45 (abstract).

147. Campbell, E.J.M., Godfrey, S., Clark, T.J.H. *et al.* (1969) The effect of muscular paralysis induced by tubocurarine on the duration and sensation of breath holding during hypercapnia. *Clin. Sci.*, **36**, 323–8.

148. Banzett, R.B., Lansing, R.W., Brown, R. *et al.* (1990) 'Air hunger' from increased PCO_2 persists after complete neuromuscular block in humans. *Respir. Physiol.*, **81**, 1–18.

149. Freedman, S. and Campbell, E.J.M. (1970) The ability of normal subjects to tolerate added inspiratory loads. *Respir. Physiol.*, **10**, 213–35.

150. Campbell, E.J.M. and Howell, J.B.L. (1963) The sensation of breathlessness. *Br. Med. Bull.*, **19**, 36–40.

151. Eisele, J., Trenchard, D., Burki, N. and Guz, A. (1969) The effect of chest wall block on respiratory sensation and control in man. *Clin. Sci.*, **35**, 23–33.

152. Remmers, J.E. (1970) Inhibition of inspiratory activity by intercostal muscle afferents. *Respir. Physiol.*, **10**, 358–83.

153. Manning, H.L., Basner, R., Ringler, J. *et al.* (1991) Effect of chest wall vibration on breathlessness in normal subjects. *J. Appl. Physiol.*, **71**, 175–81.

154. Gandevia, S.C. and Macefield, G. (1989) Projection of low threshold afferents from human intercostal muscles to the cerebral cortex. *Respir. Physiol.*, **77**, 201–14.

155. Killian, K.J., Mahutte, C.K., Howell, J.B.L. and Campbell, E.J.M. (1980) Effect of timing, flow, lung volume and threshold pressures on resistive load detection. *J. Appl. Physiol.*, **49**, 958–63.

156. Killian, K.J., Gandevia, S.C., Summers, E. and Campbell, E.J.M. (1984) Effect of increased lung volume on perception of breathlessness, effort and tension. *J. Appl. Physiol.*, **57**, 686–91.

157. Killian, K.J., Bucens, D.D., and Campbell, E.J.M. (1982) The effect of patterns of breathing on the perceived magnitude of added loads to breathing. *J. Appl. Physiol.*, **52**, 578–84.

158. Gandevia, S.C., Killian, K.J., and Campbell, E.J.M. (1981) The effect of respiratory muscle fatigue on respiratory sensations. *Clin. Sci.*, **60**, 463–6.

159. Bradley, T.D., Chartrand, D.A., Fitting, J.W. *et al.* (1986) The relation of inspiratory effort sensation to fatiguing patterns of the diaphragm. *Am. Rev. Respir. Dis.*, **134**, 1119–24.

160. Clague, J.E., Carter, J., Pearson, M.G. and Calverley, P.M.A. (1993) Physiological determinants of inspiratory effort sensation during CO_2 rebreathing in normal subjects. *Clin. Sci.*, **85**, 637–42.

161. Chonan, T., Mulholland, M.B., Cherniack, N.S. and Altose, M.D. (1987) Effect of voluntary constraining of thoracic displacement

during hypercapnia. *J. Appl. Physiol.*, **63**, 1822–8.

162. Sharp, J.T., Druz, W.S., Moisan, T. *et al.* (1980) Postural relief of dyspnea in severe COPD. *Am. Rev. Respir. Dis.*, **122**, 201–11.

163. Celli, B.R., Rassulo, J. and Make, B. (1986) Dyssynchronous breathing during arm but not leg exercise in patients with chronic airflow obstruction. *N. Engl. J. Med.*, **314**, 1485–90.

164. Ward, M.E., Eidelman, D., Stubbing, D.G. *et al.* (1988) Respiratory sensation and pattern of respiratory muscle activation during diaphragm fatigue. *J. Appl. Physiol.*, **65**, 2181–9.

165. Leblanc, P., Bowie, D.M., Summers, E. *et al.* (1986) Breathlessness and exercise in patients with cardiorespiratory disease. *Am. Rev. Respir. Dis.*, **133**, 21–5.

166. Zechman, F.W., Muza, S.R., Davenport, P.W. *et al.* (1985) Relationship of transdiaphragmatic pressure and latencies for detecting added inspiratory loads. *J. Appl. Physiol.*, **58**, 236–43.

167. Davenport, P.W., Friedman, W.A., Thompson, F.J. and Franzen, O. (1986) Respiratory-related cortical potentials evoked by inspiratory occlusion in humans. *J. Appl. Physiol.*, **60**, 1843–8.

168. Murphy, K., Mier, A., Adams, L., and Guz, A. (1990) Putative cerebral cortical involvement in the ventilatory response to inhaled CO_2 in conscious man. *J. Physiol. (Land.)*, **420**, 1–18.

169. Xu, F., Taylor, R.F., McLarney, T. *et al.* (1993) Respiratory load compensation. 1 Role of the cerebrum. *J. Appl. Physiol.*, **74**, 853–8.

170. Adams, L., Lane, R., Shea, S.A. *et al.* (1985) Breathlessness during different forms of ventilatory stimulation: a study of mechanisms in normal subjects and respiratory patients. *Clin. Sci.*, **69**, 663–72.

171. Chonan, T., Mulholland, M.B., Leitner, J. *et al.* (1990) Sensation of dyspnea during hypercapnia, exercise and voluntary hyperventilation. *J. Appl. Physiol.*, **68**, 2100–6.

172. Lane, R., Adams, L. and Guz, A. (1990) The effects of hypoxia and hypercapnia on perceived breathlessness during exercise in humans. *J. Physiol. (Lond.)*, **429**, 579–93.

173. Lane, R., Adams, L. and Guz, A. (1990) Acidosis and breathlessness in normal subjects. *Eur. Respir. J.*, **3**, 142S.

174. Lane, R., Cockcroft, A. and Guz, A. (1987) Voluntary isocapnic hyperventilation and breathlessness during exercise in normal subjects. *Clin. Sci.*, **73**, 519–23.

175. Robinson, R.W., White, D.P. and Zwillich, C.W. (1987) Relationship of respiratory drives to dyspnea and exercise performance in chronic obstructive pulmonary disease. *Am. Rev. Respir. Dis.*, **136**, 1084–90.

176. Swinburn, C.R., Wakefield, J.M. and Jones, P.W. (1984) Relationship between ventilation and breathlessness during exercise in chronic obstructive airways disease is not altered by prevention of hypoxaemia. *Clin. Sci.*, **67**, 515–9.

177. Mak, V.H.F., Bugler, J.R., Roberts, C.M. and Spiro, S.G. (1993) Effect of arterial oxygen desaturation on six minute walk distances, perceived effort and perceived breathlessness in patients with airflow limitation. *Thorax*, **48**, 33–8.

178. Spence, D.P.S., Hay, J.G., Carter, J. *et al.* (1993) Oxygen desaturation and breathlessness during corridor walking in chronic obstructive pulmonary disease: effect of oxitropium bromide. *Thorax*, **48**, 1145–50.

179. Stubbing, D.G., Killian, K.J. and Campbell, E.J.M. (1983) Weber's law and resistive load detection. *Am. Rev. Respir. Dis.*, **127**, 5–7.

180. Gottfried, S.B., Redline, S. and Altose, M.D. (1985) Respiratory sensation in chronic obstructive pulmonary disease. *Am. Rev. Respir. Dis.*, **132**, 954–9.

181. Gottfried, S.B., Altose, M.D., Kelsen, S.G. *et al.* (1978) The perception of changes in airflow resistance in normal subjects and patients with chronic airways obstruction. *Chest*, **73**, 286–8.

182. O'Donnell, A.E. and Webb, K.A. (1993) Exertional breathlessness in patients with chronic airflow limitation. *Am. Rev. Respir. Dis.*, **148**, 1351–7.

183. Noseda, A., Schmerber, J., Prigogine, T. and Yernault, J.C. (1993) How do patients with either asthma or COPD perceive acute bronchodilation? *Eur. Respir. J.*, **6**, 636–44.

184. Petrof, B.J., Calderini, E. and Gottfried, S.B. (1990) Effect of CPAP on respiratory effort and dyspnea during exercise in severe COPD. *J. Appl. Physiol.*, **69**, 179–88.

185. O'Donnell, D.E., Sanii, R., Gresbrecht, G. and Younes, M. (1988) Effect of continuous positive airway pressure on respiratory sensation in patients with chronic obstructive pulmonary disease during submaximal exercise. *Am. Rev. Respir. Dis.*, **138**, 1185–91.

186. Burki, N.K. (1979) Breathlessness and mouth occlusion pressure in patients with chronic obstruction of the airways. *Chest*, **76**, 527–31.

187. Dillard, T.A., Hnatiuk, O.W. and McCumber, T.R. (1993) Maximum voluntary ventilation. Spirometric determinants in chronic obstructive pulmonary disease patients and normal subjects. *Am. Rev. Respir. Dis.*, **147**, 870–5.

188. Morgan, A.D., Peck, D.F., Buchanan, D.E., and McHardy, G.J.R. (1983) Effect of attitudes and beliefs on exercise tolerance in chronic bronchitis. *Br. Med. J.*, **286**, 171–3.

189. Mador, J.M., and Tobin, M.J. (1991) Effect of alterations in mental activity on the breathing pattern in healthy subjects. *Am. Rev. Respir. Dis.*, **144**, 481–7.

190. Clark, T.J.H., and Cochrane, G.M. (1970) Effect of personality on alveolar ventilation in patients with chronic airways obstruction. *Br. Med. J.*, **1**, 273–5.

191. Hudgel, D.W. and Kinsman, R.A. (1983) Interactions among behavioural style, ventilatory drive and load recognition. *Am. Rev. Respir. Dis.*, **128**, 246–8.

192. Clague, J.E., Carter, J., Pearson, M.G. and Calverley, P.M.A. (1992) Effort sensation, chemoreceptors and breathing pattern during inspiratory resistive loading. *J. Appl. Physiol.*, **73**, 440–5.

193. Oliven, A., Kelsen, S.G., Deal, E.C. and Cherniack, N.S. (1985) Respiratory pressure sensation. Relationship to changes in breathing pattern in patients with chronic obstructive lung disease. *Am. Rev. Respir. Dis.*, **132**, 1214–8.

194. Nishimura, N., Suzuki, A., Yoshioka, A. *et al.* (1992) Effect of aminophylline on brain tissue oxygen tension in patients with chronic obstructive lung disease. *Thorax*, **47**, 1025–9.

195. Bardsley, P.A. (1993) Chronic respiratory failure in COPD: is there a place for a respiratory stimulant? *Thorax*, **48**, 781–4.

196. Moser, K.M., Luchsinger, P.C., Adamson, J.S. *et al.* (1973) Respiratory stimulation with intravenous doxapram in respiratory failure: a double-blind co-operative study. *N. Engl. J. Med.*, **288**, 427–31.

197. Calverley, P.M.A., Robson, R.H., Wraith, R.H. *et al.* (1983) The ventilatory effect of doxapram in normal man. *Clin. Sci.*, **65**, 65–9.

198. Powles, A.C., Tuxen, D.V., Mahood, C.B., *et al.* (1983) The effect of intravenously administered almitrine, a peripheral chemoreceptor agonist, on patients with chronic air-flow obstruction. *Am. Rev. Respir. Dis.*, **127**, 284–9.

199. Connaughton, J.J., Douglas, N.J., Morgan, A.D. *et al.* (1985) Almitrine improves oxygenation when both awake and asleep in patients with hypoxia and carbon dioxide retention caused by chronic bronchitis and emphysema. *Am. Rev. Respir. Dis.*, **132**, 206–10.

200. MacNee, W., Connaughton, J.J., Rhind, G.B. *et al.* (1986) A comparison of the effects of almitrine or oxygen on pulmonary arterial pressure and right ventricular ejection fraction in hypoxic chronic bronchitis and emphysema. *Am. Rev. Respir. Dis.*, **134**, 559–65.

201. Watanabe, S., Kanner, R.E., Cutiilo, A.G. *et al.* (1989) Long term effects of almitrine bis-methylate in patients with hypoxic chronic obstructive pulmonary disease. *Am. Rev. Respir. Dis.*, **140**, 1269–73.

202. Bardsley, P.A., Howard, P., De Backer, W. *et al.* (1991) Two years' treatment with almitrine bismethylate in patients with hypoxic chronic obstructive pulmonary disease. *Eur. Respir. J.*, **4**, 308–10.

203. Skatrud, J.B. and Dempsey, J.A. (1983) Relative effectiveness of acetazolamide versus medroxyprogesterone acetate in the correction of chronic carbon dioxide retention. *Am. Rev. Respir. Dis.*, **127**, 405–12.

204. Guyatt, G., Keller, J., Singer, J. *et al.* (1992) Controlled trial of respiratory muscle training in chronic airflow limitation. *Thorax*, **47**, 598–602.

205. Smith, K., Cook, D., Guyatt, G.H. *et al.* (1992) Respiratory muscle training in chronic airflow limitation: a meta-analysis. *Am. Rev. Respir. Dis.*, **145**, 533–9.

206. Macklem, P.T. (1986) The clinical relevance of respiratory muscle research. J. Burns Amberson Lecture. *Am. Rev. Respir. Dis.*, **134**, 812–5.

207. Hill, N.S. (1993) Non-invasive ventilation. Does it work, for whom and how? *Am. Rev. Respir. Dis.*, **147**, 1050–5.

208. Calverley, P.M.A. (1992) Domiciliary ventilation in chronic obstructive pulmonary disease. *Thorax*, **47**, 334–6.

209. Braun, N.M.T. and Marino, W.D. (1984) Effect of daily intermittent rest of respiratory muscles in patients with severe chronic airflow limitation (CAL). *Chest*, **85**, 593–605.

210. Cropp, A. and Dimarco, A.F. (1987) Effect of intermittent negative pressure ventilation on respiratory muscle function in patients with severe chronic obstructive pulmonary disease. *Am. Rev. Respir. Dis.*, **135**, 1056–61.

211. Gutierrez, M., Beroiza, T., Contreras, G. *et al.* (1988) Weekly cuirass ventilation improves blood gases and inspiratory muscle strength in patients with chronic airflow limitation and hypercarbia. *Am. Rev. Respir. Dis.*, **138**, 617–23.

212. Zibrak, J.D., Hill, N.S. and Federman, E.C. (1988) Evaluation of intermittent long term negative pressure ventilation in patients with severe chronic obstructive lung disease. *Am. Rev. Respir. Dis.*, **138**, 1515–8.

213. Celli, B., Lee, H., Criner, G. *et al.* (1989) Controlled trial of external negative pressure ventilation in patients with severe chronic airflow limitation. *Am. Rev. Respir. Dis.*, **140**, 1251–6.

214. Ambrosino, N., Montagna, T., Nava, S. *et al.* (1990) Short term effect of intermittent negative pressure ventilation in chronic obstructive lung disease patients with respiratory failure. *Eur. Respir. J.*, **3**, 502–8.

215. Scano, G., Gigliotti, F., Duranti, R. *et al.* (1990) Changes in ventilatory muscle function with negative pressure ventilation in chronic obstructive lung disease. *Chest*, **97**, 322–7.

216. Strumpf, D.A., Millman, R.P., Carlisle, C.A. *et al.* (1991) Nocturnal positive-pressure ventilation via nasal mask in patients with severe chronic obstructive pulmonary disease. *Am. Rev. Respir. Dis.*, **144**, 1234–9.

217. Elliot, M.W., Mulvey, D.A., Moxham, J. *et al.* (1991) Domiciliary nocturnal intermittent positive pressure ventilation in COPD: Mechanisms underlying changes in arterial blood gas tensions. *Eur. Respir. J.*, **4**, 1044–52.

218. Elliot, M.W., Simonds, A.K., Carroll, M.P. *et al.* (1992) Domiciliary nocturnal nasal intermittent positive pressure ventilation in hypercapnic respiratory failure due to chronic obstructive lung disease. *Thorax*, **47**, 337–41.

219. Udwadia, Z.F., Santis, G.K., Steven, M.H. and Simonds, A.K. (1992) Nasal ventilation to facilitate weaning in patients with chronic respiratory insufficiency. *Thorax*, **47**, 715–8.

220. Branthwaite, M.A. (1991) Assisted ventilation 6 – Non-invasive and domiciliary ventilation: positive pressure techniques. *Thorax*, **46**, 208–12.

221. Mitchell-Heggs, P., Murphy, K., Minty, K. *et al.* (1980) Diazepam in the treatment of dyspnoea in the 'pink puffer' syndrome. *Q. J. Med.*, **193**, 9–20.

222. Woodcock, A.A., Gross, E. and Geddes, D.M. (1981) Drug treatment of breathlessness: Contrasting effects of diazepam and promethazine in pink puffers. *Br. Med. J.*, **283**, 343–5.

223. Supinksi, G., Dimarco, A., Bark, H. *et al.* (1990) Effect of codeine on the sensations elicited by loaded breathing. *Am. Rev. Respir. Dis.*, **141**, 1516–21.

224. Woodcock, A.A., Gross, E.R., Gellert, A. *et al.* (1981) Effects of dihydrocodeine, alcohol and caffeine on breathlessness and exercise tolerance in patients with chronic obstructive lung disease and normal blood gases. *N. Engl. J. Med.*, **305**, 1611–6.

225. Johnson, M.A., Woodcock, A.A. and Geddes, D.M. (1983) Dihydrocodeine for breathlessness in 'pink puffers'. *Br. Med. J.*, **276**, 675–7.

226. Light, R.W., Muro, J.R., Sato, R.I. *et al.* (1989) Effects of oral morphine on breathlessness and exercise tolerance in patients with chronic obstructive pulmonary disease. *Am. Rev. Respir. Dis.*, **139**, 126–33.

227. Akiyama, Y., Nishimura, M., Kobayashi, S. *et al.* (1993) Effects of naloxone on the sensation of dyspnea during acute respiratory loading in normal subjects. *J. Appl. Physiol.*, **74**, 590–5.

228. Eiser, N., Denman, W., West, E. and Luce, P. (1991) Oral diamorphine: lack of effect on dyspnoea and exercise tolerance in the 'pink puffer' syndrome. *Eur. Respir. J.*, **4**, 926–31.

229. Woodcock, A.A., Gross, E.R., and Geddes, D.M. (1981) Oxygen relieves breathlessness in 'pink puffers'. *Lancet*, **i**, 907–9.

230. Davidson, A.C., Leach, R., George, R.J.D. and Geddes, D.M. (1988) Supplemental oxygen and exercise ability in chronic obstructive airways disease. *Thorax*, **43**, 965–71.

231. Leach, R.M., Davidson, A.C., Chinn, S. *et al.* (1992) Portable liquid oxygen and exercise ability in severe respiratory disability. *Thorax*, **47**, 781–9.

232. Schwartzstein, R.M., Lahire, K., Pope, A. *et al.* (1987) Cold facial stimulation reduces breathlessness induced in normal subjects. *Am. Rev. Respir. Dis.*, **136**, 58–61.

W. MacNee

11.1 PULMONARY CIRCULATION

Pulmonary arterial hypertension is the major cardiovascular complication of chronic obstructive pulmonary disease (COPD). It is associated with the development of right ventricular hypertrophy ('cor pulmonale')[1], and with a poor prognosis [2]. Progress in understanding pulmonary vascular disease in COPD has been retarded by the lack of non-invasive methods to study the structure and function of the pulmonary circulation and the right ventricle, and by the limited treatment which is available. This chapter provides an overview of the pulmonary circulation in patients with COPD. It deals with the physiology of the normal adult pulmonary vasculature, the pathophysiology of the pulmonary vasculature in COPD, the natural history of pulmonary hypertension in COPD and its influence on right ventricular function. The controversial areas of so-called 'cor pulmonale', 'right heart failure', the syndrome of fluid retention and therapy for pulmonary vascular disease in patients with hypoxic COPD will also be discussed.

11.1.1 THE NORMAL PULMONARY CIRCULATION

(a) Structure

The pulmonary circulation exists to perfuse, rather than nourish the lungs. Cumming,

Horsfield and co-workers [3,4,5] using post-mortem casts, described 17 branching orders of the human pulmonary arterial system, confusingly defining the different generations from the alveoli to the main pulmonary artery, in the opposite direction to flow. The ratio of the number of vessels from one order to that of the higher order, the branching ratio is relatively constant at 3.0. The diameter ratio is also constant at 1.6 and the average length ratio is 1.5. These dimensions have important implications for the resistance of the pulmonary vasculature.

The structure of the wall of the large pulmonary arteries, which consists of smooth muscle inserting into short elastic fibers, seems to be designed to allow distensibility of the vessel, rather than active constriction or dilatation [6]. However, the early animal work of Von Euler and co-workers [7,8] demonstrated the potential for large pulmonary arteries to constrict and thus increase the pulmonary vascular resistance. The small muscular pulmonary arteries appear to be the major site of changes in resistance in response to changes in pulmonary vascular tone. The presence of medial thickening in the small arteries will potentiate the increase in resistance of flow which results from active constriction, and lessen the ability of the vessels to passively distend. Thus, under these conditions, the small arteries will contribute even more to the resistance to blood flow [9].

Chronic Obstructive Pulmonary Disease. Edited by Dr P. Calverley and Professor N. Pride. Published in 1995 by Chapman & Hall, London. ISBN 0 412 46450 0

The terminal branches of the pulmonary arteries have a wider bore and a thinner wall than the corresponding systemic arteries. Unlike the systemic circulation, where arterioles have a coat of circular smooth muscle and are the vessels which contribute most to the systemic vascular resistance, pre-capillary muscularized arterioles are not present in the pulmonary circulation. This means that these vessels contribute less to the total vascular resistance in the pulmonary circulation. Moreover, the small pulmonary arterioles can respond to changes in blood volume by passively changing their caliber, and can thus act as a reservoir for blood.

Scanning electron microscopy shows that the pulmonary capillary bed consists of a large number (estimated to be 10^{11}) of seg-ments, of varying diameters and lengths (Fig. 11.1). The mean dimensions of the capillary segments have been estimated by Weibel in post-mortem lungs to be 5 μm in diameter and 11 μm in length [10]. These dimensions have been recently confirmed in resected human lungs [11]. Hence the pulmonary capillaries are smaller in diameter than the systemic capillaries, and also smaller than circulating blood cells, particularly neutrophils (average diameter 7 μm) [12]. This leads to trapping or sequestration of neutrophils within the normal pulmonary capillary bed [13]. The pulmonary capillaries do not have contractile cells nor smooth muscle in their walls, and therefore change their dimensions passively. A reduction in capillary diameter can be produced by swelling of the

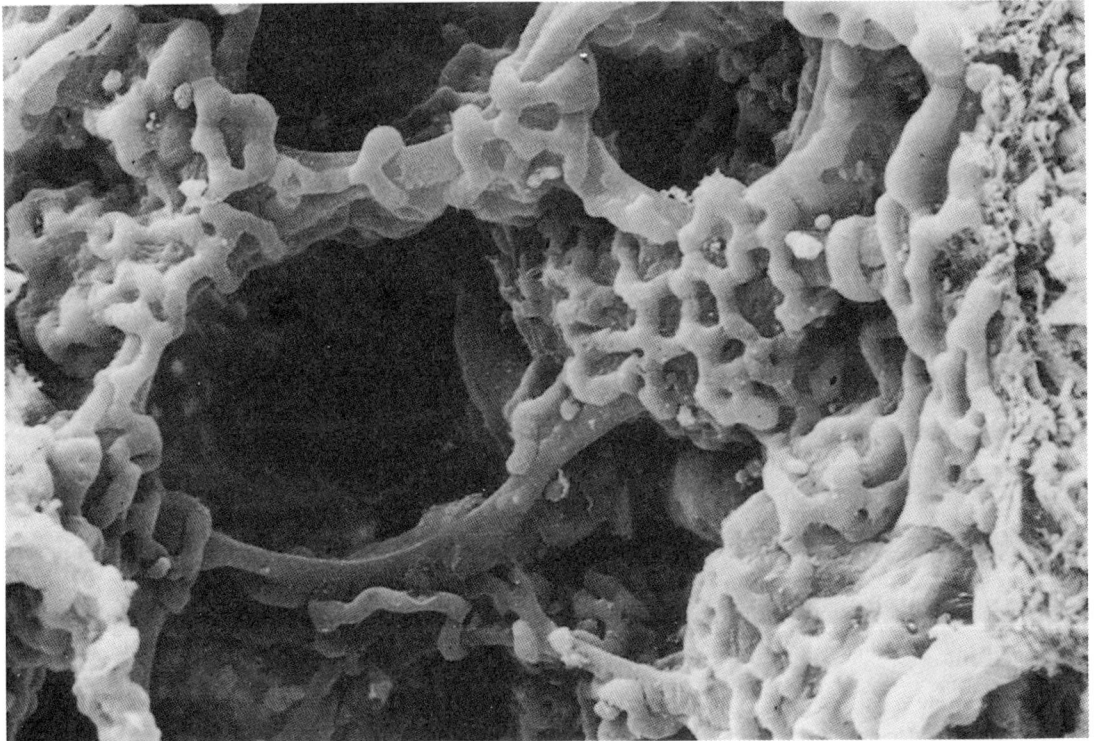

Fig. 11.1 Scanning electron micrograph of the human lung showing alveolar walls containing the intermeshing capillary segments. (Kindly produced and supplied by Dr Peter Jeffery, Department of Pathology, National Heart and Lung Institute, London.)

endothelial cells, perivascular transudates [14] or increase in alveolar [15], or pleural pressure [16], and the capillaries can distend in response to an increase in local blood volume. The pulmonary alveolar–capillary surface area in man, at rest is of the order of 50–70 m^2 at FRC, and increases to 90 m^2 at 75% of total lung capacity [17]. Further increases in the alveolar–capillary surface area can occur during exercise, without producing an inequality between alveolar ventilation and pulmonary capillary perfusion [18].

(b) Function

A perfusion pressure of only 10 mmHg is needed to distribute the cardiac output within the pulmonary vasculature at rest. The normal pulmonary circulation is therefore a low-pressure, low-resistance system, with a low vasomotor tone since vasodilators which reduce systemic vascular pressures have little effect on the normal resting pulmonary arter-

ial pressure [19–21]. The pulmonary vascular resistance is less than 1/10th of the resistance of the systemic circulation. Considerable increases in cardiac output do not increase pulmonary arterial pressure in normal subjects [22] because underperfused pulmonary vessels are recruited, particularly in the Zone I of West [23] (Fig. 11.2). There may even be a fall in pulmonary vascular resistance during exercise in normal subjects [24] (Table 11.1). In clinical practice the pulmonary vascular resistance is calculated as follows:

$$\begin{array}{l}\text{Pulmonary}\\\text{vascular}\\\text{resistance}\\(\text{mmHg}/\text{l}/\text{min})\end{array} = \dfrac{\begin{array}{l}\text{Mean}\\\text{pulmonary}\\\text{arterial}\\\text{pressure}\end{array} - \begin{array}{l}\text{Pulmonary}\\\text{capillary wedge}\\\text{pressure}\\(\text{mmHg})\end{array}}{\text{Cardiac output (l/min)}}$$

In the simple equation above pressure and flow are treated as constant, but in fact they are pulsatile, hence the time-averaged values of each variable should be used in the calculation of their ratio. Traditionally, in many studies, pulmonary vascular resistance is

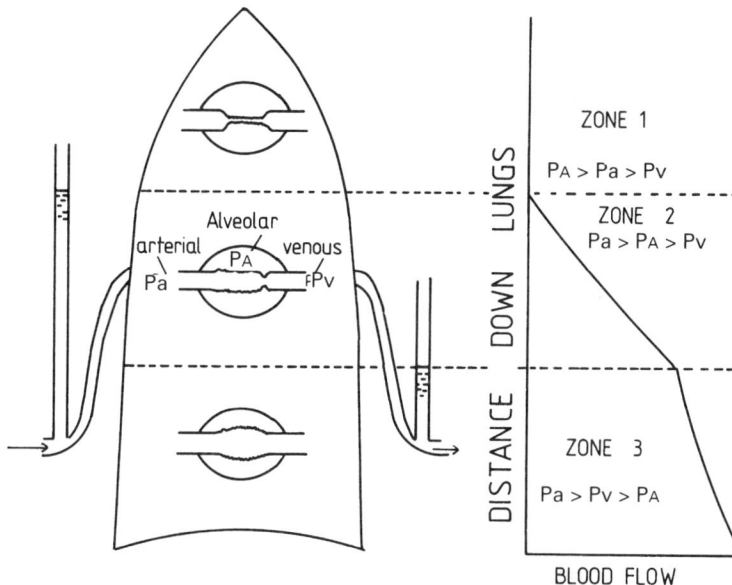

Fig. 11.2 Diagrammatic representation of the zones of West; see text for explanation.

Table 11.1   Comparison of pulmonary and systemic hemodynamic variables during rest and exercise in a normal adult man

	Rest (sitting)	Exercise
Oxygen consumption (ml/min)	300	2000
Cardiac output (l/min)	6.3	16.2
Heart rate (beats/min)	70	135
Stroke volume (ml/beat)	90	120
Intravascular pressure (mmHg)		
Pulmonary artery pressure	20/10	30/11
Mean	14	20
Pulmonary arterial wedge pressure	8	10
Brachial arterial pressure	120/70	155/78
Mean	88	112
Right atrial pressure, mean	5	1
Resistances (mmHg/l/min)		
Pulmonary vascular resistance	0.95	0.62
Systemic vascular resistance	13.2	6.9

From Murray, J.F. (1986) [24].

expressed as dynes.s.cm^{-5} by multiplying the above expression by 80. Calculation of the pulmonary vascular resistance is often further oversimplified by simply dividing the mean pulmonary arterial pressure by the cardiac output, which is called the total pulmonary vascular resistance. This does not take the pulmonary capillary wedge pressure into account. However, in normal subjects, pulmonary capillary wedge pressure is low, but this may not be true in disease. Moreover, in patients with COPD the wedge pressure may not accurately reflect the left atrial pressure [25].

Other important factors which determine the pulmonary vascular resistance include the cross-sectional area of the small muscular pulmonary arteries and the blood viscosity [26] as seen from the Poiseuille equation:

$$P = \frac{8.n.1\ Q}{\pi\ r^4}$$

$$R = P/Q = \frac{8.n.1}{\pi\ r^4}$$

where P is the pressure drop in N/m^2; n is the coefficient of viscosity in N/s/m^2; l is the length of the vessel in cm; Q is the flow as m^3/s; r is the radius of the vessel in cm. The re-sistance depends on the viscosity of blood and the length of the vessel and is inversely proportional to the 4th power of the radius of the vessel. Thus small changes in the vessel radius have a large effect on the resistance. This applies to conditions of streamlined flow, which seems applicable as calculation of the Reynolds numbers in the pulmonary vessels make turbulence unlikely, except in some subjects during peak blood velocity [26]. However, the pulmonary circulation consists of distensible vessels rather than rigid tubes. Increasing the flow of blood through a distensible tube causes the tube to dilate by increasing the transmural pressure. This increase in caliber will reduce flow and so the relationship between driving pressure and flow is no longer rectilinear, as in a rigid tube, but curvilinear.

The transmural pressure within the pulmonary vasculature is influenced by the alveolar pressure and this is particularly true for the pulmonary capillaries, which pass through the alveolar septae (Fig. 11.1). The influence of alveolar pressure on flow in the pulmonary microcirculation can be explained by considering a Starling resistor consisting of rigid tubes (the 'arterial and venule') entering and leaving a rigid chamber filled with air (the 'alveolus'), and joined within the chamber by a flexible tube (the 'capillary'). Thus by increasing the gas pressure in the chamber the flexible tube becomes compressed and imposes a resistance to flow through the tube. West and colleagues [23] described three conditions using this model to explain the vertical distribution of blood flow in the lungs (Fig. 11.2). An upper region of the lungs, Zone I where alveolar gas pressure (PA) exceeds both the pulmonary arterial (Pa) and the pulmonary venous pressure (Pv), produces compression of the capillaries and thus no flow. In the mid zone of the lungs (Zone 2), arterial pressure exceeds alveolar pressure, which in turn is greater than the venous pressure. Here flow depends on the difference between the arterial and alveolar pressure, the so-called 'waterfall' effect and not on the difference between arterial and venous pressures. In the lowest lung zone (Zone 3), where arterial pressure exceeds the venous pressure, which is in turn greater than the alveolar pressure, flow is dependent on the arterial–venous pressure difference.

An increase in the surface area of pulmonary capillaries can arise from a combination of a change in the diameter of perfused vessels and a change in the number of parallel paths which are being perfused, that is the recruitment of previously under-perfused vessels. A practical demonstration of this recruitment comes from direct measurements of the relationship between pressure and flow in the pulmonary vasculature, which were made in the early 1950s during cardiac catheterization and balloon occlusion of a pulmonary artery, usually on the right [27]. Using this technique the flow through the left lung could be doubled, while left atrial pressure remained constant. In normal supine man under these conditions the relationship between pressure and flow remains linear, so that the pulmonary vascular resistance remains unchanged [28,29]. This is not the case in the upright position, where the more dependent blood vessels, in a partly collapsed

state, may expand in response to an increase in flow, reducing the pulmonary vascular resistance [30]. Thus changes in pulmonary vascular resistance are not necessarily an accurate reflection of active changes in vascular caliber in the pulmonary circulation, unless all of the other passive mechanisms affecting caliber have been taken into account. This has led to the use of pulmonary arterial pressure/flow curves, and pulmonary vascular resistance/flow curves to detect active changes in pulmonary vascular caliber [31].

Thus during supine exercise, in normal man [24,32] (Table 11.1), the pulmonary arterial pressure may rise by 3–4 mmHg, the increase in systolic pressure generally exceeding that of the diastolic pressure, which may not change. After exercise, pulmonary arterial pressure often falls below the previous resting values [33,34]. Pulmonary vascular resistance either remains unchanged, or falls during supine exercise [35,36], as a result of passive dilatation of under-perfused vessels.

11.1.2 THE PULMONARY CIRCULATION IN CHRONIC OBSTRUCTIVE PULMONARY DISEASE

(a) Pathology

In patients with COPD and hypoxemia pathologic changes characteristically occur in the peripheral arteries [37–39]. The intima of the small pulmonary arteries develop new accumulations of vascular smooth muscle cells which are laid down longitudinally along the length of the vessels [39]. However, more recent studies have also shown that intimal thickening is an early event associated with worsening airflow limitation [40,41]. Medial hypertrophy in the muscular pulmonary arteries and less commonly fibrinoid necrosis in these vessels has also been reported in patients with COPD and pulmonary arterial hypertension [42]. Thus structural changes may be more important than hypoxic vasoconstriction in the development of sustained pulmonary hypertension in patients with COPD [41].

Pulmonary thrombosis may also occur in patients with COPD, possibly due to peripheral airway inflammation [43]. Pathologic changes in the small airways of patients with COPD have been associated with the pulmonary vascular changes which occur with pulmonary hypertension in post-mortem studies [44,45]. However, a more recent study in patients undergoing lung resection, who had a wide range of emphysema and peripheral airways inflammation, did not confirm these findings [40]. This study showed that there was a stepwise increase in arterial wall thickening comparing non-smokers and smokers with mild to moderate emphysema. While all three vessel layers increased in size, the arterial intima increased out of proportion to either the changes in the media or the adventitia. This confirms an earlier study by Hale and colleagues [45] which demonstrated intimal thickening in muscular pulmonary arteries in post-mortem lungs from a smoking population.

Chronic hypoxemia produces right ventricular hypertrophy in animal studies [46,47]. Recent data also indicate a relationship between the usual arterial pressure of oxygen in a group of patients receiving long-term oxygen therapy and the degree of right ventricular hypertrophy [43], confirming several other animal and human studies [48]. However, there appears to be no significant relationship between the weight of the right ventricle and the extent of emphysema in post-mortem lungs [49,50].

(b) Factors contributing to the development of pulmonary arterial hypertension

The increase in pulmonary arterial pressure in patients with COPD [36,51–53] was previously thought to be due to a reduction in the pulmonary vascular bed [54]. However, it is now known that the development of pulmonary arterial hypertension in patients with COPD results from a combination of several factors.

(i) Disruption of the pulmonary vascular bed

Although loss of vessels contributes to the pulmonary hypertension in thromboembolic disease [55], destruction of alveolar vessels occurs in emphysema, which is typically associated with a normal pulmonary arterial pressure. The lack of a significant correlation between right ventricular hypertrophy and total alveolar surface area [49,50] (which reflects the size of the capillary bed), suggests that loss of capillary bed *per se* is not an important determinant of pulmonary hypertension in COPD.

Previous studies have suggested that the pulmonary arterial pressure is raised in the 'bronchitic' and normal in the 'emphysematous' type of patient with COPD [56] when measured at rest, despite greater destruction of the vascular bed in emphysema. However, quantification of emphysema in life is difficult [57,58]. More recently measurements of lung density using CT scanning [59], which correlate with morphometric measurements of the size of distal airspaces [60], have shown that a similar degree of emphysema occurs in patients with the so-called 'pink and puffing' or 'emphysematous' type of COPD as in the 'blue and bloated' or 'bronchitic' type [61]. Furthermore, there is no correlation between pulmonary arterial pressure or pulmonary vascular resistance and the extent of emphysema, as measured by CT scanning in patients with COPD, although a weak, but significant correlation can be demonstrated between the stroke volume and the extent of emphysema [61].

(ii) Abnormal blood gas tensions

Alveolar hypoxia is a potent pulmonary vasoconstrictor in animals [46] and in normal subjects [47,63]. The mean pulmonary arterial pressure rises between 5–10 mmHg in response to breathing 12–14% O_2 with little change in cardiac output. The correlation between pulmonary arterial pressure and

SaO_2 in patients with COPD was first reported by Harvey *et al.* [62] and has been confirmed by many other authors [64–72]. Breathing supplemental oxygen, even in high concentrations produces a variable, and often trivial fall in pulmonary arterial pressure in patients with COPD [73–75]. Despite normalization of the PaO_2, normal values of pulmonary arterial pressure are rarely achieved in such patients. However, breathing oxygen in high concentrations increases the $PaCO_2$ in some studies of COPD patients [67,73–75], with associated acidemia, which may induce pulmonary vasoconstriction. Moreover, pulmonary hypertension is only partially relieved when mountain dwellers exposed to chronic hypoxia are given oxygen acutely, and normal levels of pulmonary arterial pressure are achieved only after residence at low altitude for 6 weeks [76].

A positive correlation has also been demonstrated between the arterial $PaCO_2$ and the pulmonary arterial pressure [67,77]. However, in studies where $PaCO_2$ was raised by increasing the inspired carbon dioxide concentration in patients with COPD, although pulmonary arterial pressure rose, this may not have been a direct vasoconstrictor effect of carbon dioxide, since cardiac output also increased [78,79]. Hence, pulmonary vascular resistance increased while patients breathed hypercapnic gas mixtures in only one of these studies [78]. Thus the pulmonary vasoconstrictor effect of carbon dioxide in patients with COPD is not particularly strong. In addition an increase in the inspired CO_2 concentration may also result in changes in lung mechanics, produced by the hyperventilation and induced by the rise in $PaCO_2$ [80]. However, an increase in $PaCO_2$ potentiates the hypoxic vasoconstrictor response in the pulmonary circulation in normal subjects [81].

Acute changes in hydrogen ion concentration produce inconsistent effects on pulmonary arterial pressure in patients with COPD [77,82–84]. An infusion of sodium bicarbonate, enough to reduce arterial pH to 7.5, did not affect the pulmonary arterial pressure or the cardiac output in normal subjects [85]. Although induction of an alkalemia in patients with COPD did not change the pulmonary arterial pressure, there was a substantial increase in cardiac output, suggesting that pulmonary vasodilatation had occurred [82]. However, the curvilinear relationship between pressure and flow in the pulmonary circulation in patients with COPD makes the interpretation of these changes more difficult. Similarly inconsistent effects on pulmonary hemodynamics have been reported when the arterial hydrogen ion concentration was increased acutely by an intravenous infusion of hydrochloric acid in patients with COPD [83,84], or over a 5–7 day period by giving ammonium chloride by mouth [85]. However, hypoxia and acidemia have synergistic effects on pulmonary vasoconstriction in patients with COPD, so that for a given SaO_2, mean pulmonary arterial pressure is higher with increasing arterial hydrogen ion concentrations [82]. Peripheral edema in patients with COPD and hypoxemia is rare in those who do not, in addition, have hypercapnia [86].

(iii) Abnormal pulmonary mechanics

At least one study has demonstrated a correlation between pulmonary arterial pressure and FEV_1 in patients with COPD [80]. Changes in airways resistance may augment pulmonary vascular resistance in patients with COPD by affecting alveolar pressure. Harris and co-workers demonstrated in normal man that the linear relationship between pressure and flow in the pulmonary circulation when alveolar pressure is normal, changes when alveolar pressure is increased so that the relationship is steeper initially, and is curvilinear as the pressure increases (Fig. 11.3). Thus when alveolar pressure is increased in normal subjects the relationship between pressure and flow in the pulmonary circulation resembles the relationship in patients with COPD during normal tidal

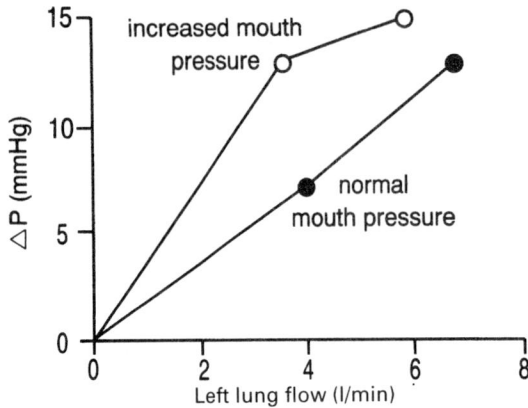

Fig. 11.3 The effect of alveolar pressure on the relation between mouth pressure and flow in the normal recumbent human pulmonary circulation studied by the technique of unilateral pulmonary arterial occlusion. See test for full explanation. (Redrawn from Harris *et al.* (1968) [80].)

breathing (see later) [54,80]. This effect may be particularly seen when airways resistance and ventilation increase during acute exacerbations of COPD. In normal subjects, hyperventilation does not affect the pulmonary circulation significantly; but in severe COPD, hyperventilation increases both pulmonary arterial and pulmonary capillary wedge pressures, without changing cardiac output, so that the pulmonary vascular resistance rises due to a reduction in vessel caliber [80]. Moreover, the amplitude of the respiratory swing of the pulmonary arterial pressure during exercise in patients with COPD (which is related to changes in intrathoracic pressure) correlates with the pulmonary arterial pressure [87]. However in less severely disabled patients with COPD, hyperventilation does not affect pulmonary vascular resistance significantly [88].

(iv) Increased cardiac output

In contrast to the situation in normal subjects [34] (Table 11.1), in patients with COPD, where the vascular bed may be restricted, a

small increase in flow, such as occurs during mild exercise, may significantly increase pulmonary arterial pressure [89].

(v) Blood volume changes

Abraham and colleagues [90] studied the effects of expansion of the blood volume on the pulmonary arterial pressure in patients with COPD. Hypoxia produced an increase in pulmonary arterial pressure associated with a small increase in cardiac index, and thus pulmonary vascular resistance increased; infusion of albumin increased pulmonary arterial pressure, but with a greater increase in cardiac index, and thus pulmonary vascular resistance fell. These data do not support the hypothesis that an increase in blood volume is a major factor in the development of pulmonary hypertension in COPD. Indeed, there is no significant correlation between pulmonary arterial pressure and the plasma or total blood volume in such patients [91]. Moreover pulmonary blood volume, measured by various techniques, is either normal [92] or low [93] in patients with COPD.

(vi) Increased blood viscosity

Patients with COPD who are hypoxemic develop secondary polycythemia which increases the blood viscosity. Reducing packed cell or blood volume, and hence plasma viscosity in patients with COPD, produces a small reduction in pulmonary arterial pressure, without changing cardiac output, and thus pulmonary vascular resistance falls slightly [28]. Arterial blood gas values are not affected by this treatment [28] which has also been confirmed in a more recent study [94].

The inter-relationship between the factors described above is complex. However, restriction of the vascular bed, as in emphysema, together with diffuse constriction of the extra-alveolar vessels, due to hypoxemia, and luminal narrowing as a result of changes in the vessels walls, may all contribute to the increase in pulmonary vascular resistance, in patients with COPD which occurs particularly on exercise, since the ability to recruit underperfused vessels is compromised. Thus patients with a restricted vascular bed respond to exercise as though they started at the bend of the normal pressure/flow relationship (Fig. 11.4), so that pressure rises dramatically with an increase in cardiac output. Hypoxic vasoconstriction and structural changes in the vessels reduce the pulmonary vascular reserve further. At this stage pulmonary arterial pressure becomes elevated at rest and the pressure/flow relationship is shifted upwards and to the left so that a small increase in flow produces a large increase in pressure over the entire range of cardiac output (Fig. 11.4). Changes in plasma viscosity and alterations in pulmonary mechanics may also contribute to the pulmonary arterial hypertension in patients with more severe COPD. The relative influence of each of these factors on the development of pulmonary hypertension is difficult to quantify and in any case varies between individuals.

(c) The endothelium

Although the factors discussed above all contribute to the development of pulmonary hypertension in patients with COPD, the underlying mechanism remains unclear [95]. Many vasodilators such as glyceryl trinitrate and sodium nitroprusside produce their response through the release of a vasodilator substance from endothelial cells, so called endothelium-derived relaxing factor (EDRF) which is now thought to be nitric oxide (NO) or a nitroso compound which releases NO [96,97]. The stimulus for the release of NO from the luminal surface of endothelial cells appears to be increased blood flow and subsequent increase in shear stress [98]. Nitric oxide causes vasodilatation by stimulating guanylate cyclase which increases the second messenger cyclic guanosine monophosphate within vascular smooth muscle [99]. Since NO is a vasodilator this suggested that it may have a role in the modulation of pulmonary vascular tone. Moreover, NO is released from endothelial cells and thickening and proliferation occurs in the intima, of which the endothelium forms a part, in response to chronic hypoxia, both in animal studies [100], and in patients with COPD [38–41] lending further support for a central role of endothelium in regulating the pulmonary circulation [101,102]. Endothelium-dependent relaxation due to EDRF (NO) has been shown in isolated pulmonary artery rings in man [103–105]. Preventing NO production in isolated vascular rings either by removing the endothelium [106,107] or biochemically by pre-treatment with an L-arginine analog which prevent the formation of NO [108,109] increases the response to vasoconstrictors. These studies suggest a mechanism where NO is released as a 'brake' to oppose a potentially excessive rise in pulmonary vascular tone. However, whether NO release *in vivo* has a role in main-

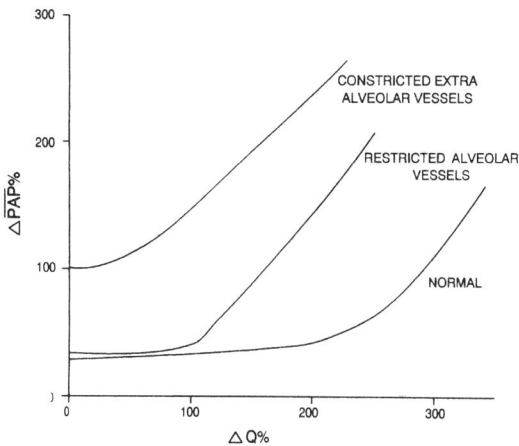

Fig. 11.4 Relationship between pressure and flow in normal, restricted and constricted pulmonary vascular beds. The vertical axis indicates percentage change in mean pulmonary arterial pressure ($\Delta\overline{PAP}\%$) and the horizontal axis shows the percentage change in cardiac output ($\Delta Q\%$); 100% = normal basal level.

taining the normally low pulmonary vascular tone remains speculative. Inhibition of NO synthesis enhances the vasoconstrictor effect of acute hypoxia [110] suggesting that hypoxia increases rather than blunts NO release and probably act as a chemical mechanism to counteract excessive hypoxic vasoconstriction.

Endothelium-dependent vasodilatation is impaired in animals chronically exposed to hypoxia [111] and in isolated pulmonary arterial rings from patients undergoing heart–lung transplantation for end-stage COPD [107] when compared with control patients. This impairment may result from a reduction in NO synthesis or release by the effect of hypoxia on NO synthase [112]. Thus the normal 'braking' mechanism which reduces the rise in pulmonary vascular tone in response to vasoconstrictors may be lacking in COPD. Furthermore this reduction in endothelium-dependent relaxation may be related to the structural changes which affect the intima and media of the pulmonary arteries in patients with COPD [107]. Indeed it has been hypothesized that NO itself may have an inhibitory effect on cell proliferation in the pulmonary vasculature and thus may not only affect the pulmonary vasomotor tone but may also have a role in the vascular remodelling which occurs in hypoxic COPD [112].

(d) Pulmonary hemodynamics

Studies of pulmonary hemodynamics in patients with COPD indicate that pulmonary arterial pressure may be normal, or only slightly elevated when measured at rest [56,113], but may rise to abnormally high levels during exercise [36,51,52,114]. By contrast, as discussed above, exercise in normal subjects produces only a small increase in pulmonary arterial pressure, the increase being greater in subjects over the age of 50 years [33,51,52]. The relationship between pressure and flow in the pulmonary circulation in patients with COPD can be studied

using the technique of balloon occlusion of the right pulmonary artery, as described previously in normal subjects [27–30]. In patients with COPD the initial part of the relation is steeper than normal indicating increased resistance [30]. However, by contrast with normal subjects, at higher flow rates the relation between pressure and flow is curvilinear (Fig. 11.5). Thus resistance decreases, due to distension of vessels at high flow rates, which were narrower than normal at low flow rates. These vessels may be narrowed due to vasoconstriction or from compression from outwith the vessel wall.

Patients with mild COPD, without severe hypoxemia or hypercapnia, have a normal or low cardiac output [1,114–119]. Right atrial and right ventricular end-diastolic pressures are normal and pulmonary arterial pressure may be normal or slightly elevated, but it is inappropriately high for the level of the cardiac output. Pulmonary vascular resistance is therefore normal, or only slightly elevated when measured at rest, but may rise markedly during exercise [36,51]. Patients

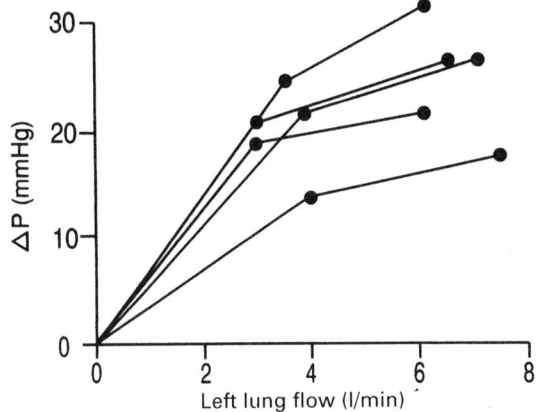

Fig. 11.5 Relation between pressure and flow in the pulmonary circulation in five patients with COPD studied by the technique of occluding the right pulmonary artery. ΔP, mean pulmonary arterial pressure–pulmonary capillary wedge pressure. (Redrawn from Harris *et al.* (1968) [30].)

with COPD stop exercising at a lower level of cardiac output and maximal O_2 consumption than normal subjects, but the slope of the relationship between oxygen consumption and cardiac output is normal [118,119]. Thus the limitation to exercise in patients with COPD is not cardiovascular, but results from changes in pulmonary mechanics. Right ventricular end-diastolic pressure and right ventricular stroke work are normal at rest in mild COPD and increase during exercise, due to an increase in pressure work against a higher pulmonary arterial pressure [118].

As airflow limitation and arterial blood gas abnormalities worsen, particularly when chronic hypoxemia and hypercapnia develop, pulmonary hypertension may be present at rest, and worsens with exercise. However, even in patients with severe COPD, the pulmonary arterial pressure is rarely very elevated. Naeije [120] measured pulmonary arterial pressure in 74 patients with severe, but clinically stable COPD who had all previously presented with an episode of acute on chronic respiratory failure and almost half had a previous episode of peripheral edema. These patients had severe airflow limitation (FEV_1 25.7 ± 1% of predicted, mean ± SD) with hypoxemia (mean 43 mmHg, range 23–67 mmHg) and the majority were hyper-

capnic ($PaCO_2$ mean 51 mmHg, range 33–68 mmHg). However, pulmonary arterial pressure was only modestly raised, with a mean of 35 mmHg in this group (Table 11.2).

11.1.3 THE EFFECTS OF PULMONARY HYPERTENSION IN COPD

Pathologically, primary airway disease and emphysema usually co-exist in most patients with COPD; those patients with predominant chronic airway disease, or mainly emphysema, form the minority at the extremes of the clinical spectrum [121–123]. The notion of two clinical patterns of patients with COPD has been attributed to Dornhurst [124]. The 'blue and bloated' type [125], also known as 'type B' [126] or 'non-fighter' [127] was thought to characterize the 'bronchial type' of disease [121]. Such patients had hypoxemia, hypercapnia and secondary polycythemia, and developed pulmonary hypertension relatively early in the course of the disease. Right ventricular hypertrophy or cor pulmonale ensues and repeated episodes of 'right heart failure', occur often during acute episodes of respiratory failure. In contrast, the 'pink and puffing' variety [125], also known as 'type A' [126] or 'fighters' [127] were thought to represent the emphysematous type [121], character-

Table 11.2 Hemodynamics and blood gases in 74 patients with COPD and 32 normal subjects

Variables	COPD		Normals	
	Mean	Range	Mean	Range
PaO_2, mmHg	43	23–67	91	75–105
$PaCO_2$, mmHg	51	33–68	38	32–43
$\dot{Q}$ l/min/m^2	3.8	2.3–5.8	3.6	2.6–4.5
Pra, mmHg	3	0–21	5	2–9
Ppa, mmHg	35	15–78	13	8–20
Ppw, mmHg	6	0–19	9	5–14
PVRI, dyne/sec/cm^5/m^2	660	231–1377	58	40–200
RVSWI, g/m	16	5–29	6	3–18

From Naeije, R. (1992), [120].
a, arterial; $\dot{Q}$ cardiac output; Pra, right atrial pressure; Ppa, mean pulmonary arterial pressure; Ppw, pulmonary artery wedge pressure; PVRI, pulmonary vascular resistance index; RVSWI, right ventricular stroke work index.

ized by severe breathlessness, but relatively normal blood gas tensions and thus no pulmonary hypertension, right ventricular hypertrophy or 'heart failure', at least until the later stages of the disease. The hypothesis that the 'pink puffer' has largely emphysema, and the 'blue bloater' represented a patient with predominantly chronic bronchitis, was perpetuated in several studies in the 1960s [128–132]. However, accurate diagnosis of emphysema requires a pathological assessment [133]. Thurlbeck [134] showed that the degree of mucus gland hypertrophy, indicative of chronic bronchitis, was similar in patients, whatever the clinical pattern of the disease, and that more than 50% of patients with the 'blue and bloated' clinical pattern had severe emphysema. These pathologic observations have been confirmed in an autopsy study from the National Institutes of Health, Nocturnal Oxygen Therapy Trial (NOTT) [135] which showed a complete overlap of the amount of mucus gland hypertrophy and emphysema in the two clinical types. Studies using CT scanning support this notion by demonstrating no significant correlation between pulmonary arterial pressure and CT measurements of emphysema [61]. However, the NOTT autopsy study showed that the 'blue bloaters' had heavier right ventricles than the 'pink puffers', and the degree of the right ventricular hypertrophy correlated with the extent of disease in the small airways [135].

(a) The natural history of untreated pulmonary hypertension

Numerous studies have shown that the level of pulmonary hypertension is moderate and progresses slowly in patients with COPD [115,136–140]. Weitzenblum and colleagues [139] studied the changes in pulmonary arterial pressure in a group of patients with COPD, over an average of 5 years, and found a mean increase in the pulmonary arterial pressure of only 3 mmHg/year. The change in pulmonary arterial pressure over this period was greater than 5 mmHg in only 33% of these patients. This sub-group of patients had baseline spirometry, arterial blood gas tensions and pulmonary hemodynamics which were similar to the group as a whole, but had progressive hypoxemia and hypercapnia, whereas those whose pulmonary arterial pressure remained stable showed no change in their arterial blood gas values. These data indicate the importance of worsening hypoxemia in the progression of pulmonary hypertension. This view is supported by the results of the MRC long-term oxygen trial [141] in which pulmonary arterial pressure rose by 3 mmHg/year in the untreated group, whereas the treated group showed no change in their pulmonary arterial pressure. However, not all studies support this view. Boushey and North [115] reported a mean increase in pulmonary arterial pressure of only 7% in 136 patients with COPD, studied over an average interval of 25 months, associated with a 6% increase in cardiac output, whilst Schrijen and colleagues [137] found no significant deterioration in pulmonary hemodynamics in a group of patients with COPD followed over three years, even when the pulmonary arterial pressure was elevated when first measured. However, in this study [137] 30% of the patients demonstrated a fall in systemic arterial pressure over time, which was thought to result from the peripheral vasodilatory effect of hypercapnia.

Despite the slow progression of pulmonary arterial hypertension in patients with COPD its presence implies a poor prognosis. Weitzenblum and co-workers [142] showed that patients whose pulmonary arterial pressure (Ppa) was normal (Ppa <20 mmHg had a 72% four-year survival compared with a 49% survival in those with an elevated pulmonary arterial pressure (Fig. 11.6a), a finding confirmed by others [143]. Burrows and colleagues [126] followed 50 patients with chronic airways obstruction over 7 years and showed that the hemodynamic parameter which correlated best with survival was the pulmonary vascular resistance. In this study none of the patients whose pulmonary vascular resistance exceeded 550 dynes/s/cm^5 survived for more than 3 years. However, in one study of patients with COPD with minimally raised pulmonary arterial pressure (Ppa 20–29 mmHg at rest), although mortality was 25% within three years, a similar percentage were alive after 10 years [144]. These conflicting data may relate to the duration of pulmonary hypertension in any individual patient. It is clear however, that some patients with COPD tolerate an elevated pulmonary arterial pressure remarkably well.

Weitzenblum and co-workers [142] showed that not only did pulmonary arterial pressure affect survival (Fig. 11.6a) but so did FEV$_1$ (Fig. 11.6b). France and colleagues [145] found that a number of variables correlated significantly with survival in 115 patients

Table 11.3 Factors affecting survival in 115 patients with COPD

Variable	x^{2a}	P
PaO$_2$	17.6	<0.0001
PaCO$_2$	15.7	<0.0001
Cor pulmonale	15.6	0.0001
FEV$_1$	9.5	0.002
FEV$_1$ (%predicted)	5.7	0.02
RVEF	4.5	0.03
FVC	3.0	0.08
FVC (% predicted)	1.1	0.31
LVEF	0.7	0.40

After France *et al.* (1988) [145].
[a]likelihood ratio test based on Cox survival model.
RVEF, LVEF, right and left ventricular ejection fractions respectively.

with COPD, including the PaO$_2$, PaCO$_2$, FEV$_1$ and the presence of peripheral edema (Table 11.3). Thus although numerous studies have shown an association between the presence of pulmonary arterial hypertension and prognosis in COPD, pulmonary hypertension may simply be a reflection of the severity of the disease, and may not have a direct effect on mortality.

(b) Oxygen transport in COPD

Survival in patients with COPD has also been correlated with oxygen transport and mixed venous oxygenation. In a group of 50 patients with stable COPD, survival was assessed over a four-year period, during which 27 of the 50 patients died [146]. In this study initial pulmonary hemodynamics were not significantly different between survivors and non-survivors, nor was oxygen transport or the coefficient of oxygen delivery (the ratio of oxygen delivery to oxygen consumption). However, arterial and mixed venous PO$_2$ were significantly lower in those who died. The authors concluded that tissue oxygenation had a more important influence on survival than defects of oxygen transport or delivery resulting from pulmonary hypertension. However, caution should be applied

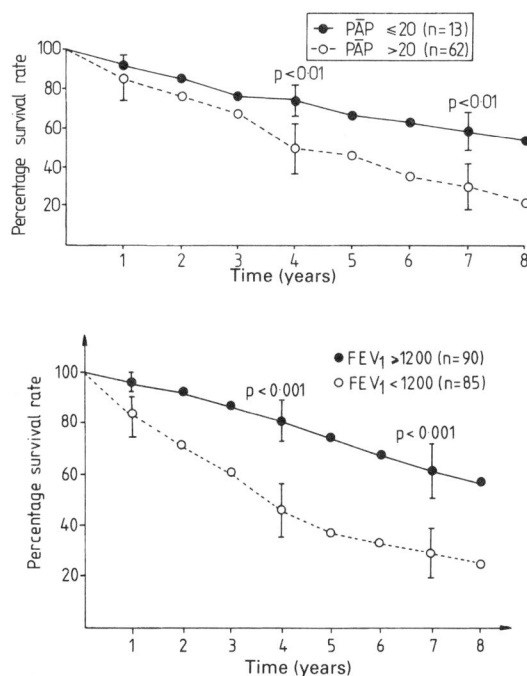

Fig. 11.6 Effect of (a) pulmonary arterial pressure, and (b) FEV$_1$ on survival in patients with COPD. (After Weitzenblum *et al.* (1981) [142].)

when interpreting these data [158] since only a small number of patients were studied and longitudinal hemodynamic or oxygen transport data were not available.

Oxygen is supplied to the tissues by two processes: first, convectional transport to the tissues in the vascular system, which is dependent on both the oxygen delivery and the oxygen consumption. The ratio of these two variables, the coefficient of oxygen delivery, was introduced by Mithoefer [147]. Second, the mixed venous oxygen tension ($P\bar{v}O_2$), which approximates the 'mean tissue oxygen tension', and is a determinant of the diffusion of oxygen into the tissues. Thus the $P\bar{v}O_2$ can be decreased by a reduction in PaO_2 due to lung disease, or due to a decrease in oxygen delivery as a result of fall in cardiac output in heart disease.

Thus in the study by Kawakami *et al.* [146], although there was an association between $P\bar{v}O_2$ and mortality, the coefficient of oxygen delivery was not different between survivors and non-survivors. By inference Tenney and Mithoefer [148] suggested that oxygen supply to the tissues is the critical factor which determines survival in such patients, and that the diffusional (mixed venous) component of tissue oxygen supply is more important than the convectional transport of oxygen in the vascular system, as measured by the coefficient of oxygen delivery.

It has been proposed in patients with COPD with decreased oxygen carriage, that maintenance of a normal, or indeed a high cardiac output may be an adaptive mechanism to maintain a normal tissue oxygen supply. Thus failure to maintain cardiac output may worsen survival [146]. It follows that vasodilators which increase oxygen delivery, by increasing cardiac output, may be beneficial in COPD [149]. Naeije [120] suggested that the increase in cardiac output induced by hypoxemia is inadequate for tissue needs in most patients with COPD and hypoxemia. In this study 61 patients with COPD were divided into two groups

depending on whether their $P\bar{v}O_2$ was greater than or less than or equal to 20 mmHg. The choice of a $P\bar{v}O_2$ of 20 mmHg was based on a study by Kasnitz *et al.* [150] which demonstrated that a $P\bar{v}O_2$ of $\leqslant 20$ mmHg in patients with COPD was associated with a uniformly fatal outcome. Despite more severe pulmonary hypertension and a lower PaO_2 in those with low values of $P\bar{v}O_2$, cardiac output was not different between the groups [120]. However, stroke–volume index was lower in those whose $P\bar{v}O_2$ was $\leqslant 20$ mmHg, and may have been insufficient for the degree of hypoxemia.

Paradoxically oxygen, when given to patients with COPD, does not always increase oxygen delivery. In a group of 35 patients presenting with acutely decompensated COPD [151], 28% oxygen, given for one hour, did not change cardiac output in 15 patients with severe hypoxemia, but oxygen delivery increased because of an increase in PaO_2. In the remaining 20 patients with lesser degrees of hypoxemia, oxygen delivery did not change because the increase in arterial oxygen content was offset by a fall in cardiac output [151]. The observation that only a proportion of patients 'respond' to oxygen therapy by increasing oxygen delivery has been confirmed in other studies of patients with both stable and decompensated COPD [152,153].

Thus in patients with COPD who develop hypoxemia one could hypothesize that an increase in cardiac output is a necessary adaptation to maintain mixed venous oxygenation, despite lower arterial oxygen saturation [154]. However, cardiac output generally remains normal or even slightly elevated in patients with COPD until very late in the course of the disease [155]. It follows that an inability to increase cardiac output in the face of worsening venous hypoxemia may be a maladaptation in COPD that adversely affects survival. This hypothesis remains unproven but has important implications for therapy directed at maintaining cardiac output and oxygen delivery [156].

11.2 CARDIAC FUNCTION

11.2.1 COR PULMONALE, RIGHT HEART FAILURE AND EDEMA: CONTROVERSIES IN DEFINITION

The term 'cor pulmonale' which was probably introduced by Paul D. White in 1931, is often misused as a synonym for 'right heart failure' secondary to pulmonary disease, or simply to indicate the presence of pulmonary hypertension in a patient with hypoxemia and COPD [157–159]. Cor pulmonale was defined by a WHO expert committee [160] as 'hypertrophy of the right ventricle resulting from diseases affecting the function and/or structure of the lungs, except when these pulmonary alterations are the result of disease that primarily affect the left side of the heart, as in congenital heart disease'. This is a pathologic rather than a functional definition, and is of limited clinical value since the diagnosis of right ventricular hypertrophy in life is imprecise [161]. The definition was revised by Behnke and colleagues [162] who replaced the term 'hypertrophy' by 'alteration in structure and function of the right ventricle'. This definition is also imprecise since it covers a spectrum of dysfunction from mild abnormality to frank right heart failure.

The problem of the definition of cor pulmonale makes comparisons between different studies difficult. Recently it has been proposed that the term cor pulmonale be abandoned in favour of a more precise description, based on objective evidence of right ventricular hypertrophy, enlargement, functional abnormality or failure [163]. A further problem is the lack of an accepted definition of heart failure [164]. Strobeck and Sonnenblick [165] suggest that heart failure could be described in two terms: 'myocardial failure' which refers to a decrease in the speed and force of the muscle contraction, which leads to 'pump failure'; 'congestive failure' on the other hand reflects the systemic response to 'pump failure', resulting in augmented sympathetic nervous system activity, renal vasoconstriction and activation of the renin–angiotensin system. Thus although myocardial failure always results in congestive failure, the reverse is not always true [166]. The European Society of Cardiology [167] defined heart failure as 'a state of any heart disease in which, despite adequate ventricular filling, the heart's output is decreased or in which the heart is unable to pump blood at a rate adequate for satisfying the requirements of the tissues with function parameters remaining within normal limits'. This definition is more applicable to the left side of the circulation. A more appropriate definition for the right ventricle is 'an inability of one or more chambers of the heart to accept and expel the venous return throughout the range of physiologic activity, without alteration of normal circulatory hemodynamics' [168]. The clinical syndrome of 'right heart failure' in chronic lung diseases has features different from those of left heart failure. The 'textbook' signs of right ventricular failure in COPD consist of raised jugular venous pressure, liver enlargement and peripheral edema but in contrast to left heart failure cardiac output is usually normal, and there is no vasoconstriction of the peripheral circulation [169].

The classic view of the development of 'heart failure' in patients with COPD is that hypoxia, in association with the other factors discussed previously, leads to pulmonary hypertension which imposes increased work on the right ventricle, leading to peripheral edema [170–172]. However, whether the edema of 'cor pulmonale' is truly 'cardiac' in origin remains the subject of debate [173–176].

11.2.2 PREVALENCE OF RIGHT VENTRICULAR HYPERTROPHY AND EDEMA

In a large European study of nearly 2000 autopsies in patients with 'lung disease', 8.9% of cases had right ventricular hypertrophy

[177]. In the UK, 40% of patients with COPD had autopsy evidence of right ventricular hypertrophy [178]. In the United States it has been estimated that 10–30% of all admissions with congestive cardiac failure are due to right ventricular hypertrophy and failure [171,179]. Considering all heart diseases 'cor pulmonale' is thought to make up 7–10% of all cases [180]. 'Cor pulmonale' in patients with COPD increases in prevalence as airflow limitation worsens, occurring in 40% of patients with an FEV_1 <1.0 l and in 70% when the FEV_1 falls to 0.6 l [2,123]. The prevalence of cor pulmonale is also higher in patients with hypercapnia, hypoxemia and polycythemia [2,123].

The development of edema in patients with hypoxic COPD is usually a late feature [181] and may appear during acute exacerbations of the condition. However, a proportion of patients, who develop pulmonary hypertension, or indeed right ventricular hypertrophy, never develop peripheral edema [182]. In two studies of 100 and of 59 patients respectively with severe COPD who were free of edema at the time of presentation, edema developed for the first time at a rate of 6% per annum over a three- to four-year follow-up period [183,184]. In a further study of 65 patients with COPD of whom 58% had moderate to severe airflow limitation, and most had hypoxemia, at least one episode of edema occurred over a follow-up period of 5.4 years, producing an incidence of 11% [138].

A large number of factors influence survival in patients with COPD. In a recent review of the literature by Hodgkin [185], age and post bronchodilator FEV_1 were the best predictors of mortality in COPD. However, several studies have shown that either the presence of pulmonary arterial hypertension or peripheral edema in patients with hypoxic COPD correlates with survival [2,142,145, 186–193]. Patients with COPD who develop peripheral edema but are not treated with long-term oxygen therapy have only a 27–33% 5 year survival [185].

11.2.3 METHODS OF ASSESSING CARDIAC FUNCTION

The majority of studies which have assessed pulmonary hemodynamics and right ventricular function in patients with COPD have employed invasive techniques since a full assessment of pulmonary hemodynamics requires measurement of pressure and flow which involves cardiac catheterization. Moreover, assessment of right ventricular function and measurement of chamber volumes is difficult because of the variable and irregular shape of the right ventricle, even in normal subjects [194]. Until recently contrast angiography was the only method to assess right ventricular volumes [195]. More recently non-invasive techniques have been employed to study patients with COPD including chest radiography, M-mode and two-dimensional echocardiography, radionuclide ventriculography and magnetic resonance imaging.

(a) Clinical assessment

The clinical signs of pulmonary hypertension or right ventricular dysfunction are often difficult to detect in patients with COPD because of hyperinflation of the chest and the slight posterior rotation of the heart in these patients [1,157,169]. The jugular venous pressure in patients with COPD is also often difficult to assess due to large swings in thoracic pressure, and pedal edema can be due to other causes, such as a hypoalbuminemia. Accentuation of the pulmonary component of the second heart sound indicates pulmonary hypertension and a systolic left parasternal heave indicates right ventricular hypertrophy or dilatation, but is often masked by hyperinflation. Extra heart sounds, or the murmur of tricuspid regurgitation, which are best heard on inspiration also suggest right ventricular dysfunction, but again may be obscured by hyperinflation. All of these signs develop relatively late in the clinical course of patients with COPD and are not sensitive indicators of pulmonary hypertension or right ventricular hypertrophy. The physiologic measurement which correlates best with pulmonary arterial hypertension in patients with COPD is the arterial oxygen saturation breathing air [72].

(b) Radiography

The width of the right descending pulmonary artery has been used to detect pulmonary arterial hypertension in patients with COPD [196,197]. Matthay and co-workers [197] in a study of 61 patients with COPD found that the widest dimension of the right descending pulmonary artery was >16 mm in 43 of 46 patients with pulmonary hypertension, whereas Chetty and colleagues [196] suggested that a right descending pulmonary artery of ≥20 mmHg discriminated best between those patients with and without pulmonary arterial hypertension. In addition a high value of the hilar cardiothoracic ratio was 95% sensitive and 100% specific for pulmonary hypertension in patients with COPD [196]. However, methods which employ plain chest radiography cannot predict the level of pulmonary arterial pressure in any individual patient, but may be useful as a screening procedure to detect pulmonary arterial hypertension.

Right ventricular hypertrophy or dilatation is also not easily discernible on a plain chest radiograph, although dilatation of the right ventricle gives the heart a globular appearance. On the lateral film encroachment of the retrosternal airspace can be a helpful sign to confirm that the enlarged silhouette is secondary to right ventricular dilatation [198,199].

(c) Electrocardiography

Electrocardiographic criteria for detecting right ventricular hypertrophy are highly specific, but have a low sensitivity. In a recent study using several ECG criteria for right ventricular hypertrophy [200] (Table 11.4), correct identification of right ventricular hypertrophy was confirmed in 75% of cases at autopsy. However, isolated right ventricular hypertrophy was present in only 53%, and only 25% of these patients had COPD [200].

Vector cardiography is no more sensitive than conventional electrocardiography [201] and techniques such as kinetocardiography [202] or orthostatic changes in CO transfer factor are of poor predictive value in patients with COPD [203].

(d) Echocardiography

Hyperinflation of the chest increases the retrosternal air space which therefore transmits sound waves poorly, making echocardiography difficult in patients with COPD. An adequate examination has been reported in 65–80% of patients with COPD [203,204]. The use of transesophageal echocardiography should improve the percentage of patients where an adequate assessment can be made [204].

Abnormal motion of the pulmonary valve, as assessed by M-mode echocardiography has been used to detect the presence of pul-

Table 11.4 ECG criteria for diagnosing RV hypertrophy

Right axis deviation greater than 100° without right bundle branch block

R or R′ ≥ S in V_1 or V_2

R < S in V_6

A + R PL ≥ 0.7

RV hypertrophy is considered to be present if one or more of the above criteria are met.

(Adapted from Lehtonen *et al.* (1988) [200].)
A, maximal R or R′ amplitude in V_1 or V_2.
R, maximal S in lead I or V_6.
PL, minimal S in V_1 or minimal R in lead I or V_6.

monary hypertension. Delayed opening of the valve, mid-systolic closure, and an increase in the ratio of right ventricular pre-ejection time to total ejection time have been reported in patients with pulmonary hypertension [205,206].

The blood velocity in the main pulmonary artery can be used to estimate the pulmonary arterial pressure [207]. The interval between the onset of right ventricular ejection and peak velocity (time to peak velocity) correlates fairly well with the mean pulmonary arterial pressure in patients with COPD ($r = 0.73$) [208]. However, a record of the flow velocity from the pulmonary valve may not be possible in 50% of patients using M-mode echocardiography [209].

The addition of doppler echocardiography has led to improved assessment of right ventricular systolic ejection flow to estimate pulmonary arterial pressure [210,211]. However, relatively few studies have been performed in patients with COPD [212].

Two other measurements can be used to estimate peak systolic pulmonary arterial pressure. They are the mean right atrial pressure and the peak systolic gradient between the right atrium and the right ventricle. The addition of these two pressures yields the systolic pulmonary arterial pressure. It is also possible to estimate the pulmonary end-diastolic pressure non-invasively by summing the mean right atrial pressure and the end-diastolic gradient between the pulmonary artery and the right ventricular out-flow tract. Right atrial pressure can be estimated from the height of the jugular venous pulse, but this correlates poorly with pressures measured at catheterization [210] in patients with COPD due to the large changes in intrathoracic pressure [207]. A fixed estimate of right atrial pressure of between 5–12 mmHg has been proposed [211], but this can lead to considerable error. A more accurate estimate of right arterial pressure can be obtained by studying the degree of collapse of the proximal inferior vena cava by echocardiography during voluntary deep inspiration [213]. However, this technique becomes inaccurate in patients with COPD since the inferior vena cava collapses spontaneously during respiration in these patients.

Measurement of the right ventricular–atrial gradient can be assessed by doppler echocardiography [214], using the regurgitant jet from the tricuspid valve [207]. Tricuspid regurgitation occurs in both normal subjects [215] and in patients with COPD [216]. The high prevalence of tricuspid regurgitation was noted as long ago as 1908 by Sir James McKenzie during his studies of external pulses using kymography [217]. He found that tricuspid insufficiency was so common that he was 'inclined to look upon the valves as being rarely able to close the orifice properly'. More recently Morrison and colleagues [216] found, in a study of 100 patients with COPD, that significant tricuspid regurgitation occurred in the majority, which could lead to an overestimation of the right ventricular ejection fraction in this group. Similarly in a recent study by Himelman and co-workers [218] tricuspid regurgitation was detected in 20 of 36 patients with COPD. The quality of the signal for detecting tricuspid insufficiency using continuous wave doppler can be improved by augmenting the signal by an intravenous infusion of saline [218,219]. However, this may be a problem in patients with COPD, where fluid overload may be already present. From the peak velocity of the tricuspid regurgitant jet (V), the modified Bernoulli equation ($P = 4V^2$) allows calculation of the peak pressure difference between the right ventricle and atrium. As indicated above the addition of this pressure gradient to the mean right atrial pressure allows calculation of the peak pulmonary arterial pressure.

Using continuous wave doppler even with intravenous saline contrast, an adequate assessment cannot be obtained in 35% of patients [220]. However, pulsed wave doppler echocardiography appears to be even more sensitive in detecting tricuspid insufficiency. Using this technique Migueres and co-workers [208] were able to assess pulmonary arterial pressure in 91% of patients with COPD. Moreover pulsed doppler echocardiography is also capable of assessing changes in pulmonary arterial pressure during exercise [208].

Numerous studies have shown correlations between echocardiographic measurements of pulmonary arterial pressure and pressures measured at cardiac catheterization [210,211, 221,222], some in patients with COPD (r = 0.98) [218].

M-mode echocardiography can also be used to measure right ventricular free wall thickness, end-diastolic dimensions and the diameter of the pulmonary artery. Detection of right ventricular hypertrophy by echocardiography is limited by the ability to differentiate the true right ventricular wall from its surrounding structures. Moreover, correlations between right ventricular wall thickness and right ventricular weight are poor even when measured at autopsy [223,224]. Measurement of right ventricular diastolic diameter by echocardiography may be useful in detecting right ventricular enlargement. This is particularly true in patients who have had previous episodes of decompensated right ventricular function, provided adequate echocardiographs can be obtained [203].

Two-dimensional (2-D) echocardiography, which has an improved accuracy over conventional M-mode techniques [209], has been used to assess right ventricular dimensions and wall thickening and hence to detect right ventricular volume overload in patients with COPD [225–228]. However, calculation of right ventricular volumes by 2-D echocardiography is fraught with problems, including the lack of a 'gold standard' by which echocardiographic measurements of volume can be assessed. Contrast angiographic measurements of right ventricular volumes involve a number of assumptions and mathematical calculations, due to the irregularity of the right ventricular cavity [195,229], which may have led to the variable correlations in the literature between volume measurements by echocardiography and contrast angiography.

Changes in right ventricular function are difficult to detect by echocardiography and doppler in patients with COPD and pulmonary arterial hypertension. Prolongation of the right ventricular pre-ejection time, and shortening of the ejection time may be present in such patients. However, right ventricular systolic time intervals are also affected by increased right ventricular preload. The position and the curvature of the intraventricular septum also gives an indication of right ventricular afterload. In the normal ventricle the interventricular septum moves to the left during systolic ejection and to the right during diastolic filling. Right ventricular volume overload tends to reverse this pattern, whereas right ventricular pressure overload displaces the septum towards the left ventricle [230].

(e) Radionuclide assessment of right ventricular ejection fraction

As discussed above contrast angiography has been used to measure right ventricular volumes, however the technique is difficult and tedious, because of the wide variability in right ventricular geometry [194,195]. Radionuclide ventriculography largely overcomes this problem and is usually performed using an intravenous injection of [99m]technetium-labelled erythrocytes or human serum albumin [231,232]. A gamma camera is used to obtain a time/activity curve, either during the first pass of the radio-tracer or by gating several points throughout the cardiac cycle once the radio-tracer has equilibrated in the blood pool [232]. Since radioactive counts acquired in this way are proportional to volume, variations in the geometric configuration of the ventricle are less important.

In the first pass technique a bolus injection of the radio-tracer is injected intravenously and followed during a few cardiac cycles as the bolus passes through the right side of the heart, to obtain time/activity curves from a region of interest around the right ventricle [233]. The right ventricular ejection fraction (RVEF) is the difference between the end-diastolic and end-systolic counts divided by the end-diastolic counts. The first pass technique allows the ventricles to be separated in time and in space (avoiding the problems of overlap between the two chambers). However, sequential measurements require repeated bolus injections of the radio-tracer and hence a larger radiation burden. Furthermore, the short acquisition time produces low counts and thus statistical uncertainty in calculating the ejection fraction. The gated equilibrium technique provides better count statistics since data from several hundred cardiac cycles are acquired [232,234]. Thus repeated measurements can be made over three hours following a single injection of a radio-tracer.

Although the reproducibility of radionuclide measurements of RVEF is good when measurements are repeated in patients with COPD studied in the same position, the reproducibility decreases when measurements are made on the same individual on different days [235]. This may reflect the inherent variably of RVEF in patients with COPD, or positional changes which result in variable ventricular and atrial overlap. The presence of tricuspid regurgitation, particularly in patients with COPD may also lead to an overestimation of the RVEF [216]. In 30 normal subjects the mean RVEF was 0.50 ± 0.09 (range 0.47–0.83) [233]. This gives a lower limit of normal (2 standard deviations below the mean) for RVEF of 0.40 when measured at rest, which increased in normal subjects during exercise by at least 0.05 [232].

[201]thallium myocardial scintigraphy has been used to diagnose right ventricular hypertrophy in patients with pulmonary arterial hypertension from various causes [236–240] including patients with COPD

[240,241]. A study by Weitzenblum and colleagues [241] in 46 patients with COPD showed that the sensitivity of [201]thallium imaging for the diagnosis of right ventricular pressure overloading was 73%. However, this is a qualitative rather than quantitative technique which has not found favor clinically, and probably has no advantage over echocardiography.

(f) Right ventricular dimensions measured by magnetic resonance imaging (MRI)

Magnetic resonance imaging is probably now the gold standard for measuring ventricular dimensions since it produces the best images of the right ventricle [242]. This technique is non-invasive and does not impose a radiation burden, but is expensive and only available in specialized centers. In preliminary studies in patients with COPD [243], the right ventricular free wall volume correlated significantly with the pulmonary arterial pressure ($r = 0.72$, $P <0.01$) and with the pulmonary vascular resistance ($r = 0.65$, $P <0.01$). Interestingly, the right ventricular free wall volume, as an estimate of wall mass correlated with the Pa_{CO_2} but not with the Pa_{O_2} [243]. This non-invasive technique can therefore be used to measure right ventricular dimensions, define right ventricular hypertrophy and to study the effect of therapeutic interventions in patients with COPD.

Recently Chappuis, Dorsaz and Rutishauser [244] developed a technique to measure right ventricular function by intravenous digital angiography, using simultaneous measurements of right ventricular volume, generated by computer from the time/volume curve during the cardiac cycle, and measurements of right ventricular pressure, using a catheter tip manometer. This sophisticated technique holds some promise for measuring right ventricular function, as does MRI imaging [245].

11.2.4 RIGHT VENTRICULAR FUNCTION

(a) In health

The differences which exist between the two ventricles in adults appear to be due to the different flow-resistance conditions in the two circulations [246,247]. The right ventricle has a concave free wall and a convex intraventricular septum producing a crescent-shaped chamber. Contraction of the right ventricle is produced by three maneuvers [116,248–250]. The longitudinal axis of the chamber shortens and the trabeculae and papillary muscles force the tricuspid valve plane downwards toward the apex. This initial contraction contributes very little toward effective ejection. Thereafter, the concave right ventricular free wall and the convex septum contract, followed by contraction of the left ventricle, which increases the curvature of the intraventricular septum. The function of right ventricular contraction appears to be to generate sufficient stroke volume to maintain adequate cardiac output, rather than to generate pressure, and operates therefore as a 'volume', rather than a 'pressure' pump [250]. In general the thin-walled right ventricle which contracts against the low pressure pulmonary circulation, is more compliant than the thicker-walled left ventricle. The geometric configuration of the right ventricle is therefore thought to be more suited to ejecting large volumes of blood, with minimal myocardial shortening. Therefore, the right ventricle can adapt to considerable variations in systemic venous return, without producing large changes in filling pressures [247,250, 251] because of the greater ratio of volume to surface area in the right, compared with the left ventricle, but is less able to cope with an acute increase in afterload [247,250,251]. This contrasts with the left ventricle which acts as a pressure pump in the high-resistance systemic circulation and has a small surface area relative to its intracavity volume [252]. An inter-dependence between the ventricles has

been suggested [253], particularly in the presence of right ventricular overload which may shift the intraventricular septum leftward and impair the contractility of the left ventricle [226]. The clinical significance of this is unknown.

(b) In COPD

Chronic pressure overload may lead to changes in the configuration, mass and function of the right ventricle. However, the effect on right ventricular function of a moderate degree of pulmonary hypertension, which slowly progresses in patients with COPD, is likely to be different from the effects of acute pulmonary hypertension, such as occurs in massive pulmonary embolism [254] or indeed the effects of the sustained 'systemic' levels of pulmonary arterial pressure which are present in patients with primary pulmonary hypertension [255]. Therefore the right ventricle may have time to adapt to the increase in pressure load in COPD.

As pulmonary hypertension develops in patients with COPD, right ventricular stroke work index increases on exercise due to an increase in pressure work. However, in patients with stable COPD, the relationship between the right ventricular stroke work index and right ventricular end-diastolic pressure suggests that although the right ventricular stroke work index is higher in these patients, they operate on an extension of the normal right ventricular function curve (Fig. 11.7) [117]. The diastolic pressure in the right ventricle can be normal, even in those patients who report episodes of peripheral edema in the past, and who have clinical evidence of right ventricular enlargement [117]. However, during exercise, right ventricular end-diastolic pressure is elevated in the majority of patients. The presence of a normal right ventricular end-diastolic pressure at rest in patients with COPD is at least presumptive evidence of a normal right ventricular end-diastolic volume [256].

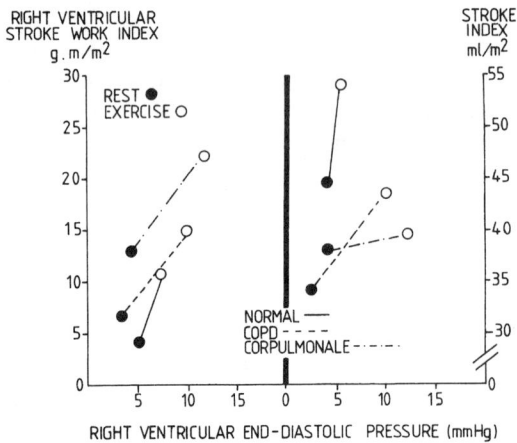

Fig. 11.7 Right ventricular stroke work index in normal subjects and patients with COPD and cor pulmonale. When stroke index (right) is related to right ventricular end-diastolic pressure, patients with cor pulmonale do not have a normal increase in stroke index during exercise, suggesting depressed right ventricular function. However, right ventricular stroke work index increases during exercise in all three groups (left), those with COPD and cor pulmonale operating on the extension of the normal right ventricular function curve. (Modified from Khaja *et al.* (1971) [118].)

Although the mean RVEF in patients with COPD (as assessed by radionuclides) is lower than in normal subjects [232,257–260], there is considerable overlap between values of RVEF in normal subjects and patients with COPD. Indeed it may be that only those patients who are edematous at the time of study have a low RVEF [176,234]. Values of the RVEF in patients with COPD are rarely as low as in patients with right ventricular infarction [261]. However, the normal increase in RVEF does not occur with exercise in such patients [258,259,262–264] suggesting that latent right ventricular dysfunction occurs in patients with COPD.

The 'right ventricular hypothesis' suggests that right ventricular function is compromised in patients with 'cor pulmonale' which influences survival [265,266]. However, there is considerable variation in the correlation

between pulmonary arterial pressure and RVEF in the literature [35,257,267–276]. Differences in the techniques used to measure RVEF may account for this variation. However, RVEF depends not only on right ventricular afterload but on ventricular contractility and preload. Moreover, pulmonary arterial pressure is not an accurate reflection of the right ventricular afterload, which is the stress or tension acting on the fibers of the right ventricular wall immediately after the onset of shortening [277], i.e. the force per unit cross-sectional area acting on the right ventricular wall [278]. The pulmonary arterial pressure has been used as an estimate of the right ventricular afterload, but this represents only a fraction of the true afterload. The pulmonary vascular resistance may be a slightly more accurate reflection of the true right ventricular afterload, but it is still an approximation. Thus measurement of RVEF should not be regarded as a non-invasive estimation of the pulmonary arterial pressure in patients with COPD.

The most important factors affecting right ventricular performance are preload, afterload, contractility and heart rate [279,280]. Ventricular preload is the force per cross-sectional area acting on the ventricular muscle fiber bundles immediately before they contract [280]. Changes in preload affect end-diastolic volume, which is an important determinant of ventricular function and is often assessed by the end-diastolic pressure/stroke volume curve [165]. End-diastolic pressure is not always an accurate substitute for end-diastolic volume, particularly in COPD [117,118].

Ventricular afterload is the instantaneous tension on the ventricular wall during active contraction [230]. It is directly related to both the intracavity pressure in the ventricle and the internal ventricular dimension, and inversely to the ventricular wall thickness. It can be measured in the left ventricle as the mean midwall circumferential wall stress and has been shown to correlate with the left ventricular ejection fraction [281]. This measurement is not possible in the right ventricle due to geometric constraints [194].

Ventricular contractility is a measure of the ability of cardiac muscle to perform stroke work, independent of changes in initial fiber length [280]. It is useful to assess changes in ventricular contractility which are independent of those caused by alterations in either preload or afterload or both [165]. It is also important to distinguish between 'myocardial contractility' and ventricular 'pump function'. Adverse loading conditions can induce the ventricle to fail as a pump without depressing myocardial contractility. Moreover, ventricular pump function may be maintained in the presence of poor myocardial contractility by favorable loading conditions. Thus ventricular failure should be subdivided into 'myocardial failure', resulting in a decrease in the speed and force of muscle contraction, which if severe leads to 'pump failure' with a low cardiac output and 'congestive failure', which consists of the systemic responses to an inadequate pump, such as augmentation of sympathetic nervous system activity, renal vasoconstriction and activation of the renin–angiotensin system. Categorizing heart failure in this way helps to explain the incongruity between the hemodynamic findings and the clinical picture in patients with COPD [249].

In patients with COPD, cardiac output is normal in the majority of subjects [282–284], even those with clinical 'congestive failure' [91,262]. The RVEF is not a good measurement of intrinsic right ventricular contractility, since it also depends on preload and afterload [285]. In order to assess the contractility or inotropic state of the right ventricle, rather than its global performance, as measured by the RVEF, it is necessary to assess a function of the ventricle which is independent of changes in preload and afterload.

New indices of contractility, reviewed by Sagawa [286] were developed initially to assess left ventricular function. These depend on the relationship between the pressure and volume of the ventricle at end-systole. Changes in the relationship between ventricular pressure and volume can be plotted as a continuous pressure–volume loop in isolated heart preparations. The end-systolic pressure–volume relationship has been shown to be independent of the initial ventricular volume [286]. For a given contractile state, an increase in afterload produces less complete emptying of the ventricle and an increase in end-systolic volume [287]. However, the end-systolic pressure–volume ratio remains constant, indicating that this relationship is also independent of changes in afterload. The relationship between end-systolic pressure and volume in the left ventricle shifts downwards and to the right in conditions of decreased contractility, such as heart failure, and upwards and to the left, increasing its slope, with increasing contractility [259,288] (Fig. 11.8). Thus this relationship defines the inotropic state of the ventricle independent of loading conditions [289]. Similar relationships have also been confirmed for the right ventricle [288]. The slope of the end-systolic pressure–volume relation describes the interaction between afterload and systolic performance and is termed the 'ventricular systolic elastance' [230]. The peak elastance (Emax) is a particularly good index of the contractile state of the ventricle [289]. The slope of the end-systolic pressure–volume relation in the right ventricle is less than that of the left ventricle resulting in a greater volume change for a given change in pressure.

Measurement of the end-systolic pressure–volume relation in the right ventricle has a number of problems. The relationship may not always be linear [290] and it may be not entirely independent of the loading conditions [291], since it may also be sensitive to changes in ventricular compliance [292]. Moreover, if measurements of right ventricular volumes are made using radionuclide ventriculography, right ventricular end-ejection and true end-systole may not always coincide [293]. Furthermore, to assess the slope of the end-

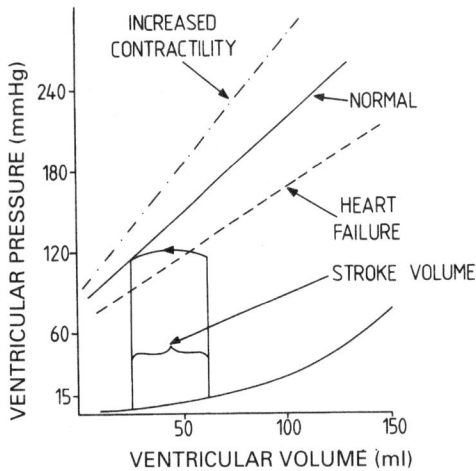

Fig. 11.8 End-systolic pressure–volume relationship is linear, but it is displaced downwards and to the right in heart failure and upwards and to the left when contractility is increased.

systolic pressure–volume relationship, measurements must be made under two or more loading conditions [294]. Allowing for these constraints simultaneous measurements of stroke volume by right heart catheterization and the thermodilution technique and RVEF by radionuclide ventriculography allow quantification of right ventricular volume, which together with simultaneous measurement of right ventricular pressure, allows measurement of the end-systolic pressure–volume relationship in patients with COPD, as an assessment of right ventricular contractility.

In a study of 20 patients with severe but stable COPD [276] who were hypoxemic, with variable degrees of hypercapnia and pulmonary arterial pressure (25 ± 9 mmHg), the mean end-systolic index was 37 ± 16 ml/m². Measurement of the right ventricular pressure–volume relation as a single point, or of the slope of this relation [295] suggest relatively well preserved right ventricular contractility, in the presence of pulmonary hypertension. In most clinically stable COPD patients the end-systolic pressure–volume ratio is displaced to the left, suggesting

normal, if not hypernormal contractility. These data have been confirmed by other workers [268]. However, Brent *et al.* [35] in a combined radionuclide/cardiac catheterization study, found right ventricular function to be depressed in COPD. This discrepancy may be due to differences in the technique used to measure RVEF. Right ventricular function is also well preserved in other forms of pulmonary hypertension [296]. Moreover in 24 patients with COPD, most of whom had pulmonary arterial hypertension, there was relatively little change in most patients in the end-systolic volume, even in the face of a large increase in right ventricular systolic pressure during exercise [276]. Other indices of right ventricular function also suggest that right ventricular function is preserved in patients with COPD and pulmonary hypertension [118,254,296].

(c) Right ventricular function in acute exacerbations

Although in most studies of patients with stable hypoxic COPD the mean pulmonary arterial pressure is 25–35 mmHg [276], during exacerbations the pulmonary arterial pressure rises to 45–70 mmHg [91,297,298] as the result of several mechanisms which include worsening hypoxia, acidosis, and changes in pulmonary mechanics. However, not every patient who develops pulmonary hypertension during an exacerbation has signs of 'right ventricular failure'. The pathophysiology of edema formation in COPD remains unresolved and is unlikely to be solely due to depressed right ventricular function as a result of chronic but mild pulmonary hypertension.

There have been relatively few studies of pulmonary hemodynamics in patients with COPD who present acutely with edema [25,91,117,299–301]. Abraham and co-workers [91] studied 8 patients with COPD presenting with acute respiratory failure, of whom six had peripheral edema. Hemodynamics were measured by cardiac catheterization on the day of admission, daily thereafter for five days and again upon recovery. This study presents the most convincing evidence of a rise in pulmonary arterial pressure during an exacerbation of COPD. However, right ventricular mechanics were not measured. In a more recent study the end-systolic and end-diastolic volumes in patients with COPD presenting acutely with edema were higher, and therefore the pressure–volume ratio was lower than in stable patients, suggesting decreased contractility in the group with edema, but with a preserved cardiac output [300]. However, this increase in ventricular volume did not appear to result from an augmented right ventricular afterload, since ventricular volumes were normal in patients with a similar level of pulmonary arterial pressure and pulmonary vascular resistance, but without peripheral edema [300]. Thus the cause of the decreased right ventricular contractility in these patients remains unresolved.

11.3 SALT, WATER AND HORMONAL BALANCE

For over 30 years doubts have been expressed over whether the edema in patients with COPD is truly 'cardiac' in origin [302,303]. Fulton and co-workers [161] noted that some patients with chronic bronchitis and emphysema who were hypoxemic and had edema in life, did not have right ventricular hypertrophy at autopsy. These early studies led Campbell and Short [86] to suggest that the sequence of events: pulmonary hypertension → right ventricular hypertrophy → right ventricular failure → venous engorgement → edema was not 'the invariable sequence in patients who become edematous, and it may in fact be uncommon.'

11.3.1 EFFECTS OF BLOOD GASES AND ACID–BASE STATUS

Although hypoxemia is invariably present in patients with COPD who have edema, hypox-

emia is present to a similar degree in patients with fibrotic lung disease, where edema is rare until the preterminal stage of the disease. Severe hypoxemia induces secondary polycythemia [304] which may contribute to the development of pulmonary arterial [305] and renal arteriolar vasoconstriction [306,307], which reduces renal function and increases acidosis through the formation of lactic acid. Hypoxemia may also promote a shift of fluid from the intra to the extracellular space [308,309] and increases the permeability of the pulmonary capillaries [310].

In a review of the literature from the 1950s, Campbell and Short [86] found only 2 cases of 150 they reviewed with chronic lung diseases, who had edema and a normal $PaCO_2$. This led them to suggest that hypercapnia was the central factor in the development of edema in hypoxic COPD. Their suggested sequence of events was: hypoventilation → respiratory acidosis → renal tubular exchange of hydrogen ion for sodium + reabsorption of bicarbonate → fluid retention → increased work of breathing → further hypoventilation producing a self-aggravating cycle for the development of edema.

Chronic hypercapnia increases the renal threshold for bicarbonate excretion, which results from an increased conversion in the renal tubular cells of carbon dioxide to HCO_3^- and H^+ by carbonic anhydrase [311]. An increase in plasma bicarbonate reduces the responsiveness of the respiratory centers to carbon dioxide, leading to a self-aggravating cycle of hypoventilation [309]. This cycle can be exacerbated by diuretics which, by reducing extracellular fluid volume, results through a process termed 'contraction alkalosis' in a further rise in HCO_3^- [312].

11.3.2 RENAL FUNCTION

Renal function in COPD has been studied from the early 1950s [302,303]. The most consistent observation in these early studies was a reduced renal blood flow in patients with

COPD and hypoxemia, particularly in those with edema [302,303,306,313,314]. This is followed by an increase in renal blood flow during the diuretic phase and a return to normal renal blood flow in convalescence [315,316]. Several mechanisms have been proposed to account for the reduction in renal blood flow. Reducing cardiac output produces a fall in renal blood flow [77]. Hypoxia and hypercapnia may also decrease renal blood flow [316], which may also fall because of an increase in pulmonary arterial and central venous pressures or volumes, which activates central blood volume receptors, enhancing the normal sympathetic activity [317]. More recent studies have also shown that effective renal plasma flow is reduced in patients who have hypercapnia [318] and is reduced further, in association with a reduction in glomerular filtration rate and sodium and water excretion [319,320], in patients with hypercapnia and edema [321]. Although hypoxemia alone is not associated with abnormal salt or water handling, the withdrawal of long-term supplemental oxygen, resulting in acute hypoxemia in patients with chronic hypercapnia reduces urinary sodium excretion [322]. Furthermore, since acute hypoxemia does not produce a fall in the fractional absorption of sodium [323], hypoxemia appears to affect glomerular rather than tubular function, which may be related to vascular autoregulation [322]. In addition, continuous oxygen therapy over a period of six days in patients with hypoxic COPD increased urinary sodium excretion [324].

The vasopressin response to changes in plasma osmolarity induced by water loading appears to be similar in normal subjects and in patients with COPD who have both hypoxemia and hypercapnia [318,319]. However, in patients who are both hypoxemic, hypercapnic and who have edema, vasopressin levels are inappropriately high for the plasma osmolarity, in some cases associated with hyponatremia [319]. These abnormalities of salt and water handling, in association with the disturbance in renal function described above, may contribute to the formation of edema in patients with advanced COPD.

The presence of edema in patients with COPD is not necessarily associated with a significant increase in body weight or total body water [325]. When a diuresis is induced in patients with COPD who have edema, body weight falls, but subsequently, during convalescence, weight increases [325]. These data may be explained by the exchange of fluid between the intra- and extracellular compartments [308]. Furthermore, total exchangeable sodium may be stable at a time when weight is fluctuating, and therefore the changes in body weight may result from changes in tissue proteins [326].

11.3.3 RENIN–ANGIOTENSIN–ALDOSTERONE SYSTEM

Several studies have shown changes in hormonal balance in patients with COPD and chronic respiratory failure. Activation of the renin–angiotensin–aldosterone system [319, 322,327,328] and elevated circulating catacholamines [322,329] occur in such patients. The activity of the renin–angiotensin–aldosterone system is increased in the majority of patients with COPD and edema [320,330–332]. A significant correlation has been shown between plasma renin and aldosterone levels and the ability to excrete sodium, free water clearance and the levels of plasma arginine vasopressin [320,321]. Furthermore, patients with COPD whose edema fails to respond to conventional treatment with oxygen and diuretics have a persistently elevated plasma renin [321]. However, interpretation of these studies is complicated by differences in blood gas values, sodium and potassium status, treatment with diuretics and long-term oxygen therapy in the patients studied.

Acute hypoxia increases plasma renin substantially in animal studies [333,334], but chronic hypoxia produces a more variable effect on plasma renin activity [335–337]. In human studies, acute hypoxemia has a variable effect on plasma renin [332,338–340] probably because of variations in sodium intake and diuretic therapy between study patients. Chronic hypoxia has been studied in healthy volunteers exposed to real or simulated high altitude, again with variable effects on the renin–angiotensin system [341–345] possibly due to variations in experimental conditions both in the degree and the duration of the hypoxemia.

Angiotensin-converting enzyme is present in the vascular bed of the lung and converts angiotensin I to angiotensin II [346,347]. Some studies of simulated or actual altitude exposure have shown that there is a dissociation in the effect of hypoxemia on plasma renin and aldosterone. Chronic hypoxia produces a variable change in plasma renin activity and in most studies a decrease in aldosterone [341,348–352]. Although initial studies suggested that this was due to a reduction in angiotensin-converting activity by hypoxemia [342,345], this is not the case in patients with COPD [353]. Indeed the relationship between plasma renin activity and plasma angiotensin II, which is an index of physiologic ACE activity, does not appear to be affected by hypoxemia and exercise in COPD patients [328]. Various mechanisms could account for a reduction in aldosterone during hypoxia, including inhibition of angiotensin-converting enzyme, intra-renal dopamine release, increased aldosterone clearance and changes in potassium and atrial natriuretic peptide.

11.3.4 ATRIAL NATRIURETIC PEPTIDE (ANP)

ANP is released from the atria and has potent natriuretic, diuretic and vasodilating properties [354]. Its release is stimulated by atrial distension [354] and circulating levels are high in patients with various edematous disorders [355–359]. Plasma ANP is elevated in patients with stable COPD [342,360,361]

and is especially high in patients with edema [362]. The inability of elevated plasma ANP to prevent edema in such patients does not result from an inability to respond to an increase in venous pressure by the release of ANP [363]. Indeed infusing ANP still results in a natriuresis in patients with hypoxic COPD [364], suggesting that the kidney is still responsive to ANP. Atrial natriuretic peptide can also suppress the renin–angiotensin– aldosterone system [365]. However, both ANP and renin levels are high in hypoxic COPD, suggesting that the effects of ANP may be overridden by a reduction in renal perfusion, producing stimulation of the renin– angiotensin system.

Atrial natriuretic peptide has a number of potential beneficial effects in preventing edema formation, including a natriuretic effect [366,367] depression of plasma renin activity [368,369] and inhibition of angiotensin II-mediated aldosterone production [365,370]. Moreover ANP produces pulmonary vasodilatation [364].

Thus a complex interaction between changes in pulmonary hemodynamics, salt, water and hormonal balance probably accounts for the clinical syndrome of edema in patients with hypoxic COPD (Fig. 11.9). However, the precise nature of these interactions is not fully understood.

11.4 VASODILATOR TREATMENT OF PULMONARY VASCULAR DISEASE

The major rationale for treating pulmonary hypertension in patients with COPD is that the presence of pulmonary hypertension reduces survival [142], as does a low mixed pulmonary venous oxygen tension [146]. Thus pulmonary vasodilators, by decreasing right ventricular afterload and allowing cardiac output to increase should improve oxygen transport, tissue oxygenation and perhaps survival, as well as improving symptoms in patients with hypoxic COPD [120,156,371,372].

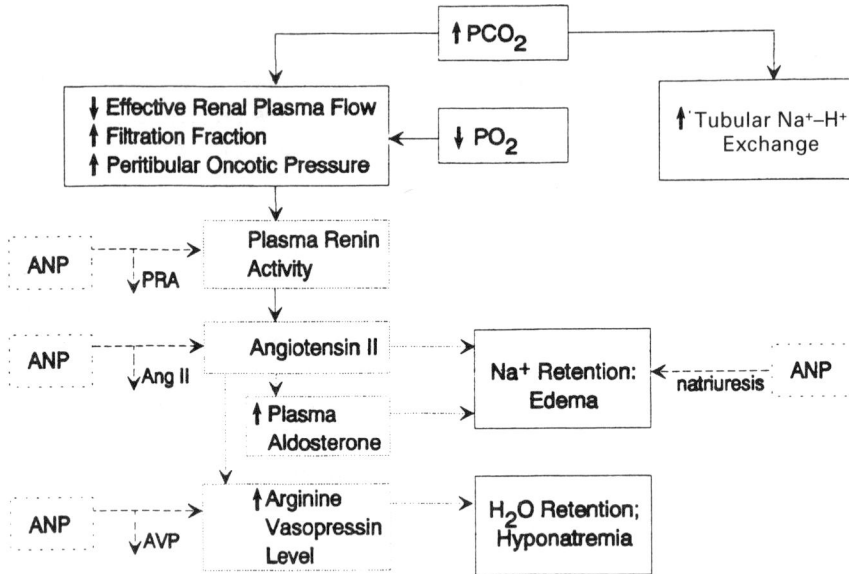

Fig. 11.9 Mechanisms of sodium and water disturbance in patients with COPD. (Modified from Farber *et al.* (1982) [320].)

The best measurement to assess outcome when treating patients with COPD and pulmonary hypertension with pulmonary vasodilators is still not clear. For example, a decrease in pulmonary vascular resistance may result from an increase in cardiac output, in the face of an unchanged, or slightly increased pulmonary arterial pressure. Moreover, the assumption that the pressure–flow relationship in the pulmonary circulation is linear and passes through the origin is questionable [30,373,374]. Furthermore, in patients with COPD the left atrial pressure, which is estimated by the pulmonary capillary wedge pressure, may not be the true outflow pressure of the pulmonary circulation [25], which may alter the interpretation of the effects of pulmonary vasodilators on pulmonary vasomotor tone. Thus pulmonary vascular resistance may not be the best variable to study the effects of a vasodilator [373,374].

Enthusiasm for treating patients with COPD and pulmonary hypertension with vasodilators arose from their apparent beneficial effects in primary pulmonary hypertension

[375]. This early enthusiasm has diminished, because of failure to sustain the acute effects of many vasodilators, the difficulty in carrying out long-term studies requiring repeated invasive measurements, the need for long-term multicenter studies of large numbers of patients to show an effect on survival, and the fact that no agent, with the exception of oxygen has been shown to cause pulmonary vasodilatation without producing systemic vasodilatation. More specific pulmonary vasodilators may become available when the mechanism of the hypoxic pulmonary vasoconstrictor response is elucidated [376]. An added complexity is the difficulty in predicting the effect which reversing vasoconstriction has on arterial oxygen tensions due to changes in ventilation and perfusion. However, a rise in cardiac output may still increase oxygen delivery to the tissues.

In spite of a lack of specificity of vasodilator drugs for the pulmonary circulation, the rarity of a reduction in pulmonary arterial pressure to normal by vasodilators in patients with COPD, and the possible deleterious effects on gas exchange, a large number of studies using these drugs have been undertaken in patients with COPD [120,372]. Most studies have assessed the acute effects of vasodilators on pulmonary hemodynamics in patients with COPD.

11.4.1 α-ADRENERGIC BLOCKERS

Phentolamine and tolazoline are non-selective α-adrenergic antagonists which reduce pulmonary arterial pressure in patients with COPD [377,378], but their clinical use is limited by side effects. Prazosin is a selective post-synaptic α_1-antagonist which reduces pulmonary arterial pressure and increases cardiac output in COPD. These effects were sustained after 8 weeks' treatment, but were associated with worsening dyspnea and a fall in SaO_2 [379]. Urapidil, a centrally acting α_1 selective antagonist reduced pulmonary arterial pressure in COPD, without changing cardiac output at rest or during exercise, an effect which did not result in an improvement in maximal oxygen consumption [380]. These studies also illustrate a further problem in comparing the studies of vasodilators in the literature, since the severity of pulmonary hypertension and the blood gas abnormalities may vary widely in different studies.

11.4.2 β-ADRENERGIC AGONISTS

β_2-Agonists given either intravenously or orally to patients with COPD produce trivial changes in pulmonary arterial pressure. However, pulmonary vascular resistance usually falls as a result of an increase in cardiac output [295,381–387]. In some studies the increase in cardiac output has been associated with a fall in oxygen saturation [295,383,387]. β_2-Agonists have also been shown to increase right ventricular ejection in most studies [295,388,389]. These drugs also have an inotropic effect, as shown by changes in the right ventricular pressure–volume relationship [295,385]. Although a fall in pul-

monary arterial pressure has been shown both acutely and over 6 weeks with the β_2-agonist pirbuterol [295] this effect was not sustained over 2 months' treatment [390].

11.4.3 CALCIUM CHANNEL BLOCKERS

The calcium channel blockers vary considerably in their effect on the pulmonary circulation, probably due to differences in the pharmacologic actions of the different drugs in this group [391]. Animal studies have shown that nifedipine can prevent or even reverse hypoxic pulmonary vasoconstriction [392–395]. A similar effect has been shown in at least one study with patients with COPD [396]. Given acutely [396–402] nifedipine reduced pulmonary vascular resistance and increased cardiac output in all but one study [402]. However, a reduction in pulmonary arterial pressure did not occur in all studies, but has been demonstrated during exercise [401,402]. Verapamil and diltiazem appear to be relatively ineffective in the pulmonary circulation [403,404].

In most studies although nifedipine causes a slight fall in SaO_2, this effect is offset by the increase in cardiac output, so that oxygen delivery increases which may improve exercise tolerance if this is limited by oxygen delivery. The deleterious effect of nifedipine on gas exchange is thought to result in part from a reduction in hypoxic vasoconstriction [399]. It has no effect on right ventricular ejection fraction in the short or the long-term [405].

In spite of a persistent pulmonary vasodilator action of nifedipine in studies of up to 9 weeks' treatment, there was no associated improvement in symptoms [398]. Other studies of between 6 weeks' and 18 months' treatment with nifedipine show no significant changes in pulmonary hemodynamics [406–408], nor any consistent long-term effect of felodipine [409]. In an uncontrolled study over 10 months' treatment the newer calcium antagonist nitrendipine produced persistent pulmonary vasodilatation in COPD but without improvement in symptoms or in survival [410]. Since nifedipine is thought to interfere with hypoxic vasoconstriction, its combination with oxygen therapy has been studied with a beneficial effect in one study [396] but not in another [397].

11.4.4 HYDRALAZINE

Since hydralazine has been used in the treatment of primary pulmonary hypertension [411] its effects have also been studied in COPD. In this case hydralazine produces a consistent increase in cardiac output, but there is considerable variation in the reduction in pulmonary artery pressure [412–417], with little effect on oxygen saturation and hence hypoxic vasoconstriction. Hydralazine has been shown to improve right ventricular function by some workers [410,415] but not by others [417]. The long-term effects of hydralazine on pulmonary hemodynamics in COPD have not been studied. Chronic dosage has been limited by the development of a systemic lupus erythematosus-like syndrome after long-term treatment in a dose of greater than 200 mg/day [418].

11.4.5 THEOPHYLLINES

Given acutely theophyllines reduce pulmonary arterial pressure and pulmonary vascular resistance without changing cardiac output [419–422]. Although theophyllines are both bronchodilators and ventilatory stimulants, they may produce a fall in oxygen saturation [421]. Theophyllines have also been shown to increase right ventricular ejection fraction acutely [423,424] with a sustained effect after three months' treatment [425].

11.4.6 ANGIOTENSIN-CONVERTING ENZYME (ACE) INHIBITORS

There was a hope that angiotensin-converting enzyme inhibitors may be a more specific

treatment for patients with hypoxic COPD and edema and that they may have beneficial effects over the long term, not only on pulmonary hemodynamics, but also on salt and water balance, exercise tolerance and survival as was found in patients with congestive cardiac failure [426]. By reducing the production of angiotensin II, ACE inhibitors may interfere with the control by angiotensin II of renal blood flow, an effect mediated through the efferent renal artery [427,428]. In addition, if ACE inhibitors interfere with hypoxic vasoconstriction, gas exchange may worsen in COPD, which has been demonstrated in preliminary studies [429]. Studies using the competitive angiotensin II antagonist saralasin to block the renin–angiotensin system have shown a beneficial effect on oxygenation, but a decrease in cardiac output in patients with various chronic pulmonary diseases, including COPD [430]. Burke and colleagues [429] found that 25 mg of captopril 3 times daily, combined with supplemental oxygen in a small group of patients with pulmonary hypertension due to COPD, reduced pulmonary arterial pressure and vascular resistance, with an associated increase in cardiac output. However, in a placebo-controlled study of 15 patients with COPD and cor pulmonale Zielinski *et al.* [431] found no significant change in either pulmonary hemodynamics or gas exchange following 25 mg of captopril and a similar negative result has been shown with a newer ACE inhibitor enalaprilat [432]. In view of the beneficial effects of captopril on salt and water balance in patients with COPD [433], long-term studies of captopril on exercise tolerance and survival in patients with COPD may be warranted.

11.4.7 OTHER VASODILATORS

Short-term acute studies with various intravenous vasodilators such as prostaglandin E_1 [434], adenosine triphosphate [435] and atrial natriuretic peptide [364] have shown a beneficial effect on pulmonary hemodynamics, with a fall in pulmonary artery pressure and pulmonary vascular resistance and an increase in cardiac output. The development of oral derivatives of these agents will be necessary before they will be therapeutically viable.

Nitric oxide (NO) is an important endogenous vasodilator. Preliminary results indicate that inhaled NO is a potent and selective pulmonary vasodilator [436,437] producing a fall in pulmonary vascular resistance from 1.9 (0.2) to 1.5 (0.2) mmHg/l/min (P <0.05) without a change in systemic vascular resistance in patients with pulmonary hypertension [437]. Whether these preliminary results will lead to an effective long-term treatment for pulmonary hypertension with no toxicity awaits further study.

The most important 'pulmonary vasodilator' used at present is domiciliary oxygen therapy which is considered in detail elsewhere (Chapter 20).

11.5 CONCLUSIONS

The hypothesis that hypoxemia resulting in pulmonary hypertension adversely affects right ventricular function and produces edema in patients with COPD and therefore subsequently reduces their survival, has not been validated by published studies. It seems unlikely therefore that treatment which directly affects cardiac function or produces pulmonary vasodilatation will have a significant long-term effect on survival in patients with pulmonary hypertension secondary to COPD. Whether such interventions have a long-term effect on exercise or symptoms also remains to be proven. It would appear that a more logical therapeutic option is to correct hypoxemia, which has proven beneficial effects on survival, or to investigate the long-term effects of more specific therapies aimed at improving salt, water and hormonal balance in these patients. It may be true that patients with COPD die with 'cor pulmonale' but they rarely die of it!

REFERENCES

1. Fishman, A.P. (1976) State of the art: chronic cor pulmonale. *Am. Rev. Respir. Dis.*, **114**, 775–94.
2. Renzetti, A.D. Jr, McClement, J.H. and Litt, B.D. (1966) The Veterans Administration co-operative study of pulmonary function. III. Mortality in relation to respiratory function in chronic obstructive pulmonary disease. *Am. J. Med.*, **41**, 115–9.
3. Cumming, G., Harding, L.K., Horsfield, K. *et al.* (1970) Morphological aspects of the pulmonary circulation and of the airways, in *Advisory Group for Aerospace Research and Development*, NATO Conference Proceedings No. 65.
4. Singhal, S., Henderson, R., Horsfield, K. *et al.* (1973) Morphometry of the human pulmonary arterial tree. *Circ. Res.*, **33**, 190–7.
5. Horsfield, K. (1978) Morphometry of the small pulmonary arteries in man. *Circ. Res.*, **42**, 593–7.
6. Heath, D., Du Shane, J.W., Wood, E.H. *et al.* (1959) Structure of the pulmonary trunk at different ages and in cases of pulmonary hypertension and pulmonary stenosis. *J. Path. Bact.*, **77**, 443–56.
7. von Euler, U.S. and Liljestrand, G. (1946) Observations on the pulmonary arterial blood pressure in the cat. *Acta Physiol. Scand.*, **12**, 301–20.
8. von Euler, U.S. and Lishajko, F. (1958) Catecholamines in the vascular wall. *Acta Physiol. Scand.*, **42**, 333–41.
9. Burton, A.C. (1954) Relation of structure to function of tissues of walls of blood vessels. *Physiol. Res.*, **34**, 619–23.
10 Weibel, E.R. (1963) *Morphometry of the Human Lung*, Springer-Verlag, Berlin, pp. 78–82.
11. Beyers, N., Doerschuk, C.M., Coxson, H. *et al.* (1989) Neutrophil volume and capillary segment diameter in the rabbit, the dog and the human. *Am. Rev. Respir. Dis.*, **139**, A297.
12. Schmid-Schonbein, G.W., Shih, Y.Y. and Chien, S. (1985) Morphometry of human leukocytes. *Blood*, **56**, 866–75.
13. MacNee, W. and Selby, C. (1990) Neutrophil kinetics in the lungs. *Clin. Sci.*, **79**, 97–107.
14. Drinkler, C.K. (1945) *Pulmonary Oedema and Inflammation*, Harvard University Press, Cambridge.
15. Robotham, J.L., Lixfeld, W., Holland, L. *et al.* (1978) Effects of respiration on cardiac performance. *J. Appl. Physiol.*, **44**, 703–9.

16. Thomas, L.J., Griffo, Z.J. and Roose, A. (1961) Effect of negative-pressure inflation of the lung on pulmonary vascular resistance. *J. Appl. Physiol.*, **16**, 451–6.

17. Weibel, E.R. and Gomez, D.M. (1962) The architecture of the human lung. *Science*, **137**, 577–85.

18. Bainbridge, F.A. (1931) *The Physiology of Muscular Exercise*, 3rd edn (Rewritten by A.V. Bock and D.B. Dill), Longmans & Green, London.

19. Knapp, E. and Gureiner, R. (1977) Reduction of pulmonary hypertension by nitroprusside. *Int. J. Clin. Pharmacol. Ther. Toxicol.*, **15**, 75–80.

20. Pace, J.B. (1978) Pulmonary vascular response to sodium nitroprusside in anaesthetised dogs. *Anesth. Analg. Cleveland*, **57**, 551–7.

21. Weir, E.K., Reeves, J.T. and Grover, R.E. (1975) Prostaglandin E, inhibits the pulmonary vascular pressor response to hypoxia and prostaglandin F 2. *Prostaglandins*, **10**, 623–31.

22. Harris, P. and Heath, D. (1986) Normal variations in pressure and flow, in *The Human Pulmonary Circulation*, 3rd edn, (eds P. Harris and D. Heath), Churchill Livingstone, Edinburgh, pp. 149–60.

23. West, J.B., Dollery, C.T. and Naimark, A. (1964) Distribution of blood flow in isolated lung: relation to vascular and alveolar pressures. *J. Appl. Physiol.*, **19**, 713–24.

24. Murray, J.F. (1986) *The Normal Lung*, Saunders, Philadelphia.

25. Lockhart, A., Tzareva, M., Nader, F. *et al.* (1969) Elevated pulmonary artery wedge pressure at rest and during exercise in chronic bronchitis – fact or fancy? *Clin. Sci.*, **37**, 503–17.

26. Harris, P. and Heath, D. (1986) Resistance, in *The Human Pulmonary Circulation*, 3rd edn, (eds P. Harris and D. Heath), Churchill Livingstone, Edinburgh, pp. 122–35.

27. Carlen, S.E., Hansen, H.E. and Nordenstöm, B. (1951) Temporary unilateral occlusion of the pulmonary artery. *J. Thorac. Surg.*, **22**, 527–36.

28. Segel, N. and Bishop, J.M. (1966) The circulation in patients with chronic bronchitis and emphysema at rest and during exercise with special reference to the influence of change in blood viscosity and blood volume on the pulmonary circulation. *J. Clin. Invest.*, **45**, 1555–68.

29. Widimsky, J. (1970) Pressure, flow and volume changes in the lesser circulation during pulmonary artery occlusion in healthy subjects and patients with pulmonary hypertension. *Prog. Respir. Res.*, **5**, 224–36.

30. Harris, P., Segel, N. and Bishop, J.M. (1968) The relation between pressure and flow in the pulmonary circulation in normal subjects and in patients with chronic bronchitis and mitral stenosis. *Cardiovasc. Res.*, **2**, 73–83.

31. Fishman, A.P. (1961) Respiratory gases in the regulation of pulmonary circulation. *Physiol. Rev.*, **41**, 214–80.

32. Sancetta, S.M. and Rakita, L. (1957) Response of pulmonary artery pressure and total pulmonary resistance of untrained, convalescent man to prolonged mild steady state exercise. *J. Clin. Invest.*, **36**, 1138–49.

33. Donald, K.W., Bishop, J.M., Cumming, G. *et al.* (1955) The effect of exercise on the cardiac output and circulatory dynamics of normal subjects. *Clin. Sci.*, **14**, 37–73.

34. Slonin, M.B., Rabin, A., Balchum, O.J. *et al.* (1954) The effect of mild exercise in the supine position on the pulmonary arterial pressure of five normal human subjects. *J. Clin. Invest.*, **33**, 1022–30.

35. Brent, B.N., Berger, H.J., Matthay, R.A. *et al.* (1982) Physiologic correlates of right ventricular ejection fraction in chronic obstructive pulmonary disease. A combined radionuclide hemodynamic study. *Am. J. Cardiol.*, **50**, 255–62.

36. Riley, R.L., Himmelstein, A., Morley, H.L. *et al.* (1948) Studies of the pulmonary circulation at rest and during exercise in normal individuals and in patients with chronic pulmonary disease. *Am. J. Physiol.*, **152**, 372–82.

37. Hasleton, P.S., Heath, D. and Brewer, D.B. (1968) Hypertensive pulmonary vascular disease in states of chronic hypoxia. *J. Pathol. Bacteriol.*, **95**, 431–40.

38. Lamb, D. (1990) Pathology of COPD, in *Respiratory Medicine*, (eds R.A.L. Brewis, G.J. Gibson and D.M. Geddes), Baillière-Tindall, London, pp. 497–507.

39. Wilkinson, M., Langhorn, C.A., Heath, D. *et al.* (1988) A pathophysiological study of 10 cases of hypoxic cor pulmonale. *Q. J. Med.*, **66**, 65–85.

40. Wright, J.L., Lawson, L., Paré, P. *et al.* (1983) The structure and function of pulmonary vasculature in mild chronic obstructive pulmonary disease; the effect of oxygen on exercise. *Am. Rev. Respir. Dis.*, **128**, 702–7.

41. Magee, F., Wright, J.L., Wiggs, B.R. *et al.* (1988) Pulmonary vascular structure and function in chronic obstructive pulmonary disease. *Thorax*, **43**, 183–9.

42. Dunhill, M.S. (1960) Fibrinoid necrosis in the branches of the pulmonary artery and chronic non-specific lung disease. *Br. J. Dis. Chest*, **54**, 355–60.

43. Calverley, P.M.A., Howatson R., Flenley, D.C. and Lamb, D. (1992) Clinicopathological correlations in hypoxic cor pulmonale. *Thorax*, **47**, 494–8.

44. Bignon, J., Khourg, F., Even, P. *et al.* (1969) Morphometric study in chronic obstructive broncho-pulmonary disease. Pathologic, clinical and physiologic correlations. *Am. Rev. Respir. Dis.*, **99**, 669–95.

45. Hale, K.A., Niewoehner, D.E. and Cosio, M.G. (1980) Morphologic changes in the muscular pulmonary arteries: Relationship to cigarette smoking, airway disease and emphysema. *Am. Rev. Respir. Dis.*, **122**, 273–8.

46. Abraham, A.S., Kay, J.M., Cole, R.B. *et al.* (1971) Haemodynamic and pathological study of the effect of chronic hypoxia and subsequent recovery of the heart and pulmonary vasculature of the rat. *Cardiovasc. Res.*, **5**, 95–102.

47. Fishman, A.P. (1976) Hypoxia and its effects on the pulmonary circulation. How and where it acts. *Circ. Res.*, **38**, 221–31.

48. Moret, P.R. (1980) Hypoxia and the heart, in *Hearts and Heart-like Organs*, (ed. G.H. Bourne), Academic Press, New York, Vol. 2, pp. 338–87.

49. Hicken, P., Brewer, D. and Heath, D. (1966) The relation between the weight of the right ventricle of the heart and the internal surface area and the number of alveoli in the human lung in emphysema. *J. Pathol. Bacteriol.*, **92**, 529–46.

50. Hicken, P., Heath, D. and Brewer, D. (1966) The relation between the weight of the right ventricle and the percentage of abnormal air space in the lung in emphysema. *J. Pathol. Bacteriol.*, **92**, 519–28.

51. Hickam, J.B. and Cargill, W.H. (1948) Effect of exercise on cardiac output and pulmonary arterial pressure in normal persons and in patients with cardiovascular disease and pulmonary emphysema. *J. Clin. Invest.*, **27**, 10–23.

52. Mahler, D.A., Brent, B.N., Loke, J. *et al.* (1984) Right ventricular performance and central circulatory hemodynamics during upright exercise in patients with chronic obstructive pulmonary disease. *Am. Rev. Respir. Dis.*, **130**, 722–9.

53. Limt, P.K. and Brownlee, W.E. (1968) Pulmonary haemodynamics in obstructive lung diseases. *Dis. Chest*, **53**, 113–7.

54. Gurtner, H.P. Walser, P. and Fassler, B. (1975) Normal values for pulmonary haemodynamics at rest and during exercise in man. *Prog. Resp. Res.*, **9**, 295–315.

55. Wilhelmsen, L., Selander, S., Sonderholm, B. *et al.* (1963) Recurrent pulmonary embolism. *Medicine*, **42**, 335–55.

56. Mounsey, J.P.D., Ritzman, L.W., Selverstone, N.H. *et al.* (1952) Circulatory changes in severe pulmonary emphysema. *Br. Heart J.*, **14**, 153–72.

57. Weitzenblum, E., Roeslin, N., Hirth, C. *et al.* (1970) A comparative study of clinical and functional data between chronic bronchitis and primary emphysema. *Respiration*, **27**, 493–510.

58. Thurlbeck, W.M. and Simon, G. (1978) Radiographic appearance of the chest in emphysema. *Am. J. Roentogen.*, **130**, 429–40.

59. MacNee, W., Gould, G. and Lamb D. (1991) Quantifying emphysema by CT scanning: clinicopathological correlates, in *Pulmonary Emphysema: The Rational for Therapeutic Intervention* (eds G. Weinbaum, R.E. Giles and R.D. Krell), *Ann. N.Y. Acad. Sci.*, **624**, pp. 179–194.

60. Gould, G.A., MacNee, W., McLean, A. *et al.* (1988) CT measurements of lung density in life can quantitate distal airspace enlargement – an essential defining feature of human emphysema. *Am. Rev. Respir. Dis.*, **137**, 380–92.

61. Biernacki, W., Gould, G.A., Whyte, K.F. *et al.* (1989) Pulmonary hemodynamics, gas exchange and the severity of emphysema as assessed by quantitative CT scan in chronic bronchitis and emphysema. *Am. Rev. Respir. Dis.*, **139**, 1509–15.

62. Harvey, R.M., Ferrer, M.I., Richards, D.W. *et al.* (1951) Influence of chronic pulmonary disease on the heart and circulation. *Am. J. Med.*, **10**, 719–38.

63. Fishman, A.P., Fritts, H.W. and Cournand, A. (1960) Effects of acute hypoxia and exercise on the pulmonary circulation. *Circulation*, **22**, 204–15.

64. Dymond, D.S., Elliot, A., Stone, D. *et al.* (1981) Factors that affect the reproducibility of measurements of left ventricular function from first pass radionuclide ventriculograms. *Circulation*, **65**, 311–22.

65. Emirgil, C., Sobol, B.J. and Herbert, W.H. (1971) Routine pulmonary function studies as a key to the status of the lesser circulation in chronic obstructive pulmonary disease. *Am. J. Med.*, **50**, 191–9.

66. Fowler, N.O., Westcott, R.N., Scott, R.G. *et al.* (1952) The cardiac output in chronic cor pulmonale. *Circulation*, **6**, 888–93.

67. Horsfield, K., Segel, N. and Bishop, J.M. (1968) The pulmonary circulation in chronic bronchitis at rest and during exercise breathing air and 80% oxygen. *Clin. Sci.*, **34**, 473–83.

68. Millard, J. and Reid, L. (1974) Right ventricular hypertrophy and its relationship to chronic bronchitis and emphysema. *Br. J. Dis. Chest*, **68**, 103–10.

69. Whitaker, W. (1954) Pulmonary hypertension in congestive heart failure complicating chronic lung disease. *Q. J. Med.*, **23**, 57–72.

70. Williams, J.F. and Behuke, R.H. (1964) The effect of pulmonary emphysema upon cardiopulmonary haemodynamics at rest and during exercise. *Ann. Intern. Med.*, **60**, 824–42.

71. Yu, P.N., Lovejoy, F.W., Joos, H.A. *et al.* (1953) Studies of pulmonary hypertension I. Pulmonary circulatory haemodynamics in patients with pulmonary emphysema at rest. *J. Clin. Invest.*, **32**, 130–7.

72. Bishop, J.M., and Cross, K.W. (1981) Use of other physiological variables to predict pulmonary arterial pressure in patients with chronic respiratory disease – a multicentre study. *Eur. Heart J.*, **2**, 509–17.

73. Wilson, R.H., Hoseth, W. and Dempsey, M.G. (1955) The effects of breathing 99.6% oxygen on pulmonary vascular resistance and cardiac output in patients with pulmonary emphysema and chronic hypoxia. *Ann. Intern. Med.*, **42**, 629–37.

74. Kitchen, A.H., Lowther, C.P. and Mathews, M.D. (1961) The effects of exercise and breathing oxygen-enriched air on the pulmonary circulation in emphysema. *Clin. Sci.*, **21**, 93–106.

75. Aber, G.M., Harris, A.M. and Bishop, J.M. (1964) Effect of acute changes in inspired oxygen concentration on cardiac, respiratory and renal function in patients with chronic obstructive airways disease. *Clin. Sci.*, **26**, 133–43.

76. Sime, F., Penaloza, D. and Ruiz, L. (1971) Bradycardia, increased cardiac output, and reversal of pulmonary hypertension in altitude natives living at sea level. *Br. Heart J.*, **33**, 647–57.

77. Aber, G.M., Bayley, T.J. and Bishop, J.M. (1963) Inter-relationships between renal and cardiac function and respiratory gas exchange in obstructive airways disease. *Clin. Sci.*, **25**, 159–70.

78. Kilburn, K.H., Asmundsson, T., Britt, R.C. *et al.* (1969) Effects of breathing 10% carbon dioxide on the pulmonary circulation of human subjects. *Circulation*, **39**, 639–53.

79. Rokseth, R. (1966) The effect of altered blood carbon dioxide tension and pH on the human pulmonary circulation. *Scand. J. Clin. Lab. Invest.*, **18**(Suppl), 90–4.

80. Harris, P., Segel, N., Green, J. *et al.* (1968) The influence of the airways resistance and alveolar pressure on the pulmonary vascular resistance in chronic bronchitis. *Cardiovasc. Res.*, **2**, 84–94.

81. Durand, J., Leroy-Ladurie, M and Ransom-Bitker, B. (1970) Effects of hypoxia and hypercapnia on the repartition of pulmonary blood flow in supine subjects. *Prog. Resp. Res.*, **5**, 156–65.

82. Enson, Y., Guintini, C., Lewis, M.L. *et al.* (1964) The influence of hydrogen ion concentration and hypoxia on the pulmonary circulation. *J. Clin. Invest.*, **43**, 1146–62.

83. Harvey, R.M., Enson, Y., Betti, R. *et al.* (1967) Further considerations of the causes of pulmonary hypertension in cor pulmonale. *Bull. Physiopathol. Resp.*, **3**, 623–32.

84. Housley, E., Clarke, S.W., Hedworth-Whitty, R.B. *et al.* (1970) Effect of acute and chronic acidaemia and associated hypoxia on the pulmonary circulation of patients with chronic bronchitis. *Cardiovasc. Res.*, **4**, 482–9.

85. Bergofsky, E.H., Lehr, D.E. and Fishman, A.P. (1962) Effect of changes in the hydrogen ion concentration on the pulmonary circulation. *J. Clin. Invest.*, **41**, 1492–501.

86. Campbell, E.J.M. and Short, D.S. (1960) The cause of oedema in 'cor pulmonale'. *Lancet*, **1**, 1184–6.

87. Weitzenblum, E., Gharbi, T.E., Vonderemme, A. *et al.* (1972) Pulmonary haemodynamic

changes during muscular exercise in non-decompensated chronic bronchitis. *Bull. Physiopath. Resp.*, **8**, 49–71.

88. Lockhart, A., Nader, F., Tzareva, M. *et al.* (1970) Comparative effects of exercise and isocapnic voluntary hyperventilation on pulmonary haemodynamics in chronic bronchitis and emphysema. *Europ. J. Clin. Invest.*, **1**, 69–76.

89. Matthay, R.A., Niederman, M.S. and Weidemann, H.P. (1990) Cardiovascular-pulmonary interaction in chronic obstructive pulmonary disease with special reference to the pathogenesis and management of cor pulmonale. *Med. Clin. North Am.*, **74**, 571–618.

90. Abraham, A.S., Hedworth-Whitty, R.B. and Bishop, J.M. (1967) Effects of acute hypoxia and hypervolemia singly and together upon the pulmonary circulation in patients with chronic bronchitis. *Clin. Sci.*, **33**, 371–80.

91. Abraham, A.S., Cole, R.B., Green, I.D. *et al.* (1969) Factors contributing to the reversible pulmonary hypertension in patients with acute respiratory failure studied by serial observations during recovery. *Circ. Res.*, **24**, 51–60.

92. Lewis, M.L., Gnoj, J., Fisher, V.J. *et al.* (1970) Determinants of pulmonary blood volume. *J. Clin. Invest.*, **49**, 170–82.

93. Raffestin, B., Valette, H., Herbert, J.L. *et al.* (1977) Pulmonary blood volume in chronic bronchitis. *Clin. Sci. Mol. Med.*, **53**, 587–93.

94. Wedzicha, J.A., Rudd, R.M., Apps, M.C.P. *et al.* (1983) Erythropheresis in patients with polycythemia secondary to hypoxic lung disease. *Br. Med. J.*, **286**, 511–4.

95. Reeves, J.T. and Voelkel, N.F. (1989) Mechanisms of chronic pulmonary hypertension: basic considerations, in *Pulmonary Circulation, Advances and Controversies*, (eds C.A. Wagenvoort and H. Denolin), Elsevier, Amsterdam, pp. 27–39.

96. Palmer, R.M.J., Ferrdge, A.G. and Moncada, S. (1987) Nitric oxide release accounts for the biological activity of endothelium-derived relaxing factor. *Nature*, **327**, 524–6.

97. Myers, P.R., Minor, R.L., Guerra, R. *et al.* (1990) Vasorelaxant properties of the endothelium-derived relaxing factor more closely resemble S-nitrosocysteine nitric oxide. *Nature*, **345**, 167–173.

98. Rubanyi, G.M., Romero, J.C. and Van Houtte, P.M. (1986) Flow induced release of endo-thelium-derived relaxing factor. *Am. J. Physiol.*, **250**, H1105–H1149.

99. Murad, F. (1986) Cyclic guanosine monophosphate as a mediator of vasodilatation. *J. Clin. Invest.*, **78**, 1–5.

100. Meyrick, B. and Reid, L. (1978) The effect of continued hypoxia on rat pulmonary arterial circulation: an ultra-structural study. *Lab. Invest.*, **38**, 188–200.

101. Ignarro, L.J. (1989) Biological actions and properties of endothelium-derived nitric oxide formed and released from artery and vein. *Circ. Res.*, **65**, 1–21.

102. Dinh-Xuan, A.T. (1992) Endothelial modulation of pulmonary vascular tone. *Eur. Resp. J.*, **5**, 757–62.

103. Thom, S., Hughes, A., Martin, G. *et al.* (1987) Endothelium-dependent relaxation of isolated human arteries and veins. *Clin. Sci.*, **73**, 547–52.

104. Greenberg, B., Rhoden, K. and Barnes, P.J. (1987) Endothelium-relaxation of human pulmonary arteries. *Am. J. Physiol.*, **252**, H434–H438.

105. Dinh-Xuan, A.T., Higenbottam, T.W., Clelland, C.A. *et al.* (1990) Acetylcholine and adenosine diphosphate cause endothelium-dependent relaxation of isolated human pulmonary arteries. *Eur. Resp. J.*, **3**, 633–8.

106. Yamaguchi, T., Rodman, D.M., O'Brian, R.F. *et al.* (1989) Modulation of pulmonary artery contraction by endothelium-relaxing factor. *Eur. J. Pharmacol.*, **161**, 259–62.

107. Dinh-Xuan, A.T., Higenbottam, T.W., Clelland, C.A. *et al.* (1991) Effect of endothelium-dependent pulmonary artery relaxation in chronic obstructive lung disease. *N. Engl. J. Med.*, **324**, 1539–47.

108. Palmer, R.M.J., Ashton, D.S. and Moncad, S. (1988) Vascular endothelial cells synthesis oxide from L-arginine. *Nature*, **333**, 664–6.

109. Crawley, D.E., Liu, S.F., Evans, T.W. *et al.* (1990) Inhibitory role of endothelium-derived relaxing factor in rat and human pulmonary arteries. *Br. J. Pharmacol.*, **101**, 166–70.

110. Liu, S.F., Crawley, D.E., Barnes, P.J. *et al.* (1991) Endothelium-derived relaxing factor inhibits hypoxic pulmonary vasoconstriction in rats. *Am. J. Respir. Dis.*, **143**, 32–7.

111. Adnot, S., Raffestin, B., Addahibi, S. *et al.* (1991) Loss of endothelium-dependent relaxant activity in the pulmonary circulation of

rats exposed to chronic hypoxia. *J. Clin. Invest.*, **87**, 155–62.

112. Moncada, S., Palmer, R.M.J., and Higgs, E.A. (1987) Prostacyclin and endothelial-derived relaxing factor: biological interactions and significance, in *Thrombosis and Haemostasis*, (eds M. Verstraete, J. Verrmylen and R.H. Lijnen), University Press, Leuven, Belgium, pp. 597–618.

113. Borden, C.W., Wilson, R.H.G., Ebert, R.V. *et al.* (1950) Pulmonary hypertension in chronic pulmonary emphysema. *Am. J. Med.*, **8**, 701–9.

114. Berglund, E. (1972) Haemodynamics of the right ventricle in chronic lung disease. *Bull. Physiol.-Pathol. Resp.*, **8**, 1417–22.

115. Boushy, J.F., North, L.B. (1977) Haemodynamic changes in chronic obstructive pulmonary disease. *Chest*, **72**, 565–70.

116. Burrows, B., Kettel, L.J., Niden, A.H. *et al.* (1972) Patterns of cardiovascular dysfunction in chronic obstructive lung disease. *N. Engl. J. Med.*, **286**, 912–8.

117. Jezek, V., Schrijen, F and Sadoul, P. (1973) Right ventricular function and pulmonary haemodynamics during exercise in patients with chronic obstructive broncho-pulmonary disease. *Cardiology*, **58**, 20–31.

118. Khaja, F. and Parker, J.O. (1971) Right and left ventricular performance in chronic obstructive lung disease. *Am. Heart J.*, **82**, 319–27.

119. Harris, P. and Heath, D. (1977) Pulmonary haemodynamics in chronic bronchitis and emphysema, in *The Human Pulmonary Circulation*, 3rd edn, (eds P. Harris and D. Heath), Churchill Livingstone, Edinburgh, pp. 522–44.

120. Naeije, R. (1992) Should pulmonary hypertension be treated in chronic obstructive pulmonary disease? in *The Diagnosis and Treatment of Pulmonary Hypertension* (eds E.K. Weir, S.L. Archer and J.T. Reeves), Futura, New York, pp. 209–39.

121. Burrows, B., Fletcher, C.M., Heard, B.E. *et al.* (1966) Emphysematous and bronchial types of chronic airways obstruction: clinicopathological study of patients in London and Chicago. *Lancet*, **1**, 830–5.

122. Burrows, B., Strauss, R.H. and Nider, A.H. (1965) Chronic obstructive lung disease III. Inter-relationships of pulmonary function data. *Am. Rev. Respir. Dis.*, **91**, 861–8.

123. Mitchell, R.S., Vincent, T.N. and Filley, G.F. (1964) Chronic obstructive broncho-pulmonary disease IV. The clinical and physiological differential of chronic bronchitis and emphysema. *Am. J. Med. Sci.*, **247**, 513–7.

124. Dornhorst, A.C. (1955) Respiratory insufficiency. *Lancet*, **1**, 1185–7.

125. Scadding, J.G. (1963) Meaning of diagnostic terms in bronchopulmonary disease. *Br. Med. J.*, **2**, 1425–30.

126. Burrows, B., Niden, A.H., Fletcher, C.M. *et al.* (1964) Clinical types of chronic obstructive lung disease in London and in Chicago. *Am. Rev. Respir. Dis.*, **90**, 14–27.

127. Robin, E.D. and O'Neill, R.P. (1963) The fighter versus the non-fighter. Control of ventilation in chronic obstructive pulmonary disease. *Arch. Environ. Health*, **7**, 125–9.

128. Filley, G.F. (1967) Emphysema and chronic bronchitis: clinical manifestations and their physiologic significance. *Med. Clin. North Am.*, **51**, 283–92.

129. Filley, G.F., Beckwitt, H.J., Reeves, J.T. *et al.* (1968) Chronic obstructive bronchopulmonary disease II. Oxygen transport in two clinical types. *Am. J. Med.*, **44**, 26–38.

130. College of General Practitioners (1961) Chronic bronchitis in Great Britain. *Br. Med. J.*, **2**, 973–9.

131. Mitchell, R.S., Maisel, J.C., Dart, G.A. *et al.* (1974) The accuracy of the death certificate in reporting cause of death in adults: with special reference to chronic bronchitis and emphysema. *Am. Rev. Respir. Dis.*, **104**, 844–50.

132. Richards, D.W. (1960) Pulmonary emphysema: etiologic factors and clinical forms. *Ann. Intern. Med.*, **53**, 1105–20.

133. Snider, G.L., Kleinerman, J., Thurlbeck, W.M. *et al.* (1985) The definition of emphysema. Report of the National Heart Lung and Blood Institute, Division of Lung Diseases Workshop. *Am. Rev. Respir. Dis.*, **132**, 182–5.

134. Thurlbeck, W.M. (1976) Chronic airflow obstruction in lung disease, in *Major Problems in Pathology* (ed. J.L. Bennington), Saunders, London, pp. 350–444.

135. Jamal, K., Fleetham, J.A. and Thurlbeck, W.M. (1990) Cor pulmonale: correlation with central airway lesions, peripheral airway lesions, emphysema, and control of breathing. *Am. Rev. Respir. Dis.*, **141**, 1172–7.

136. Sadoul, P., Schrijen, F., Uffholtz, T. *et al.* (1968) Evolution clinique de 195 pulmonares soumis

a un catheterisme du coeur droit entre 1957 et 1965. *Bull. Physiopathol Resp.*, **4**, 225–40.

137. Schrijen, F., Uffholtz, H., Polu, J.M. *et al.* (1978) Pulmonary and systemic haemodynamic evaluation in chronic bronchitis. *Am. Rev. Respir. Dis.*, **117**, 25–31.

138. Weitzenblum, E., Hirth, C., Parini, J.P. *et al.* (1978) Clinical, functional and pulmonary haemodynamic course of patients with COPD followed up over 3 years. *Respiration*, **36**, 1–9.

139. Weitzenblum, E., Loiseau, A., Hirth, C. *et al.* (1979) Course of pulmonary haemodynamics in patients with chronic obstructive pulmonary disease. *Chest*, **75**, 656–62.

140. Weitzenblum, E., Sautegeau, A., Ehrhart, M. *et al.* (1984) Long-term course of pulmonary arterial pressure in chronic obstructive pulmonary disease. *Am. Rev. Respir. Dis.*, **130**, 993–8.

141. Medical Research Council Working Party (1981) Long-term domiciliary oxygen therapy in chronic hypoxic cor pulmonale complicating chronic bronchitis and emphysema. *Lancet*, **1**, 681–6.

142. Weitzenblum, E., Hirth, C., Ducolone, A. *et al.* (1981) Prognostic value of pulmonary artery pressure in chronic obstructive pulmonary disease. *Thorax*, **36**, 752–8.

143. Massin, N., Westphal, J.L., Schrijen, F. *et al.* (1979) Valeur prognostique du bilon hemodynamic des bronchiteux chronique. *Bull. Europ. Physiopathol. Resp.*, **15**, 821–37.

144. Ourednik, A. and Susa, Z. (1975) How long does the pulmonary hypertension last in chronic obstructive bronchopulmonary disease? *Prog. Resp. Res.*, **9**, 24–8.

145. France, A.J., Prescott, R.J., Biernacki, W. *et al.* (1988) Does right ventricular function predict survival in patients with chronic obstructive pulmonary disease? *Thorax*, **43**, 621–6.

146. Kawakami, Y., Kishi, F., Yamamoto, H. *et al.* (1983) Relation of oxygen delivery, mixed venous oxygenation and pulmonary haemodynamics to progress in chronic obstructive pulmonary disease. *N. Engl. J. Med.*, **308**, 1046–9.

147. Mithoefer, J.C., Holford, F.D. and Keighley, J.F.H. (1974) The effect of oxygen administration on mixed venous oxygenation in chronic obstructive pulmonary disease. *Chest*, **66**, 122–32.

148. Tenney, S.M. and Mithoefer, J.C. (1982) The relationship of mixed venous oxygenation to oxygen transport: with special reference to

high altitude and pulmonary disease. *Am. Rev. Respir. Dis.*, **125**, 474–9.

149. Kawahami, Y., Terai, T., Yamamato, H. *et al.* (1982) Exercise and oxygen inhalation in relation to prognosis of chronic obstructive pulmonary disease. *Chest*, **81**, 182–8.

150. Kasnitz, P., Druger, G.L., Yorra, F. *et al.* (1976) Mixed oxygen tension and hyperlactatemia. Survival in severe cardiopulmonary disease. *JAMA*, **236**, 570–4.

151. Degaute, D., Domenighetti, G., Naeije, R. *et al.* (1981) Oxygen delivery in acute exacerbation of chronic obstructive pulmonary disease. Effects of controlled oxygen therapy. *Am. Rev. Respir. Dis.*, **124**, 26–30.

152. Corriveau, M.L., Rosen, B.J. and Dolan, G.F. (1989) Oxygen transport and oxygen consumption during supplemental oxygen administration in patients with chronic obstructive pulmonary disease. *Am J. Med.*, **87**, 633–7.

153. Bergofsky, E.H. (1963) Tissue oxygen delivery and cor pulmonale in chronic obstructive pulmonary disease with and without heart failure. *Am. J. Cardiol.*, **11**, 477–82.

154. Bergofsky, E.H. (1983) Tissue oxygen delivery and cor pulmonale in chronic obstructive pulmonary disease. *N. Engl. J. Med.*, **308**, 1092–4.

155. Finlay, M., Middleton, H.C., Peake, M.D. *et al.* (1983) Cardiac output, pulmonary hypertension, hypoxaemia and survival in patients with chronic obstructive airways disease. *Eur. J. Respir. Dis.*, **64**, 252–63.

156. Howard, P. (1983) Drugs or oxygen for hypoxic cor pulmonale? *Br. Med. J.*, **287**, 1159–60.

157. McFadden, E.R. and Braunwald, E. (1980) Cor pulmonale and pulmonary thromboembolism, in *Heart Disease* (ed. E. Braunwald), Saunders, Philadelphia, pp. 1643–80.

158. Hooper, R.G. (1987) Chronic right heart failure: Pulmonary considerations, in *The Right Heart* (ed. R.L. Fisk), Davis, Philadelphia, pp. 181–90.

159. Wiedemann, H.P. and Matthay, R.A. (1989) The management of acute and chronic cor pulmonale, in *Heart–Lung Interactions in Health and Disease* (eds. S.M. Scharf and S.S. Cassidy), Dekker, New York, pp. 915–82.

160. World Health Organization (1963) Chronic cor pulmonale. A report of the expert committee. *Circulation*, **27**, 594–8.

161. Fulton, R.M., Hutchinson, E.C. and Jones, A.M. (1952) Ventricular weight in cardiac hypertrophy. *Br. Heart J.*, **14**, 413–20.

162. Behnke, R.H., Blount, S.G., Bristo, W. *et al.* (1970) Primary prevention of pulmonary heart disease. *Circulation*, **41**, A17–A23.

163. Jezek, V. and Morpurgo, M. (1992) Right heart failure in chronic lung disease. Where are we now? in *Current Topics in Rehabilitation: Right Ventricular Hypertrophy and Function in Chronic Lung Disease* (eds V. Jezek, M. Morpurgo and R. Tramarin), Springer-Verlag, Verona, pp. 1–9.

164. Denolin, H. (1992) Clinical diagnosis of right heart failure in chronic obstructive lung disease in *Current Topics in Rehabilitation: Right Ventricular Hypertrophy and Function in Chronic Lung Disease* (eds. V. Jezek, M. Morpurgo and R. Tramarin), Springer-Verlag, Verona, pp. 97–9.

165. Strobeck, J.E. and Sonnenblick, E.H. (1985) Pathophysiology of heart failure, in *The Ventricle*, (eds H.J. Levine and W.H. Gaasch), Martinus Nijhoff, Boston, pp. 209–24.

166. Taylor, S.H. (1988) Cardiovascular consequences of heart failure. *Eur. Heart J.*, **9** (Suppl H), 41–7.

167. Denolin, H., Kuhn, H., Krayenbuehl, H.P. *et al.* (1983) The definition of heart failure. *Eur. Heart J.*, **4**, 445–8.

168. Friedberg, C.K. (1966) *Diseases of the Heart*, 3rd edn, Saunders, Philadelphia.

169. Rubin, L.J. (1984) *Pulmonary Heart Disease*, Martinus Nijhoff, Boston.

170. Ferrer, M.I. (1975) Cor pulmonale: present day status. *Am. Heart J.*, **89**, 657–64.

171. Rubin, L.L. (1984) Pulmonary hypertension secondary to lung disease, in *Pulmonary Hypertension* (eds E.K. Weir and J.T. Reeves), Futura, New York, pp. 291–320.

172. Lupi-Herrera, E., Sandoval, J., Seoane, M. *et al.* (1982) Behaviour of the pulmonary circulation in chronic obstructive pulmonary disease. *Am. Rev. Respir. Dis.*, **126**, 509–14.

173. Thomas, A.J. (1972) Chronic pulmonary heart disease. *Br. Heart J.*, **34**, 653–7.

174. Leading article (1975) Oedema in cor pulmonale. *Lancet*, **2**, 1289–90.

175. Richens, J.M. and Howard, P. (1982) Oedema in cor pulmonale. *Clin. Sci.*, **62**, 255–9.

176. MacNee, W. (1988) Right ventricular function in cor pulmonale. *Cardiology*, **75** (Suppl 1), 30–40.

177. Vogt, P. and Ruttner, J.R. (1977) Das cor pulmonale aus pathologisch-anatomischer sicht. *Schweiz. Med. Wochenschr.*, **107**, 549–53.

178. Heath, D., Brewer, D. and Hicken, P., (1968) in *Cor Pulmonale in Emphysema*, (ed. D. Heath), Springfield, pp. 1–37.

179. Intersociety Commission for Heart Disease Resources: Primary prevention of pulmonary heart disease (1970) *Circulation*, **41**, A17–A23.

180. Feldman, N.T. and Ingram, R.H. Jr. (1978) Chronic cor pulmonale, in *The Heart, Arteries, and Veins* (eds J.W. Hurst, R.B. Logue, R.C. Schlant and N.K. Wenger), McGraw-Hill, New York, pp. 1485–98.

181. Berbel, L.N. and Miro, R.E. (1983) Pulmonary hypertension in the pathogenesis of cor pulmonale. *Cardiovasc. Rev.*, **4**, 356–63.

182. Diener, C.F. and Burrows, B. (1975) Further observations on the course and prognosis of chronic obstructive lung disease. *Am. Rev. Respir. Dis.*, **111**, 719–24.

183. Jones, N.L., Burrows, B. and Fletcher, C.M. (1967) Serial study of 100 patients with chronic airway obstruction in London and Chicago. *Thorax*, **22**, 327–35.

184. Bates, D.V., Knott, J.M.S. and Christie, R.V. (1956) Respiratory function in emphysema in relation to prognosis. *Q. J. Med.*, **25**, 137–57.

185. Hodgkin, J.E. (1990) Prognosis in chronic obstructive pulmonary disease. *Clin. Chest Med.*, **11**, 555–69.

186. Boushy, S.F., Adhikari, P.K., Sakamoto, A. *et al.* (1964) Factors affecting prognosis in emphysema. *Dis. Chest*, **45**, 402–11.

187. Kanner, R.E., Renzett, A.D., Stanish, W.M. *et al.* (1983) Predictors of survival in subjects with chronic airflow limitation. *Am. J. Med.*, **74**, 249–55.

188. Kawakami, Y. (1985) Prognostic factors in COPD: The importance of pulmonary hemodynamic variables. *Pract. Cardiol.*, **11**, 124–37.

189. Kok-Jensen, A., Sorenson, E. and Damsgaard, T. (1974) Prognosis in severe chronic obstructive pulmonary disease. *Scand. J. Respir. Dis.*, **55**, 120–8.

190. Mitchell, R.S., Webb, N.F. and Filley, G.F. (1964) Chronic obstructive bronchopulmonary disease, III. Factors influencing prognosis. *Am. Rev. Respir. Dis.*, **89**, 878–96.

191. Sahn, S.A., Nett, L.M. and Petty, T.L. (1980) Ten-year follow-up of a comprehensive rehabilitation program for severe COPD. *Chest*, **77** (suppl), 311–4.

192. Simpson, T. (1968) Chronic bronchitis and emphysema with special reference to prognosis. *Br. J. Dis. Chest*, **62**, 57–69.

193. Traver, G.A., Cline, M.G. and Burrows, B. (1979) Predictors of mortality in chronic obstructive pulmonary disease. *Am. Rev. Respir. Dis.*, **119**, 895–902.

194. Arcilla, R.A., Tsai, P., Thilenus, O. *et al.* (1971) Angiographic method for volume estimation of the right and left ventricles. *Chest*, **60**, 446–54.

195. Gentzler, R., Briselli, M. and Gault, J. (1974) Angiographic estimation of right ventricular volume in man. *Circulation*, **4**, 1–55.

196. Chetty, K.G., Brown, S.E. and Leight, R.W. (1982) Identification of pulmonary hypertension in chronic obstructive pulmonary disease from routine chest radiographs. *Am. Rev. Respir. Dis.*, **126**, 338–41.

197. Matthay, R.A., Schwarz, M.I., Ellis, J.H. *et al.* (1981) Pulmonary artery hypertension in chronic obstructive pulmonary disease: Chest radiographic assessment. *Invest. Radiol.*, **16**, 95–100.

198. Kirch, E. (1955) Die pathologische anatomie des cor pulmonale. *Verh. Dtsch. Ges. Kreislaufforsch*, **21**, 163–81.

199. Konstam, M.A., and Pandian, N. (1988) Assessment of right ventricular function, in *The Right Ventricle* (eds M.A. Konstam and J.M. Isner). Kluwer, Boston, pp. 1–15.

200. Lehtonen, J., Sutinen, S., Ikaheimo, P *et al.* (1988) Electrocardiographic criteria for the diagnosis of right ventricular hypertrophy verified at autopsy. *Chest*, **93**, 839–42.

201. Moccetti, T. and Morpurgo, M. (1977) Contribution of vector cardiography to the diagnosis of chronic cor pulmonale, in *Cor Pulmonale Cronicum* (ed. S. Daum), European Society for Clinical Respiratory Physiology and European Society of Cardiology, Munchen, pp. 299–314.

202. Bancroft, W.H. and Eddleman, E.E. (1967) Methods and physical characteristics of the kinetocardiographic and apexcardiographic systems for recording low-frequency precordial motion. *Am. Heart J.*, **73**, 756–64.

203. Weitzenblum, E., Zielinski, J. and Bishop, J.M. (1983) The diagnosis of 'cor pulmonale' by non-invasive methods: a challenge for pulmonologists and cardiologists. *Bull. Europ. Physiopath. Resp.*, **19**, 423–6.

204. Marchandise, B., De Bruyne, B., Delaunois, L. *et al.* (1987) Non-invasive prediction of pulmonary hypertension in chronic obstructive pulmonary disease by echocardiography. *Chest*, **91**, 361–5.

205. Berger, H.J. and Matthay, R.A. (1981) Noninvasive radiographic assessment of cardiovascular function in acute and chronic respiratory failure. *Am. J. Cardiol.*, **47**, 950–62.

206. Matthay, R.A. and Berger, H.J. (1983) Noninvasive assessment of right and left ventricular function in acute and chronic respiratory failure. *Crit. Care Med.*, **11**, 329–38.

207. Schiller, N.B. and Sahn, D.J. (1992) Pulmonary pressure measurement by doppler and two-dimensional echocardiography in adult and paediatric populations, in *The Diagnosis and Treatment of Pulmonary Hypertension*, (eds E.K. Weir, S.L. Archer and J.T. Reeves), Futura, New York, pp. 41–59.

208. Migueres, M., Escamilla, R., Coca, F. *et al.* (1990) Pulsed doppler echocardiography in the diagnosis of pulmonary hypertension and COPD. *Chest*, **98**, 280–5.

209. Morpugo, M., Saviotti, M., Dickele, M.C. *et al.* (1984) Echocardiographic aspect of pulmonary arterial hypertension in chronic lung disease. *Bull. Europ. Physiopath. Resp.*, **20**, 251–5.

210. Yock, P.J. and Popp, R.L. (1984) Non-invasive estimation of right ventricular systolic pressure by doppler ultrasound in patients with tricuspid regurgitation. *Circulation*, **70**, 657–62.

211. Masuyama, T., Kodama, K., Kitabatake, A. *et al.* (1986) Continuous wave doppler echocardiographic detection of pulmonary regurgitation and its application to noninvasive estimation of pulmonary arterial pressure. *Circulation*, **74**, 484–92.

212. Danchin, N., Cornette, E.A., Henriquez, A. *et al.* (1987) Two-dimensional echocardiographic assessment of the right ventricle in patients with chronic obstructive lung disease. *Chest*, **92**, 229–33.

213. Kirchir, B., Himelman, R.B. and Schiller, M.B. (1988) Right atrial pressure estimation in respiratory behaviour of the inferior vena cava. *Circulation*, **78** II, 550 (2196).

214. Stevenson, G., Kawabori, I. and Guntheroth, W. (1981) The validation of doppler diagnosis of tricuspid regurgitation. *Circulation*, **64**, 255.

215. Berger, M., Hect, S., Van Tos, H.A. *et al.* (1989) Pulse and continuous wave doppler echocardiographic assessment of valvular regurgitation in normal subjects. *J. Am. Coll. Card.*, **13**, 1540–5.

216. Morrison, D.A., Ovitt, T. and Hammermeister, K.E. (1988) Functional tricuspid regurgitation and right ventricular dysfunction in pulmonary hypertension. *Am. J. Cardiol.*, **62**, 108–12.

217. McKenzie, J. (1908) *Diseases of the Heart.* Oxford Medical Publishing, London, pp. 229.

218. Himelman, R.B., Stulbarg, K., Kircher, B. *et al.* (1989) Non-invasive evaluation of pulmonary arterial pressure during exercise by saline enhanced doppler echocardiography in chronic pulmonary disease. *Circulation*, **79**, 863–71.

219. Beard, J.T. and Byrd, B.F. (1988) Saline contrast enhancement of trivial doppler tricuspid regurgitation signals for estimating pulmonary artery pressure. *Am. J. Cardiol.*, **62**, 486–8.

220. Laaban, J.P., Diebold, B., Raffoul, H. *et al.* (1988) Non-invasive estimation of systolic pulmonary arterial pressure (Pps) using continuous wave doppler ultrasound in COPD. *Am. Rev. Respir. Dis.*, **137**, 150.

221. Berger, M., Haimowtz, A., Van Tosh, A. *et al.* (1985) Quantitative assessment of pulmonary hypertension in patients with tricuspid regurgitation using continuous wave Doppler. *J. Am. Coll. Cardiol.*, **6**, 359–65.

222. Currie, P.J., Seward, J.B., Chan, K.L. *et al.* (1985) Continuous wave Doppler determination of right ventricular pressure: a simultaneous Doppler catheterization study in 127 patients. *J. Am. Coll. Cardiol.*, **6**, 750–6.

223. Mitchell, R.S., Stanford, R.E., Silvers, G.W. *et al.* (1976) The right ventricle in chronic airway obstruction: a clinico-pathologic study. *Am. Rev. Respir. Dis.*, **11**, 147–54.

224. Murphy, M.I. (1987) The pathology of the right heart in chronic hypertrophy and failure, in *The Right Heart* (ed. R.L. Fisk), Davis, Philadelphia, pp. 159–69.

225. Bommer, W., Weinert, L., Neumann, A. *et al.* (1979) Determination of right atrial and right ventricular size by two-dimensional echocardiography. *Circulation*, **60**, 91–100.

226. Niederman, M.S. and Matthay, R.A. (1986) Cardiovascular function in secondary pulmonary hypertension *Heart & Lung*, **15**, 341–51.

227. Starling, M.R., Crawford, M.H., Sorensen, S.G. *et al.* (1982) Two-dimensional echocardiographic technique evaluating right ventricular size and performance in patients with obstructive lung disease. *Circulation*, **66**, 612–20.

228. Watanabe, T., Katsum, E., Matsukubo, H. *et al.* (1982) Estimation of right ventricular volume with two-dimensional echocardiography. *Am. J. Cardiol.*, **49**, 1946–53.

229. Ferlinz, J. (1977) Measurements of right ventricular volumes in man from single plain cine-angiograms. *Am. Heart J.*, **94**, 87–90.

230. Konstam, M.A. and Levine, H.A. (1988) Effects of afterload and preload on right ventricular systolic performance, in *The Right Ventricle* (eds M.A. Konstam and J.M. Isner), Kluwer, Boston, pp. 17–35.

231. Berger, H.J., Matthay, R.A., Loke, J. *et al.* (1978) Assessment of cardiac performance with quantitative radionuclide angiography: right ventricular ejection fraction with reference to findings in chronic obstructive pulmonary disease. *Am. J. Cardiol.*, **41**, 897–905.

232. Maddahi, J., Bermon, D.S., Matsuoka, D.T. *et al.* (1979) A new technique for assessing right ventricular ejection fraction using rapid multiple gated equilibrium cardiac blood pool scintigraphy. *Circulation*, **60**, 581–9.

233. Xue, Q.F., MacNee, W., Flenley, D.C. *et al.* (1983) Can right ventricular performance be assessed by gated equilibrium ventriculography? *Thorax*, **38**, 486–93.

234. MacNee, W., Xue, Q.F., Hannan, W.J. *et al.* (1983) Assessment by radionuclide angiography of right and left ventricular function in chronic bronchitis and emphysema. *Thorax*, **38**, 494–500.

235. Wathen, C.G., Hannan, W.J., Flenley, D.C. *et al.* (1988) Reproducibility of radionuclide right ventricular ejection fraction (RVEF) in chronic bronchitis and emphysema (COLD). *Clin. Sci.*, **74** (Suppl 18), 60P.

236. Cohen, H.A., Baird, M.G., Rouleau, J.R. *et al.* (1976) Thallium 201 myocardial imaging in patients with pulmonary hypertension. *Circulation*, **54**, 790–5.

237. Kondo, M., Kubo, A., Yamazaki, H. *et al.* (1978) Thallium 201 myocardial imaging for evaluation of right ventricular overloading. *J. Nucl. Med.*, **19**, 1197–203.

238. Khaja, F., Alam, M., Goldstein, S. *et al.* (1979) Diagnostic value of visualization of the right ventricle using Thallium 201 myocardial imaging. *Circulation*, **59**, 182–8.

239. Ohsuzu, F., Handa, S., Kondo, M. *et al.* (1980) Thallium 201 myocardial imaging to evaluate

right ventricular overloading. *Circulation*, **61**, 620–5.

240. Berger, H., Wackers, F., Mahler, D. *et al.* (1980) Right ventricular visualisation on Thallium 201 myocardial images in chronic obstructive pulmonary disease: relationship to right ventricular function and hypertrophy (abstract). *Circulation*, **62**, III: 103.

241. Weitzenblum, E., Moyses, B., Dickele, M. *et al.* (1984) Detecting right ventricular pressure overloading by Thallium-201 myocardial scintigraphy: results in 57 patients with chronic respiratory diseases. *Chest*, **85**, 164–9.

242. Longmore, D.B., Klipstein, R.H., Underwood, S.R. *et al.* (1988) Dimensional accuracy of magnetic resonance studies of the heart. *Lancet*, **1**, 1360–2.

243. Turnbull, L.W., Ridgeway, J.P., Biernacki, W. *et al.* (1990) Assessment of the right ventricle by magnetic resonance imaging in chronic obstructive lung disease. *Thorax*, **45**, 597–601.

244. Chappuis, E., Dorsaz, P.A. and Rutishauser, W. (1989) New method for the assessment of right ventricular function by intravenous digital angiography. First International Workshop on New Trends in Cardiovascular Therapy and Technology, Genoa, (abstr) 25P.

245. Smith, M.A., Ridgway, J.P., Brydon, J.W.E. *et al.* (1986) ECG-gated T1 images of the heart. *Phys. Med. Biol.*, **3**, 771–8.

246. Brecker, G.A. and Galletti, P.M. (1963) Functional anatomy of cardiac pumping, in *Handbook of Physiology. Circulation, vol. II*, (eds A.F. Hamilton and P. Dow), *American Physiological Society*, Washington DC, pp. 759–98.

247. Laks, M.M., Garner, D. and Swan, H.J.C. (1967) Volumes and compliances measured simultaneously in the right and left ventricles of the dog. *Circ. Res.*, **20**, 565–9.

248. Rushmer, R. (1976) Functional anatomy and control of the heart, in *Cardiovascular Dynamics*, 4th edn, Saunders, Philadelphia, pp. 89–98.

249 Morpurgo, M. and Jezek, V. (1992) Evaluation of right heart failure: controversies in definition and methods of evaluation, in *Current Topics in Rehabilitation. Right Ventricular Hypertrophy and Function in Chronic Lung Disease*, (eds V. Jezek, M. Morpurgo and R. Tramarin), Springer-Verlag, Verona, pp. 79–95.

250. Furey, S.A., Zieska, H.A. and Levy, M.N. (1984) The essential function of the right ventricle. *Am. Heart J.*, **107**, 404–10.

251. Fishman, A.P. (1980) Cor pulmonale: General aspects, in *Pulmonary Diseases and Disorders*, McGraw-Hill, New York, pp. 853–82.

252. Abel, R.L. (1965) Effects of alterations in peripheral resistance on left ventricular function. *Proc. Soc. Exp. Biol. Med.*, **120**, 52–6.

253. Bahler, R.C. (1977) Does increased work of the right ventricle diminish left ventricular function? *Chest*, **72**, 551–2.

254. Stein, P.D., Sabbah, N.H., Anbe, D.T. *et al.* (1979) Performance of the failing and non-failing right ventricle of patients with pulmonary hypertension. *Am. J. Cardiol.*, **44**, 1050–5.

255. Wagenvoort, C.A. and Wagenvoort, N. (1970) Primary pulmonary hypertension; a pathological study of the lung vessels in 156 clinically diagnosed cases. *Circulation*, **42**, 1163–84.

256. Bristow, J.D., Morris, J.F. and Kloster, F.E. (1966) Haemodynamics of cor pulmonale. *Proc. Cardiovasc. Dis.*, **9**, 239–58.

257. Ellis, J.H., Kirch, D. and Steele, P.P. (1977) Right ventricular ejection fraction in severe chronic airway obstruction (Abstr) *Chest*, **71** (Suppl), 281–2.

258. Olvey, S.K., Reduto, L.A., Stevens, P.M. *et al.* (1980) First pass radionuclide assessment of right and left ventricular ejection fraction in COPD. *Chest*, **78**, 4–9.

259. Matthay, R.A. and Berger, H.J. (1981) Cardiovascular performance in chronic obstructive pulmonary disease. *Med. Clin. North Am.*, **65**, 489–520.

260. Slutsky, R., Hooper, W., Gerber, K. *et al.* (1980) Assessment of right ventricular function at rest and during exercise in patients with coronary artery disease. *Am. J. Cardiol.*, **45**, 63–71.

261. Tobinick, E., Schelbert, H.R., Henning, H. *et al.* (1978) Right ventricular ejection fraction in patients with acute anterior and inferior infarction assessed by radionuclide angiography. *Circulation*, **57**, 1078–84.

262. MacNee, W. (1992) Clinical importance of right ventricular function in pulmonary hypertension, in *The Diagnosis and Treatment of Pulmonary Hypertension* (eds E.K. Weir, S.L. Archer and J.T. Reeves), Futura, New York, pp. 13–40.

263. Berger, H.J., Matthay, R.A., Davies, R.A. *et al.* (1979) Comparison of exercise right ventricular performance in chronic obstructive pulmonary disease and coronary artery disease: non-invasive assessment by quantitative radionuclide angiocardiography. *Invest. Radiol.*, **14**, 342–53.

264. MacNee, W., Morgan, A.D., Wathen, C.G. *et al.* (1985) Right ventricular performance during exercise in chronic obstructive pulmonary disease. *Respiration*, **48**, 206–11.

265. Morrison, D.A. (1987) Pulmonary hypertension in chronic obstructive pulmonary disease. The right ventricular hypothesis. *Chest*, **92**, 387–9.

266. Klinger, J.R. and Hill, N.S. (1991) Right ventricular dysfunction in chronic obstructive pulmonary disease. Evaluation and management. *Chest*, **99**, 715–23.

267. Dahlstrom, J.A. (1983) Simultaneous assessment of right ventricular ejection fraction and central haemodynamics at rest and during exercise in patients with pulmonary hypertension. *Clin. Physiol.*, **3**, 267–79.

268. Burghuber, O.C. and Bergmann, H. (1988) Right ventricular contractility in chronic obstructive pulmonary disease. A combined radionuclide and haemodynamic study. *Respiration*, **53**, 1–12.

269. Winzelberg, G.G., Boucher, C.A., Pohost, G.M. *et al.* (1981) Right ventricular function in aortic and mitral valve disease. Relation of gated first pass radionuclide angiography to clinic and haemodynamic findings. *Chest*, **79**, 520–8.

270. Korr, K.S., Grandsman, E.J., Winkler, M.L. *et al.* (1982) Hemodynamic correlates of right ventricular ejection fraction measured with gated radionuclide angiography. *Am. J. Cardiol.*, **49**, 71–7.

271. Friedman, B.J. and Holman, B.L. (1978) Scintigraphic prediction of pulmonary arterial systolic pressure by regional right ventricular ejection fraction during the second half of systole. *Am. J. Cardiol.*, **50**, 1114–9.

272. Morrison, D.A., Sorenson, S., Caldwell, J. *et al.* (1982) The normal right ventricular response to supine exercise. *Chest*, **82**, 686–91.

273. Marmor, A.T., Mijiritsky, Y., Plich, M. *et al.* (1986) Improved radionuclide method for assessment of pulmonary artery pressure. *Chest*, **89**, 64–9.

274. Mahler, D.A., Brent, B.N., Loke, J. *et al.* (1984) Right ventricular performance and central circulatory hemodynamics during upright exercise in patients with chronic obstructive pulmonary disease. *Am. Rev. Respir. Dis.*, **130**, 722–9.

275. Burghuber, O.C., Bergman, H., Silberbauer, K. *et al.* (1984) Right ventricular performance in chronic airflow obstruction. *Respiration*, **45**, 124–30.

276. Biernacki, W., Flenley, D.C., Muir, A.L. *et al.* (1988) Pulmonary hypertension and right ventricular function in patients with COPD. *Chest*, **94**, 1169–75.

277. Caro, C.G., Pedley, T.J., Schroter, R.C. *et al.* (1981) *The Mechanics of the Circulation*, Oxford University Press, Oxford, pp. 213–4.

278. Braunwald, E., Sonnenblick, E.H. and Ross, J. Jr. (1984) Contraction of the normal heart, in *Heart Disease* (ed. E. Braunwald), Saunders, Philadelphia, pp. 409–47.

279. Green, J.F. (1987) *Fundamental Cardiovascular and Pulmonary Physiology*, Lea & Febiger, Philadelphia, pp. 45–55.

280. Goerke, J. and Mines, A.H. (1988) *Cardiovascular Physiology*, Raven Press, New York, pp. 99–152.

281. Gunther, S. and Grossman, W. (1979) Determinants of ventricular function in pressure overload hypertrophy in man. *Circulation*, **59**, 679–88.

282. Weber, K.T. and Janicki, J.S. (1986) Pulmonary hypertension, in *Cardiopulmonary Exercise Testing: Physiological Principles and Clinical Applications*, Saunders, Philadelphia, pp. 220–34.

283. Shaw, D.R., Grover, R.F., Reeves, J.T. *et al.* (1965) Pulmonary circulation in chronic bronchitis and emphysema. *Br. Heart J.*, **27**, 674–83.

284. Light, R.W., Mintz, H.M., Linden, G.S. *et al.* (1984) Hemodynamics of patients with severe chronic obstructive pulmonary disease during progressive upright exercise. *Am. Rev. Respir. Dis.*, **130**, 391–5.

285. Altschule, M.D. (1986) Limited usefulness of the so-called ejection fraction measurement in clinical practice. *Chest*, **90**, 134–5.

286. Sagawa, K. (1981) The end-systolic pressure volume relation to the ventricle; definition, modifications and clinical use. *Circulation*, **63**, 1223–7.

287. Weber, K.T., Janick, I., Schroff, S. *et al.* (1981) Contractile mechanics and interaction of right and left ventricles. *Am. J. Cardiol.*, **47**, 686–95.

288. Maughan, W.L. and Oikawa, P.Y. (1989) *Right Ventricular Function*, (ed. S.M. Scharf), Dekker, New York, pp. 179–220.

289. Weber, K.T., Janicki, J.S. and Shroff, S.J. (1986) The heart as a mechanical pump, in *Cardio-ulmonary Exercise Testing*, (eds K.T. Weber and J.S. Janicki), Saunders, Philadelphia, pp. 34–56.

290. Noble, M.I.M. (1988) The pressure-volume relationship of the intact heart, in *Starling's Law of the Heart Revisited*, (eds H.E.D.J. ter Keurs and M.I.M. Noble), Kluwer, Dordrecht, pp. 126.

291. Redington, A.N., Gray, H.H. and Hodson, M.E. (1988) Characterisation of the normal right ventricular pressure–volume relation by biplane angiography and simultaneous micromanometer pressure measurements. *Br. Heart J.*, **59**, 23-30.

292. Parmley, W.W. (1985) Mechanics of ventricular muscle, in *The Ventricle*, (eds H.J. Levine and W.H. Gaasch), Martinus Nijhoff, Boston, pp. 41–62.

293. Sagawa, R., Sunagawa, K. and Maughan, W.L. (1985) Ventricular end-systolic pressure–volume relations, in *The Ventricle*, (eds H.J. Levine and W.H. Gaasch), Martinus Nijhoff, Boston, pp. 79–103.

294. Wasserman, K. (1988) New concepts in assessing cardiovascular function. *Circulation*, **78**, 1060–71.

295. MacNee, W., Wathen, C.G., Hannan, W.J. *et al.* (1983) Effects of pirbuterol and sodium nitroprusside on pulmonary haemodynamics in hypoxic cor pulmonale. *Br. Med. J.*, **287**, 1169–72.

296. Wroblewski, E., James, F., Spann, J.F. *et al.* (1981) Right ventricular performance in mitral stenosis. *Am. J. Cardiol.*, **47**, 51–6.

297. Herles, F., Jezek, V. and Daum, S. (1968) Site of pulmonary resistance in cor pulmonale in chronic bronchitis. *Br. Heart J.*, **30**, 654–60.

298. Zapol, W.M. and Snider, M.T. (1977) Pulmonary hypertension in severe acute respiratory failure. *N. Engl. J. Med.*, **296**, 476–80.

299. Lejeune, P., Mols, P., Naeije, R. *et al.* (1984) Acute hemodynamic effects of controlled oxygen therapy in decompensated chronic obstructive pulmonary disease. *Crit. Care Med.*, **12**, 1032–5.

300. MacNee, W., Wathen, C.G., Flenley D.C. *et al.* (1988) The effects of controlled oxygen therapy on ventricular function in acute and chronic respiratory failure. *Am. Rev. Respir. Dis.*, **137**, 1289–95.

301. Aber, G.M. and Bishop, J.M. (1965) Serial changes in renal function arterial gas tensions and the acid base state in patients with chronic bronchitis and oedema. *Clin. Sci.*, **28**, 511–25.

302. Fishman, A.P., Maxwell, M.H., Crowder, C.H. *et al.* (1951) Kidney function in cor pulmonale. Particular consideration of changes in renal haemodynamics and sodium excretion during variations in the level of oxygenation. *Circulation*, **3**, 703–21.

303. Davies, C.E. (1951) The effect of treatment on the renal circulation in heart failure. *Lancet*, **2**, 1052–7.

304. Weil, J.V., Jamieson, G., Brown, D.W. *et al.* (1968) The red cell mass/arterial oxygen relationship in normal man. *J. Clin. Invest.*, **47**, 1627–39.

305. Palevsky, H.I. and Fishman, A.P. (1990) Chronic cor pulmonale: etiology and management. *JAMA*, **263**, 2347–53.

306. Kilburn, K.H. and Dowell, A.R. (1971) Renal function in respiratory failure. Effects of hypoxia, hyperoxia, and hypercapnia. *Arch. Intern. Med.*, **127**, 754–62.

307. Baudouin, S.V., Bott, J., Wald, A. *et al.* (1992) Short term effects of oxygen on renal haemodynamics in patients with hypoxic chronic obstructive airways disease. *Thorax*, **47**, 550–4.

308. Semple, Pd'A., Watson, W.S., Beastall, G.H. *et al.* (1983) Endocrine and metabolic studies in unstable cor pulmonale. *Thorax*, **38**, 45–9.

309. Turino, G.M., Goldring, R.M. and Heinemann, H.O. (1970) Water, electrolytes and acid-base relationships in chronic cor pulmonale. *Prog. Vasc. Dis.*, **12**, 467–83.

310. Kinasewitz, G.T., Groome, J.L., Marchall, R.P. *et al.* (1986) Effect of hypoxia on permeability of pulmonary endothelium of canine visceral pleura. *J. Appl. Physiol.*, **61**, 554–60.

311. Polak, A., Haynie, G.D., Hays, R.M. *et al.* (1961) Effects of chronic hypercapnia on electrolyte and acid-base equilibrium. 1 Adaptation. *J. Clin. Invest.*, **40**, 1223–37.

312. Cannon, P.J., Heinemann, H.O., Albert, M.S. *et al.* (1965) 'Contraction' alkalosis after diuresis of edematous patients with ethacrynic acid. *Ann. Intern. Med.*, **62**, 979–90.

313. Stuart-Harris, C.H., MacKinnon, J., Hammond, J.D.S. *et al.* (1956) The renal circulation in chronic pulmonary disease and pulmonary heart failure. *Q. J. Med.*, **25**, 389–405.

314. Platts, M.M., Hammond, J.D.S. and Stuart-Harris, C.H. (1960) A study of cor pulmonale in patients with chronic bronchitis. *Q. J. Med.*, **29**, 559–74.

315. Richens, J.M. and Howard, P. (1982) Oedema in cor pulmonale. *Clin. Sci.*, **62**, 255–9.
316. Harris, P. and Heath, D. (1986) The influence of respiratory gases on the pulmonary circulation, in *The Human Pulmonary Circulation* (eds P. Harris and D. Heath), Churchill Livingstone, Edinburgh, pp. 456–83.
317. Zehr, J.E., Hasbargen, J.A. and Kurz, K.D. (1976) Reflex suppression of renin secretion during distension of cardiopulmonary receptors in dogs. *Circ. Res.*, **38**, 232–9.
318. Farber, M.O., Bright, T.P., Strawbridge, R.A. *et al.* (1975) Impaired water handling in chronic obstructive lung disease. *J. Lab. Clin. Med.*, **85**, 41–9.
319. Farber, M.O., Kiblawi, S.S.O., Strawbridge, R.A. *et al.* (1977) Studies on plasma vasopressin and the renin-angiotensin-aldosterone system in chronic obstructive lung disease. *J. Lab. Clin. Med.*, **90**, 373–80.
320. Farber, M.O., Roberts, L.R., Weinberger, M.H. *et al.* (1982) Abnormalities of sodium and H₂O handling in chronic obstructive lung disease. *Arch. Intern. Med.*, **142**, 1326–30.
321. Farber, M.O., Weinberger, M.H., Robertson, G.L. *et al.* (1984) Hormonal abnormalities affecting sodium and water balance in acute respiratory failure due to chronic obstructive lung disease. *Chest*, **85**, 49–54.
322. Reihman, D.H., Farber, M.O., Weinberger, M.H. *et al.* (1985) Effect of hypoxemia on sodium and water excretion in chronic obstructive lung disease. *Am. J. Med.*, **78**, 87–94.
323. Ackerman, G.L. and Arruda, A.L. (1983) Acid base and electrolyte imbalance in respiratory failure. *Med. Clin. North Am.*, **67**, 646–56.
324. Mannix, E.T., Dowdeswell, I., Carlowe, S. *et al.* (1990) The effect of oxygen on sodium excretion in hypoxaemic patients with obstructive lung disease. *Chest*, **97**, 840–4.
325. Campbell, R.H.A., Brand, H.L., Cox, J.R. *et al.* (1975) Body weight and body water in chronic cor pulmonale. *Clin. Sci. Mol. Med.*, **49**, 323–35.
326. Daugherty, R.M. Jr, Scott, J.B. and Haddy, F.J. (1967) Effects of generalized hypoxemia and hypercapnia on forelimb vascular resistance. *Am. J. Physiol.*, **213**, 1111–4.
327. Colice, G.L. and Ramirez, G. (1985) The effect of furosemide during normoxemia and hypoxemia. *Am. Rev. Respir. Dis.*, **133**, 279–85.
328. Raff, H. and Levy, S.A. (1986) Renin-angiotensin-aldosterone and ACTH-cortisol control during hypoxemia and exercise in patients with chronic obstructive lung disease. *Am. Rev. Respir. Dis.*, **133**, 369–99.
329. Hendriksen, J., Christensen, N.J., Kok-Jensen, A. *et al.* (1980) Increased plasma noradrenaline concentration in patients with chronic obstructive lung disease: relation to haemodynamics and blood gases. *Scand. J. Clin. Lab. Invest.*, **40**, 419–27.
330. Tomaszewski, J., Kowalewski, J., Wozniak, K. *et al.* (1975) Plasma renin activity in patients with chronic cor pulmonale syndrome. *Pol. Med. Sci. Hist. Bull.*, **18**, 207–11.
331. Anderson, W.H., Datta, J. and Samols, E. (1976) The renin-angiotensin-aldosterone system in patients with acute respiratory failure. *Chest*, **69** (Suppl), 309–11.
332. Colice, G.L. and Ramirez, G. (1985) Effect of hypoxemia on the renin-angiotensin-aldosterone system in humans. *J. Appl. Physiol.*, **58**, 724–30.
333. Liang, C.S. and Gavras, H. (1978) Renin-angiotensin system inhibition in conscious dogs during acute hypoxemia. Effects on systemic hemodynamics, regional blood flows, and tissue metabolism. *J. Clin. Invest.*, **62**, 961–70.
334. Weismann, D.N. and Williamson, H.E. (1981) Hypoxaemia increases renin secretion rate in anaesthetised newborn lambs. *Life Sci.*, **29**, 1887–93.
335. Gould, A.B. and Goodman, S.A. (1970) The effect of hypoxia on the renin-angiotensinogen system. *Lab. Invest.*, **22**, 443–7.
336. Martin, A., Baulan, D., Basso, N. *et al.* (1982) The renin-angiotensin-aldosterone system in rats of both sexes subject to chronic hypobaric hypoxia. *Arch. Int. Physiol. Biochim.*, **90**, 129–33.
337. Raff, H., and Fagin, K.D. (1984) Measurement of hormones and blood gases during hypoxia in conscious cannulated rats. *J. Appl. Physiol.*, **56**, 1426–30.
338. Tuffley, R.E., Rubenstein, D., Slater, J.D.H. *et al.* (1970) Serum renin activity during exposure to hypoxia. *J. Endocrinol.*, **48**, 497–510.
339. Heyes, M.P., Farber, M.O., Manfredi, F. *et al.* (1982) Acute effects of hypoxia on renal and endocrine function in normal individuals. *Am. J. Physiol.*, **243**, R265–70.
340. Ashack, R., Farber, M.O., Weinberger, M.H. *et al.* (1985) Renal and hormonal responses to acute hypoxia in normal individuals. *J. Lab. Clin. Med.*, **106**, 12–6.

341. Maher, J.T., Jones, L.G., Hartley, L.H. *et al.* (1975) Aldosterone dynamics during graded exercise at sea level and high altitude. *J. Appl. Physiol.*, **39**, 18–22.
342. Milledge, J.S. and Catley, D.M. (1982) Renin, aldosterone, and converting enzyme during exercise and acute hypoxia in humans. *J. Appl. Physiol.*, **52**, 320–32.
343. Milledge, J.S., Catley, D.M., Williams, E.S. *et al.* (1983) Effect of prolonged exercise at altitude on the renin-aldosterone system. *J. Appl. Physiol.*, 44, 413–8.
344. Frayser, R., Rennie I.D., Gray G.W. *et al.* (1975) Hormonal and electrolyte response to exposure to 17500 ft. *J. Appl. Physiol.*, **38**, 636–42.
345. Milledge, J.S., Catley, D.M., and Ward, M.P. (1983) Renin-aldosterone and angiotensin converting enzyme during prolonged altitude exposure. *J. Appl. Physiol.*, **55**, 699–702.
346. Block, E.R. and Stalcup, J.A. (1982) Metabolic functions of the lung. Of what clinical relevance? *Chest*, **81**, 215–23.
347. Pitt, B.R. (1984) Metabolic functions of the lung and systemic vasoregulation. *Fed. Proc.*, **43**, 2574–7.
348. Ayres, P.J., Hurter, R.C. and Williams, E.S. (1961) Aldosterone excretion and potassium retention in subjects living at high altitude. *Nature*, **191**, 78–80.
349. Slater, J.D.H., Tuffley, R.E., Williams, E.S. *et al.* (1969) Control of aldosterone secretion during acclimatization to hypoxia in man. *Clin. Sci.*, **37**, 327–41.
350. Hogan, R.P., Kotchen, T.A., Boyd, A.E. *et al.* (1973) Effect of altitude on renin-aldosterone system and metabolism of water and electrolytes. *J. Appl. Physiol.*, **35**, 385–90.
351. Sutton, J.R., Viol, G.W., Gray, G.W. *et al.* (1977) Renin, aldosterone, electrolyte, and cortisol responses to hypoxic decompression. *J. Appl. Physiol.*, **43**, 421–4.
352. Keynes, R.J., Smith, G.W., Slater, J.D.H. *et al.* (1982) Renin and aldosterone at high altitude in man. *J. Endocrinol.*, **92**, 131–40.
353. Neilly, J.B., Clark, C.J., Tweddel, A. *et al.* (1987) Transpulmonary angiotensin II formation in patients with chronic stable cor pulmonale. *Am. Rev. Respir. Dis.*, **135**, 891–5.
354. Yamaji, T., Ishibishi, M., Takaku, F. *et al.* (1985) Atrial natriuretic factor in human blood. *Clin. Invest.*, **76**, 1705–9.
355. Cody, R.J. (1990) Atrial natriuretic factor in oedematous disorders. *Ann. Rev. Med.*, **41**, 377–82.
356. Nakaoka, H., Imataka, K., Amano, M. *et al.* (1985) Plasma levels of atrial natriuretic factor in patients with congestive heart failure. *N. Engl. J. Med.*, **313**, 892–3.
357. Tikkanen, I., Fyhrquist, F., Metsarinne, K. *et al.* (1985) Plasma atrial natriuretic peptide in cardiac disease and during infusion in healthy volunteers. *Lancet*, **2**, 66–9.
358. Hartter, E., Weissel, M., Stummvoll, H.K. *et al.* (1985) Atrial natriuretic peptide concentrations in blood from right atrium in patients with severe right-heart failure. *Lancet*, **2**, 93–4.
359. Raine, A.E.G., Erne, P., Burgisser, E. *et al.* (1986) Atrial natriuretic peptide and atrial pressure in patients with congestive heart failure. *N. Engl. J. Med.*, **315**, 533–7.
360. Burghuber, O.C., Hartter, E., Punzengruber, C. *et al.* (1988) Human atrial natriuretic peptide secretion in precapillary pulmonary hypertension. Clinical study in patients with COPD and interstitial fibrosis. *Chest*, **92**, 31–7.
361. Winter, R.J.D., Davidson, A.C., Treacher, D. *et al.* (1989) Atrial natriuretic peptide concentrations in hypoxic secondary pulmonary hypertension: relation to henodynamic and blood gas variables and response to supplemental oxygen. *Thorax*, **44**, 58–62.
362. Skwarski, K., Lee, M., Turnbull, L. and MacNee, W. (1993) Atrial natriuretic peptide in stable and decompensated chronic obstructive pulmonary disease. *Thorax*, **48**, 730–5.
363. Carlone, S., Palange, P., Mannix, E.T. *et al.* (1989) Atrial natriuretic peptide, renin and aldosterone in obstructive lung disease and heart failure. *Am. J. Med. Sci.*, **298**, 243–8.
364. Adnot, S., Andrivet, P., Chabrier, P.E. *et al.* (1989) Atrial natriuretic factor in chronic obstructive lung disease with pulmonary hypertension. Physiological correlates and response to peptide infusion. *J. Clin. Invest.*, **83**, 986–93.
365. Anderson, J.V., Struthers, A.D., Payne, N.N. *et al.* (1986) Atrial natriuretic peptide inhibits the aldosterone response to angiotensin II in man. *Clin. Sci.*, **70**, 507–12.
366. Richards, A.M., McDonald, D., Fitzpatrick, M.A. *et al.* (1988) Atrial natriuretic hormone has biological effects in man at physiological

plasma concentrations. *J. Clin. Endocrinol. Metab.*, **67**, 1134–9.

367. Anderson, J.V., Donckier, J., Payne, N.N. *et al.* (1987) Atrial natriuretic peptide: evidence of action as a natriuretic hormone at physiological plasma concentrations in man. *Clin. Sci.*, **72**, 305–12.

368. Burnett, J.C., Granger, J.P. and Opgenorth, T.J. (1984) Effects of synthetic atrial natriuretic factor on renal function and renin release. *Am. J. Physiol.*, **247**, F863–F866.

369. Sangella, G.A., Markandu, N.D., Shore, A.C. *et al.* (1986) Plasma natriuretic peptide: its relationship to changes in sodium intake and plasma renin activity and aldosterone in man. *Clin. Sci.*, **71**, 299–305.

370. Atarashi, K., Mulrow, P.J. and Franco-Saenz, R. (1985) Effects of atrial peptides on aldosterone production. *J. Clin. Invest.*, **76**, 1807–11.

371. Howard, P. and Sugget, A.J. (1983) Cor pulmonale, in *Cardiology* (eds P. Slight and J. Vann Jones) Heinemann, London.

372. Whyte, K.F. and Flenley, D.C. (1988) Can pulmonary vasodilators improve survival in cor pulmonale due to hypoxic chronic bronchitis and emphysema? *Thorax*, **43**, 1–8.

373. Versprille, A. (1984) Pulmonary vascular resistance: a meaningless variable. *Intens. Care Med.*, **10**, 51–3.

374. McGregor, M. and Sniderman, A. (1985) On pulmonary vascular resistance: the need for more precise definition. *Am. J. Cardiol.*, **55**, 217–21.

375. Reeves, J.T. (1980) Hope in primary pulmonary hypertension. *N. Engl. J. Med.*, **302**, 112–3.

376. Voelkel, N.F. (1986) Mechanisms of hypoxic pulmonary vasoconstriction. *Am. Rev. Respir. Dis.*, **133**, 1186–95.

377. Gould, L., Zahir, M., Martino, A. *et al.* (1971) Haemodynamic effects of phentolamine in chronic obstructive pulmonary disease. *Br. Heart J.*, **33**, 445–50.

378. Widimsky, J., Kasalicky, J., Valach, A. *et al.* (1960) Effect of priscol on the pulmonary circulation in cor pulmonale. *Br. Heart J.*, **22**, 571–8.

379. Vik-Mo, H., Walde, N., Jentoft, H. *et al.* (1985) Improved haemodynamics but reduced arterial blood oxygenation, at rest and during exercise after long-term oral prazosin therapy in chronic cor pulmonale. *Eur. Heart J.*, **6**, 1047–53.

380. Adnot, S., Andrivet, P., Piquet, J. *et al.* (1988) The effects of urapidil therapy on hemodynamics and gas exchange in exercising patients with chronic obstructive pulmonary disease and pulmonary hypertension. *Am. Rev. Respir. Dis.*, **137**, 1068–74.

381. Koziorowski, A., Zielinski, J., Maszczyk, Z. *et al.* (1972) Effect of salbutamol on pulmonary circulation, ventilation and gas exchange in patients with chronic obstructive airways disease. Preliminary report. *Bull. Physiopathol. Respir.*, **8**, 611–6.

382. Stockley, R.A., Finnegan, P. and Bishop, J.M. (1977) Effect of intravenous terbutaline on arterial blood gas tensions, ventilation and pulmonary circulation in patients with chronic bronchitis and cor pulmonale. *Thorax*, **32**, 601–5.

383. Teule, G.J.J. and Majid, P.A. (1980) Haemodynamic effects of terbutaline in chronic obstructive airways disease. *Thorax*, **35**, 536–42.

384. Jones, R.M., Stockley, R.A. and Bishop, J.M. (1982) Early effects of intravenous terbutaline on cardiopulmonary function in chronic obstructive bronchitis and pulmonary hypertension. *Thorax*, **37**, 746–50.

385. Brent, B.N., Mahler, D., Berger, H.J. *et al.* (1982) Augmentation of right ventricular performance in chronic obstructive pulmonary disease by terbutaline; a combined radionuclide and hemodynamic study. *Am. J. Cardiol.*, **50**, 313–9.

386. Peacock, A., Busst, C., Dawkins, K. *et al.* (1982) Response of pulmonary circulation to oral pirbuterol in chronic airflow obstruction. *Br. Med. J.*, **287**, 1178–80.

387. Lockhart, A., Lissac, J., Salmon, D. *et al.* (1967) Effects of isoproterenol on the pulmonary circulation in obstructed airways disease. *Clin. Sci.*, **32**, 177–87.

388. Winter, R.J.D., Langford, J.A. and Rudd, R.M. (1984) Effects of oral and inhaled salbutamol and oral pirbuterol on right and left ventricular function in chronic bronchitis. *Br. Med. J.*, **288**, 824–5.

389. Mols, P., Ham, H., Naeije, R. *et al.* (1988) How does salbutamol improve the ventricular performance in patients with chronic obstructive pulmonary disease. *J. Cardiovasc. Pharmacol.*, **12**, 127–33.

390. Biernacki, W., Prince, K., Whyte, K. *et al.* (1989) The effect of six months of daily treatment with the beta-2 agonist pirbuterol on

pulmonary hemodynamics in patients with chronic hypoxic cor pulmonale receiving long-term oxygen therapy. *Am. Rev. Respir. Dis.*, **139**, 492–7.

391. Opie, L.H. (1984) Calcium antagonists. Mechanisms, therapeutic indications and reservations: a review. *Q. J. Med.*, **53**, 1–16.

392. McMurty, I.F., Davidson, A.B. and Reeve, S.J.T. (1976) Inhibition of hypoxic pulmonary vasoconstriction by calcium antagonists in isolated rat lungs. *Circ. Res.*, **38**, 99–104.

393. Kennedy, T. and Summer, W. (1982) Inhibition of hypoxic pulmonary vasoconstriction by nifedipine. *Am. J. Cardiol.*, **50**, 864–8.

394. Young, T.E., Lundquist, L.J., Chelser, E. *et al.* (1983) Comparative effects of nifedipine, verapamil and diltiazem on experimental pulmonary hypertension. *Am. J. Cardiol.*, **51**, 195–200.

395. Stanbrook, H.S., Morris, K.G. and McMurty, I.F. (1984) Prevention of hypoxic pulmonary hypertension by calcium antagonists. *Am. Rev. Respir. Dis.*, **130**, 81–5.

396. Kennedy, T.P., Michael, J.R., Huang, C.K. *et al.* (1984) Nifedipine inhibits hypoxic pulmonary vasoconstriction during rest and exercise in patients with chronic obstructive pulmonary disease. *Am. Rev. Respir. Dis.*, **129**, 544–51.

397. Simmoneau, G., Escourrou, P., Duroux, P. *et al.* (1981) Inhibition of hypoxic pulmonary vasoconstriction by nifedipine. *N. Engl. J. Med.*, **304**, 1582–5.

398. Sturani, C., Bassein, L., Schiavina, M. *et al.* (1983) Oral nifedipine in chronic cor pulmonale secondary to severe chronic obstructive pulmonary disease. Short and long term haemodynamic effects. *Chest*, **84**, 135–42.

399. Melot, C., Halleman, R., Naieje, R. *et al.* (1984) Deleterious effect of nifedipine on pulmonary gas exchange in chronic obstructive pulmonary disease. *Am. Rev. Respir. Dis.*, **130**, 612–6.

400. Gaucher, L.R., Payen, D.M., Minsart, P.J. *et al.* (1984) Effects of nifedipine on pulmonary arterial hypertension in patients with respiratory insufficiency without acute failure. *Respiration*, **45**, 443–9.

401. Muramoto, A., Caldwell, J., Albert, R.K. *et al.* (1985) Nifedipine dilates the pulmonary vasculature without producing symptomatic systemic hypotension in upright resting and exercising patients with pulmonary hypertension secondary to chronic obstructive pulmonary disease. *Am. Rev. Respir. Dis.*, **132**, 963–6.

402. Singh, H., Ebejer, M.J., Higgins, D.A. *et al.* (1985) Acute haemodynamic effects of nifedipine at rest and during maximal exercise in patients with chronic cor pulmonale. *Thorax*, **40**, 910–4.

403. Brown, S., Linden, G.S., King, R.R. *et al.* (1983) Effects of verapamil on pulmonary haemodynamics during hypoxaemia, at rest, and during exercise in patients with chronic obstructive pulmonary disease. *Thorax*, **38**, 840–4.

404. Clozel, J.P., Delorme, N., Battistella, P. *et al.* (1987) Hemodynamic effects of intravenous diltiazem in hypoxic pulmonary hypertension. *Chest*, **91**, 171–5.

405. Mookherjee, S., Ashutosh, K., Dunsky, M. *et al.* (1988) Nifedipine in chronic cor pulmonale: acute and relatively long-term effects. *Clin. Pharmacol. Ther.*, **44**, 289–96.

406. Saadjian, A.Y., Philip-Joet, F., Vestri, R. *et al.* (1988) Long-term treatment of chronic obstructive lung disease by nifedipine: an 18 month haemodynamic study. *Eur. Respir. J.*, **1**, 716–20.

407. Agostoni, P., Doria, E., Galli, C. *et al.* (1989) Nifedipine reduces pulmonary pressure and vascular tone during short- but not long-term treatment of pulmonary hypertension in patients with chronic obstructive pulmonary disease. *Am. Rev. Respir. Dis.*, **139**, 120–5.

408. Philip-Joet, F., Saadjian, A., Vestri, R. *et al.* (1986) One year follow-up study of nifedipine in the treatment of secondary pulmonary hypertension (abstract) *Eur. J. Respir. Dis.*, **69** (suppl 146), A128.

409. Bratel, T., Hedenstierna, G., Nyquist, O. *et al.* (1986) Long term treatment with a new calcium antagonist, felodipine, in chronic obstructive lung disease. *Eur. J. Respir. Dis.*, **68**, 351–61.

410. Rubin, L.J. and Moser, K. (1986) Long term effects of nitrendipine on haemodynamics and oxygen transport in patients with cor pulmonale. *Chest*, **89**, 141– 5.

411. Rubin, L.J. and Peter, R.H. (1980) Oral hydralazine therapy for primary pulmonary hypertension. *N. Engl. J. Med.*, **302**, 69–73.

412. Rubin, L.J. and Peter, R.H. (1981) Hemodynamics at rest and during exercise

after oral hydralazine in patients with cor pulmonale. *Am. J. Cardiol.*, **47**, 116–22.

413. Brent, B.N., Berger, H.J., Matthay, R.A. *et al.* (1983) Contrasting acute effects of vasodilators (nitroglycerin, nitroprusside and hydralazine) on right ventricular performance in patients with chronic obstructive pulmonary disease and pulmonary hypertension: A combined radionuclide-hemodynamic study. *Am. J. Cardiol.*, **51**, 1682–9.

414. Keller, C.A., Shepard, J.W., Chun, D.S. *et al.* (1984) Effects of hydralazine on hemodynamics, ventilation, and gas exchange in patients with chronic obstructive pulmonary disease and pulmonary hypertension. *Am. Rev. Respir. Dis.*, **130**, 606–11.

415. Rubin, L.J., Handel, F. and Peter, R.H. (1982) Effects of oral hydralazine on right ventricular end-diastolic pressure in patients with right ventricular failure. *Circulation*, **65**, 1369–73.

416. Lupi-Herrera, E., Seoane, M. and Verdejo, J. (1984) Hemodynamic effect of hydralazine in advanced, stable chronic obstructive pulmonary disease with cor pulmonale. *Chest*, **85**, 156–63.

417. Tuxen, D.V., Powles, A.C.P., Mathur, P.N. *et al.* (1984) Detrimental effect of hydralazine in patients with chronic obstructive pulmonary disease and pulmonary hypertension. *Am. Rev. Respir. Dis.*, **129**, 388–95.

418. Rudd, P. and Blaschke, T.F. (1985) Antihypertensive agents and the drug therapy of hypertension, in *Goodman and Gilman's The Pharmacological Basic of Therapeutics* 7th edn (eds A. Goodman-Gilman, L.A. Goodman, T.W. Rall and F. Murad), Macmillan, New York, pp. 795–6.

419. Parker, J.O., Ashekian, P.B., Di Giorgi, S. *et al.* (1967) Haemodynamic effects of aminophylline in chronic obstructive pulmonary disease. *Circulation*, **35**, 365–72.

420. Parker, J.O., Kelkar, K. and West, R.O. (1966) Haemodynamic effects of aminophylline in cor pulmonale. *Circulation*, **33**, 17–25.

421. Jezek, V., Ourednik, A., Stepanek, J. *et al.* (1970) The effect of aminophylline on the respiration and pulmonary circulation. *Clin. Sci.*, **38**, 549–54.

422. Leeman, M., Lejeune, P., Melot, C. *et al.* (1987) Reduction in pulmonary hypertension and in airway resistances by enoximone (MDL 17,043) in decompensated COPD. *Chest*, **91**, 662–6.

423. Matthay, R.A. (1985) Effects of theophylline on cardiovascular performance in chronic obstructive pulmonary disease. *Chest*, **88** (Suppl), 1125–75.

424. Matthay, R.A., Berger, H.J., Loke, J. *et al.* (1978) Effects of aminophylline upon right left ventricular performance in chronic obstructive pulmonary disease. *Am. J. Med.*, **65**, 903–10.

425. Matthay, R.A., Berger, H.J., Davies, R. *et al.* (1982) Improvement in cardiac performance by oral long-acting theophylline in chronic obstructive pulmonary disease. *Am. Heart J.*, **104**, 1022–6.

426. The CONCENSUS trial study group (1987) Effects of enalapril on mortality in severe congestive heart failure; results of the co-operative North Scandinavian enalapril survival study (CONCENSUS). *N. Engl. J. Med.*, **316**, 1429–35.

427. Hall, J.E., Coleman, T.G., Guyton, A.C. *et al.* (1981) Control of glomerural filtration rate by circulating angiotensin II. *Am. J. Physiol.*, **241**, R190–R197.

428. Packer, M., Lee, W.H. and Kessler, P.D. (1986) Preservation of glomerular filtration rate in human heart failure by activation of the renin-angiotensin system. *Circulation*, **74**, 766–74.

429. Burke, C.M., Harte, M., Duncan, J. *et al.* (1985) Captopril and domiciliary oxygen in chronic airflow obstruction. *Br. Med. J.*, **290**, 1251.

430. Mookherjee, S., Ashutosh, K., Smulyan, V. *et al.* (1983) Arterial oxygenation and pulmonary function with saralasin in chronic lung disease. *Chest*, **83**, 842–7.

431. Zielsinki, J., Hawrylkiewicz, I., Goreika, D. *et al.* (1986) Captopril effects on pulmonary and systemic haemodynamics in chronic cor pulmonale. *Chest*, **90**, 562–5.

432. Neilly, J.B., Carter, R., Morton, J.T. *et al.* (1987) Acute hemodynamic, hormonal and gas exchange effects of enalaprilat (MK 422) in stable cor pulmonale. *Am. Rev. Respir. Dis.*, **135**, A515.

433. Farber, M.O., Weinberger, M.H., Robertson, G.L. *et al.* (1987) The effects of angiotensin-converting enzyme inhibition on sodium handling in patients with advanced chronic obstructive pulmonary disease. *Am. Rev. Respir. Dis.*, **136**, 862–6.

434. Naeije, R., Melot, C., Mols, P. *et al.* (1982) Reduction in pulmonary hypertension by prostaglandin E$_1$ in decompensated chronic

obstructive pulmonary disease. *Am. Rev. Respir. Dis.*, **125**, 1–5.

435. Gaba, S.J.M., Bourgouin-Karaouni, D., Dujols, P. *et al.* (1986) Effects of adenosine triphosphate on pulmonary circulation in chronic obstructive pulmonary disease. *Am. Rev. Respir. Dis.*, **134**, 1140–4.

436. Frostell, C., Fratacci, M.D., Wain, J.C. *et al.* (1991) Inhaled nitric-oxide, a selective pulmonary vasodilator reversing hypoxic pulmonary vasoconstriction. *Circulation*, **83**, 2038–47.

437. Pepke-Zaba, J., Higenbottom, T.W., Dinh-Xuan, A.T. *et al.* (1991) Inhaled nitric oxide is the cause of selective vasodilatation in pulmonary hypertension. *Lancet*, **338**, 1173–4.

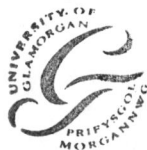

SLEEP

SLEEP 12

N.J. Douglas

12.1 INTRODUCTION

In the 1950s, Robin and colleagues found that expired carbon dioxide tension rose by 10 mmHg during sleep in 7 patients with 'emphysema and chronic hypercapnia' and that 4 of the 7 had Cheyne–Stokes respiration during sleep [1,2]. In the early 1960s, studies using an early ear oximeter showed that arterial oxygen saturation fell during sleep in all the COPD patients studied, and the authors noted that the lowest oxygen saturations during sleep were recorded in those whose saturations were also lowest when awake [3]. All this had been reported before the sleep apnea syndrome was recognized [4] in 1966. However, the great interest in breathing during sleep stimulated by the sleep apnea syndrome has resulted in increased attention being paid to breathing and oxygenation during sleep in patients with COPD.

Studies in which arterial blood gas tensions were monitored in sleeping patients with COPD demonstrated that the most severe hypoxemia and hypercapnia occurred during rapid eye movement (REM) sleep [5–8] (Fig. 12.1). The development of accurate and progressively less obtrusive oximeters has allowed continuous measurement of arterial oxygenation in sleeping patients with COPD. Douglas *et al.* [9] reported that 23 of 28 episodes in which arterial oxygen saturation fell by more than 10% occurred during REM

sleep (Fig. 12.2) and that during such episodes arterial oxygen tension fell to as low as 26 mmHg. Similar observations have subsequently been made by others [10–14]. The most severe hypoxemia occurs during episodes of REM sleep in which there are frequent eye movements [15] (Fig. 12.3). During such hypoxemic episodes, arterial carbon dioxide tension also rises, but the nocturnal rise in carbon dioxide tension is usually relatively small [16].

12.2 MECHANISMS OF HYPOXEMIA DURING SLEEP IN COPD

The major cause of REM hypoxemia in patients with COPD is hypoventilation but there are probably also contributions from a reduction in functional residual capacity and alterations in ventilation/perfusion matching.

12.2.1 HYPOVENTILATION

Ventilation is lower during sleep than wakefulness in both normal subjects [17] and patients with COPD [14]. There is a relatively small decline in ventilation from wakefulness to non-REM sleep, but during REM sleep, there is intermittent marked hypoventilation [17] which is most severe during periods of intense eye movements [19]. This drop in ventilation is largely caused by a decrease in tidal volume. It is important to recognize that this

Chronic Obstructive Pulmonary Disease. Edited by Dr P. Calverley and Professor N. Pride. Published in 1995 by Chapman & Hall, London. ISBN 0 412 46450 0

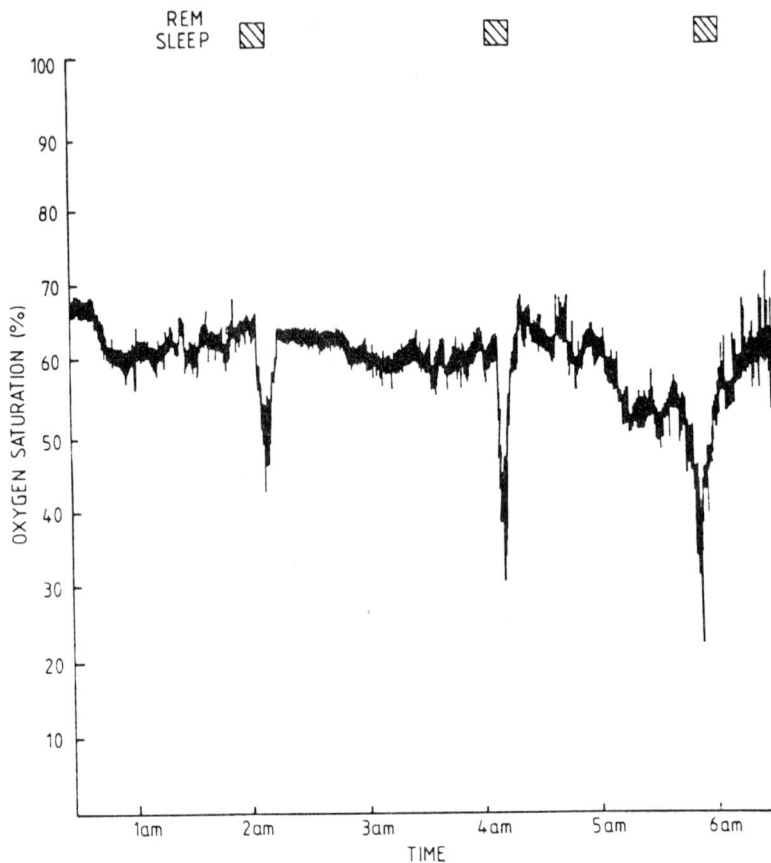

Fig. 12.1 Oxygen saturation throughout the night in a patient with COPD, the shaded areas representing rapid eye movement sleep.

hypoventilation is *not* associated with apneas [18–21].

Although ventilation has not been accurately measured during sleep in patients with COPD, the thoraco-abdominal movement during REM sleep is similar to that in normal subjects [13]. In normal subjects, it has been estimated that alveolar ventilation during REM sleep falls to around 60% of the level during wakefulness [17,19]. As patients with COPD have raised physiologic dead spaces, the rapid shallow breathing during REM sleep may produce an even greater decrease in alveolar ventilation. It has been calculated that this could account for all of the REM hypoxemia observed in patients with COPD [22].

There are many factors which combine to produce hypoventilation during sleep. In normal subjects, ventilation falls during non-REM sleep, despite an increase in respiratory drive as assessed by mouth occlusion pressure [23,24]. This suggests that the increase in upper airways resistance which occurs during non-REM sleep [24,26] may contribute to the non-REM hypoventilation. This effect will be augmented because the ventilatory response to added resistance is impaired during non-REM sleep [24,27]. The increase in upper airways resistance is, however, unlikely to be a major factor in the additional hypoventilation and hypoxemia of REM sleep, because upper airways resistance is not greater in

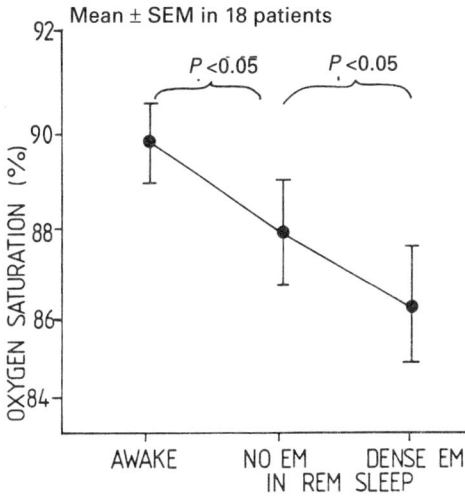

Fig. 12.2 The effect of sleep stage on oxygen saturation in 18 patients with COPD where rapid eye movement sleep is divided into periods with no eye movements (no EM) or periods with frequent eye movements (dense EM). (Data redrawn from George *et al.* (1987) [15].)

response to added resistance appears to be similar between non-REM and REM sleep [24,27]. However, during REM sleep, there is marked alteration of brain stem function. In animals during REM sleep, there is phasic activity of respiratory neurones [28] and it seems probable that similar fluctuations in respiratory output may be a major determinant of the highly variable level of ventilation found during REM sleep in man.

There is also hypotonia of postural muscles during REM sleep [29] and this affects the intercostal muscles, resulting in a decreased contribution from the ribcage to ventilation [20]. In hyperinflated COPD patients, this ribcage flaccidity will result in grossly inefficient ventilation as the flattened diaphragm will then pull in the lower chest wall, further decreasing ventilation during REM sleep. In addition, the postural hypotonia during REM sleep also involves the accessory muscles of respiration [30] which may be important in maintaining ventilation in patients with COPD. This may explain why hyperinflated patients with COPD tend to be more hypoxemic during REM sleep than

REM than non-REM sleep, at least in normal subjects [26]. In addition, although few measurements have been made, the ventilatory

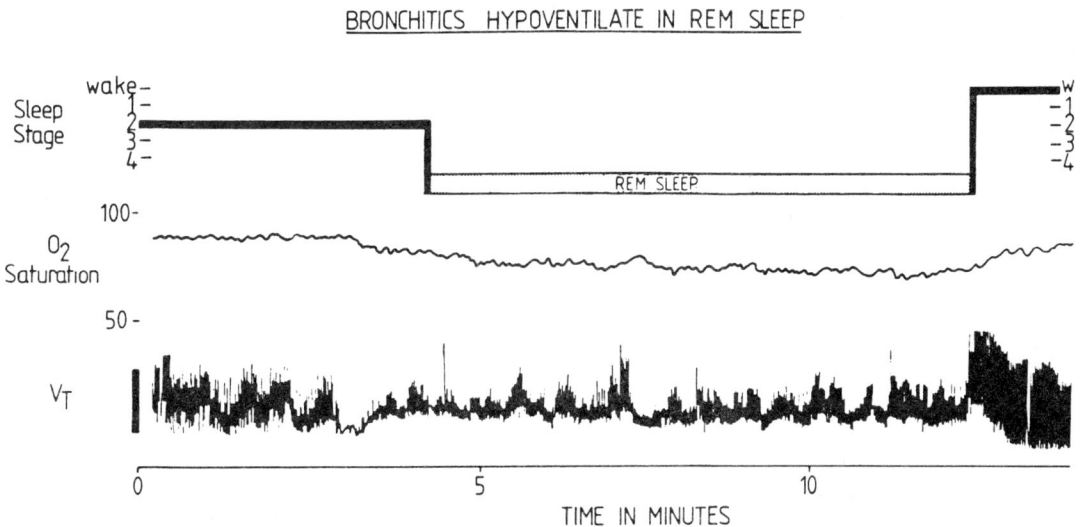

Fig. 12.3 Changes in oxygen saturation and 'tidal volume' in a patient with COPD during an episode of rapid eye movement (REM) sleep. (Data redrawn from Fletcher *et al.* (1983) [21].)

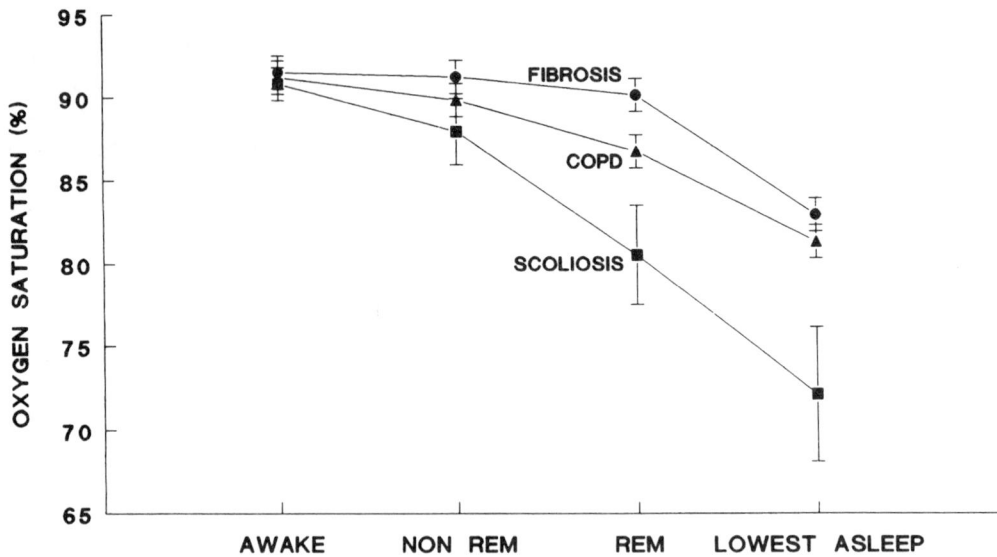

Fig. 12.4 Mean ± SEM oxygen saturation awake, during non-REM sleep, during REM sleep and at the lowest oxygen saturation recorded during sleep in patients with pulmonary fibrosis (○) COPD (Δ) and kyphoscoliosis (□). (Drawn from data in reference [31].)

hypo-inflated patients with fibrotic lung disease [31] (Fig. 12.4).

The body's normal defence mechanism to hypoxemia would be to increase ventilation. However, during REM sleep, there is marked reduction of the ventilatory responses both to hypoxia [32,33] and hypercapnia [34,35]. This, therefore, permits REM hypoxemia to occur.

12.2.2 DECREASE IN FUNCTIONAL RESIDUAL CAPACITY

Functional residual capacity decreases during REM sleep in normal man [26]. Similar changes have been reported in patients with COPD [14] but this study used surface inductive plethysmography which may not be accurate during sleep [36]. A recent preliminary report [37] which used horizontal body plethysmography found no decrease in FRC during REM sleep in patients with COPD.

12.2.3 VENTILATION/PERFUSION IMBALANCE

The importance of the reported ventilation/perfusion mismatch during REM sleep as a cause of hypoxemia in patients with COPD [6,7,21] is difficult to assess. The data on which this assumption is based depend largely on the existence of a steady state of gas transfer which does not occur during REM hypoxemia in COPD [22]. However, the marked hypoventilation which occurs during REM sleep must result in alterations in ventilation/perfusion matching. This conclusion is supported by the fact that cardiac output is maintained during the hypoventilation, indicating changes in overall ventilation/perfusion matching [21,22]. However, current technology does not allow the relative importance of $\dot{V}/\dot{Q}$ matching changes during this unsteady state to be adequately assessed.

12.2.3 COPD COMBINED WITH THE SLEEP APNEA/HYPOPNEA SYNDROME

Both COPD and the sleep apnea/hypopnea syndrome are relatively common conditions [38–40]. Thus, the two conditions will coexist in some patients by chance alone. There is no doubt that the two conditions do coexist in some patients [41–43], but most studies performed in patients referred to respiratory clinics have not found an increased frequency of sleep apnea/hypopnea syndrome in patients with COPD compared to the normal population [11–15]. However, a recent study from Australia has suggested that many patients with hypercapnic COPD have an increased frequency hypopneas [44], a finding at variance with the observations from ourselves and others in Europe and North America [11–15].

12.2.4 MECHANISMS OF HYPOXEMIA DURING SLEEP IN COPD: CONCLUSIONS

Hypoventilation is the main cause of hypoxemia during REM sleep in patients with COPD. In addition, however, there may be contributions from impairment of ventilation/perfusion matching and possibly also from a reduction in functional residual capacity. In a small minority of patients with COPD, there may also be coexisting obstructive sleep apnea/hypopnea syndrome.

12.3 CONSEQUENCES OF HYPOXEMIA DURING SLEEP IN COPD

REM sleep hypoxemia has significant cardiovascular and neurophysiologic sequelae in patients with COPD. In addition, REM hypoxemia may also have hematological effects and may contribute to nocturnal death.

12.3.1 CARDIAC DYSRHYTHMIAS

Patients with COPD have an increased rate of ventricular ectopics during sleep [45]. How-ever, no correlation could be found between ventricular ectopic frequency and oxygen saturation in a study of 42 patients with COPD, except in 6 of the 20 patients in whom oxygen saturation fell below 80% [46]. There was a non-significant trend for nocturnal oxygen therapy to reduce nocturnal ectopic frequency in COPD patients [45]. There is no evidence that such ventricular ectopics are of clinical importance.

12.3.2 HEMODYNAMICS

Pulmonary arterial pressure rises during REM sleep in patients with COPD as oxygenation falls [8,9,47]. For example in 12 patients with COPD, mean pulmonary arterial pressure rose from 37 to 55 mmHg as the mean arterial oxygen tension fell from 56 to 43 mmHg [8]. There is an inverse correlation between oxygen saturation and mean pulmonary arterial pressure with an average 1 mmHg rise in pulmonary arterial pressure per % fall in SaO_2 [47]. During these episodes of REM pulmonary hypertension, cardiac output increases little, if at all [21,22].

The long-term significance of these episodes of REM sleep pulmonary hypertension is unknown. However, in rats, intermittent hypoxemia induced by breathing 12% oxygen for as little as 2 h each day for 4 weeks led to a significant increase in right ventricular mass [48] (Fig. 12.5). It thus seems probable that the intermittent REM hypoxemia seen in patients with COPD may have a similar effect on the human myocardium. Two studies have suggested that the short-term consequences of REM sleep hypoxemia on the myocardium in patients with COPD may be similar to those of maximal exercise when assessed either in terms of myocardial oxygen consumption [49] or left ventricular ejection [50].

Pulmonary hemodynamics have been compared in patients with COPD who desaturate at night to at least 85%, with more than 5 min

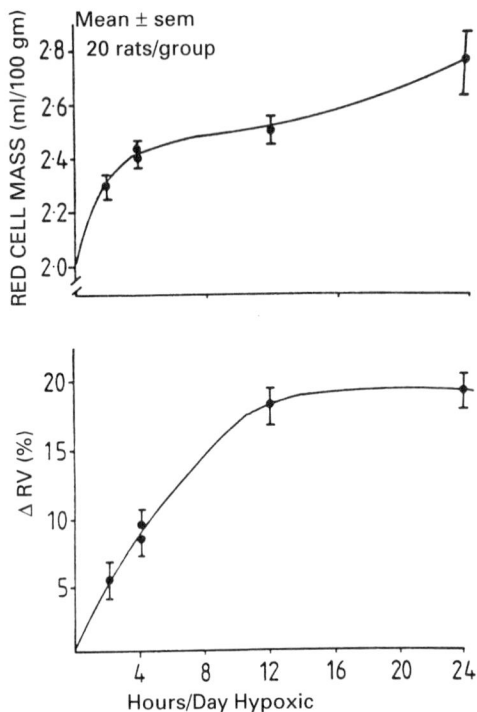

Fig. 12.5 Percentage change in right ventricular mass (ΔRV%) and changes in red cell mass in rats spending the number of hours per day indicated over a 28-day period breathing 12% oxygen. The two points at the four hour time point represents results obtained in rats spending a single 4-hour period and rats spending 8 thirty minute periods per day breathing 12% oxygen, the latter to simulate transient sleep hypoxemia. (Data redrawn from Moore-Gillon and Cameron (1985) [48].)

12.3.3 POLYCYTHEMIA

Intermittent hypoxemia in rats results in elevation of red cell mass [48] (Fig. 12.5). Thus, nocturnal desaturation in patients with COPD might also stimulate erythropoiesis. Morning erythropoietin levels have been found to be raised in some patients with COPD [53,54]. A recent report has suggested that patients whose oxygen saturation fall below 60% at night may have progressive rises in serum erythropoietin during the night [54] but that more minor degrees of hypoxemia are not associated with measurable elevation of erythropoietin levels.

12.3.4 QUALITY OF SLEEP

Both symptomatic enquiry [56] and objective assessment with polysomnography [13,56–58] show that patients with COPD sleep poorly compared to normal subjects. Although COPD patients frequently arouse from sleep during episodes of desaturation [57], the extent of sleep disruption appears to be at least as great in non-desaturating COPD patients [58]. Thus, it may not be the desaturation *per se* which causes the sleep disruption. Despite the subjective and objective evidence of impaired sleep quality, there is no evidence of objective daytime sleepiness in patients with COPD when tested using the multiple sleep latency test [59].

spent below 90%, with those patients who did not desaturate [51]. The desaturating patients had significantly higher daytime pulmonary arterial pressures and red cell masses than the non-desaturators. While the excess nocturnal hypoxemia may explain these findings, the desaturator group had significantly lower daytime oxygen tensions which could thus have contributed to these hemodynamic and hematologic differences.

12.4 DEATH DURING SLEEP IN COPD

Deaths in patients with COPD occur more often at night than in age-matched controls, and nocturnal death has been reported to be particularly common in COPD patients who are hypoxemic and hypercapnic [60]. In hypoxemic patients with COPD, nocturnal death is more common in those breathing air than in those receiving nocturnal oxygen therapy [61]. However, care must be taken not to equate nocturnal death with death during sleep.

12.5 CONSEQUENCES OF COPD COMBINED WITH SAHS

Patients who have the combination of COPD and SAHS are more likely to develop pulmonary hypertension [62], right heart failure [42,63] and CO_2 retention [64] than patients with either condition alone. This seems likely to be due to their having two separate causes for nocturnal hypoxemia, and thus developing more severe nocturnal hypoxemia than would have occurred if they had had only one of these conditions.

12.6 PREDICTION OF NOCTURNAL OXYGENATION

It has been known for over 30 years that the patients with COPD who are most hypoxic when awake are those who become the most hypoxemic during sleep [3]. This has since been widely confirmed by others [13,65,66] and several equations have been derived to predict the extent of nocturnal hypoxemia. Although each is statistically significant [13,65,66], their clinical applicability is limited as there is marked scatter around the regression lines, especially in the most hypoxemic patients (Fig. 12.6). Such equations, however, do show that the extent of nocturnal hypoxemia is related not only to the level of daytime oxygenation, but also to daytime arterial carbon dioxide tension [65,66] and to the duration of REM sleep [66]. There has been considerable recent attention paid to the concept of 'nocturnal desaturators' [67], who have daytime arterial oxygen tensions of >60 mmHg but desaturate to some extent during sleep. Such patients have significantly lower daytime arterial oxygen tensions and higher arterial carbon dioxide tensions than those who do not desaturate and thus from the above regression relationships [13,65,66] would be expected to desaturate more than the non-desaturators.

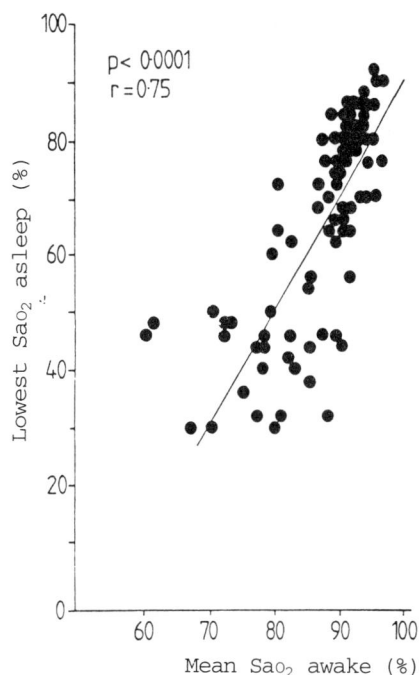

Fig. 12.6 Relationship between mean oxygen saturation during wakefulness and lowest nocturnal oxygenation during sleep in 97 patients with severe COPD. (Data redrawn from Connaughton *et al.* (1988) [66].)

12.7 CLINICAL VALUE OF STUDIES OF BREATHING AND OXYGENATION DURING SLEEP IN PATIENTS WITH COPD

Overnight sleep studies could theoretically be of benefit in patients with COPD by detecting unsuspected cases of SAHS, by detecting clinically important excess hypoxemia during sleep in some patients, or by guiding selection of which patients might benefit from nocturnal oxygen therapy and/or what oxygen concentration such patients should inspire at night. These latter two roles will be discussed in section 12.8.

Although no large studies have been carried out, there is as yet no convincing evidence that the prevalence of SAHS is increased in patients with COPD [13]. When SAHS coexists with COPD, the typical symptoms of SAHS [68,69] are present and current evidence suggests that sleep studies do not yield unsuspected cases of SAHS [66], provided an initial sleep history has been taken. Thus, the symptoms of SAHS should be sought in all patients with COPD, and if major symptoms exist, a clinical sleep study should be performed.

Oxygenation during sleep can be predicted from arterial blood gas tensions measured during wakefulness [13,65,66]. However, all such predictions leave considerable unexplained residual variance, but it is unclear whether this variance is of clinical importance. It has been claimed that measurements of nocturnal oxygenation in such patients can be a useful guide to treatment [70]. To establish the clinical importance of this variability between patients in the extent of sleep-related hypoxemia, Connaughton and colleagues [66] studied the relationship between nocturnal oxygen saturation and survival in 97 patients with COPD. Both mean nocturnal SaO_2 and the lowest SaO_2 during sleep were significantly related to survival, the patients with the lowest nocturnal oxygenation having the worst prognosis. However, neither nocturnal measure was a significantly better predictor of survival than the easier and cheaper measurements of oxygenation when awake or vital capacity [66].

These investigators also studied the significance of the scatter around the regression relationship between measurements of oxygen saturation and PCO_2 when awake with oxygen saturation during sleep. Those patients who had excess nocturnal hypoxemia – the term used to describe those patients whose oxygen saturation during sleep was lower than that predicted from their oxygen saturation and arterial carbon dioxide tension during wakefulness – had similar survivals at a median of 70 months to those who became less hypoxemic at night relative to their awake oxygenation and $PaCO_2$ (Fig. 12.7).

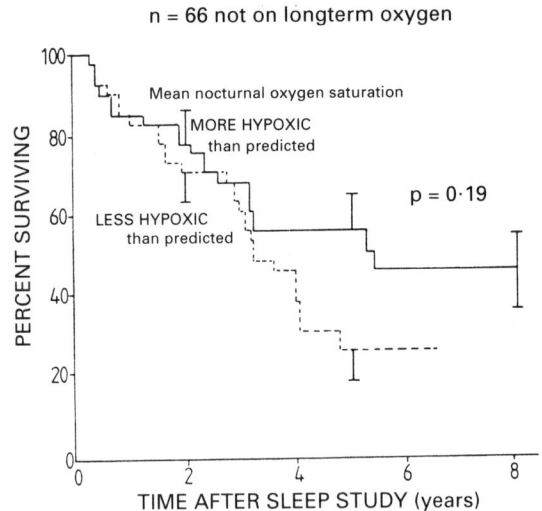

Fig. 12.7   Effect of nocturnal oxygenation on survival in 66 patients with COPD indicating the survival of those who were less hypoxic than predicted and those more hypoxic than predicted from the regression equation between oxygen saturation awake and mean nocturnal oxygen saturation. (Figure reproduced from [63] with permission.)

Fletcher *et al.* [71] reported lower survival in 'desaturators' than non-desaturators. However, these groups were not matched for awake oxygenation which was significantly lower in the desaturators (67 vs 75 mmHg; $P < 0.0001$).

Thus, it seems that there is no clinical value in performing routine polysomnography in patients with COPD. The only patients with COPD in whom I currently perform clinical sleep studies are those with symptoms of SAHS or, occasionally, those who have cor pulmonale or polycythemia but whose daytime arterial oxygen tension is >8 kPa. In these situations, it is imperative to perform full polysomnography as overnight oximetry is extremely difficult to interpret [72] particularly in hypoxemic patients.

12.8 TREATMENT OF NOCTURNAL HYPOXEMIA IN COPD

Oxygen therapy improves oxygenation in sleeping patients with COPD [9,57,73], although mild desaturation will occur during REM sleep. The only firm evidence as to which patients benefit from domiciliary oxygen therapy remains the Nocturnal Oxygen Therapy Trial [74] and the Medical Research Council study [75], both of which showed that home oxygen therapy prolonged life in hypoxemic patients with COPD. However, in both studies the patient selection and choice of inspired oxygen concentration was entirely guided by daytime oxygenation. These studies were carried out on relatively hypoxemic patients who would be expected to become markedly hypoxemic at night. As the period of oxygen administration always included the night, it is tempting to conclude that at least some of the benefit of oxygen therapy was due to blunting of the pulmonary arterial pressure rise during REM sleep [76].

Two recent studies have attempted to answer the difficult question of whether measurement of nocturnal oxygenation should be used to guide oxygen therapy [71,77]. In a multicenter parallel group study, nocturnal oxygen therapy did not help survival in 'desaturators' [71]. Fletcher and colleagues [77] compared survival and physiologic measurements in a group of 38 patients with COPD who 'desaturated' at night. Unfortunately, only 16 patients completed the 3 year protocol, and only 7 of these received nocturnal oxygen therapy. There was no significant effect of nocturnal oxygen therapy on survival, hospitalization or hematological variables, but the patients who received nocturnal oxygen therapy had a lesser rise in pulmonary arterial pressure than the controls. The clinical significance of this observation requires further assessment. Certainly, my present policy is only to give oxygen therapy to patients with significant daytime hypoxemia.

Occasionally, patients will experience symptomatic carbon dioxide retention on nocturnal oxygen therapy, and this is often identified by morning headaches. This seems to be particularly a problem in patients with coexisting SAHS [73] and I do perform polysomnography on patients who develop morning headaches on oxygen.

Some [56,73] but not all [57,78] studies have reported that correction of nocturnal hypoxemia improves sleep quality in patients with COPD. The inconsistency of this finding may have resulted from differing severities of daytime hypoxemia and also from the lack of familiarization nights and of randomization in some of the studies [57,73]. It seems probable that severely hypoxemic patients with COPD do sleep better on nocturnal oxygen therapy although this conclusion needs further testing.

12.8.1 PROTRIPTYLINE

In an uncontrolled study, Series *et al.* [79] reported that protriptyline 20 mg daily improved nocturnal oxygenation in COPD, presumably by suppressing REM sleep. However, all patients experienced dryness of the mouth and 6 of the 11 patients also complained of dysuria. A subsequent non-randomized non-blinded trial [80] suggested that protriptyline may improve daytime arterial oxygen and carbon dioxide tension in patients with COPD, but again the side-effects were common causing cessation of therapy within 10 weeks in 4 of 14 patients.

12.8.2 MEDROXYPROGESTERONE ACETATE

Medroxyprogesterone acetate improved arterial oxygen tension and reduced arterial carbon dioxide tension during both wakefulness and non-REM sleep in 5 of 17 hypercapnic patients with COPD [12]. However, a double-blind controlled trial found no such beneficial effect [81]. Furthermore, MPA may cause troublesome side-effects including impotence in many patients.

12.8.3 ALMITRINE

Almitrine is an investigational drug which can raise arterial oxygen tension in patients with COPD. In a randomized double-blind study, two weeks of almitrine 50 mg twice daily improved oxygenation during sleep in patients with COPD without altering sleep quality [82]. This finding was subsequently confirmed by others [83,84].

It was hoped that the combination of almitrine plus nocturnal oxygen therapy might produce greater improvements in oxygenation and right heart pressure than the use of either agent alone. However, this hope has not been fulfilled. There was no additional benefit in nocturnal oxygenation with the combination of the two therapies and there was a tendency for pulmonary arterial pressure to be higher in almitrine plus oxygen than when on oxygen alone [85].

In addition, neither the dosage of almitrine [86] nor the importance of the peripheral neuropathy that has been associated with its use has as yet been established.

12.8.4 ACETAZOLAMIDE

Acetazolamide improved arterial oxygen tension both when awake and when asleep in 5 patients with COPD, but it did not alter arterial PCO_2 during sleep in 2 of the patients [87]. However, paresthesia, nephrolithiasis and acidosis may limit tolerance of this drug.

12.8.5 THEOPHYLLINE

Neither oral [88] nor intravenous [89] theophylline has been found to improve overnight oxygenation in patients with COPD.

12.8.6 NEGATIVE PRESSURE VENTILATION

Negative pressure ventilation has been reported to reduce arterial carbon dioxide tension and increase respiratory muscle strength in some patients with COPD [90,91]. However, negative pressure ventilation results in increased upper airways obstruction and sleep disturbance [92] and thus cannot be recommended in patients with COPD.

12.8.7 INTERMITTENT POSITIVE PRESSURE VENTILATION BY NASAL MASK

Nocturnal IPPV via nasal mask was originally developed for use in patients with kyphoscoliosis or neuromuscular disorders [93–96]. However, some patients with COPD find this technique acceptable, and it also has the theoretical advantage over long-term oxygen therapy of reducing carbon dioxide tension. There are relatively few data as yet available on the use of nasal IPPV in patients with COPD. Medium-term studies [95,97] suggest that this technique might be useful in a minority of COPD patients but long-term data, particularly data comparing the effect on survival of nasal IPPV with long-term oxygen therapy, is required before this promising technique can be widely advocated as first line therapy.

12.8.8 HYPNOTICS

Although hypnotics are often used to treat sleep disturbance in patients with COPD, they should not be used in hypercapnic patients in case ventilatory responses are further inhibited and acute on chronic ventilatory failure precipitated. Benzodiazepines have been reported to increase sleep duration in some [98–100] but not all [101] studies performed in eucapnic patients with COPD, but the frequency and severity of desaturation may increase [98]. Thus, even in eucapnic patients, hypnotics should only be used with great caution.

12.8.9 ALCOHOL

Alcohol ingestion before sleep may aggravate nocturnal hypoxemia [102] and ventricular ectopic frequency [103] in COPD patients. Recent evidence suggests that heavy alcohol consumption by COPD patients may lead to hypercapnic respiratory failure [44] and right heart failure [104] and to an increase in irregular breathing during sleep [44]. These data require confirmation and clarification, and in particular, it is not clear whether any effect of alcohol may be due to heavy drinkers being overweight. However, the two studies do suggest that alcohol consumption should be discouraged in COPD patients, and this may particularly apply to alcohol consumption in the evening which has been shown to contribute to the development of apneas and hypopneas during sleep.

12.9 TREATMENT OF COPD COMBINED WITH SAHS

There is relatively little evidence about how best to treat patients who have both COPD and the sleep apnea/hypopnea syndrome. A non-randomized study has shown that patients with both conditions improve their daytime arterial blood gas tensions and pulmonary arterial pressures only when their SAHS is adequately treated, the treatment in that study being tracheostomy [43] (Fig. 12.8). The patients who declined tracheostomy had no improvement in their blood gas tensions even though 9 of the 10 received domiciliary oxygen therapy. Thus, it is reasonable to conclude that it is important to recognize coexisting SAHS in such patients and to treat it aggressively, and currently this would usually mean with continuous positive airway pressure therapy with or without supplemental oxygen. It is possible that nocturnal nasal IPPV or bilevel positive pressure ventilatory support might be useful alternatives.

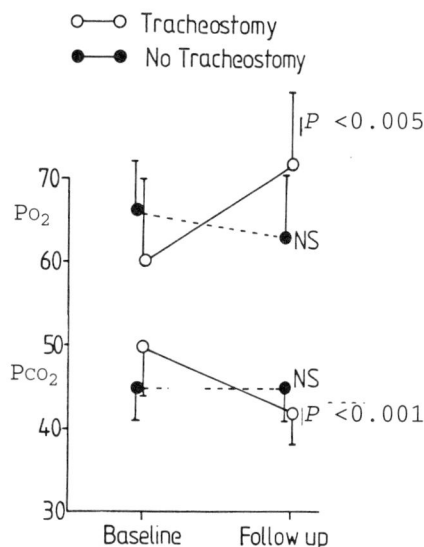

Fig. 12.8 Arterial oxygen and carbon dioxide tensions during the daytime in two groups of patients who had both COPD and the sleep apnea/hypopnea syndrome. In those who accepted tracheostomy, arterial blood gas tensions improved at follow-up whereas there was no such change in those who declined tracheostomy. (Data redrawn from reference [43].)

12.10 BREATHING DURING SLEEP IN COPD: CONCLUSIONS

Patients with COPD become hypoxemic during sleep, especially during REM sleep. There is no conclusive evidence that measurement of nocturnal hypoxemia in breathing patterns in individual patients provides prognostic information which adds significantly to the more simple measurement of oxygenation and lung function made during wakefulness. In small minority of COPD patients, SAHS may coexist and any COPD patient with a history suggestive of SAHS should have full polysomnography. Those found to have SAHS should be treated aggressively. Domiciliary oxygen therapy is the current treatment of choice in COPD patients who are hypoxemic by day and night, although the roles of respiratory stimulants and of nocturnal IPPV may grow.

REFERENCES

1. Robin, E.D., Whaley, R.D., Crump, C.H. *et al.* (1957) The nature of the respiratory acidosis of sleep and of the respiratory alkalosis of hepatic comas (abstract). *J. Clin. Invest.*, **36**, 924.
2. Robin, E.D. (1958) Some interrelations between sleep and disease. *Arch. Intern. Med.*, **102**, 669–75.
3. Trask, C.H and Cree, E.M. (1962) Oximeter studies on patients with chronic obstructive emphysema, awake and during sleep. *N. Engl. J. Med.*, **266**, 639–42
4. Gastaut, H., Tassinari, C.A. and Duron, B. (1966) Polygraphic study of the episodic diurnal and nocturnal (hypnic and respiratory) manifestations of the Pickwick syndrome. *Brain Res.*, **1**, 167–86
5. Pierce, A.K., Jarrett, C.E., Werkle, G. *et al.* (1966) Respiratory function during sleep in patients with chronic obstructive lung disease. *J. Clin. Invest.*, **45**, 631–6.
6. Koo, K.W., Sax, D.S. and Snider, G.L. (1975) Arterial blood gases and pH during sleep in chronic obstructive pulmonary disease. *Am. J. Med.*, **58**, 663–70.
7. Leitch, A.G., Clancy, L.J., Leggett, R.J.E. *et al.* (1976) Arterial blood gas tensions, hydrogen ion, and electroencephalogram during sleep in patients with chronic ventilatory failure. *Thorax*, **31**, 730–5.
8. Coccagna, G. and Lugaresi, E. (1978) Arterial blood gases and pulmonary and systemic arterial pressure during sleep in chronic obstructive pulmonary disease. *Sleep*, **1**, 117–24.
9. Douglas, N.J., Calverly, P.M.A., Leggett, R.J.E. *et al.* (1979) Transient hypoxemia during sleep in chronic bronchitis and emphysema. *Lancet*, **i**, 1–4.
10. Wynne, J.W., Block, A.J., Hemenway, J. *et al.* (1979) Disordered breathing and oxygen desaturation during sleep in patients with chronic obstructive lung disease (COLD). *Am. J. Med.*, **66**, 573–9
11. Fleetham, J.A., Mezon, B., West, P. *et al.* (1980) Chemical control of ventilation and sleep arterial oxygen desaturation in patients with COPD. *Am. Rev. Respir. Dis.*, **122**, 583–9
12. Skatrud, J.B., Dempsey, J.A., Iber, C. *et al.* (1981) Correction of CO_2 retention during sleep in patients with chronic obstructive pulmonary disease. *Am. Rev. Respir. Dis.*, **124**, 260–8.
13. Catterall, J.R., Douglas, N.J., Calverly, P.M.A. *et al.* (1983) Transient hypoxemia during sleep in chronic obstructive pulmonary disease is not a sleep apnea syndrome. *Am. Rev. Respir. Dis.*, **128**, 24–9.
14. Hudgel, D.W., Martin, R.J., Capehart, M. *et al.* (1983) Contribution of hypoventilation to sleep oxygen desaturation in chronic obstructive pulmonary disease. *J. Appl. Physiol.*, **55**, 669–77.
15. George, C.F., West, P. and Kryger, M.H. (1987) Oxygenation and breathing pattern during phasic and tonic REM in patients with chronic obstructive pulmonary disease. *Sleep*, **10**, 234–43.
16. Midgren, B. and Hansson, L. (1987) Changes in transcutaneous PCO_2 with sleep in normal subjects and in patients with chronic respiratory diseases. *Eur. J. Respir. Dis.*, **71**, 384–387.
17. Douglas, N.J., White, D.P., Pickett, C.K. *et al.* (1982) Respiration during sleep in normal man. *Thorax*, **37**, 840–4.
18. Aserinsky, E. (1965) Periodic respiratory pattern occurring in conjunction with eye movements during sleep. *Science*, **150**, 763–6.
19. Gould, G.A., Gugger, M., Molloy, J. *et al.* (1988) Breathing pattern and eye movement density during REM sleep in man. *Am. Rev. Respir. Dis.*, **138**, 874–7.
20. Millman, R.P., Knight, H., Kline, L.R. *et al.* (1988) Changes in compartmental ventilation in association with eye movements during REM sleep. *J. Appl. Physiol.*, **65**, 1196–202.
21. Fletcher, E.C., Gray, B.A. and Levin, D.C. (1983) Non-apneic mechanisms of arterial oxygen desaturation during rapid-eye movement sleep. *J. Appl. Physiol.*, **54**, 632–9.
22. Caterall, J.R., Calverley, P.M.A., MacNee, W. *et al.* (1985) Mechanism of transient nocturnal hypoxemia in hypoxic chronic bronchitis and emphysema. *J. Appl. Physiol.*, **59**, 1698–703.
23. White, D.P. (1986) Occlusion pressure and ventilation during sleep in normal humans. *J. Appl. Physiol.*, **61**, 1279–87.
24. Gugger, M., Molloy, J., Gould, G.A. *et al.* (1989) Ventilatory and arousal responses to added inspiratory resistance during sleep. *Am. Rev. Respir. Dis.*, **140**, 1301–7.
25. Lopes, J.M., Tabachnik, E., Muller, N.L. *et al.* (1983) Total airway resistance and respiratory muscle activity during sleep. *J. Appl. Physiol.*, **54**, 773–7.

26. Hudgel, D.W., Martin, R.J., Johnson, B. *et al.* (1984) Mechanics of the respiratory system and breathing pattern during sleep in normal humans. *J. Appl. Physiol.*, **56**, 133–7.

27. Wiegand, L., Zwillich, C.W. and White, D.P. (1988) Sleep and the ventilatory response to resistive loading in normal men. *J. Appl. Physiol.*, **64**, 1186–95.

28. Orem, J. (1980) Medullary respiratory neuron activity: relationship to tonic and phasic REM sleep. *J. Appl. Physiol.*, **48**, 54–65.

29. Tabachnik, E., Muller, N.L., Bryan, A.C. *et al.* (1981) Changes in ventilation and chest wall mechanics during sleep in normal adolescents. *J. Appl. Physiol.*, **51**, 557–64.

30. Johnson, M.W. and Remmers, J.E. (1984) Accessory muscle activity during sleep in chronic obstructive pulmonary disease. *J. Appl. Physiol.*, **57**, 1011–17.

31. Midgren, B. (1990) Oxygen desaturation during sleep as a function of the underlying respiratory disease. *Am. Rev. Respir. Dis.*, **141**, 43–6.

32. Douglas, N.J., White, D.P., Weil, J.V. *et al.* (1982) Hypoxic ventilatory response decreases during sleep in normal men. *Am. Rev. Respir. Dis.*, **125**, 286–9.

33. Berthon-Jones, M. and Sullivan, C.E. (1982) Ventilatory and arousal responses to hypoxia in sleeping humans. *Am. Rev. Respir. Dis.*, **125**, 632–639.

34. Douglas, N.J., White, D.P., Weil, J.V. *et al.* (1982) Hypercapnic ventilatory response in sleeping adults. *Am. Rev. Respir. Dis.*, **126**, 758–62.

35. Berthon-Jones, M. and Sullivan, C.E. (1984) Ventilation and arousal responses to hypercapnia in normal sleeping adults. *J. Appl. Physiol.*, **57**, 59–67.

36. Whyte, K.F., Gugger, M., Gould, G.A. *et al.* (1991) Accuracy of the respiratory inductive plethysmograph in measuring tidal volume during sleep. *J. Appl. Physiol.*, **71**, 1866–71.

37. Ballard, R.D. and Clover, C.W. (1992) Influence of sleep on respiratory function in emphysema. *Am. Rev. Respir. Dis.*, **145**, A769.

38. Franceschi, M., Zamproni, P., Crippa, D. *et al.* (1982) Excessive daytime sleepiness: a 1-year study in an unselected in-patient population. *Sleep*, **5**, 239–47.

39. Lavie, P. (1983) Incidence of sleep apnea in a presumably healthy, working population: a significant relationship with excessive daytime sleepiness. *Sleep*, **6**, 312–18.

40. Stradling, J.R. and Crosby, J.H. (1991) Predictors and prevalence of obstructive sleep apnoea and snoring in 1001 middle aged men. *Thorax*, **46**, 85–90.

41. Guilleminault, C., Cummiskey, J. and Motta, J. (1980) Chronic obstructive airflow disease and sleep studies. *Am. Rev. Respir. Dis.*, **122**, 397–406.

42. Bradley, T.D., Rutherford, R., Grossman, R.F. *et al.* (1985) Role of daytime hypoxemia in the pathogenesis of right heart failure in the obstructive sleep apnea syndrome. *Am. Rev. Respir. Dis.*, **131**, 835–9.

43. Fletcher, E.C., Schaaf, J.W., Miller, J. *et al.* (1987) Long-term cardiopulmonary sequelae in patients with sleep apnea and chronic lung disease. *Am. Rev. Respir. Dis.*, **135**, 525–33.

44. Chan, C.S., Bye, P.T.P., Woolcock, A.J. *et al.* (1990) Eucapnia and hypercapnia in patients with chronic airflow limitation: the role of the upper airway. *Am. Rev. Respir. Dis.*, **141**, 861–5.

45. Flick, M.R. and Block, A.J. (1979) Nocturnal versus diurnal cardiac arrhythmias in patients with chronic obstructive pulmonary disease. *Chest*, **75**, 8–11.

46. Shepard, J.W., Garrison, M.W., Grither, D.A. *et al.* (1985) Relationship of ventricular ectopy to nocturnal oxygen desaturation in patients with chronic obstructive pulmonary disease. *Am. J. Med.*, **78**, 28–34.

47. Boysen, P.G., Block, A.J., Wynne, J.W. *et al.* (1979) Nocturnal pulmonary hypertension in patients with chronic obstructive pulmonary disease. *Chest*, **76**, 536–42.

48. Moore-Gillon, J.C. and Cameron, I.R. (1985) Right ventricular hypertrophy and polycythemia in rats after intermittent exposure to hypoxia. *Clin. Sci.*, **69**, 595–9.

49. Shepard, J.W., Schweitzer, P.K., Keller, C.A. *et al.* (1984) Myocardial stress: exercise versus sleep in patients with COPD. *Chest*, **86**, 366–74.

50. Levy, P.A., Guilleminault, C., Fagret, D. *et al.* (1991) Changes in left ventricular ejection during REM sleep on exercise in chronic obstructive pulmonary disease in sleep apnoea syndrome. *Eur. Respir. J.*, **4**, 347–50.

51. Fletcher, E.C., Luckett, R.A., Miller, T. *et al.* (1989) Pulmonary vascular hemodynamics in chronic lung disease patients with and

without oxyhemoglobin desaturation during sleep. *Chest*, **95**, 757–64.

52. Miller, M.E., Garcia, J.F., Cohen, R.A. *et al.* (1981) Diurnal levels of immunoreactive erythropoietin in normal subjects and subjects with chronic lung disease. *Br. J. Haemotol.*, **49**, 189–200.

53. Wedzicha, J.A., Cotes, P.M. and Empey, D.W. (1985) Serum immuno-reactive erythropoietin and hypoxic lung disease with and without polycythemia. *Clin. Sci.*, **69**, 413–22.

54. Fitzpatrick, M.F., Mackay, T., Whyte, K.F. *et al.* (1993) Nocturnal desaturation and serum erythropoietin: a study in patients with chronic obstructive pulmonary disease and normal subjects. *Clin. Sci.*, **84**, 319–24.

55. Cormick, W., Olsen, L.G., Hensley, M.J. *et al.* (1986) Nocturnal hypoxemia and quality of sleep in patients with chronic obstructive lung disease. *Thorax*, **41**, 846–54.

56. Calverley, P.M.A., Brezinova, V., Douglas, N.J., *et al.* (1982) The effect of oxygenation on sleep quality in chronic bronchitis and emphysema. *Am. Rev. Respir. Dis.*, **126**, 206–10.

57. Fleetham, J., West, P., Mezon, B. *et al.* (1982) Sleep, arousals and oxygen desaturation in chronic obstructive pulmonary disease. *Am. Rev. Respir. Dis.*, **126**, 429–33.

58. Brezinova, V., Catterall, J.R., Douglas, N.J., *et al.* (1982) Night sleep of patients with chronic ventilatory failure and age-matched controls. Number and duration of EEG episodes of intervening wakefulness and drowsiness. *Sleep*, **5**, 123–30.

59. Orr, W.C., Shamma-Othman, Z., Levin, D. *et al.* (1990) Persistent hypoxemia and excessive daytime sleepiness in chronic obstructive pulmonary disease. *Chest*, **97**, 583–5.

60. McNicholas, W.T. and Fitzgerald, M.X. (1984) Nocturnal deaths in patients with chronic bronchitis and emphysema. *Br. Med. J.*, **289**, 878.

61. Douglas, N.J. (1990) Breathing during sleep in patients with respiratory disease, in *Obstructive Sleep Apnea Syndrome*, (eds C. Guilleminault and M. Partinen), Raven Press, New York, pp. 37–48.

62. Weitzenblum, E., Krieger, J., Apprill, M. *et al.* (1988) Daytime pulmonary hypertension in patients with obstructive sleep apnea syndrome. *Am. Rev. Respir. Dis*, **138**, 345–9.

63. Whyte, K.F. and Douglas, N.J. (1991) Peripheral edema in the sleep apnea/hypopnea syndrome. *Sleep*, **14**, 354–6.

64. Bradley, T.D., Rutherford, R., Lue, F. *et al.* (1986) Role of diffuse airway obstruction in the hypercapnia of obstructive sleep apnea. *Am. Rev. Respir. Dis.*, **134**, 920–4.

65. McKeon, J.L., Muree-Allan, K. and Saunders, N.A. (1988) Prediction of oxygenation during sleep in patients with chronic obstructive lung disease. *Thorax*, **43**, 312–7.

66. Connaughton, J.J., Catterall, J.R., Elton, R.A., *et al.* (1988) Do sleep studies contribute to the management of patients with severe chronic obstructive pulmonary disease? *Am. Rev. Respir. Dis.*, **138**, 341–4.

67. Fletcher, E.C., Miller, J., Devine, G.W. *et al.* (1987) Nocturnal oxyhemoglobin desaturation in COPD patients with arterial oxygen tension above 60 mmHg. *Chest*, **92**, 604–8.

68. Guilleminault, C., van den Hoed, J. and Mitler, M.M. (1978) Clinical overview of the sleep apnea syndromes, in *Sleep Apnea Syndromes*, (ed C. Guilleminault and W.C. Dement), Alan R. Liss, New York, pp. 1–12.

69. Whyte, K.F., Allen, M.B., Jeffrey, A.A. *et al.* (1989) Clinical features of the sleep apnoea/hypopnoea syndrome. *Q. J. Med.*, **72**, 659–66.

70. Phillipson, E.A. and Remmers, J.E., (Chairmen) (1989) Indications and standards for cardiopulmonary sleep studies. *Am. Rev. Respir. Dis.*, **139**, 559–68.

71. Fletcher, E.C., Donner, C.F., Midgren, B. *et al.* (1992) Survival in COPD patients with a daytime PaO_2 > 60 mmHg with and without nocturnal oxyhemoglobin desaturation. *Chest*, **101**, 649–55.

72. Douglas, N.J., Thomas, S. and Jan, M.A. (1992) Clinical value of polysomnography. *Lancet*, **339**, 347–50.

73. Goldstein, R.S., Ramcharan, V., Bowes, G. *et al.* (1984) Effect of supplemental nocturnal oxygen on gas exchange in patients with severe obstructive lung disease. *N. Engl. J. Med.*, **310**, 425–9.

74. Nocturnal Oxygen Therapy Trial Group (1980) Continuous or nocturnal oxygen therapy in hypoxemic chronic obstructive lung disease: a clinical trial. *Ann. Intern. Med.*, **93**, 391–8.

75. Medical Research Council Working Party Report. (1981) Long-term domiciliary oxygen therapy in chronic hypoxic cor pulmonale

complicating chronic bronchitis and emphysema. *Lancet* i, 681–6.

76. Fletcher, E.C. and Levin, D.C. (1984) Cardiopulmonary hemodynamics during sleep in subjects with chronic obstructive pulmonary disease: the effect of short and long-term oxygen. *Chest* **85**, 6–14.

77. Fletcher, E.C., Luckett, R.A., Goodnight-White, S. *et al.* (1992) A double-blind trial of nocturnal supplemental oxygen for sleep desaturation in patients with chronic obstructive pulmonary disease and a daytime PaO_2 above 60 mmHg. *Am. Rev. Respir. Dis.*, **145**, 1070–6.

78. McKeon, J.L., Murree-Allen, K. and Saunders, N.A. (1989) Supplemental oxygen and quality of sleep in patients with chronic obstructive lung disease. *Thorax*, **44**, 184–8.

79. Series, F., Cormier, Y. and La Forge, J. (1989) Changes in day and in night time oxygenation with protriptyline in patients with chronic obstructive lung disease. *Thorax*, **44**, 275–9.

80. Series, F. and Cormier, Y. (1990) Effects of protriptyline on diurnal and nocturnal oxygenation in patients with chronic obstructive pulmonary disease. *Ann. Intern. Med.*, **133**, 507–11.

81. Dolly, F.R. and Block, A.J. (1983) Medroxyprogesterone acetate in COPD: effect on breathing and oxygenation in sleeping and awake patients. *Chest*, **84**, 394–8.

82. Connaughton, J.J., Douglas, N.J., Morgan, A.D. *et al.* (1985) Almitrine improves oxygenation when both awake and asleep in patients with hypoxia and carbon dioxide retention caused by chronic bronchitis and emphysema. *Am. Rev. Respir. Dis.*, **132**, 206–10.

83. Daskalopoulou, E., Patakas, D., Tsara, V. *et al.* (1990) Comparison of almitrine bismesylate and medroxyprogesterone acetate on oxygenation during wakefulness and sleep in patients with chronic obstructive lung disease. *Thorax*, **45**, 666–9.

84. Gothe, B., Cherniack, N.S., Bachandrt, R.T. *et al.* (1988) Long-terrm effects of almitrine bismesylate on oxygenation during wakefulness and sleep in chronic obstructive pulmonary disease. *Am. J. Med.*, **84**, 436–43.

85. Ruhle, K.H., Kempf, P., Mossinger, B. *et al.* (1988) Einfluss von almitrin einem chemorezeptoren stimulator, auf die nachtliche hyperkapnie und dem pulmonarteriellen druck unter O_2 atmung bei chronisch obstruktiver lungenerkrankung. *Prax. Clin. Pneumol.*, **42**, 411–4.

86. Howard, P. (1989) Hypoxia, almitrine and peripheral neuropathy. *Thorax*, **44**, 247–50.

87. Skaturd, J.B. and Dempsey, J.A. (1983) Relative effectiveness of acetazolamide versus medroxyprogesterone acetate in correction of carbon dioxide retention. *Am. Rev. Respir. Dis.*, **127**, 405–12.

88. Martin, R.J. and Pak, J. (19922) Overnight theophylline concentrations and effects on sleep and lung function in chronic obstructive pulmonary disease. *Am. Rev. Respir. Dis.*, **145**, 540–4.

89. Ebden, P. and Vathenen, A.S. (1987) Does aminophylline improve nocturnal hypoxia in patients with chronic airflow obstruction? *Eur. J. Respir. Dis.*, **71**, 384–7.

90. Braun, N.M.T. and Marino, W.D. (1984) Effectively daily intermittent rest of respiratory muscles in patients with severe chronic airflow limitation. *Chest*, **85**, 59S–60S.

91. Crop, A.J. and Di Marco, A.F. (1987) Effects of intermittent negative pressure ventilation on respiratory muscle function in patients with severe chronic obstructive pulmonary disease. *Am. Rev. Respir. Dis.*, **135**, 1056–61.

92. Levy, R.D., Cosio, M.G., Gibbons, L. *et al.* (1992) Induction of sleep apnoea with negative pressure ventilation in patients with chronic obstructive lung disease. *Thorax*, **47**, 612–5.

93. Ellis, E.R., Bye, P.T.P., Bruderer, J.W. *et al.* (1987) Treatment of respiratory failure during sleep in patients with neuromuscular disease. *Am. Rev. Respir. Dis.*, **135**, 148–52.

94. Kerby, G.R., Mayer, L.S. and Pringleton, S.K. (1987) Nocturnal positive pressure ventilation via mask. *Am. Rev. Respir. Dis.*, **135**, 738–40.

95. Carroll, N. and Branthwaite, M.A. (1988) Control of nocturnal hypoventilation by nasal intermittent positive pressure ventilation. *Thorax*, **43**, 349–53.

96. Ellis, E.R., Grunstin, R.R., Chan, S. *et al.* (1988) Noninvasive ventilatory support during sleep improves respiratory failure in kyphoscoliosis. *Chest*, **94**, 811–5.

97. Elliot, M.W., Simonds, A.K., Carroll, M.P. *et al.* (1992) Domiciliary nocturnal nasal intermittent positive pressure ventilation in hypercapnic respiratory failure due to chronic

obstructive lung disease: effects on sleep and quality of life. *Thorax*, **47**, 342–8.

98. Block, A.J., Dolly, F.R. and Slayton, P.C. (1984) Does flurazepam ingestion affect breathing and oxygenation during sleep in patients with chronic obstructive lung disease? *Am. Rev. Respir. Dis.*, **129**, 230–3.

99. Wedzicha, J.A., Wallis P.J.W., Ingram, D.A. *et al.* (1988) Effect of diazepam on sleep in patients with chronic airflow obstruction. *Thorax*, **43**, 729–30.

100. Midgren, B., Hansson, L., Skeidsvoll, H. *et al.* (1989) The effects of nitrazepam and fluni-trazepam on oxygen desaturation during sleep in stable hypoxemic non hypercapnic COPD. *Chest*, **95**, 765–8.

101. Cummiskey, J., Guilleminault, C., Rio, G.D. *et al.* (1983) The effects of flurazepam on sleep studies in patients with chronic obstructive pulmonary disease. *Chest*, **84**, 143–7.

102. Easton, P.A., West, P., Meatherall, R.C. *et al.* (1987) The effect of excessive ethanol ingestion on sleep in severe chronic obstructive pulmonary disease. *Sleep*, **10**, 224–33.

103. Dolly, F.R. and Block, A.J. (1983) Increased ventricular ectopy and sleep apnea following ethanol ingestion in COPD patients. *Chest*, **83**, 469–72.

104. Jalleh, R., Fitzpatrick, M.F., Jan, M.A. *et al.* (1993) Alcohol and cor pulmonale in chronic bronchitis and emphysema. *Br. Med. J.*, **306**, 374.

CLINICAL AND LABORATORY ASSESSMENT

13

M.G. Pearson and P.M.A. Calverley

Although the definition of COPD in clinico-pathologic terms presents continuing difficulties (Chapter 1), the identification of symptomatic patients is more straight-forward. The pathologic changes of inflammation and distortion of the small airways and patchy loss of the alveolar walls antedate the onset of symptoms, even those of mucus hypersecretion in regular smokers. The identification of these presymptomatic individuals is difficult but by the time the patient recognizes their symptoms, there is physiologic evidence of airflow limitation and there may be abnormal physical signs. However, these signs may be undramatic, and are not always present. This chapter will review the clinical and laboratory findings which favor a diagnosis of COPD, consider some of its different clinical presentations and look at the practical aspects of achieving a diagnostic formulation on which treatment can be based.

13.1 SYMPTOMS IN COPD

The principal symptoms of which patients complain are breathlessness on exertion, wheeze and cough (usually with sputum) [1]. Of these, breathlessness is the most important and disabling and the one most likely to lead the patient to seek medical help. However, it is not usually the first to appear as a significant amount of ventilatory capacity has to be lost before respiratory disability is

noticeable [2]. The clinical picture of COPD will vary both over time as the severity increases and with the ability of the patient to adapt to his or her limitations. Only some of the features below will apply to individual patients at any one point in time.

13.1.1 COUGH

In 75% of COPD patients cough either precedes the onset of breathlessness or appears simultaneously with it [3]. Cough productive of sputum occurs in up to 50% of cigarette smokers [3,4] and maybe present within 10 years of starting to smoke. In COPD the cough is usually worse in the morning but seldom disturbs the patient's sleep and is often dismissed as a 'smokers cough' of little importance. Its significance was recognized in early attempts to define COPD [5] and the MRC symptom questionnaire used cough and sputum production as the defining characteristics of clinical chronic bronchitis [6]. However, occupational studies have shown that cough relates to increases in inhaled dust burden rather than changes in lung function [7], whilst most longitudinal studies in COPD have found no association between mortality and symptoms of cough and/or sputum production [2] (Chapter 4). When cigarette smokers stop smoking cough diminishes or disappears in 94% of them [8,9] but abnormalities in lung function persist. Thus cough

Chronic Obstructive Pulmonary Disease. Edited by Dr P. Calverley and Professor N. Pride. Published in 1995 by Chapman & Hall, London. ISBN 0 412 46450 0

is a marker of the processes leading to disability but does not produce disabling symptoms in the early stages of disease [10].

Whether cough in COPD is a normal physiologic response to increased mucus production or is itself pathologic is not known. Studies in asthmatic patients suggest that cough threshold is reduced possibly because of the release of airway inflammatory mediators [11,12] but comparable data in COPD [9] are lacking. Sputum production is increased in COPD but mucociliary clearance (as assessed by radio-isotope methods) is reduced [13] due to direct ciliotoxicity [14] and possibly increases in sputum viscosity. Interpretation of total sputum clearance is difficult without allowing for the variations in the frequency of cough. Thus Loudon and co-workers using objectively recorded cough counts detected an average of 120 coughs during 8 hours overnight recording compared with just 23 coughs per night in patients being treated for tuberculosis [15]. However, nocturnal cough frequency does not appear to be increased in stable COPD [16]. The variability in cough threshold, total sputum volume and the ability to swallow, rather than expectorate sputum, between individual patients, make it hard to interpret sputum production objectively. None the less, sputum purulence is a reasonably reliable sign of endobronchial infection which merits antibiotic treatment.

When severe airflow obstruction is present, recurrent coughing bouts can be severe enough to produce 'cough syncope' [17] and 'cough fractures' of the ribs [18]. These events probably share a common mechanism with high intrathoracic pressures being developed during coughing, in patients whose relatively long mechanical time constants prevent adequate pulmonary deflation before the next cough begins.

13.1.2 WHEEZING

This complaint is difficult to evaluate because of its intermittent nature and limitations in patient understanding. It is usually associated with wheezes audible on auscultation but this feature is not universal. Some patients can produce convincing wheeze from their larynx as do those with factitious asthma [19]. Whether this is a psychologic problem or is an attempt to modify expiratory airflow is unknown. Wheeze is not specific to COPD. It is due to turbulent airflow through larger airways narrowed from any cause, e.g. smooth muscle contraction, anatomic distortion or the presence of excess secretion. Although the IPPB trial found the presence of wheezing to be commoner in those patients showing a bronchodilator response the interpretation of these data is difficult [20] (see below). We could not confirm this relationship in our on-going study of over 200 patients assessed with nebulized beta agonists and oral corticosteroids. The presence of wheezing is believed to be a pointer against the diagnosis of COPD but we found that in our series of moderate to severe patients 83% reported that they wheezed on most days, whilst wheeze on auscultation was present in 66% of patients.

13.1.3 BREATHLESSNESS

The physiologic basis of breathlessness is reviewed in Chapter 10. This is the symptom associated with the worst prognosis, greatest disability and largest loss of lung function over time [2]. In early COPD, behavior can be modified to limit breathlessness, e.g. not talking when walking, using a car for short journeys. The gradual increase in background respiratory impedance over the years makes detection of further acute changes harder and patients may alter their breathing pattern to minimize the sensation of breathlessness. Thus a greater degree of inspiratory effort can be tolerated for the same level of discomfort [21]. How rapidly this adaptive behavior occurs is not known but many patients presenting to their physicians have substantially reduced ventilatory capacity, often less than

50% of predicted. By the time the FEV_1 has fallen to 30% or less predicted (equivalent to an FEV_1 of about 1 l) and the VO_2 max is less than 15 ml/kg/min, the patient is breathless on minimal exertion [22]. However, it is difficult to accurately grade symptoms such as breathlessness from simple spirometric percentages, as hyperinflation which develops at a variable rate as FEV_1 declines, and pulmonary hypertension, especially on exercise, will both affect exercise tolerance. The wide range of breathlessness intensity perceived at any given level of lung function is illustrated by data from Wolkove and colleagues using a 10 point Borg scale. They found that for any given level of lung function impairment there was a range of scoring of 5 or more points [23]. Moreover mental state is a crucial determinant of the severity of perceived breathlessness in COPD [24]. For example, occupational medicolegal claimants have a significantly higher level of symptoms for each level of lung impairment than do patients with no claim to support [25].

The terms used by patients to describe breathlessness vary widely. Specific clusters of symptoms have been reported in COPD and in asthma, but may be modified by local experience. Thus in Liverpool, men complain of 'blowing for tugs' when describing their breathlessness, meaning 'wheezing as loudly as a ship's horn calling for tugs to help the ship into its docking berth'. The degree of breathlessness may be recorded by relating it to specific tasks, e.g. shopping or climbing stairs or can be formally quantified using one of the several scales developed to assess breathlessness. The MRC scale is simple and has been extensively used as an epidemiologic tool. It is still a valuable means of describing population behavior but is too insensitive to detect clinically important changes in symptoms. Short-term assessments with category scales such as the Borg scale or with visual analog scales are helpful in monitoring the progress of specific symptoms but a more global view is obtained by detailed questionnaire based studies such as the baseline dyspnea index and transitional dyspnea index [26].

In severe COPD, orthopnea can occur reflecting the increased diaphragmatic activity required to maintain lung volume when supine [27], but some patients, especially those with marked increases in FRC, complain of breathlessness worse on leaning forward which is relieved by lying flat [28]. Again this reflects particular chest wall configuration patterns of respiratory muscle activation.

13.1.4 OTHER SYMPTOMS

Chest pain is a common complaint in COPD but is not usually related to the disease itself. Ischemic heart disease is frequent in any population of heavy smokers and may be difficult to distinguish from symptoms of gastroesophageal reflux. Acid reflux occurs in up to 40% of COPD patients [29] presumably due to impairment of the pinch-cock mechanism at the esophageal hiatus secondary to hyperinflation and/or methylxanthine therapy [30]. COPD patients often complain of chest tightness during exacerbations which is not pleuritic and for which no cause is found. Possible explanations include intercostal muscle ischemia due to the increased work of respiration or trapped air under pressure in poorly ventilated peripheral areas of lung. Dull persistent pain especially if accompanied by increasing breathlessness or fixed wheezing raises the possibility of a central bronchial neoplasm whilst acute pleurisy and dyspnea require that pulmonary embolism, pneumothorax or pneumonia be urgently excluded.

Ankle swelling may simply reflect immobility but if there is pitting edema and an elevated JVP, this raises the possibility of cor pulmonale. The difficulties associated with this commonly used term are reviewed in Chapter 11. Hemoptysis, especially if it occurs as streaks of blood in purulent phlegm, may be due simply to airway inflammation [31]. However, this can never be assumed until bronchoscopy and a CT scan have excluded bronchial carcinoma or bronchiectasis.

Anorexia and weight loss often occur in advanced disease and are a marker of a worse prognosis. The cause is unclear but reduction in calorie intake and hypermetabolism have been suggested [32,33] (Chapter 21). Psychiatric morbidity is high in COPD reflecting the social isolation the disease produces, its chronicity and the neurologic effects of hypoxemia [34,35]. Sleep quality is impaired in advanced disease, more so in the pink and puffing than the blue and bloated patients [36] and this may contribute to impaired neuropsychiatric performance. Recent data in hypoxemic hypercapnic COPD patients suggest a specific pattern of cognitive deterioration characterized by an impaired verbal memory test, well preserved visual attention and diffuse worsening of other functions. These changes cannot be explained by age or associated vascular dementia [37].

13.2 SOCIAL HISTORY

Smoking is the principle cause of COPD in industrial countries (Chapter 5) and the diagnosis should always be made with great caution in non-smokers even when the history and physiology appear to be typical. It is useful to assess life time smoking habits in terms of pack-years; 1 pack-year being equivalent to smoking 20 cigarettes per day for 1 year. This overcomes the problems of different durations and intensities of cigarette smoking but there is still considerable variation in the effects of apparently equivalent exposures on lung function which is illustrated in Fig. 13.1 [38]. In general the greater the cumulative exposure, the worse the decline in FEV_1 but a very susceptible light smoker (1–20 pack-years) can have much worse lung function than a 'resistant' heavy smoker (61–80 pack-years). A similar spectrum of response is seen

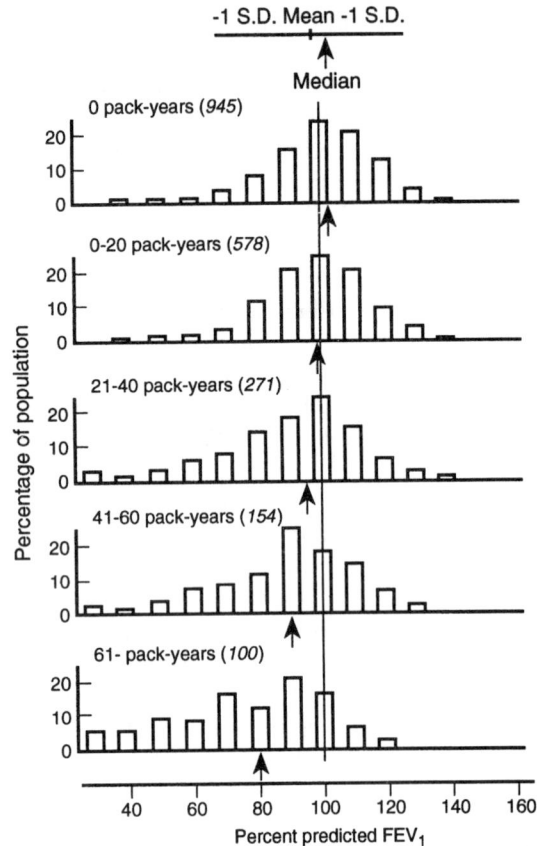

Fig. 13.1 The 'dose-related' effects of cigarette smoking in a population sample expressed as the percentage distribution of predicted FEV_1 for subjects divided by pack-years of smoking. Figures in brackets refer to the number in each sample and solid arrows to the median FEV_1 values. Mean and median FEV_1 fall as cigarette consumption increases but the individual change is still very variable and spirometry can be normal despite heavy tobacco exposure (reproduced with permission from reference [38].)

pathologically but patients can be assured that most smokers of 40 pack years or more have pathologic evidence of emphysema even if this is not yet affecting their pulmonary physiology [39]! Some of this variability presumably reflects differences in puff size, cigarette type and the accuracy of the patient's own assessment of their cigarette consumption but most represents the differences in susceptibility between individuals [40].

There may be additive effects from occupational dust or home exposures [41]. Love and Miller in a longitudinal study of coal miners reported that both smoking and years of dust exposure contributed to the fall in FEV_1 in a ratio of 3:1 [42]. Separating out the relative effects of cigarette smoke and dust exposure is difficult and controversial. However, the UK Industrial Injuries Advisory Committee has recently concluded that coal miners with radiographic pneumoconiosis and airflow limitation should be compensated by the State for the airflow limitation irrespective of whether or not they have smoked cigarettes.

13.3 PHYSICAL SIGNS IN COPD

Unlike other respiratory diseases the most useful physical signs in COPD are those obtained by careful inspection rather than palpation or auscultation. They are qualitative rather than quantitative and support a diagnosis made from the history and investigations rather than being specific in their own right.

Many patients are distressed by minimal exertion and may appear tachypneic at rest. 'Nicotine-stained' fingers (a common misnomer since it is tar that stains) may bely the stated smoking habits while definite central cyanosis indicates significant hypoxemia. However, the assessment of cyanosis may be influenced by the background lighting and secondary polycythemia (Chapter 20). Overall nutrition, especially muscle mass, may be reduced whilst finger clubbing suggests bronchiectasis or a pulmonary tumour.

It is important to observe the breathing pattern. Symptomatic patients will often have a prolonged expiratory phase and some will purse their lips in expiration. Patients adopting pursed lip breathing at rest usually have a severely reduced FEV_1, and pulmonary hyperinflation, i.e. an increase in resting FRC,

but the physiologic basis of this sign is still obscure. Lip pursing may reduce expiratory airway collapse or slow the breathing frequency [43]. Pursed lip breathing when taught to patients as part of respiratory rehabilitation (Chapter 21) is reported to improve oxygenation [44]. Use of the accessory muscles, principally the sternomastoids, at rest suggests advanced disease and/or a clinical exacerbation. When the patient leans forward and supports themself on a chair or handrail this fixes the shoulder girdle and allows the muscles such as the pectorals and latissimus dorsi to be used for increased rib cage movement [45,46]. Breathing frequency is usually more than 16/min even when rested and becomes rapid and shallow with exertion. Some patients can develop 'respiratory alternans' when they breathe alternately with predominantly rib cage and then predominantly diaphragmatic (abdominal) movements. This is best documented in normal subjects during external-resistive breathing but may be seen in patients in the intensive care unit [47,48].

Patients with advanced COPD develop progressive hyperinflation with an increased AP chest diameter but the stage in the natural history when this change starts is not well defined. Several mechanical consequences follow from these changes in lung volume. The ribs become more horizontal and since the tracheal position is fixed by the mediastinum there appears to be a shortening of the trachea, i.e. the distance between the cricoid cartilage and xiphisternal notch is less than three finger breadths, often less than one. Moreover the trachea appears to descend with each inspiration. The diaphragm becomes more horizontal and acts to pull in the lower ribs during inspiration – Hoover's sign (Chapter 9). This is associated with a widened xiphisternal angle and apparent abdominal protuberance as the abdominal contents are displaced forwards. Some patients may be alarmed by this apparent 'weight gain' until it is explained to them. As the diaphragm descends the liver is displaced and may be palpable below the costal margin.

Low frequency vesicular breath sounds are thought to originate from turbulent flow in the central airways attenuated by passage through the natural filters of the lung and chest wall [49]. These sounds are typically reduced in intensity in COPD producing the 'silent' chest found in advanced disease. This has been related to regional changes in ventilation and perfusion [50]. Recent observations suggest that breath sound intensity can be reproducibly recorded and when airflow is standardized there is no significant difference between COPD patients and observations in normal subjects [51]. Wheezes are often present but their clinical significance has not been systematically studied [52]. Similarly a few scanty crackles may be heard but can usually be easily distinguished from the coarse crackles of bronchiectasis and the persistent late inspiratory fine crackles of fibrosis or left heart failure.

Cardiovascular examination may reveal pitting edema, tricuspid regurgitation or elevation of the jugular venous pressure all of which point to pulmonary hypertension. Although assessment of the jugular venous pressure can be difficult in patients with prominent accessory muscle activity, it remains one of the best clinical signs of right ventricular overload. When these signs are present, patients should be assessed with blood gases as potential candidates for long-term oxygen therapy (Chapter 20).

13.4 CLINICAL SIGNIFICANCE OF SYMPTOMS AND SIGNS

Attempts to identify COPD patients on the basis of symptoms and signs alone have been disappointing. In a study examining the specificity of a range of markers of COPD, independent observers picked out a heavy smoking history and those already with a diagnosis of COPD, and the only additional diagnostic information came from the reduc-

tion in the intensity of breath sounds [53]. In a similar exercise Bohadana and colleagues found breath sound intensity during auscultation to be related to the FEV_1 and the specific airways conductance [54]. Both studies show the considerable variation in the criteria adopted for diagnosis even in skilled hands. When the diagnosis has been made, symptoms and signs have been suggested as potential predictors of response to bronchodilator therapy. Wardman and colleagues described a six-item combination with some predictive value but the work has not been replicated [55]. In our own study of 211 patients we could not identify any symptom or sign, either singly or in combination, that could predict the response to either bronchodilators or oral corticosteroids in the short or long term.

13.5 CLINICAL PRESENTATION

Patients reach their doctors by a variety of routes. Although some may be identified when relatively asymptomatic by abnormal spirometry in a health screening program, most accept their cough and reduced exercise tolerance as part of being a smoker and have relatively advanced disease by the time they first seek attention. Since the lung damage takes time to develop, most patients are in their sixth decade or older at first presentation. In our own study of 211 COPD patients we found that although all complained of breathlessness and had spirometric airflow obstruction (FEV_1/FVC <60%), only 82% admitted to wheezing and 73% to having a cough. In spite of an average smoking history of 37 pack-years, only 64% fulfilled the MRC definition of chronic bronchitis which may in part reflect the fact that only 33% were still smoking by the time they presented to hospital for assessment. Patients described how their wheeze or their cough was worst at specific times of day but there was no discernible pattern to this and nor did it have bearing on their later response to bronchodilators or to an oral steroid trial [56]. Thus symptoms and history can suggest the diagnosis of COPD but cannot define either treatment or prognosis.

Whilst this is the usual pattern of patients seen in hospital outpatient clinics, two less common variants are worth noting. The first is patients with advanced disease confirmed by markedly impaired spirometry who insist that they were fully active until the time of a relatively recent intercurrent infection. It seems likely that such patients have been compensating well for their increasing airflow limitation until a final, relatively trivial, rise in respiratory impedance has been enough to provoke a host of symptoms. How many of these changes are psychologic or physiologic is not clear. Second, some patients present with fluid retention, persistent hypoxemic hypercapnia and relatively well preserved nutrition. The relationship of this presentation to abnormal ventilatory control, respiratory muscle function and the pulmonary circulation have already been touched on elsewhere (Chapters 9, 10, 11). Table 13.1 lists some typical features found in these patients, although the frequency of this particular presentation appears to be declining. None the less they are important to identify as their mortality rate is approximately twice that of 'pink and puffing' patients with equivalent degrees of airflow obstruction [57].

13.6 MEASUREMENTS

13.6.1 DIAGNOSTIC IMAGING

This topic is considered elsewhere (Chapter 14). Good quality postero-anterior and lateral chest radiographs are essential in order to exclude other diagnoses, e.g. bronchial tumour, pneumothorax and possibly bronchiectasis. Large emphysematous bullae may be identified which if they occupy more than one-third of the hemithorax on a plain radiograph should be considered for surgical

Table 13.1 Clinical and physiologic features of 'pink and puffing' and 'blue and bloated' patients

	'Pink and puffing'	*'Blue and bloated'*
Synonym	Type A	Type B
Clinical	Dyspneic at rest Thin Hyperinflated	Less dyspneic Obese Edematous
Gas exchange Kco PaO$_2$ resting PaCO$_2$ resting PaO$_2$ exercise	 Low/normal >60 mmHg <50 mmHg Reduced	 Normal <60 mmHg >50 mmHg, usually Variable
Total lung capacity	Moderate increase	Small increase
Static lung compliance	Normal/high	Normal
Pulmonary artery pressure	Normal	Modest elevation
Red cell mass	Normal–low	High

These represent extreme ends of a spectrum of disease with many patients lying between these extremes. In general, clinic spirometry is equally disturbed in both groups whilst argument persists about the amount of macroscopic emphysema present within their lungs. Classically this is more obvious in the 'pink and puffing' patients but not all studies support this view.

resection (Chapter 22). A standard CT scan is of limited value, providing qualitative rather than quantitative information. Measurements of CT lung density have been correlated with the severity of emphysema but this and MRI scanning are still primarily of research interest [58]. Ventilation–perfusion scanning can be difficult to interpret in patients with severe airflow obstruction and can lead to an erroneous diagnosis of pulmonary embolism.

13.6.2 PHYSIOLOGIC ASSESSMENT

The cardinal feature of COPD is obstruction to forced expiratory airflow [59,60] (Chapter 7). The degree of airflow obstruction cannot be predicted from the symptoms or signs and can only be quantified by making measurements. Even in asthma nearly 30% of non-respiratory specialist physicians fail to measure the changing lung function [61] and a similar pattern was observed when physicians were asked to evaluate a hypothetical COPD case history [62]. This may reflect custom but it is also true that some clinicians find it difficult to relate undergraduate respiratory physiology to the practical tests presently available. In this section we will consider what these tests are, how they should be performed and what abnormalities are likely in COPD.

The earliest changes in COPD affect the alveolar walls and small airways and the increased peripheral airways resistance may precede detectable change in the static volume pressure curve of the lung (Chapter 2). A variety of specialized physiologic tests devised to study these early changes are discussed fully elsewhere (Chapter 7). However, these tests are difficult to perform, have high coefficients of variation and are only really valid when elastic recoil is normal and there is no proximal airway limitation, conditions that are seldom met even in mild COPD.

As the disease progresses, spirometric values begin to fall and end expiratory volumes begin to rise. The work required of the inspiratory muscles increases and breathing pattern changes, attempting to minimize respiratory discomfort. The reduced alveolar surface area is reflected in a reduced DLCO, and changes in the pulmonary circulation coupled with ventilation–perfusion mismatching lead to hypoxia. Finally in very severe disease the combination of ventilation–perfusion mismatching, circulatory changes and compromised musculature leads to hypercapnia and sometimes cor pulmonale.

Thus as the disease progresses the number of physiologic tests showing abnormality rises but no single variable can characterize the whole process. An approximate relationship between the clinical presentation and the physiologic abnormality is shown in Table 13.2 whilst the most commonly reported indices, their physiologic basis and their derangement in COPD are summarized in Tables 13.3 and 13.4.

(a) 'Dynamic' or spirometric tests

Volumetric spirometers record volume by displacement and derive flow by differentiation of the volume–time record. Since volume is recorded directly as the primary measurement, the accuracy of the volume is high and the device can never overestimate. The disadvantage of volume-based spirometers is a small resistance that has to be overcome in order to move the recording apparatus. Thus there are subtle but predictable differences between flow–volume loops generated on such machines as compared to the flow-based devices [63]. Clinically the differences are too small to be important. The flow-based spirometers (pneumotachographs, turbine spirometers and others) record pressure changes with time, assume that the relationship between pressure and flow is linear and then integrate the flow–time signal to obtain volume. The accuracy of these devices has been greatly improved by computers which

Table 13.2 Schematic relationship between disease progression, symptoms and physiologic test results

Clinical state	Results of measurements
Stage 1 No symptoms No abnormal signs	Abnormalities reported on specialized tests, e.g. frequency dependence of compliance, closing volume and N_2 slope increased, volume of helium iso-flow increased, elastic recoil reduced Of limited value for practical patient management
Stage 2 'Smokers' cough' but no breathlessness No abnormal signs	Abnormalities as in stage 1 plus small reductions in FEV_1, FEV_1/VC ratio and other indices of expiratory airflow
Stage 3 Breathlessness (± wheeze) on exertion, cough (± sputum) and some abnormal signs	Reduction in FEV_1 often to less than 50% predicted. Variable increases in FRC Reductions in DLCO Some patients hypoxemic but normocapnic
Stage 4 Breathless on minimal exertion. Wheeze and cough prominent Clinical evidence of hyperinflation usual plus cyanosis and polycythemia in some	Severe airflow limitation (FEV_1 <30% predicted) Marked hyperinflation (RV and FRC) Wide range of DLCO Reduced maximum inspiratory pressures Hypoxia usual and hypercapnia in some

can correct for the non-linearity between pressure and flow which is most marked at low flows. There is one important caveat. They require more care in calibration and can be wrongly calibrated to yield either falsely low or high results.

The first major attempt to standardize spirometry came with the American Thoracic Society's 'Snowbird' workshop which produced technical guidelines that spirometers should meet [64] and also made recommendations about how to perform the test. These were revised by the ATS in 1987 [65] and 1991 [66,74] and it is to these standards that most equipment manufacturers are producing spirometers. Separately, European guidelines on lung function were produced in 1983 [67]

and revised in 1993 [68]. Good quality spirometry depends more upon the care and training of the supervising technicians than on any differences between equipment [69].

It is important to inspect the volume–time tracings and ensure:

- that there are at least three technically satisfactory readings
- that there is a smooth expiratory trace without irregularities that suggest either variable submaximal effort or coughing
- that a least two recordings are within 100 ml or 5% of the other, and
- that a volume plateau has been reached. This can take 15 or more seconds in severe COPD

Table 13.3 Dynamic or spirometric tests

Name	Test	Physiologic basis	Results	Comment
FEV_1	Forced expiratory volume in first second from TLC	During a forced expiration the driving pressure is sufficient that at any given lung volume, the airflow is limited by the cross-sectional area of the flow limiting segment of the airways. Reproducible because depends more on airway dimensions than on test effort	Always ↓, often very low	Reproducible to ±200 ml, always abnormal in COPD so that COPD usually defined in terms of FEV_1/VC ratio
FVC	Forced expiratory volume from TLC to RV (see also VC)		Normal or mildly ↓	Nearly as reproducible as FEV_1 but can be underestimated if expiration not continued for up to 15 seconds
PEF	Peak expiratory flow from TLC		Usually ↓	The most effort dependent of the 3 – may be relatively preserved compared to FEV_1. Less sensitive and less reproducible (±60 l/min) but easily repeated
Flow-volume loop	Maximum expiration from TLC, followed by maximum inspiration to TLC; usually preceded by a tidal breathing loop	As above for the expiratory phase. Inspiration more dependent on effort airway dimensions	Characteristic shape of expiratory phase (Fig. 13.2)	Many measurements can be calculated from the loop, but none have better predictive power than FEV1 and FVC. Shape of loop may indicate airway collapsibility

These are the most important lung function measurements simple, quick, highly reproducible and surprisingly sensitive. Note that a reduced FEV_1/VC ratio is an important defining characteristic of airways obstruction.

Table 13.4 Static Lung Volumes

Name	Test	Physiologic basis	Results	Comment
TLC	Total lung capacity – lung volume at maximum inspiration	Depends on size and balance between maximum inspiratory pressure and elastic recoil of the respiratory system	Normal or ↑	Respiratory muscles adapt to a high TLC and work more efficiently. Reproducible ±5%
VC	Slow or relaxed vital capacity. Maximum volume of gas expired slowly from TLC to RV (or vice versa) (slow or relaxed vital capacity)	Depends on the different factors influencing the TLC and RV	Usually ↓	Can be preserved if both TLC and RV increase in parallel. Usually larger than FVC because less air trapping. Simple and reproducible. Relates well to self-paced walking distance
FRC	Functional residual capacity – lung volume at the end of tidal breath (elastic equilibrium volume) should be measured when relaxed – sensitive to changes in breathing pattern	Volume at which lung elastic recoil exactly balances outward chest wall recoil. Dynamic effects very important in COPD	Usually ↑	Affected by small reductions in lung elasticity (Pel). Limited reproducibility clinically (±10%), FRC increases dynamically as respiratory rate increases
RV	Residual volume – volume of air remaining in lungs at end expiration	Depends on the balance of expiratory pressure and the outward recoil of the chest wall at low lung volumes and the collapsibility of the airways	Raised, often markedly	Reproducible to ±10%, a measure of hyperinflation due to early airway closure. Some airways may begin to close during tidal breathing in severe COPD. Raised by bronchospasm/pulmonary edema

Representative traces are shown in Fig. 13.2

The greatest errors arise from submaximal efforts, and are not likely to be detected unless the actual traces are checked [69] (Fig. 13.2). The FVC can be significantly underestimated if a full expiration is not performed [70,71]. Both the ATS and European standards advocate that vital capacity should be measured either from a relaxed expiration or from an inspiratory maneuver whenever possible. If this is not possible, the physician should be aware that the forced maneuver is a potential underestimate. Recent work suggests that the ATS criteria should be modified so that a maximum expiratory effort is made in the first part of the maneuver and then a 'relaxed' expiration be encouraged when expiratory airflow falls to less than 200 ml/s [71]. Further modifications of the testing criteria suitable for COPD are likely in the coming

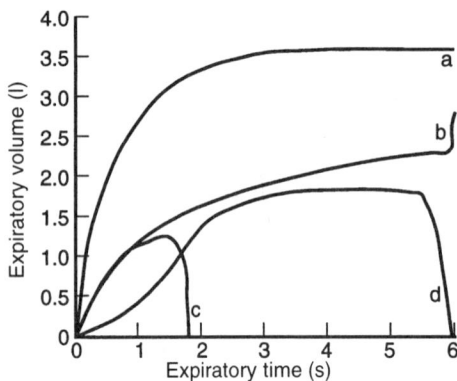

Fig. 13.2 A volume/time plot of a forced expiratory maneuver on a typical display which only shows 6 seconds on the X axis. a, Health with FEV_1 2.7 l and FVC 3.6 l – the curve plateaus at 3.5 seconds. b, A good sustained expiratory effort in COPD with an FEV_1 of 1.2 l. A further 0.45 l have been expired after 6 seconds to make a total FVC of 2.7 l. c, Good initial effort in the same patient to give an FEV_1 of 1.15 l but stopping expiration at 1.5 seconds means no FVC can be recorded. d, In the same COPD patient showing a poor effort, not sustained for even 6 seconds, resulting in falsely low volumes. To be acceptable, curves must be smooth and convex upwards throughout.

years as large multicenter studies based on FEV_1 measurements such as the Lung Health Study, Euroscop and ISOLDE all begin to report their data [72]. This may create problems for those who use computerized recording systems which set end of test criteria based on the 1987 ATS recommendations.

The most recent guidelines [66,68] recommend that the best FEV_1 and best FVC should be reported from at least three acceptable tracings even if the values do not come from the same expiratory effort. However, computerized systems utilizing data from the flow–volume loop usually report the FEV_1 and FVC from the best loop (defined as the loop with the largest sum of FEV_1 and FVC).

Individual values can be interpreted by comparison with a predicted value based on the subject's age, sex, height and race. Thus for example, Negroes have lung volumes that are 13% less than Caucasians with Asians being an intermediate range. European laboratories usually use the European Community Coal and Steel values (ECCS) [73] now revised [65]. In North America each laboratory is encouraged to establish its own reference range. Using different published US equations can result in a 10% difference in the predicted value and hence a 10% variability in spirometry expressed as percent predicted [74,75].

For FEV_1 and FVC the lower limit of normal equates to about 80% of the predicted value. However, the standard deviation from the predicted equation is the same for all ages and sizes and is not proportional to the FEV_1 or FVC. This has led to the suggestion that results be expressed as the number of 'residual standard deviations' below the normal value [76]. Although this concept is statistically sound, it is uncertain whether clinicians will adopt it widely.

Although spirometry is recorded from a forced expiratory maneuver, the results obtained are largely independent of the effort used because the determining factors in the size of the FEV_1 are the dynamic cross-sectional area of the flow limiting segments within the airways. These flow limiting segments change during expiration with changing lung volume, elastic recoil pressure and the extent of airway disease. Thus the FEV_1 is in effect a proxy measurement of overall airway narrowing (Chapter 7) and hence has proved to be the most robust general marker of pathology and prognosis in COPD. Alternatively, results may be interpreted in terms of the FEV_1 alone (e.g. as percent predicted) to indicate how advanced the disease is, and by repeating observations over time to assess progress. A rapid decline in FEV_1 indicates a worse prognosis.

Spirometry before and after bronchodilators may yield clinically useful information about potential treatment (see later) whilst the FEV_1 can be used to predict the potential peak exercise ventilation. The conventional equation of $FEV_1 \times 35$ probably underestimates peak voluntary ventilation at least in moderate COPD [77] and a better alternative is $(18.9 \times FEV_1) + 19.7$ l/min [78]. Finally FEV_1 can be used as a guide to potential disability assessment as seen in Table 13.5a. It has also been related to symptom intensity although the level of symptoms associated with a particular degree of lung function is always higher in patients involved in medicolegal claims (Table 13.5b) [79].

(b) Tests of flow in relation to volume

The graphic display of flow and volume provides a complementary approach to the usual volume–time plot and adds some information about lung mechanics in COPD especially when the tidal volume loop is considered in relation to the maximum flow volume envelope. The configuration of this latter may suggest significant effort independent of expiratory airflow limitation even during tidal breathing. Figure 13.3 shows the flow volume loop in severe COPD illustrating the airway collapse which begins after the first 200–300 ml have been expelled from the

Table 13.5a   Disability and lung function

Obstructive abnormality: The FEV_1/VC ratio must be below the normal range

	FEV_1 expressed as % predicted
May be a physiological variant	>101
Mild	70–100
Moderate	60–69
Moderately severe	50–59
Severe	35–49
Very severe	<35

Date modified from reference [74].

Table 13.5b

Mean FEV_1		Dyspnea grade
l	*% predicted*	*(0–4)*
3.2	95	0
2.4	62	1
1.8	45	2
1.2	35	3
0.75	–	4

Data modified from reference [79].

trachea and upper airway and continues throughout expiration. Quiet, non-forced breathing may result in better flows. A number of measurements have been made from the flow volume curve including FEF_{50}, FEF_{75} and FEF_{75-85}. All have problems of reproducibility such that values must fall to below 50% of predicted to be outside the normal range. The flows in the latter part of the expiratory curve were thought to be an indicator of small airway function, but at least one long-term study has shown that all the clinically useful information resides in the FEV_1 and the FVC [80].

There are technical reasons why flow measurements made at iso-volume are so variable. Volume calculated from flow at the mouth makes no allowance for the effect of thoracic gas compression during expiration. Hence there are small, but systematic, differences between tests performed on a spirometer and those recorded with a body plethysmograph. More importantly, if the FVC changes between two tests, after an intervention (e.g. bronchodilator) or because of too short a forced expiratory time, then the reported flow indices will have been derived at different ab-

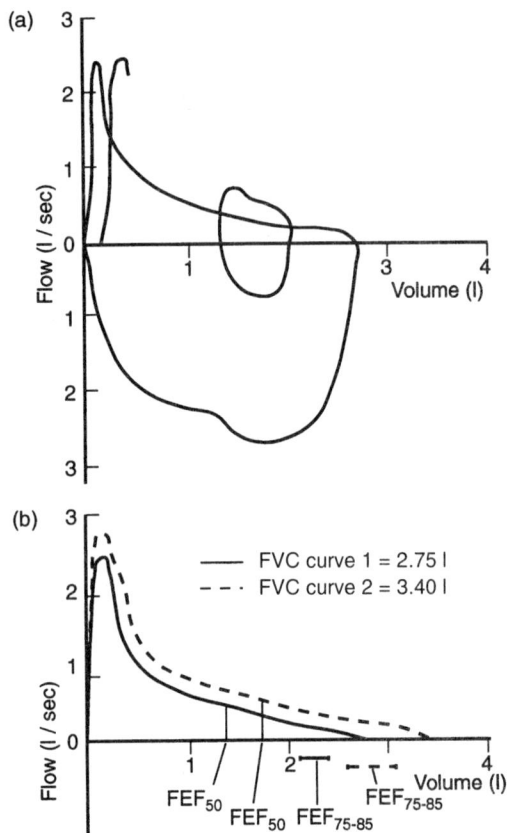

Fig. 13.3 (a) Flow–volume loop in severe COPD showing a relatively preserved PEF followed by a rapid diminution in flow as airways collapse. Inspiratory flows better preserved. Flow during tidal breathing (low effort) exceeds that during forced expiration. (b) Expiratory flow volume curve before (—) and after (---) bronchodilator. TLC has been assumed constant for the purpose of illustration. Changed FVC leads to flow measurements being made at different absolute lung volumes.

solute lung volumes. They will not therefore be strictly comparable since each relates to a different set of mechanical and geometric factors (Fig. 13.3b).

(i) Peak expiratory flow

This can be read from the flow–volume loop or measured independently with a hand-held peak flow meter. These use a linear scale but the instruments are not in fact linear with respect to flow [82] and so not directly comparable to data from plethysmography. The value of these instruments lies in the ease with which repeated measurements can be made at home. Although the importance of diurnal variability as a reliable defining characteristic in asthma is now well established [83–85], the same is not necessarily true in COPD. Most patients show little daily change in PEF but caution should be exercised in interpreting the absolute levels of PEF with the FEV_1. During the first part of expiration air is rapidly expelled from the trachea and main airways before more distal airway collapse limits further increases in expiratory flow. Thus the initial PEF may markedly overestimate the FEV_1. Single measurements of PEF are very variable and changes of 60 l/min are within the natural variability of the measurement [86]. Although serial PEF values can give information similar to the FEV_1 [87] the PEF is not a sensitive measure for detecting the small treatment changes typical in COPD, and an isolated PEF recording is a poor alternative to spirometry in the diagnosis of COPD.

(c) 'Static tests of lung mechanics

(i) Lung volumes

The determinants of TLC, RV and FRC are given in Table 13.4. These measures indicate the severity of hyperinflation, i.e. the progressive rise in FRC, usually accompanied by increases in RV due to loss of pulmonary elastic recoil and airway collapse. In addition a dynamic component due to breathing pattern is now recognized (Chapter 7). This latter is particularly important during exercise and is not readily predictable from data obtained during tidal breathing. Hyperinflation is a major determinant of symptoms such as breathlessness as it increases the elastic work of breathing and reduces inspiratory capacity. Several methods have been developed to assess lung volume:

1. Helium dilution during rebreathing – this is long established and widely available, but in COPD poorly ventilated areas of lung (including bullae) do not have time to equilibrate properly with the inspired helium and so the measured total lung volume is an underestimate of the true value.
2. Helium dilution during a single breath – this is calculated during the measurement of DLCO (see below) but is even more subject to underestimates than the above.
3. Body plethysmography – this relies on the accurate measurement of small fluctuations in mouth and box pressure during gentle panting against a closed shutter and uses Boyle's Law to calculate lung volumes. It measures all trapped air within the thorax including that in poorly ventilated areas and usually produces higher readings than helium dilution testing. However, artefacts due to delayed equilibration of pressure between the alveoli and the mouth will accentuate any trend to overestimation [88]. The panting frequency adopted can increase these effects [89] as can the 'shunt compliance' of the upper airways. This latter problem can be reduced by supporting the cheeks with both hands [90].
4. X-ray planimetry. This apparently cheap means of deriving lung volume data from routine radiographs has now been quantified and computerized [91]. However, to obtain accurate data requires careful standardization of both the radiographic maneuver and the subsequent X-ray measurements. There are reports that the values obtained are valid [92] but we found in COPD and normal subjects wide discrepancies with both helium dilution and body box results. In individuals the 95% confidence intervals were up to 2 l either way [93].

The demonstration of changes in FRC, residual volumes and possibly TLC add support to the diagnosis of COPD and may help to explain why a patient is particularly symptomatic with apparently modest spirometric limitation. Changes in lung volumes after bronchodilators provide an alternative means of assessing response [94,95] but are more time consuming than routine spirometry. A potential refinement of this approach has been to seek changes in 'trapped gas volume', i.e. the difference between the lung volumes measured by plethysmography and helium dilution methods [96]. This corresponds to the 'slow ventilating' compartment described by physiologists in the 1950s and 1960s. Changes in 'trapped gas volume' were claimed to be an indicator of response to bronchodilator and to relate to performance. However, the initial report has never been replicated and methodologic problems and the difficulty of subtracting one inherently variable number from another make its routine use undesirable [97].

(ii) Maximum respiratory pressure generation

The measurement of maximum inspiratory and expiratory pressures is gaining in popularity as an end-point in respiratory rehabilitation programmes (Chapter 21). Normal values have been defined [98] but these measurements are still not routinely available in many laboratories. Their physiologic basis is discussed fully elsewhere (Chapter 9). The test equipment is now relatively inexpensive but several practical issues

324 *Clinical and laboratory assessment*

should be considered. Care is needed to ensure the patient seals their lips around the mouth piece and some practice is required to obtain reproducible results. Maximum efforts are normally reached within five attempts but the patient soon tires if the test is prolonged beyond this. The development of simple more portable instruments may make mouth pressure assessment more clinically valuable [99].

13.6.3 BRONCHODILATOR REVERSIBILITY TESTING

Reversibility can be defined as an improvement in an index of airflow obstruction and/or relevant functional variable in response to an active treatment which is greater than that likely to have occurred by chance. The assessment of reversibility is recognized as being an essential part of the management of COPD [59]. Despite this, there is little agreement about which test should be used, what doses and types of drug to use and what a positive result signifies [101]. Reversibility can be assessed in terms of changes in symptoms (e.g. breathlessness) or exercise performance (e.g. self-paced walking tests) but is usually done using either FEV_1 or PEF. Several factors can determine the outcome of reversibility testing.

(a) Limitations of the measurement

The coefficient of variation for FEV_1 is reported to be less than 5% in normal subjects [102]. In fact the variability is independent of baseline FEV_1 and of similar absolute size whatever the FEV_1. Tweedale, Alexander and McHardy [102] found that the standard deviation of repeated measurements on the same day was 102 ml. This means that only if a change in FEV_1 exceeds 170 ml can it be considered to have arisen other than by chance. Both the ATS [65] and European guidelines [68] recommend that changes should only be

considered significant if they exceed an absolute volume of 200 ml. Our own data strongly support this [103,104].

(b) Response criteria

The commonest approach in the past has been to define a response in terms of the percentage change from the initial value, e.g. a rise of 15%. However, in subjects with a low FEV_1 a 20% rise may still be within the range of spontaneous variability due to the measurement. To overcome this the ERS recommended that a response be defined as an increase in FEV_1, greater than both 15% of baseline and 200 ml [68], an approach adopted in some physiologic studies [103,105]. The ATS suggest a significant change of both 200 ml and a 12% change in FEV_1 as a percent of the predicted normal value [65]. A third approach is to express the change as a percentage of the potential possible change, i.e. (predicted–baseline) [86]. For most patients the differences in approach are relatively unimportant [104] but need to be clearly stated before comparing data.

(c) Change in baseline airway caliber

If on the test day, a patient has a relatively high level of airway smooth muscle tone and hence a low FEV_1, there is a greater chance of a 200 ml plus change in FEV_1 occurring than on another day when resting tone happens to be lower and the initial FEV_1 higher. Thus about one-third of those who are graded responders on day 1 may be classed as nonresponders on day 2 and vice versa [20]. Differences in drug deposition due to altered airway caliber may contribute to this variability [106]. It is possible that use of the postbronchodilator FEV_1 to monitor progress will remove any confounding effects of varying airway smooth muscle tone and allow more accurate monitoring of long-term deterioration in lung function.

(d) Choice of drug and dosage

A small dose of bronchodilator from a metered dose inhaler will cause fewer subjects to have a significant response than would repeated doses from the MDI or a larger dose by nebulizer [107]. Adding a second drug will further increase the FEV_1 and response rate of some patients [108]. Given the uncertainties above it is difficult to make definitive statements about the relative efficacy of β-agonist and anticholinergic agents [104]. The balance of the evidence suggests that ipratropium is more likely to elicit a bronchodilator response than salbutamol (Chapter 17). β-Agonists have the advantage of a quicker onset of action (15 min vs 45 min), leading to a shorter test time. However, which single drug or combination should be used remains unclear because there are few data relating laboratory tests to treatment outcome.

(i) Corticosteroids

The role of corticosteroids in acute and stable disease is reviewed in Chapter 18.

Many clinicians give a short course of oral steroids, in addition to the short acting bronchodilator tests, to identify potential steroid responsive COPD patients. The commonest dosages used in studies have been 30 mg prednisolone or 0.6 mg/kg/day and the commonest trial period is two weeks. All the problems of defining a response described above apply to oral steroid trials but there are no published studies of reproducibility. Our own data using 30 mg prednisolone for 2 weeks and defining a response as a 200 ml or greater rise in FEV_1, showed that 44/211 consecutive referrals were oral steroid responsive (21%). All but three also responded to bronchodilators. We were unable to identify either singly or in combination any part of clinical history, examination or laboratory tests that would predict the response and avoid the need for trial of steroids.

The time before a response to oral prednisolone occurs has not been examined in COPD but Weir *et al.* suggested that 6 weeks was required before a response could be expected if inhaled corticosteroids were used [109] although their studies did use a mixture of end-points involving changes in FEV_1, FVC and PEF [110]. Patients with a positive response to β-agonists whether from a metered dose inhaler [111] or a nebulizer [56], are more likely to subsequently respond to oral prednisolone. Nebulized anticholinergic drugs can identify a few additional cases [104]. In our series a small number of steroid responsive patients were not identified whichever bronchodilator was used, but the improvement in FEV_1 after oral corticosteroids in this group was small, normally being less than 250 ml. A response to oral steroids could not be predicted from the appearance of the flow–volume loop, lung volumes, DLCO or atopic status [112]. In one placebo-controlled study inhaled beclomethasone produced small but significant improvements in lung function (ΔFEV_1 48 ml) which were not increased further by oral prednisolone [113]. These beneficial effects of corticosteroids in COPD are supported by at least one meta-analysis [114].

(e) Clinical significance

The usual hope is that acute bronchodilator trials will identify patients likely to have a reduction in symptoms and improvement in exercise tolerance after treatment. However, this is not the case, at least in severe COPD (Chapter 17). Hay *et al.* showed that 80 μg of oxitropium bromide increased exercise tolerance and reduced symptoms by approximately 13% in 32 patients with stable COPD [103]. Responses were similar whether or not patients had been shown beforehand to be reversible to bronchodilator. Berger and Smith showed similar changes in self-paced walking distance after orciprenaline in patients with fixed airflow obstruction [115] whilst both Corris *et al.* [116] and Spence *et al.* [117] found similar functional improvements even in patients unresponsive to oral cortico-steroids. Thus acute bronchodilator testing using spirometry is not an appropriate way of selecting patients likely to have a symptomatic response [118]. Whether other tests or spirometric criteria would be more sensitive/specific has not been systematically examined but our own data are not encouraging.

However, there are potential benefits in establishing the reversibility status. Data from the IPPB study suggested that those patients with the least bronchodilator response were most likely to lose lung function rapidly over time even allowing for other risk factors [57] a finding supported by data from Holland [119]. We have found that patients with a positive corticosteroid trial have a more favorable prognosis over 5 years even allowing for age and cigarette consumption than those who do not [120]. Improvement in lung function over time was greater in the group of patients treated with inhaled steroids but greatest in those who had already demonstrated a response to oral corticosteroids.

13.6.4 GAS TRANSFER FACTOR

The diffusing capacity for carbon monoxide is a measure of the passive transfer of gas across the alveolar membrane and into the blood. Its size reflects the alveolar surface area but changes in the blood component must not be overlooked. Thus an increase in pulmonary capillary blood volume, e.g. during pulmonary edema, an increased pulmonary blood flow, e.g. on exercise or with a left to right cardiac shunt or a raised hemoglobin, e.g. polycythemia will lead to higher values. Conversely, anemia or a high carboxyhemoglobin level will depress the measured DLCO.

At present there are several different methods by which this measurement can be made, each yielding rather different answers in COPD patients. The method described by Ogilvie and colleagues in 1957 recorded the rate of carbon monoxide uptake during a 10-second breath-hold and related this to the alveolar volume derived by adding the inspired volume to the residual volume measured in a separate helium dilution test [121]. More widely used is the single breath modification suggested by Mitchell and Renzetti who used helium dilution during the single breath maneuver to calculate alveolar volume [122]. This will underestimate alveolar volume in severe COPD and produce a lower value for the DLCO measurement. Although this was accepted by the ATS and initial European guidelines the most recent European revision [68] has advocated reversion to the original method especially in patients with COPD. The method of calculation can completely change the result for a given patient. Thus, for example, a man with bullous emphysema may have an inspiratory capacity of 3 liters during the single breath maneuver and a residual volume of 2 liters from the single breath helium dilution but 4.5 liters from the multiple breath dilution. The alveolar volume in one method is 5 liters and in the other 7.5 which could represent a DLCO of 60% predicted against 90%. One way around this dilemma is to report diffusing capacity as the KCO, i.e. DLCO divided by alveolar volume, which effectively represents diffusion per unit lung volume. Although an attractive idea, the prediction equations are not well documented and the European statement [68] does not even recommend a standard prediction set. Confusion is likely to remain until the international standards are in agreement.

There is little doubt that DLCO values are below normal in many patients with COPD and this has been related to the presence of macroscopic emphysema [58,123]. However, the correlation between the severity of COPD and the reduction of DLCO in individual patients is relatively poor. None the less at least one study has reported a significant inverse relationship between DLCO and three year survival [124]. Those patients with a KCO of less than 70% predicted have a mortality of over 80% compared with 30% of those with a KCO of more than 70% predicted. However, earlier studies did not observe this large effect [57, 125], whilst a more recent study reported a DLCO rise even when the underlying disease was progressing [126], possibly due to the subtle changes in ventilation–perfusion matching in the lungs of ex-smokers.

In summary a low DLCO is suggestive of a significant degree of alveolar damage probably due to emphysema, but a normal DLCO does not exclude the diagnosis of COPD.

13.6.4 TESTS OF GAS EXCHANGE

The modern approach to gas exchange in COPD is discussed in Chapter 8. However, many clinicians find it difficult to apply logarithmic dispersions of ventilation and perfusion to bedside problems and still rely on the rather simpler concepts of the three-compartment model described by Riley and Cournand [127]. This considers the lung as three theoretical compartments; one in which there is 'ideal' ventilation but no perfusion (physiologic dead space), a second with both 'ideal' ventilation and perfusion and the third in which there is 'ideal' perfusion but no ventilation.

In practice compartment one includes a contribution from units of above average $\dot{V}_A/\dot{Q}$ dispersion and the anatomic dead space. Within the physiologic dead space (V_D) all the ventilation is wasted and the ventilation to perfusion ratio is infinity. The size of V_D can be calculated from the mixed expired ($P_{E_{CO_2}}$) and arterial (Pa_{CO_2}) carbon dioxide tensions and the tidal volume.

Thus: $V_D = V_T (1 - [P_{E_{CO_2}}/Pa_{CO_2}])$

Physiologic dead space is useful conceptually but is of less value clinically. The calculation of the dead space to tidal volume ratio V_D/V_T is useful during exercise as a measure of the general effectiveness of ventilation and gas exchange. The concept can be used to understand what determines the level of arterial CO_2 in an individual.

Thus: $Pa_{CO_2} = V_{CO_2}/V_A \times k$

where V_A is the alveolar ventilation and K is a constant.

Alveolar ventilation is $f \times (V_T - V_D)$ giving the revised equation:

$$Pa_{CO_2} = \frac{V_{CO_2} \times k}{f \times (V_T - V_D)}$$

When metabolic CO_2 production is constant, i.e. at rest with no fever and no parenteral feeding, any reduction in breathing frequency or tidal volume (e.g. from ventilation depressing drugs) or rise in physiologic dead space (e.g. during exacerbations of COPD) will elevate the Pa_{CO_2}. Most COPD patients maintain their CO_2 tension within the normal range, despite a large physiologic dead space until the airflow obstruction is severe (e.g. FEV_1 less than 1.2 l). An elevated Pa_{CO_2} without a mechanical explanation (i.e. low FEV_1) should prompt a search for an additional cause, e.g. sleep apnea or neuromuscular disease.

The third theoretical compartment has no ventilation, i.e. a $\dot{V}_A/\dot{Q}$ ratio of zero. The partially saturated pulmonary arterial blood behaves as though it passes through this compartment unchanged. If the saturation of the systemic mixed venous blood and the arterial blood are known then the proportion of cardiac output passing through this theoretical compartment can be calculated (the venous admixture fraction). In practice the measurements and calculations necessary mean that formal shunt fraction assessment is confined to the research laboratory and to the intensive care unit where oxygen delivery must be optimized.

Since nitrogen plays no part in gas exchange, it follows that the non-nitrogen part of the inhaled gas mixture can be considered separately. A simple equation can be derived relating the arterial blood gas tensions, the inspired oxygen concentration and the alveolar–arterial oxygen difference ((A–a)D): Thus:

$$FIO_2 = PO_2 + PCO_2/0.8 + (A–a)D$$

where FIO_2 is the inspired O_2 tension oxygen

PO_2 and PCO_2 are the arterial blood gas tensions

(A–a)D is the alveolar–arterial oxygen difference

Since the percentage of oxygen in air is very close numerically to the partial pressure of oxygen in air expressed in kPa, the various factors can be related with simple mental arithmetic. For example the alveolar–arterial oxygen difference in a normal person breathing air could be

21 = 13.3 + 5.2/0.8 + (A–a)D
so the (A–a)d = 1.2 kPa

Or in severe COPD, breathing 24% O_2

24 = 7.3 + 7.6/0.8 + (A–a)D
so the (A–a)d = 7.2 kPa

When the PaO_2 is above 8 kPa then a raised (A–a)D is a surrogate measure of an increased venous admixture. When the PaO_2 is less than 8, small changes in PaO_2 correspond to larger changes in oxygen fraction and this simple estimation will underestimate the true level of physiologic shunting.

(a) Arterial blood gases

The methodology of taking arterial blood for blood gases and some aspects of interpretation of the results are dealt with in Chapter 8. Arterial blood gas measurement is an essential part of the assessment of COPD to confirm the degree of hypoxia, assess if hypercapnia is present and, in the acutely ill patient, detect pH changes. These are dynamic measurements and change rapidly in unstable patients. However, it may take 30

minutes for a change in inspired oxygen concentration to become fully apparent in the PO_2 because of the prolonged time constants for alveolar gas equilibration. In the stable patient, resting hypoxemia is prognostically important, although the absolute oxygen tension is less important than the fact that it is below 7.5 kPa. In contrast hypercapnia has less predictive power and survival is improved in patients receiving domiciliary oxygen despite small increase in CO_2 tensions during treatment [128,129]

13.6.5 PULSE OXIMETRY AND TRANSCUTANEOUS TENSIONS

The advent of relatively inexpensive and reliable non-invasive oximeters has aided the assessment of arterial oxygenation [131]. These devices measure oxygen saturation reliably down to approximately 75% but are sensitive to changes in the COHB level which may be elevated in chronic smokers [132]. They should not replace blood gases as the first measurement in a patient, but once the initial gas tensions are known a pulse oximeter is a valuable tool with which to monitor progress during an acute episode, or overnight. However, oxygen saturation measures take no account of CO_2 tension and can lull the unwary into a false sense of security that results in deteriorating acid–base status. At present it is better to make repeated estimates of blood gas tensions if necessary by inserting an arterial cannula than to place undue reliance on saturation measurements at least when dealing with acutely sick patients. Measurement of transcutaneous oxygen and CO_2 tensions have still to find a useful place in adult practice as particular care is needed to obtain a stable and reliable signal [133]. These devices require a biologic calibration for each individual and tend to record CO_2 tensions which are higher than the true arterial values although this can be allowed for. Since they operate at temperatures higher than 37°C there is always the risk of thermal injury if they are used for prolonged periods.

(a) Acid–base status

Arterial pH and bicarbonate measurements are normally reported at the same time as gas tensions and provide complementary information. Unfortunately acid–base physiology generates confusion easily but this has been lucidly reviewed in several recent texts [134,135]. A major problem is the logarithmic nature of the pH scale and most people (including ourselves) find the negative logarithm to the base 10 of the hydrogen ion concentration a difficult concept with which to grapple. It is much easier to think in terms of the modified Henderson equation: $[H^+] = k \times$ PCO_2/HCO_3^- where H^+ = concentration of hydrogen ions, k is a constant, HCO_3^- bicarbonate concentration and PCO_2 is arterial CO_2 tensions. Thus increases in CO_2 tension, which are usually rapid, can be compensated by renal conservation of bicarbonate, a relatively slow process. Once any two variables are known the third can be calculated. It is useful to think about, and with serial data plot out, the changes in $[H^+]$ concentration (pH) and PCO_2 on a non-logarithmic diagram (Fig. 13.4). The version we use is that of Flenley [136] which incorporates data derived from carefully characterized patients with acute and chronic respiratory acidosis, the latter being compensated by increased levels of bicarbonate as well as data from patients with chronic stable metabolic acidosis and

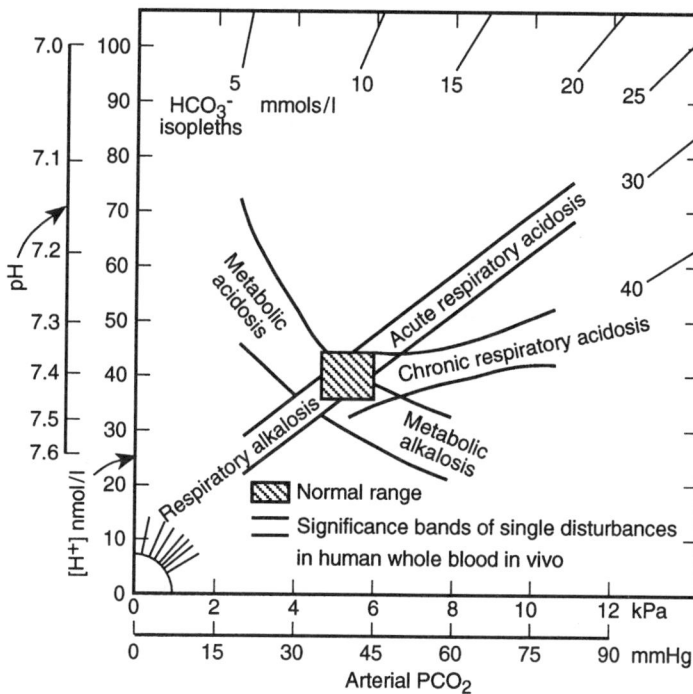

Fig. 13.4 A non-logarithimic acid–base diagram derived from the measured acid–base status of patients within the 5 abnormal bands illustrated and of normal subjects (hatched box). This plot of CO_2 tension against hydrogen ion concentration (pH) allows the likely acid–base disturbance and calculated by carbonate value (obtained from the relevant isopleth) to be rapidly determined whilst changes during treatment can be plotted serially for each patient (after reference [136] with permission).

alkalosis. The position of the PCO_2/H^+ point within these boundaries indicates how much of any acid–base problem results from acute changes in CO_2 tension and how much from coexisting metabolic or chronic respiratory derangements. Many hypoxemic COPD patients have a normal pH despite their elevated $PaCO_2$ due to chronic HCO_3 conservation and they lie within the chronic respiratory acidosis band. Although this is at best a semi-quantitative approach it removes many of the problems found in the practical management of acid–base chemistry.

13.6.6 EXERCISE TESTS

Of all the more complex procedures exercise testing is the most frequently performed and potentially most informative. Several different protocols have been devised and the test chosen should be specific for the information desired. Before considering the practical issues of exercise testing it is worth briefly reviewing those aspects of exercise physiology relevant to patients with COPD. The relationship of exercise to respiratory muscle function and gas exchange have already been considered and the whole topic has been reviewed in detail elsewhere [137, 138].

Exercise is associated with an increasing oxygen consumption and CO_2 production due to substrate use by skeletal muscle. An integrated cardiorespiratory response is needed to ensure adequate oxygen delivery, CO_2 removal and maintenance of blood gas homeostasis. Despite some early doubts [139] COPD patients have the same oxygen consumption for a given level of external work as do normal subjects. However, their dead space ventilation is higher and so a larger minute ventilation is needed to maintain CO_2 tension constant. For many patients expiratory airflow is limited within the tidal volume range and the only way to increase minute ventilation is to increase inspiratory flow and/or shift the end expiratory position [140–142]. The former requires more work from the already disad-

vantaged inspiratory muscles whilst the latter produces progressive pulmonary hyperinflation which worsens both symptoms and the work of breathing. The ability of some subjects to apparently exceed their maximum flow volume envelope during tidal breathing, especially in exercise [142] probably represents a gas compression artefact together with possible bronchodilatation during exercise and the effects of non-uniform lung emptying.

The respiratory muscles cope with the increased mechanical load by reducing abdominal volume due to tonic abdominal muscle contraction and so optimizing diaphragmatic performance [143]. Both the expiratory intercostal muscle activity and that of the abdominals is enhanced whilst inspiration is augmented by the use of the accessory muscles. There is still a healthy debate about whether exercise is limited in these circumstances by the development of inspiratory muscle fatigue or whether the patient stops before this process has a chance to become established [144–146]. Like normal subjects tidal volume and frequency increase progressively with exercise. The increase in tidal volume is limited by the reduced FEV_1, the former rising to approximately 50% of the vital capacity and further increases in ventilation must be by a raised respiratory frequency, although this may worsen the V_D/V_T ratio and the shorter expiratory time makes it even harder to maintain tidal volume. Normal subjects increase their respiratory duty cycle (T_I/T_{TOT}) during exercise but COPD patients cannot [140,147], mainly due to the relatively fixed expiratory time.

The effects on blood gas tensions are variable. Some types of exercise are more likely to induce oxygen desaturation than others. Thus COPD patients walking on a treadmill develop greater degrees of oxygen desaturation than they do when performing cycle exercise, possibly because the latter is associated with a greater degree of lactic acidosis and a high overall minute ventilation [148]. In some patients large falls in oxygen tension occur due to the effects of mixed venous PO_2 on low ventilation perfusion units [149,150]. The effects of different regional changes in pulmonary artery pressure further complicate the picture. Changes in arterial CO_2 tension are much less marked because of the greater buffering capacity of the blood as well as the non-steady state nature of most exercise protocols.

In general the cardiovascular responses are reasonably appropriate with total cardiac output being normal for any given workload [151]. However, increases in stroke volume are less in severe COPD possibly because of the effects of pulmonary hyperinflation and pulmonary hypertension whilst the heart rate response is proportionately greater than in healthy subjects [151]. Despite these preserved cardiovascular responses, metabolic acidosis develops in severe COPD patients at lower work rates [152]. Determination of the anaerobic threshold is particularly difficult in these patients.

Exercise is normally stopped by a combination of breathlessness and leg weakness. The latter is a surprisingly frequent symptom particularly in the less severely disabled COPD patient. Thus Killian and colleagues studying 97 COPD patients during progressive cycle exercise found that in 40% exercise was limited by dyspnea but in 25% leg effort was more troublesome than dyspnea, the remainder rating both symptoms to be equally troublesome [153]. This prevalence of leg fatigue emphasizes the role of general debility in COPD [154] and this provides a potentially useful target for rehabilitation programs (Chapter 21)[154].

Three forms of exercise testing are available and they are complementary rather than competitive in nature.

(a) Progressive symptom limited exercise

Although the protocol employed, particularly the rate of workload increase, varies between laboratories and some investigators use tread-mill rather than cycle ergometry, the overall objective is to assess cardiorespiratory performance as workload is increased in a steady ramp-like fashion. The patient is encouraged to maintain the exercise until symptoms terminate the test and symptom scoring of breathlessness during the test provides useful information along with the more conventional metabolic ventilatory and cardiac variables (Table 13.6). A number of criteria for defining a maximum test are available, the most commonly applied being a heart rate in excess of 85% predicted or a ventilation greater than 90% predicted. More conventional desaturation criteria are hard to apply in patients who are already hypoxemic and particular caution is needed in interpreting end tidal gas tensions in COPD patients. We have found that simultaneous automatic monitoring of ECG for ST segment depression and blood pressure to ensure an appropriate cardiovascular response greatly increases the usefulness of the test protocol.

At present data from cycle ergometry are largely of diagnostic rather than therapeutic or prognostic value. Results have good between-day reproducibility [155] and are invaluable in trying to determine how much functional limitation is due to coexisting cardiac or psychological factors. Typical examples of the different types of test are given in Fig. 13.5.

(b) Steady state exercise

Exercising at a sustainable percentage of maximum capacity for 3 to 6 minutes allows the measurement of blood gas tensions and so the calculation of the VD/VT and the cardiac shunt. Although of intellectual interest this is now seldom performed clinically in COPD patients.

(c) Self-paced exercise tests

These are simple to perform and can yield information about more sustained exercise

Table 13.6 Variables measured during cycle ergometry

Term	Recording	COPD	Comment
Work (W)	Measured in watt or k pond meters per minute	Reduced	A common denominator in exercise tests, related to aerobic work capacity
Oxygen consumption ($\dot{V}O_2$) (ml/min)	Calculated from mixed expired oxygen content – needs correction if FIO_2 increased	Reduced	A common denominator of exercise capacity linearly related to ventilation below the anaerobic threshold. $\dot{V}O_2$ max is recorded at the maximum workload achieved.
Carbon dioxide production ($\dot{V}CO_2$) (ml/min)	Calculated from mixed expired CO_2 tension	Reduced	Related to ventilation at all workloads
Heart rate (beats/min)	Usually from chest leads of ECG	Normal for the $\dot{V}O_2$ achieved unless coexisting cardiac problem	Useful to monitor 12-lead ECG during exercise to detect occult cardiac ischemia
Oxygen pulse (ml/beat)	Amount of O_2 extracted per heartbeat	Usually normal	A surrogate for stroke volume provided SaO_2 normal
Minute ventilation ($\dot{V}E$) (l/min)	Usually expired ventilation ($\dot{V}E$) – may be measured cumulatively or averaged from 'instantaneous minute ventilation' of each breath	Reduced, often Substantially	Often related to predicted values based on $FEV_1 \times 35$ – this does not allow for effects of MIP (see text)
Tidal volume (VT)	Volume of each breath – may be measured by pneumo tachograph or turbine spirometer	Normal or reduced	Rapid shallow breathing is common and may increase dead space
Respiratory frequency (f)	Derived from the timed ventilation	Often increased	Rapid shallow breathing is common and may increase dead space

Table 13.6 *Cont'd.*

Ventilatory equivalent (V_E/V_{O_2})	Derived from ventilation V_{O_2} at a specified level of ventilation or at V_E max	Increased due to ventilation of high V/Q units	Values of 40 are seen – normal
Oxygen saturation (Sa_{O_2})	Assessed non-invasively by pulse oximetry	Usually falls rapidly with exercise but some hypoxemic patients may maintain or increase Sa_{O_2} with exercise	Cycle ergometry underestimates desaturation as compared to treadmill exercise. A hidden cause of polycythemia
Breathlessness	Assessed by visual analog or Borg scales	Increased at every level of ventilation. Significant inter-subject variability	Less reproducible in exercise than during CO_2 rebreathing. Limits exercise in 40% of cases

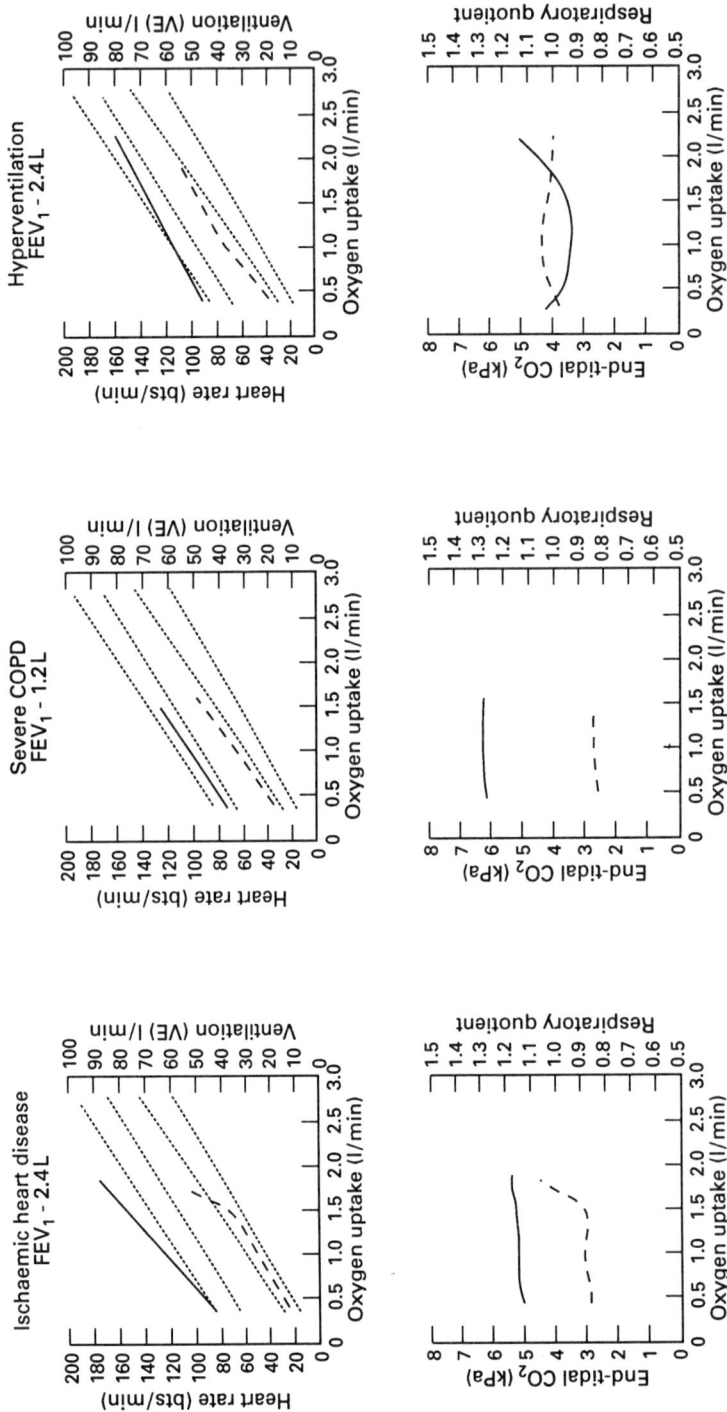

Fig. 13.5 Different responses to exercise in three different clinical situations. In myocardial dysfunction (left panel), the heart rate is increased at each work-load to compensate for its inability to increase stroke volume (lower O_2 pulse). The ECG showed ST segment depression of 2.1 mm at the end of the test which was terminated because the patient noted chest pain and maximum predicted heart rate was reached. Anaerobic threshold occurs early at a workload less than 70% predicted maximum. Arterial oxygen desaturation occurs above the anaerobic threshold as the vascular system fails deliver enough oxygen to satisfy the demands of the skeletal musculature. Ventilatory responses at each workload are entirely normal.

In COPD (central panel), the cardiac function may be entirely normal, but the minute ventilation (V_E) is disproportionately high at each work load. The test finished because of breathlessness at which point the patient was breathing at 51 l/min which is 123% of his predicted maximum ventilation. The ventilatory equivalent is high reflecting the increased physiological dead space and the tidal volume never rises above 1.1 l reflecting the low resting FEV_1. Despite the increased ventilation at each workload the $PetCO_2$ remains normal with a tendency to rise as the test progresses indicating a relative alveolar hypoventilation, resulting in mild progressive oxygen desaturation. The RQ remains less than unity since the man fails to reach an anaerobic threshold.

In the right hand panel are the results of a 55-year-old man who presented with breathlessness on 'any' exercise and chest tightness – sometimes at rest. The cardiac responses are normal. Ventilation (particularly respiratory frequency) increases rapidly as exercise commences, the ventilatory equivalent is high, the end-tidal CO_2 falls and the RQ is artificially high. As exercise progresses the relative alveolar hyperventilation becomes less marked. The patient reached 84% of his predicted maximum VO_2 and stopped because of lightheadness and tired legs. The ability to exercise to an acceptable workload without cardiac or respiratory limitation and without desaturation suggests that this man's problem is not cardiorespiratory structural damage but an inappropriate pattern of breathing.

performance which itself may be more relevant to everyday life. Here the patient determines the intensity of exercise rather than having it imposed externally. McGavin and colleagues [156] advocated a 12-minute test in which patients were instructed to walk as far as they could along a measured distance in a hospital corridor. Stops were permitted if necessary, instructions to patients were standardized and the result recorded as the total distance in metres. The test was reasonably reproducible (coefficient of variation 8%) [157] but others have subsequently showed that a 6-minute walk is as reproducible and easier to perform [158]. Attempts to shorten this to 2 minutes have led to a loss of reproducibility [159].

Apart from the lack of metabolic data there are two important limitations to these walking tests. First there is an effect of familiarization such that after the first one or two walks the patient will perform consistently better. One paper has suggested that as many as four walks on successive days are needed before a plateau is reached [159] but the protocol adopted was atypical and others have not found any significant change once two practice walks have been performed [103]. Second the test is only applicable to patients with severe COPD (i.e. an FEV_1 of less than 1.5 l) since milder patients would not be sufficiently stressed by walking and tend to plateau at around 600 metres in 6 minutes. There is a crude relationship between FEV_1 and walking distance [156,160] but if a more restricted population, e.g. FEV_1 less than 1 l, is studied this disappears and other factors including the level of breathlessness [161], severity of hyperinflation [162] and patient motivation [24] become dominant. Oxygen desaturation occurs frequently during corridor walking [163] and some have related this exercise-induced desaturation to the DLCO [164], although this finding has not been universal. An alternative to self-paced walking is a shuttle walking test [165] where walking speed is dictated by an audible signal and is

increased with each minute. This appears to be reproducible and to avoid the need for a practice walk. Further experience will be needed to evaluate this more thoroughly.

Walking tests provide an attractive means of monitoring the results of treatment in rehabilitation program. However, it is not clear whether practice walks are needed on every occasion once the patient has been familiarized with the test and this limits their value as a test for monitoring long-term progress.

13.6.7 OTHER COMPLEX TESTS

These involve more equipment, are more time consuming, may be more invasive and are needed to answer specific subsidiary questions rather than being part of the routine patient evaluation.

(a) Measurement of esophageal and gastric pressure

This is readily done by swallowing an esophageal ballon catheter and this is needed if the volume–pressure curve is to be measured and static compliance calculated. Catheter positioning and response characteristics affect these results as does the amount of esophageal pressure artefact, a common feature when the patient is supine. If a gastric balloon is also swallowed, the trans-diaphragmatic pressure can be calculated by subtraction and this can be useful if symptoms are disproportionate to spirometric testing. Values for maximum trans-diaphragmatic pressures vary with the technique employed [166] especially the amount of abdominal activation [167]. Diaphragm function can be more simply assessed using the unoccluded sniff method, normal ranges for which are available [168].

(b) Pulmonary artery catheterization

This is now often done in the ITU to assess gas exchange, the degree of pulmonary hypertension and possibly the adequacy of left ventricular function as indicated by the wedge pressure (Chapter 11). Although popular as a research tool in the investigation of the pulmonary vascular consequences of chronic hypoxemia and initially advocated as a guide to prognosis in long-term oxygen treatment [169,170], more recent data suggest that acute trials of oxygen in chronically hypoxic COPD patients are of little value in predicting the long-term pulmonary vascular response or mortality experience [171].

(c) Sleep studies

As noted elsewhere there is no role at present for full polysomnography in the assessment of the typical COPD patient even if hypoxemic by day (Chapter 12). Overnight oximetry is a useful way of assessing the adequacy of supplementary oxygen therapy but there are no data to show that this refinement improves the prognosis of these patients.

13.6.8 OTHER NON-PHYSIOLOGICAL ASSESSMENTS

A range of other investigations can give useful additional information in COPD and are readily available.

(a) Hematology

The important abnormality here is polycythemia. This should be suspected when the hematocrit is elevated (greater than 52% in men, 47% in women) and/or the hemoglobin is raised (greater than 18 g/dl in men, 16 g/dl women). However, some caution is needed since these values represent the combined effects of increases in red cell mass and plasma volume. Although changes in the latter parallel the former, plasma volume can be reduced by diuretics, dehydration and cigarette smoking producing spurious polycythemia (Fig. 13.6). Although desirable,

routine measurement of red cell mass by radio-isotopes is difficult and most treatment is guided by the simple indirect measurements. Red cell mass can be elevated as part of a myeloproliferative disorder or more commonly due to chronic hypoxia with or without cigarette smoking. Smoker's polycythemia was recognized by Smith and Landaw who described elevated red cell masses in 12 of 22 heavy smokers [172]. Variations in red cell mass were well correlated with mean carboxyhemoglobin exposure in a large group of hypoxic COPD patients [173], and along with chronic hypoxia, smoking was thought to explain the polycythemia via its effects on oxygen delivery to the kidney. Other important stimuli to polycythemia include nocturnal desaturation [174] and exercise [117] which can add substantially to the overall hypoxic stimulus during the day. In contrast intercurrent infection depresses red cell production [175]. Given the many factors which influence tissue oxygen delivery it is not surprising that the relationship between polycythemia and chronic hypoxemia is a complex one [176].

Identifying polycythemia is important as increased blood viscosity predisposes to vascular events and there is some evidence that venesection improves exercise performance [177,178]. The best method for venesection is uncertain as is the time course of any resulting benefit. While erythropheresis and plasma replacement is elegant and safe [179], most clinicians rely on the removal of the occasional unit of blood and its replacement with Dextran to try and limit rebound hyperviscocity. Generally this process is repeated over several days until the hematocrit falls below 60% although there are no data to support the choice of this particular level.

Other hematological changes are worth noting. Chronic hypoxemic patients often have raised MCV values. This cannot be accounted for by vitamin deficiencies or

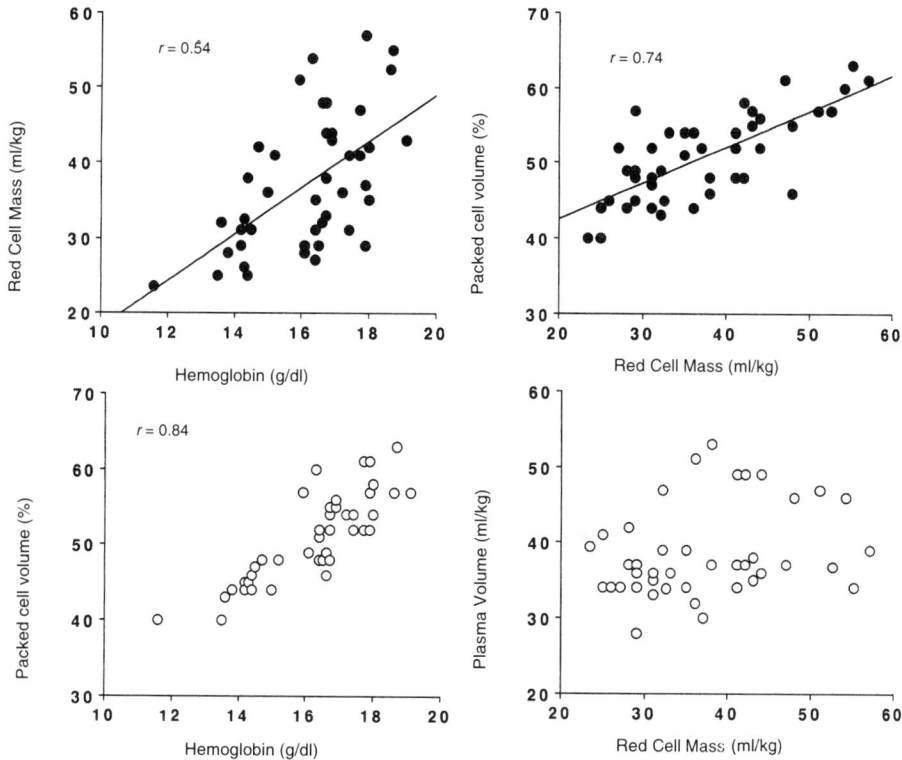

Fig. 13.6 Relationship between hemoglobin, packed cell volume, red cell mass (RCM) and plasma volume (PV) (measured radio-isotopically) in 43 patients with stable hypoxemic COPD (mean FEV_1 0.92 l, PaO_2 less than 7.5 kPa). Although there is a relationship between hemoglobin and red cell mass (top left panel) this is relatively weak and individuals with hemoglobin of 18 g/dl may have a normal to greatly increased RCM. Packed cell volume is a better guide, values of 50% or more indicating significant polycythemia (top right panel). The variability of PCV and hemoglobin increases as hemoglobin rises (lower left panel). The discrepancy between RCM and hemoglobin is due to the variation in plasma volume which is unrelated to RCM and reflects other changes, e.g. diuretic therapy. Thus clinical decisions on venesection should be based on PCV, not hemoglobin, when no RCM data are available.

alcohol excess. Eosinophilia may be a marker of a potential response to oral corticosteroids, although this is an extremely infrequent finding in our hands. None the less patients with evidence of eosinophilia appear to follow a more a benign course [180]. Finally there is evidence of enhanced platelet activity in hypoxemic COPD with a reduced survival time and increase in plasma and beta thromboglobulin [181,182]. The relevance of these changes to subsequent pulmonary and systemic vascular disease is presently obscure.

(b) Biochemistry

Hypoxemic COPD patients have reduced water clearance and an activated renin–angiotensin system (Chapter 11). Moreover they receive diuretics to control peripheral edema and so reductions in serum sodium and potassium are relatively common Whether chronic β-agonist therapy produces sustained hypokalemia is more doubtful (Chapter 17). Hypophosphatemia has been reported in 17% of COPD patients compared with 5% of non-respiratory patients [183] presumably reflecting malnutrition and the effects of respiratory acidosis. This can have clinically important effects, at least in the ITU, as low phosphate impairs respiratory muscle function and prolongs ventilatory weaning [184].

(c) α_1-Antitrypsin

This is discussed in full elsewhere (Chapter 6).

(d) ECG

The ECG is abnormal in up to 75% of advanced COPD patients (Chapter 11) but the significance of these changes either for diagnosis or prognosis is dubious. Most of these reflect changes in cardiac configuration secondary to hyperinflation. Changes in the P wave are a better guide to right ventricular overload and are the most reliable pointer to increase in right ventricular mass, being abnormal in 50% of our cor pulmonale patients [185]. However, other abnormalities suggestive of cor pulmonale are disappointingly insensitive. These criteria were developed largely in patients with congenital heart disease and do not take account of the coexisting problems of hyperinflation in COPD.

13.7 DIFFERENTIAL DIAGNOSIS

Several other illnesses can be confused with or exist along with COPD and their differential diagnosis is not always easy. Many patients have pulmonary edema due to left ventricular dysfunction as well as chronic airways disease and the relative roles of each pathology may need cycle ergometry and echocardiography to resolve. However, the presence of dyspnea and angina does not mean that the latter causes the former and evidence of radiographic pulmonary edema or symptoms disproportionate to lung function should be sought before 'cardiac failure' is diagnosed. Peripheral edema and an elevated jugular venous pressure are not synonymous with

biventricular disease as previously noted. Conversely abnormal spirometry has long been recognized in severe mitral stenosis. There is evidence of mild airflow limitation in some cases [186] but reductions in vital capacity and increases in residual volume are more frequent [187] and related to disease severity [186]. The signs of valvular heart disease may be difficult to elicit in an overinflated chest and echocardiography will be needed when the clinical suspicion is high.

Less acute presentations are usually resolved by a mixture of investigations and clinical assessement. Bronchiectasis can be associated with progressively declining lung function although this is far from universal. Large volumes of purulent sputum with or without a predisposing factor, e.g. past tuberculosis, cystic fibrosis, together with CT scanning makes this differential diagnosis relatively straight forward. More taxing is bronchiolitis obliterans which can be very non-specific in its presentation. The presence of progressive airways obstruction especially in a relatively young person with a history of toxic fume exposure should always raise this diagnosis. It has been reported in patients with rheumatoid arthritis and should always be considered when COPD develops without reason in a non-smoker. Of more local interest are the unusual problems of panbronchiolitis which have been described in Japan and are associated with a distinctive pathology and progressive airflow limitation [188]. The largest and in many ways most difficult differential is that of bronchial asthma. As noted in Chapter 1 it can be very difficult and there is obviously an overlap between the features of asthma, bronchitis and emphysema. Endobronchial biopsy data may resolve this problem but at present this is still too experimental a technique for clinical purposes. The final terminology for the patient with chronic airflow obstruction will often depend upon an arbitrary decision about how large a change in FEV_1 after bronchodilator testing is really required to make the diagnosis of asthma.

Ultimately it is more important that the patient receives the correct treatment rather than the diagnostic label being modified to fit clinical preconceptions.

13.8 GENERAL ASSESSMENT OF COPD

This will always involve as detailed a history and clinical examination as the patient's condition permits. Most patients need at least one chest radiograph, ECG, full blood count and clinical chemistry but the selection of further investigations will vary with the clinical setting.

In the acute in-patient episode arterial blood gas tensions on and off supplementary oxygen give the most useful and reliable guide to severity and prognosis. It is worth trying to record baseline spirometry and repeating this as the patient's condition improves. However, more detailed assessment is not appropriate at this point.

In the out-patient clinic spirometry, preferably accompanied by a flow–volume loop, is valuable in confirming the diagnosis and assessing severity as is the measurement of lung volumes and DLCO. There is a temptation to use pulse oximetry to identify the persistently hypoxemic patient but blood gas tensions are much more informative. This test is usually confined to those patients with an FEV_1 <1.0 l or with evidence of cyanosis. Nebulized bronchodilator testing with a combination of β-agonists and anticholinergics is helpful in establishing the maximum bronchodilitation which can be achieved and relating subsequent therapy to this whilst those patients showing the largest absolute increase in FEV_1 are the ones in which some form of corticosteroid trial can be expected to yield benefits. In general corticosteroid trials are worthwhile in patients with atypical features, e.g. low cigarette consumption, high DLCO and/or a response to bronchodilators of more than 200 ml above baseline (see earlier). The validity of this approach is being tested as part of the ISOLDE long-term trial of inhaled

steroids which includes a preliminary corticosteroid assessment unlike its companion study, the Euroscop trial, in which patients are simply randomized to active or placebo inhaler. Hopefully between the two major studies it will be possible to determine whether oral steroid trials are needed or whether some other features will be likely to predict corticosteroid responsiveness. At present more complex tests are reserved to resolve specific queries.

13.9 ASSESSMENT FOR THORACIC AND NON-THORACIC SURGERY

It is difficult to offer hard and fast rules in defining surgical suitability as careful prospective studies in COPD patients are lacking, most patients being derived from a mixed population only some of whom suffer from COPD. Moreover the chance of survival and/or complications depends upon the skill of both the anesthetist and surgeon, the availability of postoperative intensive care and the surgical team's familiarity with a specific physiologic problems of COPD patients. However, certain general principles are worth noting. The risk of complications depends upon the site of surgery; thus only 2 of 330 patients undergoing lower abdominal procedures developed respiratory complications [189]. This is not surprising as the FRC falls after any operation, a change which is greater the closer the incision is to the thorax [190]. Surgery and/or anesthesia compromise the function of the respiratory muscles which tend to maintain FRC in COPD [191]. Reduced cough and mucociliary clearance consequent upon both pain and analgesic use exacerbate the tendency to atelectasis whether macro- or microscopic. Thoracotomy compounds these problems but may have to be considered in the COPD patient whose risk of developing lung cancer is at least double that of control subjects [2,192].

No single test can reliably predict the risks of postoperative complications. The role of abnormal spirometry has been reviewed on many occasions [193,194], about two-thirds of studies finding it of value in predicting outcome. A useful rule of thumb is that if the FEV_1 is >2.0 l or 50% predicted patients seldom have major complications (sensitivity 96%, negative predictive value 99%) [195,196] and this is a very useful screening test. Other indices related to gas exchange and exercise performance are useful. Thus a $PaCO_2$ >45 mmHg (6.0 kPa) has been reported as predicting a high postoperative mortality [193], whilst impaired exercise performance with a VO_2 <16 ml/kg/min is a specific (91%) but less sensitive marker of complications [197]. An additional problem in patients being considered for lung resection for lung tumors is the local effect of the tumor on ventilation and perfusion within the lung. This is seldom a problem when lobectomy is being considered but may be important when pneumonectomy is required [198]. If these defects exceed two-thirds of the total perfusion to the involved lung then the lesion is unlikely to be resectable [198,199]. Isotope scans have been used to predict postoperative pulmonary function in these patients and several groups have confirmed that ventilation and perfusion scanning can be used equivalently to predict post-operative FEV_1 using the formula

$$\text{Postoperative } FEV_1 = \text{preoperative } FEV_1 \times \frac{\text{perfusion of contralateral lung}}{\text{total perfusion}}$$

Thus the larger the scanning defect the better the postoperative lung function (but the greater the risk of incomplete resection). Such studies are still useful for patients whose lung function and symptoms postoperatively are likely to make pneumonectomy a borderline decision but many of these are now excluded on CT grounds as there is evidence of locally extensive tumor. A possible scheme of preoperative assessment for the COPD patient is shown in Fig. 13.7. This can define relatively

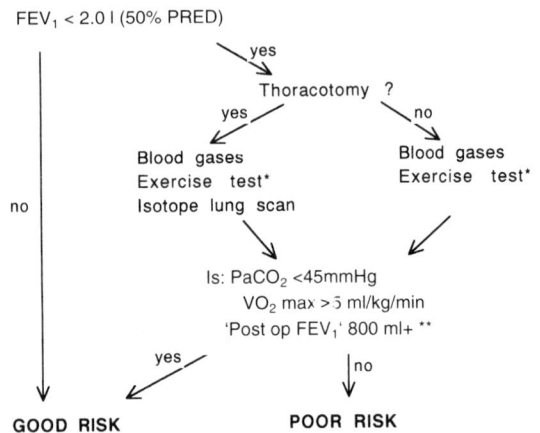

Fig. 13.7 A schematic approach to the presurgical assessment of the COPD patient. This is not relevant to the emergency situation where only blood gas tensions are likely to be available. Nonthoracic, non-abdominal surgery is relatively low risk and needs little more than spirometry. Single asterix indicates that this test provides useful additional information but is not mandatory. Other 'functional measures' such as corridor or shuttle walking may be substituted in more severe patients to give a semi-quantitative indication of severity. Double asterisks indicate this test is only relevant/appropriate in patients undergoing thoracotomy. These assessments can define groups at risk of postoperative complications but will not necessarily indicate long term functional status after surgery.

high and low risk groups but the final decision about surgery will depend upon its urgency, its chance of cure and the availability of appropriate postoperative intensive care as much as on any of these values which are helpful in predicting the perioperative complication rate and to some extent the subsequent lung function.

When elective procedures are considered simple measures are still worth emphasizing. Smoking cessation does lead to gradual improvements in mucociliary clearance and even lung function. However, the time course of these changes is long and they are unlikely to begin in less than one month of stopping smoking. Optimizing bronchodilator treatment and the use of high dose nebulized β-agonists and/or anticholinergics pre-operatively is easier to achieve although fuller assessment involving a trial of oral cortico-steroids will take up to a month to complete. Bronchodilator treatment should be combined with appropriate physiotherapy especially when significant sputum production is reported. The role of other physical therapies such as IPPB or incentive spirometry pre-operatively remain controversial whilst the benefits of prophylactic antibiotics are unproven. Time and money spent optimizing preoperative lung function is likely to be well repaid by reduced intensive care unit stays and postoperative morbidity.

REFERENCES

1. Fletcher, C.M., Peto, R., Tinker, C. and Speizer, F.C. (1976) *The natural history of Chronic Bronchitis and Emphysema*, Oxford University Press, Oxford.
2. Peto, R., Speizer, F.E., Cochrane, A.L. *et al.* (1983) The relevance of airflow obstruction but not of mucus hypersecretion to mortality from chronic lung disease: results from 20 years of prospective observation. *Am. Rev. Respir. Dis.*, **128**, 491–500.
3. Burrows, B., Niden, A.H., Barclay, W.R. and Kasik, J.E. (1965). Chronic obstructive lung disease. II. Relationship of clinical and physiologic findings to the severity of airways obstruction. *Am. Rev. Respir. Dis.*, **91**, 665–78.
4. Wynder, E.L., Lamm, F.R. and Mantel, N. (1965) Epidemiology of persistent cough. *Am. Rev. Respir. Dis.*, **91**, 679–700.
5. CIBA Guest Symposium Report (1959) Terminology, definitions and classifications of chronic pulmonary emphysema and related conditions. *Thorax*, **14**, 286–99.
6. Medical Research Council Committee on Research into Chronic Bronchitis (1966) *Instructions for Use of the Questionnaire on Respiratory Symptoms*, W.J. Holman, Devon.
7. Morgan, W.K.C. (1993) Bronchitis, airways obstruction and occupation, in *Occupational Lung Diseases* (ed. R. Parkes) Butterworths, London.
8. Brinkman, G.L., Block, D.L. and Cress, C. (1972) The effects of bronchitis on occupational pulmonary ventilation over an 11 year period. *J. Occup. Med.*, **14**, 615–20.
9. Jamal, K., Cooney, T.P., Fleetham, J.A. and Thurlbeck, W.M. (1984) Chronic bronchitis: Correlation of morphologic findings to sputum production and flow rates. *Am. Rev. Respir. Dis.*, **129**, 717–22.
10. Higgins, M.W., Keller, J.B., Landis, J.R. *et al.* (1984) Risk of chronic obstructive pulmonary disease. *Am. Rev. Respir. Dis.*, **130**, 380–5.
11. Fuller, R.W. and Jackson, D.M. (1990) Physiology and treatment of cough. *Thorax*, **45**, 425–30.
12. Choudry, N.B., Fuller, R.W. and Pride, N.B. (1989) Sensitivity of the human cough reflex: effect of inflammatory mediators prostaglandin E2, bradykinin and histamine. *Am. Rev. Respir. Dis.*, **140**, 137–41.
13. Goodman, R.M., Tergin, B.M., Lauda, J.F. *et al.* (1978) Relationship of smoking history and pulmonary function tests to tracheal mucus velocity in non-smokers, young smokers, ex-smokers and patients with chronic bronchitis. *Am. Rev. Respir. Dis.*, **117**, 205–14.
14. Zahm, J.M., Girard, F. *et al.* (1980) Mucociliary transport *in vivo* and *vitro*. Relations to sputum properties in chronic bronchitis. *Eur. J. Respir. Dis.*, **61**, 254–8.
15. Loudon, R.G. and Brown, L.C. (1967) Cough frequency in patients with respiratory disease. *Am. Rev. Respir. Dis.*, **96**, 1137–43.
16. Power, J.T., Stewart, I.C., Connaughton, J.J. *et al.* (1984) Nocturnal cough in chronic bronchitis and emphysema. *Am. Rev. Respir. Dis.*, **130**, 999–1001.
17. Aaronson, D.W., Rovner, R.N. and Patterson, R. (1970) Cough syncope: case presentation and review. *J. Allergy*, **46**, 359.
18. Irwin, R.S. and Rosen, M.J. (1977) Cough: a comprehensive review. *Arch. Intern. Med.*, **137**, 1186–91.
19. Rodenstein, D.O., Francis, D. and Stanescu, D.C. (1983) Emotional laryngeal wheezing: a new syndrome. *Am. Rev. Respir. Dis.*, **127**, 354–7.
20. Anthonisen, N.R., Wright, E.C. and the IPPB Trial Group (1986) Bronchodilator response in chronic obstructive pulmonary disease. *Am. Rev. Respir. Dis.*, **133**, 814–9.
21. Gottfried, S.B., Altose, M.D., Kelsen, S.G. and Cherniack, N.S. (1981). Perception of changes

in airflow resistance in obstructive pulmonary disorders. *Am. Rev. Respir. Dis.*, **124**, 566–70.

22. American Medical Association (1984) The respiratory system, in *Guides to the Evaluation of Permanent Impairment*, 2nd edn Chicago, pp. 85–107.

23. Wolkove, N., Dajczman, E., Colacone, A. and Kreisman, H. (1989) The relationship between pulmonary function and dyspnoea in obstructive lung disease. *Chest*, **96**, 1247–51.

24. Morgan, A.D., Peck, D.F., Buchanan, D.R. and McHardy, G.J.R. (1983) Effects of beliefs on exercise in chronic bronchitis. *Br. Med. J.*, **286**, 171–3.

25. Morgan, W.K.C. (1979) Disability or disinclination? Impairment or importuning. *Chest*, **75**, 712–5.

26. Mahler, D.A., Weinberg, D.H., Wells, C.K. and Feinstein, A.R. (1984) The measurement of dyspnea: Contents, interobserver agreement and physiologic correlates of two new clinical indices. *Chest*, **85**, 751–8.

27. Druz, W.S. and Sharp, J.T. (1982) Electrical and mechanical activity of the diaphragm accompanying body position change in severe COPD. *Am. Rev. Respir. Dis.*, **125**, 275–80.

28. Sharp, J.T., Druz, W.S., Moisan, T. *et al.* (1980) Postural relief of dyspnea in severe COPD. *Am. Rev. Respir. Dis.*, **122**, 201–11.

29. David, P., Denis, P., Nouvet, G. *et al.* (1982) Lung function and gastro-oesophageal reflux during chronic bronchitis. *Bull. Eur. Physiopathol. Respir.*, **18**, 81–6.

30. Berquist, N.E., Rachelefsky, G.S., Kadden, M. *et al.* (1981) Effect of theophylline on gastro-oesophageal reflux in normal adults. *J. Allergy Clin. Immunol.*, **67**, 407–11.

31. Pode, G. and Stradling, P. (1964) Routine radiography for haemoptysis. *Br. Med. J.*, **1**, 341–2.

32. Wilson, D.D., Rogers, R.M. and Hoftman, R.M. (1985) Nutrition and chronic lung disease. *Am. Rev. Respir. Dis.*, **132**, 1347–65.

33. Donahoe, M., Rogers, R.M., Wilson, D.D. and Pennock, B.E. (1989) Oxygen consumption of the respiratory muscles in normal and malnourished patients with chronic obstructive pulmonary disease. *Am. Rev. Respir. Dis.*, **140**, 385–91.

34. Grant, I., Heaton, R.K., McSweeny, A.J. *et al.* (1982) Neuropsychologic findings in hypo-

xemic chronic obstructive pulmonary disease. *Arch. Intern. Med.*, **142**, 1470–6.

35. McSweeney, A.J., Grant, I., Heaton, R.K. *et al.* (1982) Life quality of patients with chronic obstructive pulmonary disease. *Arch. Intern. Med.*, **142**, 473–8.

36. Calverley, P.M.A., Brezinova, V., Douglas, N.J. *et al.* (1982) The effect of oxygenation on sleep quality in chronic bronchitis and emphysema. *Am. Rev. Respir. Dis.*, **126**, 206–10.

37. Incalzi, R., Gemma, A., Marra, C. *et al.* (1993) Chronic obstructive pulmonary disease: An original model of cognitive decline. *Am. Rev. Respir. Dis.*, **148**, 418–24.

38. Burrows, B., Knudson, R.J., Cline, M.G. and Leibowitz, M.D. (1979) Quantitative relationships between cigarette smoking and ventilatory function. *Am. Rev. Respir. Dis.*, **115**, 751–60.

39. Petty, T.L., Ryan, S.F. and Mitchell, R.S. (1967) Cigarette smoking and the lungs. Relation to postmortem evidence of emphysema chronic bronchitis and black lung pigmentation. *Arch. Environ. Health*, **14**, 172–7.

40. United States Public Health Service (1984) *The health consequences of smoking. Chronic obstructive pulmonary disease: a report of the Surgeon General*. Rockville MD: US Government Printing Office. DHSS Publ. (PHS) 84–50205.

41. Humerfelt, S., Gulsvik, A., Skjaerven, R. *et al.* (1993) Decline in FEV_1 and airflow limitation related to occupational exposure in men of an urban community. *Eur. Respir. J.*, **6**, 1095–1103.

42. Love, R.G., and Miller, B.G. (1992) Longitudinal study of lung function in coal-miners. *Thorax*, **37**, 193–7.

43. Ingram, R.H. and Schilder, D.P. (1967) Effect of pursed lips expiration on the pulmonary pressure-flow relationship in obstructive lung disease. *Am. Rev. Respir. Dis.*, **96**, 381–7.

44. Tiep, B.L., Burns, M., Kao, D. *et al.* (1986) Pursed lips breathing training using ear oximetry. *Chest*, **90**, 218–21.

45 Banzett, R.B., Topulos, G.P., Leith, D.E. and Nations, C.S. (1988) Bracing arms increases the capacity of substained hyperpnea. *Am. Rev. Respir. Dis.*, **138**, 106–9.

46. Celli, B.R., Rassulo, J. and Make, B.J. (1986) Dyssynchronous breathing during arm but not leg exercise in patients with chronic airflow obstruction. *N. Engl. J. Med.*, **314**, 1485–90.

47. Tobin, M.J., Perez, W., Guenther, S.M. *et al.* (1987) Does rib cage-abdominal paradox signify respiratory muscle fatigue? *J. Appl. Physiol.*, **63**, 851–60.

48. Cohen, C.A., Zagelbaum, G., Gross, D. *et al.* (1982) Clinical manifestations of respiratory muscle fatigue. *Am. J. Med.*, **73**, 308–16.

49. Loudon, R. and Murphy, R.L.H. (1984) State of the art: Lung sounds. *Am. Rev. Respir. Dis.*, **130**, 663–73.

50. Ploysongsang, Y., Pare, J.A.P. and Macklem, P.T. (1982) Comparison of regional breath sounds with regional ventilation in emphysema. *Am. Rev. Respir. Dis.*, **126**, 526–9.

51. Schreur, H.J.W., Sterk, P.J., Vanderschoot, J. *et al.* (1992) Lung sounds intensity in patients with emphysema and in normal subjects at standardized airflows. *Thorax*, **47**, 674–9.

52. Marini, J.J., Pierson, D.J., Hudson, L.D. *et al.* (1979) The significance of wheezing in chronic airflow obstruction. *Am. Rev. Respir. Dis.*, **120**, 1069–72.

53. Badgett, R.G., Tanaka, D.J., Hunt, D.K., *et al.* (1993) Can moderate chronic obstructive pulmonary disease be diagnosed by historical and physical findings alone? *Am. J. Med.*, **94**, 188–96.

54. Bohadana, A.B., Pelsin, R. and Uffholtz, H. (1978) Breath sounds in the clinical assessment of airflow obstruction. *Thorax*, **33**, 345–51.

55. Wardman, A.G., Binns, V., Claydon, A.D. and Cooke, N.J. (1986). The diagnosis and treatment of adults with obstructive airways disease in general practice. *Br. J. Dis. Chest*, **80**, 19–26.

56. Nisar, M., Walshaw, M.J., Earis. J.E. *et al.* (1990) Assessment of airway reversibility of airway obstruction in patients with chronic obstructive airways disease. *Thorax*, **45**, 190–4.

57. Anthonisen, N.R., Wright, E.C., Hodgkin, J.E. and the IPPB Trial Group (1986) Prognosis in chronic obstructive pulmonary disease. *Am. Rev. Respir. Dis.*, **133**, 14–20.

58. Gould, G.A., MacNee, W., McLean, A. *et al.* (1988) CT measurements of lung density in life can quantitate distal airspace enlargement. *Am. Rev. Respir. Dis.*, **137**, 380–92.

59. American Thoracic Society (1987) Standards for the diagnosis and care of patients with chronic obstructive pulmonary disease (COPD) and asthma. *Am. Rev. Respir. Dis.*, **136**, 225–44.

60. Fletcher, C.M. and Pride, N.B. (1984) Definitions of emphysema, chronic bronchitis, asthma and airflow obstruction: 25 years on from the CIBA symposium. *Thorax*, **39**, 81–5.

61. Pearson, M.G., Ryland, I. and Harrison, B.D.W. (1994) A national audit of acute severe asthma in adults admitted to hospital. *Quality in Health Care*, In press.

62. Kesten, S. and Chapman, K.R. (1993) Physician perceptions and management of COPD. *Chest*, **104**, 254–8.

63. Ingram, R.H. and Schilder, D.P. (1966) Effect of gas compression on pulmonary pressure, flow and volume relationships. *J. Appl. Physiol.*, **21**, 1821–6.

64. Gardner, R.M., Baker, C.D., Broennie, A.M. *et al.* (1979) Snowbird workshop on the standardisation of spirometry. *Am. Rev. Respir. Dis.*, **119**, 831–8.

65. American Thoracic Society (1987) Standardization of spirometry – 1987 update. *Am. Rev. Respir. Dis.*, **136**, 1285–98.

66. Crapo, R.D. (1991) Spirometry: Quality control and reproducibility criteria. *Am. Rev. Respir. Dis.*, **143**, 1212–13.

67. Quanjer, P.H. (ed.) Standardised lung function testing. *Bull. Eur. Physiopathol. Respir.*, **19**(suppl.), 1–95.

68. Quanjer, P.H. (1993) Standardised lung function testing. *Eur. Respir. J.*, **6**, (suppl.16) S3–102.

69. Krowka, M.J., Enright, P.L., Rodarte, J.R. and Hyatt, R.E. (1987) Effect of effort on measurement of FEV_1. *Am. Rev. Respir. Dis.*, **136**, 829–33.

70. Hyatt, R.F., Okeson, G.C. and Rodarte, J.R. (1973) Influence of expiratory flow limitation on the pattern of lung emptying in man. *J. Appl. Physiol.*, **35**, 411–19.

71. Stoller, J.K., Basheda, S., Laskowski, D. *et al.* (1993) Trial of standard versus modified expiration to achieve end-of-test spirometry criteria. *Am. Rev. Respir. Dis.*, **148**, 275–80.

72. Enright, P.L., Johnson, L.R., Connett, J.E. *et al.* (1991) Spirometry in the Lung Health Study 1. Methods and quality control. *Am. Rev. Respir. Dis.*, **143**, 1215–23.

73. European Coal and Steel Community Recommendations (1983) *Bull. Eur. Physiopathol. Respir.*, **19**(suppl.5), 1–93.

74. American Thoracic Society (1991) Lung function testing: Selection of reference values and

interpretative strategies. *Am. Rev. Respir. Dis.,* **144**, 1202–28.

75. Hankinson, J.L. and Bang, K.M. (1991) Acceptability and reproducibility criteria of the American Thoracic Society as observed in a sample of the general population. *Am. Rev. Respir. Dis.,* **143**, 516–21.

76. Miller, M.R. and Pincock, A.C. (1988) Predicted values: how should we use them? *Thorax,* **43**, 267–9.

77. Dillard, T.A., Hnatiuk, O.W. and McCumber, R. (1993) Maximum voluntary ventilation. Spirometric determinants in chronic obstructive pulmonary disease patients and normal subjects. *Am. Rev. Respir. Dis.,* **147**, 870–5.

78. Spiro, S.G., Hahn, H.L., Edwards, R.H.T. *et al.* (1975) An analysis of the physiological strain of submaximal exercise in patients with chronic obstructive bronchitis. *Thorax,* **30**, 415–25.

79. Morgan, W.K.C. (1984) The relationship between pulmonary impairment and disability, in *Occupational Lung Disease* (eds W.K.C. Morgan and A. Seaton), Saunders, Philadelphia, pp.66–67.

80. Detels, R., Tashkin, D.P., Simmons, M.S. *et al.* (1982) The UCLA population studies of chronic obstructive respiratory disease. 5. Agreement and disagreement of tests in identifying abnormal lung function. *Chest,* **82**, 630–5.

81 Eisen, E.A., Dockery, D.W., Speizer, F.E. *et al.* (1987) The association between health status and the performance of excessively variable spirometry tests in a population based study in six US cities. *Am. Rev. Respir. Dis.,* **136**, 1371–6.

82. Miller, M.R., Dickinson, S.A. and Hitchings, D.J. (1992) The accuracy of portable peak flow meters. *Thorax,* **47**, 904–9.

83. Higgins, B.G., Britton, J.R., Chinn, S. *et al.* (1989) The distribution of peak expiratory flow variability in a population sample. *Am. Rev. Respir. Dis.,* **140**, 1368–72.

84. Higgins, B.G., Britton, J.R., Chinn, S. *et al.* (1992) Comparison of bronchial reactivity and peak expiratory flow variability measurements for epidemiological studies. *Am. Rev. Respir. Dis.,* **145**, 588–93.

85. Jamison, J.P. and McKinley, P.K. (1993) Validity of peak expiratory flow rate variability for the diagnosis of asthma. *Clin. Sci.,* **85**, 365–71.

86. Brand, P.L.P., Quanjer, P.H., Postma, D.S. *et al.* (1992) Interpretation of bronchodilator response in patients with obstructive airways disease. *Thorax,* **47**, 429–36.

87. Mitchell, D.M., Gildeh, P., Dimond, A.H. and Collins, J.V. (1986) Value of serial peak expiratory flow measurements in assessing treatment response in chronic airflow limitation. *Thorax,* **41**, 606–10.

88. Rodenstein, D.O. and Stanescu, D.C. (1982) Reassessment of lung volume measurement by helium dilution and by body plethysmography in chronic airflow obstruction. *Am. Rev. Respir. Dis.,* **126**, 1040–4.

89. Rodenstein, D.O. and Stanescu, D.C. (1983) Frequency dependence of plethysmographic volume in healthy and asthmatic subjects. *J. Appl. Physiol.,* **54**, 159–63.

90. Liistro, G., Stanescu, D., Rodenstein, D. and Veritier, C. (1989) Reassessment of the interruption technique for measuring flow resistance in humans. *J. Appl. Physiol.,* **67**, 933–7.

91. Pierce, R.J., Brown, D.J., Holmes, M. *et al.* (1979) Estimation of lung volumes from chest radiography using shape information. *Thorax,* **34**, 725–34.

92. Bernhard, H.J., Pierce, J.A., Joyce, J.W. and Bates, J.H. (1960) Roentgenographic determination of TLC. A new method evaluated in health, emphysema and congestive cardiac failure. *Am. J. Med.,* **28**, 51–60.

93. Spence, D.P.S., Ahmed, J., Sumner, A. *et al.* (1990) Is computerised x-ray planimetry a reliable measure of lung volumes in normal subjects? *Thorax,* **45**, 807.

94. Gross, N.J. and Skorodin, M.S. (1984) Role of the parasympathetic system in airway obstruction due to emphysema. *N. Engl. J. Med.,* **311**, 421–5.

95. Taylor, D.R., Buick, B., Kinney, C. *et al.* (1985) The efficacy of orally administered theophylline, inhaled salbutamol and a combination of the two in the management of chronic bronchitis with reversible airflow obstruction. *Am. Rev. Respir. Dis.,* **131**, 747–51.

96. Chrystyn, H., Mulley, B.A. and Peake, M.D. (1988) Dose reponse relation to oral theophylline in severe chronic obstructive airways disease. *Br. Med. J.,* **297**, 1506–10.

97. Spence, D.P.S., Calverley, P.M.A. and Pearson, M.G. (1991) Thoracic gas volume, a promise unfulfilled. *Am. Rev. Respir. Dis.,* **143**, A449.

98. Wilson, S.H., Cooke, N.T., Edwards, R.H.T. and Spiro, S.G. (1984) Predicted normal values for maximal respiratory pressures in Caucasion adults and children. *Thorax*, **39**, 535–8.

99. Carroll, N., Clague, J.E., Pollard, M.H. *et al.* (1992) Portable maximum respiratory pressure measurement – a comparison with laboratory techniques. *J. Med. Eng. Tech.*, **16**, 82–6.

100. Eliasson, O and De Graffe, A.C. (1985) The use of criteria of reversibility and obstruction to define patient groups for bronchodilator trials. *Am. Rev. Respir. Dis.*, **132**, 858–64.

101. Meslier, N. and Racineux, J.L. (1991) Tests of reversibility of airflow obstruction. *Eur. Respir. Rev.*, **1**, 34–40.

102. Tweedale, P.M., Alexander, F. and McHardy, G.J.R. (1987) Short term variability in FEV_1 and bronchodilator responsiveness in patients with obstructive ventilatory defects. *Thorax*, **42**, 487–90.

103. Hay, J.G., Stone, P., Carter, J. *et al.* (1992) Bronchodilator reversibility, exercise performance and breathlessness in stable chronic obstructive pulmonary disease. *Eur. Resp. J.*, **5**, 659–64.

104. Nisar, M., Earis, J.E., Pearson, M.G. and Calverley, P.M.A. (1992) Acute bronchodilator trials in chronic obstructive pulmonary disease. *Am. Rev. Respir. Dis.*, **146**, 555–9.

105. Filuk, R.B., Easton, P.A. and Anthonisen, M.R. (1985) Responses to large doses of salbutamol and theophylline in patients with chronic obstructive pulmonary disease. *Am. Rev. Respir. Dis.*, **132**, 871–4.

106. Laube, B.L., Swift, D.L., Wagner, H.N. *et al.* (1986) The effect of bronchial obstruction on central airway deposition of a saline aerosol in patients with asthma. *Am. Rev. Respir. Dis.*, **133**, 740–3.

107. Gross. N.J., Petty, T.L., Freidman, M. *et al.* (1989) Dose response to ipratropium as a nebulised solution in patients with chronic obstructive pulmonary disease. *Am. Rev. Respir. Dis.*, **139**, 1188–91.

108. van Schayck, C.P., Folgering, H., Harbers, H. *et al.* (1991) Effects of allergy and age on responses to salbutamol and ipratropium in moderate asthma and chronic bronchitis. *Thorax*, **46**, 355–9.

109. Weir, D.C., Robertson, A.S. Gove, R.I. and Burge, P.S. (1990) Time course of response to oral and inhaled corticosteroids in non-asthmatic chronic airflow obstruction. *Thorax*, **45**, 118–21.

110. Weir, D.C., Gove, R.I., Robertson, A.S. and Burge, P.S. (1990) Corticosteroid trials in non-asthmatic chronic airflow obstruction: a comparison of prednisolone and beclomethasone dipropionate. *Thorax*, **45**, 112–17.

111. Mendella, L.A., Manfreda, J., Warren, C.P.N. and Anthonisen, N.R. (1982) Steroid response in stable chronic obstructive pulmonary disease. *Ann. Intern. Med.*, **96**, 17–21.

112. Weir, D.C., Gove, R.I., Robertson, A.S. and Burge, P.S. (1991) Response to corticosteroids in chronic airflow obstruction; relationship to emphysema and airways collapse. *Eur. Respir. J.*, **4**, 1185–90.

113. Weir, D.C. and Burge, P.D. (1993) Effects of high dose inhaled beclomethasone dipropionate 750 mcg and 1500 mcg twice daily and 40 mg per day oral prednisolone on lung function, symptoms and bronchial hyperresponsiveness in patients with non-asthmatic chronic airflow obstruction. *Thorax*, **48**, 309–16.

114. Stoller, J.K., Gerbarg, Z.B. and Feinstein, A.R. (1987) Corticosteroids in stable chronic obstructive pulmonary disease. *J. Gen. Intern. Med.*, **2**, 29–35.

115. Berger, R. and Smith, D. (1988) Effect of inhaled metaproterenol on exercise performance in patients with stable 'fixed' airway obstruction. *Am. Rev. Respir. Dis.*, **138**, 624–9.

116. Corris, P.A., Neville, E., Nariman, S. and Gibson, G.J. (1983) Dose response study of inhaled salbutamol powder in chronic airflow obstruction. *Thorax*, **38**, 292–6.

117. Spence, D.P.S., Hay, J.G., Carter, J. *et al.* (1993) Oxygen desaturation and breathlessness during corridor walking in chronic obstructive pulmonary disease. *Thorax*, **48**, 1145–50.

118. Kerstjens, H.A.M., Brand, P.L.P., Quanjer, P.H. *et al.* (1993) Variability of bronchodilator response and effects of inhaled corticosteroid treatment in obstructive airways disease. *Thorax*, **48**, 722–9.

119. Postma, D.S. Gimeno, F., Van der Weele, L.Th. and Sluiter, H.J. (1985) Assessment of ventilatory variables in survival prediction of patients with chronic airflow obstruction: the importance of reversibility. *Eur. J. Respir. Dis.*, **67**, 360–8.

120. Rimmington, L.D., Spence, D.P.S., Nisar, M. *et al.* (1993) Predictors of 5 year mortality in COPD. *Am. Rev. Respir. Dis.*, **147**, A323.

121. Ogilvie, C.M., Forster, R.E., Blakemore, W.S. and Morton, J.W. (1957) A standardised breathholding technique for the clinical measurement of the diffusing capacity of the lung for carbon monoxide. *J. Clin. Invest.*, **36**, 1–17.

122. Mitchell, M.M. and Renzetti, A.D. (1968) Application of the single breath method of total lung capacity measurement to the calculation of the carbon monoxide diffusing capacity. *Am. Rev. Respir. Dis.*, **97**, 581–4.

123. McLean, A., Warren, P.M., Gillooly, M. *et al.* (1992) Microscopic and macroscopic measurements of emphysema: relation to carbon monoxide gas transfer. *Thorax*, **47**, 144–9.

124. Dubois, P., Machiels, J., Smeets, F. *et al.* (1990) CO transfer capacity as a determining factor of survival for severe hypoxaemic COPD patients under long term oxygen therapy. *Eur. Respir. J.*, **3**, 1042–7.

125. Burrows, B. and Earl, R.H. (1969) Course and prognosis of chronic obstructive lung disease. *N. Engl. J. Med.*, **280**, 397–404.

126. Watson, A., Joyce, H., Hopper, L. and Pride, N.B. (1993) Influence of smoking habits on change in carbon monoxide transfer factor over 10 years in middle aged men. *Thorax*, **48**, 119–24.

127. Riley, R.L. and Cournand, A. (1949). 'Ideal' alveolar air and the analysis of ventilation-perfusion relationships in the lungs. *J. Appl. Physiol.*, **1**, 825–47.

128. Vergeret, G., Tunon de Lara, M., Douvier, J.J. *et al.* (1986) Compliance of COPD patients with long term oxygen therapy. *Eur. J. Respir. Dis.*, **69** (Suppl.146), 421–5.

129. Baudouin, S.V., Waterhouse, J.C., Tahtamouni, T. *et al.* (1990) Long term domiciliary oxygen treatment for chronic respiratory failure revisited. *Thorax*, **45**, 195–8.

130. Nickerson, B.G., Sarkisian, C. and Tremper, K. (1988) Bias and precision of pulse oximeters and arterial oximeters. *Chest*, **93**, 515–7.

131. Severinghaus, J.W., Naifeh, K.H. and Koh, S.O. (1989) Errors in 14 pulse oximeters during profound hypoxia. *J. Clin. Monit.*, **5**, 72–81.

132. Douglas, N.J., Brash, H.M., Wraith, P.K. *et al.* (1979) Accuracy, sensitivity to carboxyhemoglobin and speed of response of the Hewlett Packard 47201A ear oximeter. *Am. Rev. Respir. Dis.*, **119**, 311–3.

133. Peabody, J.L., Willis, M.M., Gregory, G.A. *et al.* (1978) Clinical limitations and advantages of transcutaneous oxygen electrodes. *Acta Anaesthesiol. Scand.*, (Suppl.), **68**, 76–82.

134. Effros, R.M. (1988) Acid base balance, in *Textbook of Respiratory Medicine*, (eds J.F. Murray and J.A. Nadel) Saunders, Philadephia, pp. 129–48.

135. Gibson, G.J. (1984) Carbon dioxide carriage by the blood, in *Clinical Tests of Respiratory Function*, (ed. G.J. Gibson), MacMillan, London, pp. 87–99.

136. Flenley, D.C. (1971) Another non-logarithmic acid base diagram. *Lancet*, **i**, 961–5.

137. Jones, N.L. (1988) *Clinical Exercise Testing*, Saunders, Philadelphia.

138. Gallagher, C.G. (1990) Exercise and chronic obstructive pulmonary disease. *Med. Clin. North Am.*, **74**, 619–41.

139. Shuey, C.B., Pierce, A.K. and Johnson, R.L. (1969) An evaluation of exercise tests in chronic obstructive pulmonary disease. *J. Appl. Physiol.*, **27**, 256–61.

140. Dodd, D.S., Brancatisaho, T. and Engel, L.A. (1984) Chest wall mechanics during exercise in patients with severe chronic airflow obstruction. *Am. Rev. Respir. Dis.*, **129**, 33–8.

141. Leaver, D.G. and Pride, N.B. (1971) Flow volume curves and expiratory pressures during exercise in patients with chronic airways obstruction. *Scand. J. Respir. Dis.*, **52**, 23–7.

142. Stubbing, D.G., Pengelly, L.D., Morse, J.L.C. *et al.* (1980) Pulmonary mechanics during exercise in subjects with chronic airflow obstruction. *J. Appl. Physiol.*, **49**, 511–5.

143. Potter, W.A., Olaffson, S. and Hyatt, R.E. (1971) Ventilatory mechanics and expiratory flow limitation during exercise in patients with obstructive lung disease. *J. Clin. Invest.*, **50**, 910–9.

144. Pardy, R.L., Rivington, R.W., Despas, P.J. *et al.* (1981) The effect of inspiratory muscle training on exercise performance in chronic airflow limitation. *Am. Rev. Respir. Dis.*, **123**, 426–33.

145. Bazzy, A.R., Korten, J.B. and Haddad, G.G. (1986) Increase in electromyogram low frequency power in non-fatigued contracting skeletal muscle. *J. Appl. Physiol.*, **61**, 1012–17.

146. Gallagher, C.G. and Younes, M. (1986) Breathing pattern during and after maximal exercise in patients with chronic obstructive lung disease, interstitial lung disease and cardiac disease and in normal subjects. *Am. Rev. Respir. Dis.*, **133**, 581–6.

147. Scano, G., Gigliotti, F., van Meerhaeghe, A. *et al.* (1988) Influence of exercise and CO_2 on breathing pattern in patients with chronic obstructive lung disease (COLD). *Eur. Respir. J.*, **1**, 139–44.

148. Cockroft, A., Beaumont, A., Adams, L. and Guz, A. (1985) Arterial oxygen desaturation during treadmill and bicycle exercise in patients with chronic obstructive airways disease. *Clin. Sci.*, **68**, 327–32.

149. Minh, V.D., Lee, H.M., Dolan, G.F. *et al.* (1979) Hypoxemia during exercise in patients with chronic obstructive pulmonary disease. *Am. Rev. Respir. Dis.*, **120**, 787–94.

150. Dantzker, D.R. and D'Alonzo, G.E. (1986) The effect of exercise pulmonary gas exchange in patients with chronic obstructive pulmonary disease. *Am. Rev. Respir. Dis.*, **134**, 1135–9.

151. Light, R.W., Mintz, H.M., Linden, G.S. *et al.* (1984) Hemodynamics of patients with severe chronic obstructive pulmonary disease during progressive upright exercise. *Am. Rev. Respir. Dis.*, **130**, 391–5.

152. Sue, D.Y., Wasserman, K., Morrica, R.B. *et al.* (1988) Metabolic acidosis during exercise in patients with chronic obstructive pulmonary disease. *Chest*, **91**, 931–8.

153. Killian, K.J., Leblanc, P., Martin, D.H. *et al.* (1992) Exercise capacity and ventilatory, circulatory and symptom limitation in patients with chronic airflow limitation. *Am. Rev. Respir. Dis.*, **146**, 935–40.

154. Jones, N.L. and Killian, K.J., (1991) Limitation of exercise in chronic airway obstruction, in Cherniack NS (ed): *Chronic Obstructive Pulmonary Disease*, (ed. N.S. Cherniack), Saunders, Philadephia, pp. 196–206.

155. Brown, S.E., Fisher, C.E., Stausburg, D.N. and Light, R.W. (1985) Reproducibility of VO_2 max in patient with chronic airflow obstruction. *Am. Rev. Respir. Dis.*, **131**, 435–8.

156. McGavin, C.R., Gupta, S.P. and McHardy, G.J.R. (1976) Twleve minute walking test for assessing disability in chronic bronchitis. *Br. Med. J.*, **1**, 822–3.

157. Mungall, I.P.F. and Hainsworth, R. (1979) Assessment of respiratory function patients with chronic obstructive airways disease. *Thorax*, **34**, 254–8.

158. Butland, R.J.A., Gross, E.R., Pang, J. *et al.* (1982) Two, six and twelve minute walking tests in respiratory diseases. *Br. Med. J.*, **284**, 1607–8.

159. Knox, A.J., Morrison, J.F. and Muers, M.F. (1988) Reproducibility of walking test results in chronic obstructive airways disease. *Thorax*, **43**, 388–92.

160. Swinburn, C.R., Wakefield, J.M. and Jones, P.W. (1985) Performance, ventilation and oxygen consumption in three different types of exercise tests in patients with chronic obstructive airways disease. *Thorax*, **40**, 581–6.

161. O'Donnell, D.E. and Webb, K.A. (1992) Breathlessness in patients with severe chronic obstructive airways limitation: physiologic correlates. *Chest*, **102**, 824–31.

162. Morgan, A.D., Peck, D.F., Buchanan, D.R. and McHardy, G.J.R. (1983) Effect of attitudes and beliefs on exercise tolerance in chronic bronchitics. *Br. Med. J.*, **268**, 171–3.

163. Mak, V.H.F., Bugler, J.R., Roberts, C.M. and Spiro, S.G. (1993) Effect of arterial oxygen desaturation on six minute walk distance, perceived effort and perceived breathlessness in patients with airflow limitation. *Thorax*, **48**, 33–8.

164. Owens, G.R., Rogers, R.M., Pennock, B.E. and Lewis, D. (1984) The diffusing capacity as a predictor of arterial oxygen desaturation during exercise in patients with chronic obstructive pulmonary disease. *N. Engl. J. Med.*, **310**, 1218–21.

165. Singh, S.J., Morgan, M.D.L., Scott, S. *et al.* (1992) Development of a shuttle walking test of disability in patients with chronic airways obstruction. *Thorax*, **47**, 1019–24.

166. Laporta, D. and Grassino, A. (1985) Assessment of transdiaphragmatic pressure in humans. *J. Appl. Physiol.*, **58**, 1469–76.

167. Hillman, D.R., Markus, J. and Finnucane, K.E. (1990) Effects of abdominal compression on maximum transdiaphragmatic pressure. *J. Appl. Physiol.*, **68**, 2296–304.

168. Laroche, C.M., Mier, A.K., Moxham, J. and Green, M. (1988) The value of sniff esophageal pressure in the assessment of global inspiratory muscle strength. *Am. Rev. Respir. Dis.*, **138**, 598–603.

169. Ashutosh, K., Mead, G. and Dunsky, M. (1983) Early effects of oxygen administration

and prognosis in chronic obstructive pulmonary disease and cor pulmonale. *Am. Rev. Respir. Dis.*, **127**, 399–404.

170. Timms, R.M., Khaja, F.U., Williams, G.W. *et al.* (1985) Hemodynamic response to oxygen therapy in chronic obstructive pulmonary disease. *Ann. Intern. Med.*, **102**, 29–36.

171. Sliwinski, P., Hawrgliewicz, I., Gorecka, D. and Zielinski, J. (1992) Acute effects of oxygen on pulmonary artery pressure does not predict survival on long term oxygen therapy in patients with chronic obstructive pulmonary disease. *Am. Rev. Respir. Dis.*, **146**, 665–9.

172. Smith, J.R. and Landaw, S.A. (1978) Smokers' polycythemia, *N. Engl. J. Med.*, **298**, 6–10.

173. Calverley, P.M.A., Leggett, R.J.E., McElderry, L. and Flenley, D.C. (1982) Cigarette smoking and secondary polycythemia in hypoxic cor pulmonale. *Am. Rev. Respir. Dis.*, **125**, 507–10.

174. Wedzichia, J.A., Cotes, P.M., Empey, D.W. *et al.* (1985) Serum immunoreactive erythropoietin in hypoxic lung disease with and without polycythaemia. *Clin. Sci.*, **69**, 413–22.

175. Wilson, R.H., Borden, C.W. and Ebert, R.V. Adaptions to anoxia in chronic pulmonary emphysema. *Arch. Intern. Med.*, **88**, 581–90.

176. Stradling, J.R. and Lane, D.J. (1981) Development of secondary polycythaemia in chronic airways obstruction. *Thorax*, **36**, 321–5.

177. Harrison, B.D.W., Davis, J., Madgwick, R.G. and Evans, M. (1973) The effects of a therapeutic decrease in packed cell volume on the response to exercise of patients with polycythaemia secondary to lung disease. *Clin. Sci. Mol. Med.*, **45**, 833–47.

178. Chetty, K.G., Brown, S.E. and Light, R.W. (1983) Improved exercise tolerance of the polycythemic lung patient following phlebotomy. *Am. J. Med.*, **74**, 415–20.

179. Wedzicha, J.A., Cotter, F.E., Rudd, R.M. *et al* (1984) Erythropheresis compared with placebo apheresis in patients with polycythaemia secondary to hypoxic lung disease. *Eur. J. Respir. Dis.*, **65**, 579–85.

180. Burrows, B., Bloom, J.W., Traver, G.A. and Cline, M.G. (1987) The cause and prognosis of different forms of chronic airways obstruction in a sample from the general population. *N. Engl. J. Med.*, **317**, 1309–14.

181. Steele, P., Ellis, J.H., Neily, H.S. and Genton, E. (1977) Platelet survival time in patients with hypoxemia and pulmonary hypertension. *Circulation*, **55**, 660–2.

182. Cordova, C., Musca, A., Violi, F. *et al.* (1985) Platelet hyperfunction in patients with chronic airways obstruction. *Eur. J. Respir. Dis.*, **66**, 9–12.

183. Fisher, J., Magid, N., Kallman, C. *et al.* (1983) Respiratory illness and hypophosphatemia. *Chest*, **83**, 504–8.

184. Aubier, M., Murciano, D., Lecocgnic, Y. *et al.* (1985) Effect of hypophosphatemia on diaphragm contractility in patients with acute respiratory failure. *N. Engl. J. Med.*, **313**, 420–4.

185. Calverley, P.M.A., Howaston, R., Flenley, D.S. and Lewis, D. (1992) Clinicopathological correlations in cor pulmonale. *Thorax*, **47**, 494–8.

186. Rhodes, K.M. Evemy, K., Nariman, S. and Gibson, G.J. (1982) Relation between severity of mitral valve disease and routine tests in non-smokers. *Thorax*, **37**, 751–5.

187. Wood, J.E., McLeod, P., Anthonisen, N.R. and Macklem, P.T. (1971) Mechanics of breathing in mitral stenosis. *Am. Rev. Respir. Dis.*, **104**, 52–60.

188. Kitaichi, M., Nishimura, K. and Izumi, T. (1991) Diffuse panbrochiolitis, in *Lung Disease in the Tropics*, (ed. O.P. Sharma), Marcel Dekker, New York, pp. 479–510.

189. Wightman, J.A. (1968) A prospective survey of the incidence of post-operative pulmonary complications. *Br. J. Surg.*, **55**, 85–91.

190. Mittman, C. (1991) Preoperative evaluation and perioperative care, in *Chronic Obstructive Pulmonary Disease*, (ed. N.S. Cherniak), Saunders, Philadelphia, pp. 555–9.

191. Ford, G.T., Whitelaw, W.A., Rosenal, T.W. *et al.* (1983) Diaphragm function after upper abdominal surgery in humans. *Am. Rev. Respir. Dis.*, **127**, 431–5.

192. Samet, J.M., Humble, C.G. and Pathak, D.R. (1986) Personal and family history of respiratory diseases and lung cancer risk. *Am. Rev. Respir. Dis.*, **105**, 503–7.

193. Tisi, G.M. (1987) Preoperative identification and evaluation of the patient with lung disease. *Med. Clin. North Am.*, **71**, 399–412.

194. Zibrak, J.D. and O'Donnell, C.R. (1993) Indications for pre-operative pulmonary function testing. *Clinics Chest Med.*, **14**, 227–36.

195. Boushy, S.F., Billig, D.M., North, L.B. and Helgason, A.H. (1971) Clinical course related to preoperative and postoperative pulmonary

function in patients with bronchogenic carcinoma. *Chest*, **59**, 383–91.

196. Van Nostrand, D., Kjelsberg, H.O. and Humphrey, E.N. (1968) Preresectional evaluation of risk from pneumonectomy. *Surg. Gynecol. Obstet.*, **127**, 306–11.

197. Olsen, G.N. (1989) The evolving role of exercise testing prior to lung resection. *Chest*, **95**, 218–25.

198. Ellis, D.A., Hawkins, T., Gibson, G.J. and Nariman, S. (1988) The place of lung scanning in carcinoma of the bronchus. *Thorax*, **38**, 261–6.

199. Secker Walker, R.H., Alderson, P.O., Wilhelm, J. *et al.* (1974) Ventilation–perfusion scanning in carcinoma of the bronchus. *Chest*, **65**, 660–3.

IMAGING

14

A.G. Wilson

In chronic obstructive pulmonary disease (COPD) imaging techniques have made an important contribution both to the understanding of its pathophysiology and to its clinical management. Much of the information provided by imaging has been static and structural and this aspect has been emphasized with the advent of computed tomography (CT) and high resolution computed tomography (HRCT) which currently provide the most sensitive and specific means of diagnosing generalized emphysema *in vivo*. In addition a variety of dynamic imaging techniques give pathophysiologic information.

In the following section these two important aspects of imaging will be considered following a loose anatomic framework that begins with the trachea and moves peripherally to the alveoli.

14.1 TRACHEA

A well recognized but unusual association of COPD is coronal narrowing of the trachea ('saber-sheath' trachea) [1]. Its pathogenesis is unclear but may be related to abnormal intrathoracic pressure gradients generated in COPD. Coronal tracheal narrowing is essentially confined to male smokers over 50 years of age and is thought to be a feature of patients at the 'chronic bronchitis' end of the COPD spectrum. As a sign of chronic bron-

chitis it has high specificity but low sensitivity. It can be detected by chest radiography or CT (Fig. 14.1).

On the frontal chest radiograph the tracheal air column is evenly narrowed from the thoracic inlet to the main carina [1] and by definition the coronal diameter is two-thirds or less of the sagittal diameter. Compared with controls the mean coronal diameter in 60 cases was reduced to 61% and the sagittal increased to 115% giving an overall reduction in tracheal luminal area of 75% [2]. Cartilage rings are commonly calcified or ossified both pathologically and radiologically. There are limited and conflicting data on tracheal compliance [1,3]. Nevertheless it seems unlikely that saber-sheath trachea contributes significantly to airflow obstruction.

14.2 CENTRAL AIRWAYS

Airways with cartilage in their walls show a number of pathologic changes in COPD – mucus gland enlargement, smooth muscle hyperplasia, cartilage atrophy (equivocal) and inflammation [4]. Although these changes thicken the bronchial wall the overall increase is mild [4] and it is not surprising that radiologic detection of bronchial wall thickening has not proved to be a very useful sign of COPD. Apart from one or two end-on segmental bronchi close to the hilum, airways of normal subjects are invisible on a chest

Chronic Obstructive Pulmonary Disease. Edited by Dr P. Calverley and Professor N. Pride. Published in 1995 by Chapman & Hall, London. ISBN 0 412 46450 0

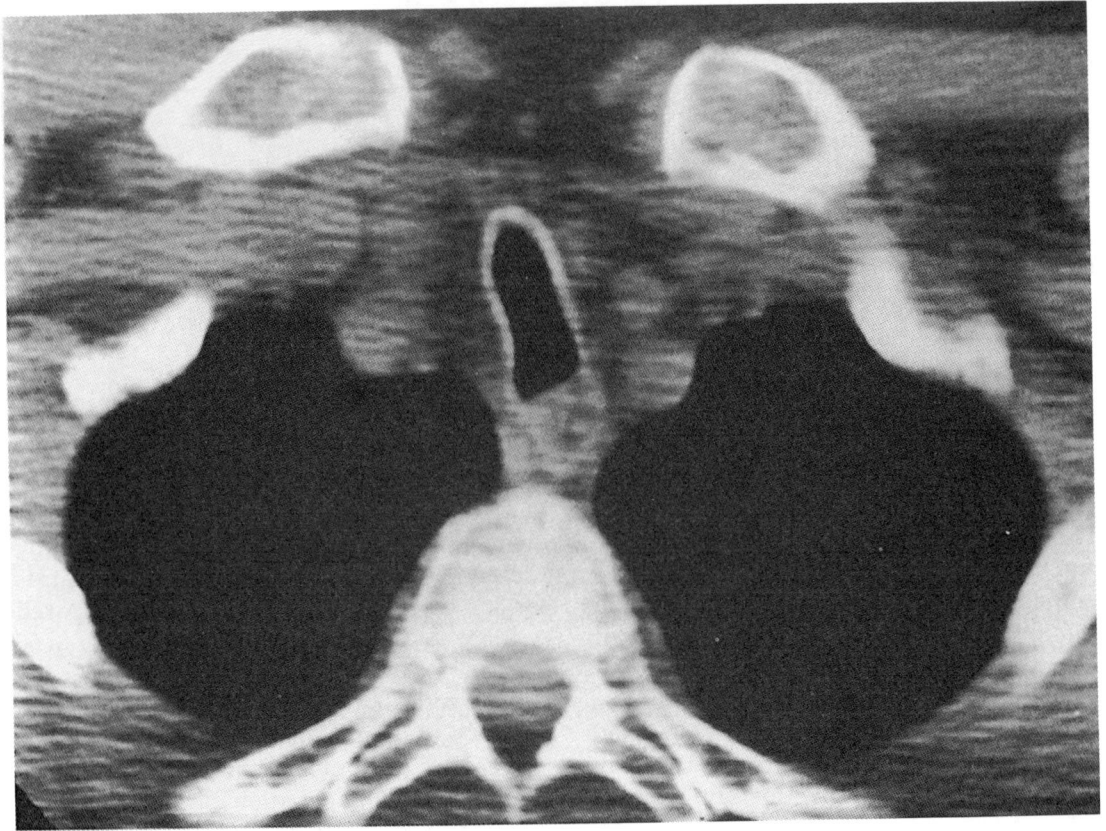

Fig. 14.1   Coronal narrowing of the trachea ('saber sheath' trachea). Sagittal and coronal diameters of the trachea are usually approximately equal. In this patient CT of the thoracic trachea shows diameters of 9 mm (coronal) and 27 mm (sagittal).

radiograph as they have walls that are too thin to resolve. In one of the three clinico-radiologic series describing chronic bronchitis [5], the authors recorded line and parallel line opacities considered to represent bronchial wall thickening in 42% of patients. This sign was not described in the other two series [6,7]. In another study, end-on airways lateral to the hilum, which are a normal finding, were studied. These were seen with similar frequency in controls and subjects with chronic bronchitis but in the latter group bronchial walls assessed subjectively appeared thicker [8]. However, a large inter-observer variation makes this a sign of dubious value. Bronchial walls assessed sub-

jectively on HRCT in 124 smokers and ex-smokers, many of whom had clinical chronic bronchitis also demonstrated mild proximal and peripheral bronchial wall thickening [9].

In normal subjects there is mild dynamic narrowing of lobar airways during a forced expiratory maneuver which is accentuated in patients with COPD. This was demonstrated by Fraser using cinebronchograms imaged during cough. He found a disproportionately large collapse of major proximal airways (diameter reduction of 49% in normals, 67% in COPD patients), particularly marked in lower lobar airways [10]. This corresponds to the level at which marked pressure drops, detected manometrically, occur in COPD during forced expiration [11]. It seems likely that such collapse is due to large transmural pressures rather than a significant increase in bronchial wall compliance. Dynamic airway collapse might have a significant effect on the efficiency of the cough mechanism.

14.3 SMALL AIRWAY DISEASE

Small airway abnormalities are an important aspect of the pathologic findings in COPD [4]. Changes consist of bronchiolar inflammation and scarring; muscle hypertrophy; goblet cell metaplasia; mucous plugging; and loss of radial attachments, all contributing in varying degrees to bronchiolar tortuosity, narrowing and obliteration.

For the purposes of this discussion the term 'small airway' covers non-cartilaginous airways, and terminal and respiratory bronchioles. Disorders may affect small airways exclusively (e.g. bronchiolitis obliterans) or as part of a more widespread process affecting the tracheobronchial tree and lung parenchyma (e.g. COPD, mineral dust exposure).

14.3.1 BRONCHIOLITIS OBLITERANS (OBLITERATIVE BRONCHIOLITIS)

Bronchiolitis obliterans is a non-specific pathologic finding that may be primary or secondary to a number of disorders or to exposure to toxic agents [12]. Two subvarieties are recognized:

(a) Bronchiolitis obliterans with organizing pneumonia (BOOP) [13]

This condition which is also called cryptogenic organizing pneumonia (COP) has a distinctive pathology that includes intraluminal inflammatory polyps in small airways and alveolar ducts and an organizing pneumonia. It is associated with a restrictive rather than an obstructive defect and will not be considered further.

(b) Bronchiolitis obliterans (*per se*)

In this condition the main histologic changes are of chronic bronchiolar inflammation and scarring (submucosal, adventitial) leading to partial or complete obliteration of small airways. This causes progressive and often disabling airflow obstruction. To avoid confusion with BOOP it has been suggested that this entity be called constrictive bronchiolitis [12] but in this discussion the established term, bronchiolitis obliterans (BO) will be used.

BO has a number of recognized precipitating factors and associations which include inhalation of toxic gases and fumes, infections (particularly viral and mycoplasmal), connective tissue disorders, graft-versus-host disease (marrow, lung and heart-lung transplants) [14,15], drugs (e.g. penicillamine), and healed diffuse alveolar damage [12]. There is also a cryptogenic variety.

In BO there is a great variety of radiologic appearances in part reflecting differing etiologies and in part disparate changes in respiratory units distal to the obstructed airways [16,17]. Both, from a clinical and radiologic viewpoint it is useful to distinguish between primary and secondary forms.

(i) Cryptogenic bronchiolitis obliterans

Patients with cryptogenic BO manifest progressive dyspnea often with a dry cough but without systemic features. Lung function tests show an obstructive defect with evidence of gas trapping and the chest radiograph is either normal or shows hyperinflation with hypovascularity, particularly peripherally in the mid-lower zones [18,19,20]. In the past bronchograms have been performed in a limited number of patients with cryptogenic disease showing obstruction to peripheral airways, lack of sidebranch filling (particularly fifth and sixth generation branches), lack of airway tapering and lack of alveolar filling [18,19]. CT shows widespread patchy areas of slightly increased and slightly

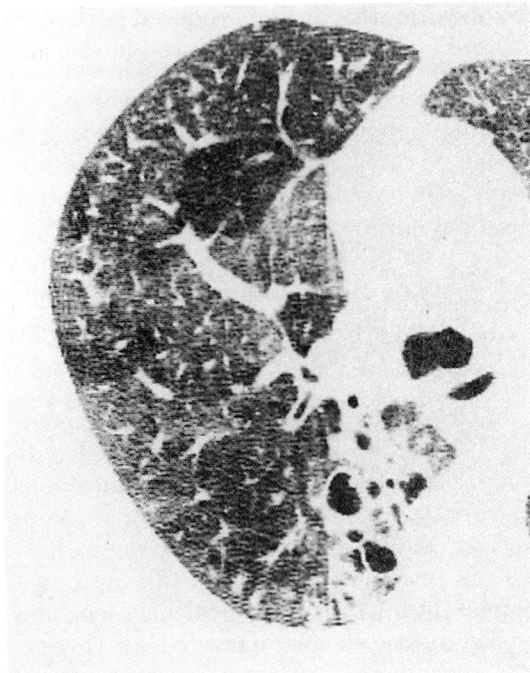

Fig. 14.2 Bronchiolitis obliterans. A high resolution CT scan shows areas of low density interspersed with areas of normal lung density. On expiration low density areas showed evidence of air trapping. Ring opacities inferomedially are due to bronchiectasis.

decreased attenuation (Fig. 14.2) accentuated by expiration [20]. Decreased attenuation is ascribed to air-trapping and reduced vascularity and increased attenuation to failure of normal alveolar expansion secondary to airway obstruction. $\dot{V}_A/\dot{Q}$ scintiscans predictably show matched defects [19].

(ii) Secondary bronchiolitis obliterans

The chest radiographic pattern in secondary BO is very variable. Thus with rheumatoid arthritis with/without penicillamine therapy the radiograph is commonly normal [19] or shows hyperinflation [21]. With inhalation of toxic fumes or gases as in silo-filler's disease the clinical and radiographic findings of BO are typically delayed by 2–5 weeks when

they manifest themselves as diffuse 1–5 mm nodulations which may in part become confluent [22,23]. In other reports of inhalation (sulfur dioxide, nitrogen dioxide) BO has been manifest by hyperinflation and a clear chest radiograph [24]. Radiographic changes in graft-versus-host disease following marrow transplantation are either absent or are those of hyperinflation [25,26]. BO due to graft-versus-host disease in heart-lung and, less commonly, lung transplants is accompanied by a range of radiographic abnormalities not all of which are necessarily related to BO itself. The most notable finding is of bronchial wall thickening and bronchiectasis sometimes accompanied by multiple small to medium-sized nodules, thin linear opacities and basal airspace shadows [27,28]. Finally, following infections the chest radiograph is either normal or shows a diffuse nodular/recticulonodular pattern, occasionally with airspace opacity due to a concomitant organizing pneumonia [17].

There are a limited number of CT studies in secondary BO. The commonest findings are of areas of reduced attenuation (Fig. 14.2) accompanied by decreased vascularity due to reduced perfusion consequent upon locally impaired ventilation [28,29]. The other striking findings in these high resolution CT studies have been bronchial dilatation particularly at segmental and subsegmental level [28,29] and the presence of branching structures in the centre of lobules representing terminal airway plugging [29].

(c) Swyer–James (MacLeod's) syndrome

The Swyer–James [30] or MacLeod's [31] syndrome is a form of BO that has special features: (i) it occurs following an insult to the developing lung – before the age of 8 years; (ii) it affects smaller bronchi as well as bronchioles; (iii) the lung supplied by abnormal airways remains inflated (by collateral air drift) and may show emphysematous changes [4]; and (iv) most importantly, it is predominantly unilateral causing a unilateral transradiancy on the chest radiograph. Patients with pathologic involvement that is patchy or bilateral are described [32] but they lack the defining radiographic sign of unilateral transradiancy. Synonyms for the syndrome include unilateral transradiancy and unilateral or lobar emphysema. The commonest antecedent event is a childhood lung infection, particularly viral (adenovirus, measles) but non-viral infections and non-infectious causes are also described. Airways from fourth generation bronchi to terminal bronchioles are scarred and have irregular or occluded lumens. The lung parenchyma is hypoplastic with reduced vascularity and sometimes panacinar emphysematous change.

The plain radiographic findings (Fig. 14.3(a)) closely mirror the pathology. The affected lung is transradiant (darker than its fellow) due principally to reduced perfusion. All ipsilateral vessels are reduced in size and number, and the hilum is small. Lung volume, reflecting a mixture of hypoplasia and emphysema is usually normal or slightly decreased. An essential feature of the Swyer–James syndrome is air trapping which is best demonstrated by a chest radiograph exposed during rapid expiration (taken 1 or 2 seconds after the start of a forced expiration maneuver). This will show mediastinal shift to the contralateral side and reduced upward movement of the ipsilateral diaphragm (Fig. 14.3(b)) In the past both pulmonary angiography and bronchography have been performed disclosing small vessels and mildly dilated, irregular airways that end at about the 6th generation with absent filling of side branches. These investigations are no longer warranted. $\dot{V}A/\dot{Q}$ scintiscans show reduced perfusion and ventilation and using xenon-133 a delayed washout from the affected lung can be demonstrated [33]. Some authors have

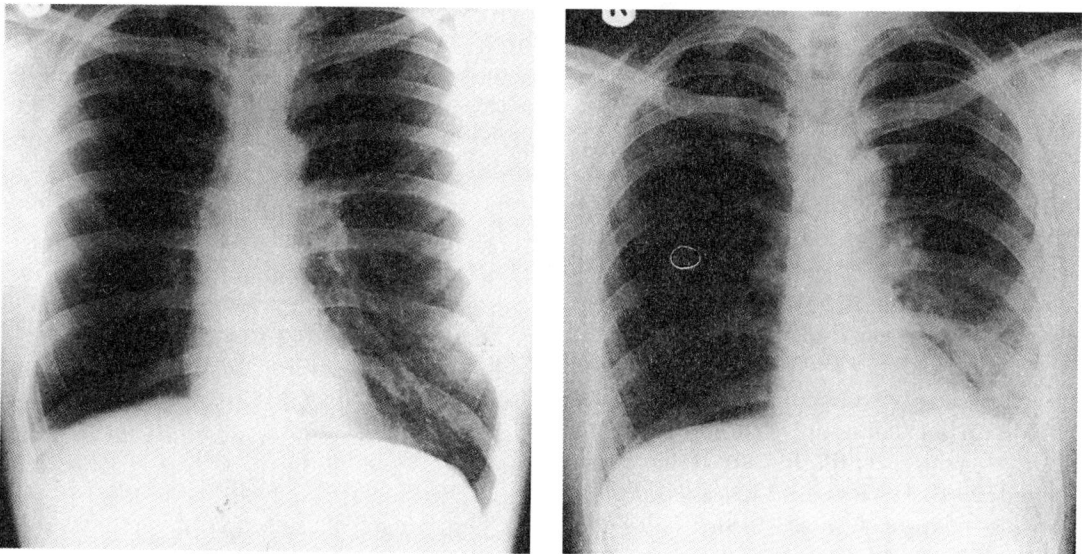

Fig. 14.3 Swyer-James syndrome (MacLeod's syndrome). A chest radiograph (a) on full inspiration shows a hypertransradiant right lung of normal volume with attenuated lung vessels and a small hilum. On expiration (b) there is evidence of air trapping on the right with modest shift of the mediastinum to the left and a left hemidiaphragm that is now higher than the right.

found $\dot{V}_A/\dot{Q}$ scintiscans useful particularly in children, allowing exclusion of primary perfusion abnormalities and compensatory emphysema [34]. Scintiscans may show similar but less extensive abnormalities on the contralateral side [34].

CT studies confirm unilateral transradiancy in some patients but in others show changes that are in fact bilateral. Hypertransradiancy is often patchy with areas of reduced CT density, both sharply and poorly marginated, interspersed with areas of normal lung [35]. Some areas of reduced density probably represent emphysema whereas others are due to small airway obstruction and air trapping, demonstrable on expiratory scans. Brochiectasis may or may not be present [35] together with post inflammatory scarring [36]. CT allows exclusion of unilateral bullous disease.

All the plain radiographic signs of the Swyer–James syndrome including air trapping can be seen with partial obstruction of a large central airway that causes hypoventilation and secondary hypoxic vasoconstriction. This possibility can be excluded by bronchoscopy or CT using 5 mm continuous sections for the central airways.

14.4 LUNG SCINTIGRAPHY IN COPD

Scintigraphic studies of lung perfusion ($\dot{Q}$) and ventilation ($\dot{V}$) are usually abnormal in COPD. The pathogenesis of these abnormalities is complex being in part related to small airway disease and in part to areas of alveolar and vascular destruction.

In clinical practice the perfusion agent employed is usually technetium 99m with a particulate carrier (commonly macro-aggregated albumin) while ventilation studies are performed with gases or, less commonly, aerosols. In the UK most studies have used krypton 81m (^{81m}Kr) whereas in the USA the favoured agent has been xenon 133 (^{133}Xe). The advantages and disadvantages of these gases has been reviewed [37]. An important difference between these two agents is in

their half-lives – 5.2 days for ^{133}Xe and 13 seconds for ^{81m}Kr. This allows ^{133}Xe to be used for tests of breath wash in, equilibrium and wash out, allowing ventilation per unit lung volume to be calculated accurately. In Great Britain ^{81m}Kr is usually used for assessing regional ventilation, counts being collected for about 90 seconds. The final image is the summation of the regional distribution of 10–20 tidal inspirations; this technique does not 'correct' for differences in lung volume in different regions.

In COPD both perfusion and ventilation scans show multiple patchy areas of absent or reduced activity (Fig. 14.4) [38]. These defects tend to be matched and are distributed fairly evenly throughout the lungs [39] except in α_1-antitrypsin deficiency where they are basally predominant [40]. In emphysema defects are non-segmental and are due to parenchymal destruction [38] and because of this they are fixed and unaffected by therapy including bronchodilators [41]. When emphysema has a predominantly central distribution scintiscans may show a characteristic area of low central activity with a preserved peripheral band of high activity – 'stripe sign' [42]. Defects on scintiscans in emphysema may correspond to areas of oligemia or bulla formation on the chest radiograph or to areas that are radiographically normal [43].

In contrast to the defects in emphysema those in type B COPD are sometimes segmental [38]. However, other workers have not confirmed this finding and have been unable to distinguish between type A and B COPD (Chapter 8) on lung scan evidence [39]. Defects in type B COPD are thought to be due to airway narrowing causing distal hypoxia and subsequent hypoxic vasoconstriction and as might be expected with this mechanism, perfusion defects are sometimes smaller than ventilation ones [38]. This thesis is supported by $\dot{V}_A/\dot{Q}$ studies using multiple inert gas-elimination techniques in which areas of low $\dot{V}_A/\dot{Q}$ were common in type B COPD [44]. An extreme example of the situation is where

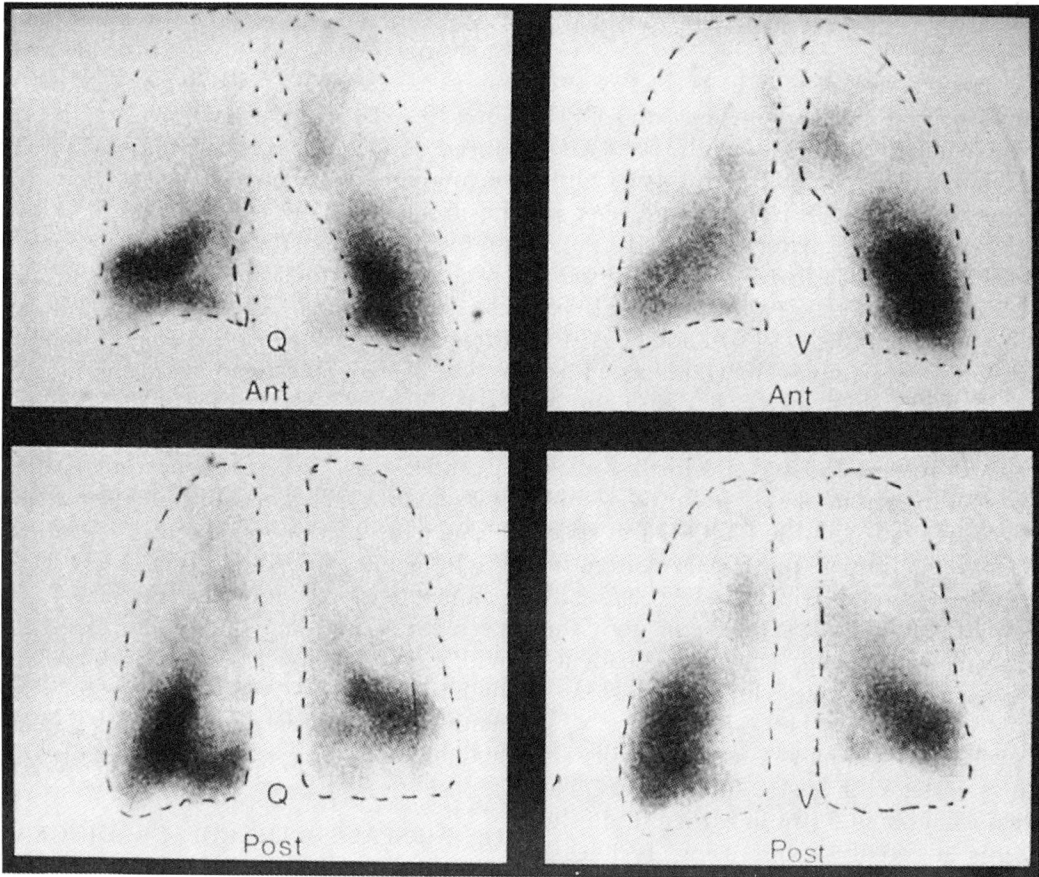

Fig. 14.4 Lung scintiscanning in generalized emphysema, probably centriacinar type. There are large defects of nondescript shape in both perfusion (Q images on left) and ventilation (V images on right) scintiscans. The defects correspond in Q and V images, i.e. they are matched, a characteristic feature of emphysema.

ventilation defects are completely mismatched (no corresponding perfusion defect) and this may sometimes be seen in acute exacerbations of type B COPD [39]. Such mismatched defects are commonly basal and on follow-up scans are seen to resolve suggesting airway narrowing on the basis of edema, inflammation or plugging rather than scarring. Such findings imply lack of hypoxic vasoconstriction. In the same study the authors noted that matched defects with one or two exceptions remained stable on follow-up scans delayed by an average of seven months.

Scintiscans performed using the long half-life agent ^{133}Xe allow an analysis of wash in and wash out characteristics of the lung. In COPD wash in is slower than normal and an equilibrium state may never be achieved [37]. Wash out is also delayed and deviates from the normal monoexponential curve. Clearance is prolonged beyond the usual 3 minutes taken to achieve background counts [45]. Several studies have shown a significant correlation between the FEV and the degree of COPD quantitated by scintiscans [39,46]. The sensitivity of scintiscans and spirometric tests in detecting COPD are generally considered to be similar [37].

Pulmonary embolism (PE) is a cause for clinical deterioration in patients with COPD. PE is commonly diagnosed with the help of $\dot{V}A/\dot{Q}$ scintiscans but their utility in COPD might be expected to be reduced. However, in a report of 83 patients with COPD and a possible PE diagnosis studied by $\dot{V}A/\dot{Q}$ scintiscan and angiography there was a scan sensitivity of 0.83 and a specificity of 0.92 for PE. False negatives were mainly seen in patients with a more than 50% summated scan defect and in those with a less than 50% overall deficit the sensitivity rose to 0.95 and specificity to 0.94 [47]. These are remarkably accurate results when compared with the PIOPED (prospective investigation of pulmonary embolism diagnosis) series in which there was a 82% sensitivity and 52% specificity for high and intermediate probability scans in 755 patients, unselected apart from a clinical suspicion of pulmonary embolism [48].

Labelled aerosols may be used in ventilation studies instead of gases. Particle size has varied from about 3 μm in earlier studies to 0.2 μm in recent studies using Technegas (^{99m}Tc-labelled carbon particles) [49]. In normal individuals gases and aerosols produce similar images [50] but in patients with COPD they produce strikingly different appearances. The pattern in COPD is markedly inhomogeneous with focal spots of high and low activity [51,52]. Focal deposition may be peripheral or central with the former tending to occur in type B COPD and the latter with dominant emphysema [51,52,53]. Reasons for the accumulation of aerosols are poorly understood though it is usually attributed to areas of narrowing with resultant flow distortion, turbulence, and inertial impaction [54]. Other authors have suggested that peripheral 'hot spots' are due to high convective flow which magnifies the maldistribution seen with inhaled gas such as ^{81m}Kr [55]. It has also been suggested that central deposition may occur at the site of dynamic expiratory narrowing [53].

With the advent of positron emission tomography (PET) a highly sophisticated technique has become available for studying the lung. Results of investigations may be produced as images or as qualitative data. The technique uses substances labelled with positron emitting isotopes (e.g. ^{11}C, ^{13}N, ^{19}Ne) and after administration by inhalation and intravenously their activity concentrations can be measured producing multiple two-dimensional images of the lung. The application of PET investigations to the lung has recently been reviewed [56]. An example of the type of information provided by PET is given by a recent report concerning patients with COPD [57]. This study looked at local tissue density, ventilation and $\dot{V}A/\dot{Q}$ ratios in the lung and showed that type A COPD was characterized by low tissue density, low peripheral vascular volume and blood flow with a high $\dot{V}A/\dot{Q}$ whereas type B COPD had high tissue density possibly related to inflammation and edema, a low ventilation and high blood flow.

14.5 AIRSPACES – THE CHEST RADIOGRAPH

Chest radiographic findings in emphysema are conventionally divided into three: hyperinflation, vascular change and bullae. There is good evidence that 'increased markings' should make a fourth [58].

Hyperinflation is indicated by a number of signs: (i) A low, flat hemidiaphragm (Fig. 14.5). Diaphragms are abnormally *low* when their border, in the midclavicular line, is at or below the anterior end of the seventh rib [59]; some authors take the sixth rib in pyknic patients [60]. Pathologic *flattening* may be assessed subjectively or, objectively, by drawing a line between the costal and cardiophrenic angles and measuring the maximum perpendicular height from this line to the border of the diaphragm (less than 1.5 cm is taken as flattened). The combination of depression and flattening is specific for emphysema whereas depression on its own

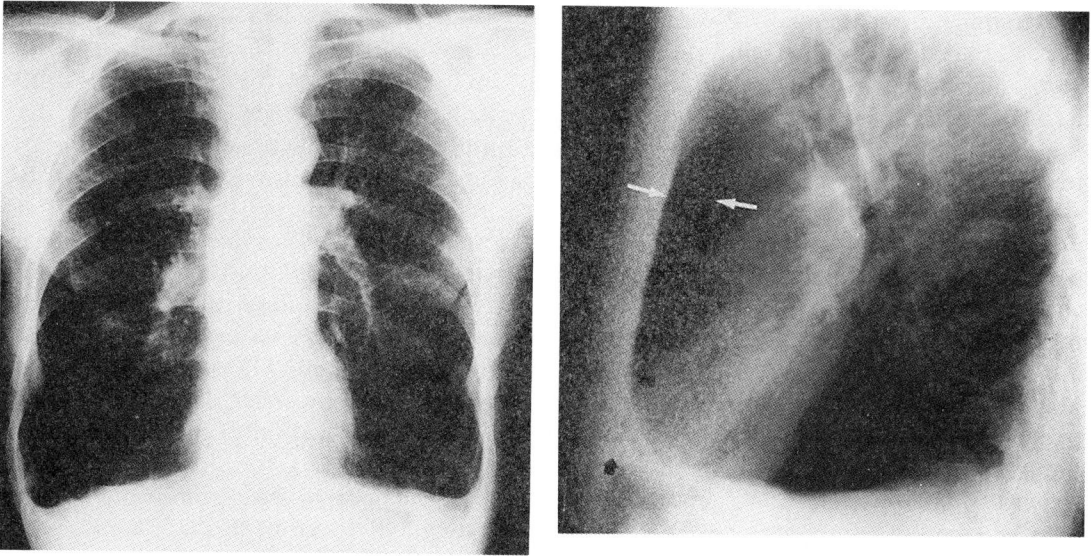

Fig. 14.5 Generalized emphysema (panacinar). (a) PA radiograph. The most important feature is that the diaphragms are low (below anterior ends of seventh ribs) and flat. Vessels are reduced in the lower zones which are transradiant because of oligemia. Obtuse costophrenic angles. (b) lateral radiograph. Again the diaphragm is low and flat (in fact mildly inverted). The retrosternal transradiancy is wide (white arrows) and inferiorly closely approaches the diaphragm (black arrows).

may be seen with overinflation in non-emphysematous conditions such as acute asthma. In severe hyperinflation, the area of apposition of the diaphragm to the rib cage may be virtually absent at TLC revealing the costal origins of the diaphragm. (ii) Increased retrosternal airspace (Fig. 14.5b), measured from the anterior aortic margin to the posterior aspect of the sternum. Critical values have ranged from 2.5 cm [61] to 4.5 cm [62], with the higher values being more specific. (iii) An obtuse costophrenic angle on the PA or lateral chest radiograph (Fig. 14.5). (iv) A retrosternal airspace with its inferior margin 3.0 cm or less from the anterior aspect of the diaphragm (Fig. 14.5b).

A number of vascular changes are described: (i) Reduction in number and size of pulmonary vessels (Fig. 14.5) and their branches especially in the middle and outer aspects of the lungs ('arterial deficiency'). Such vascular changes can be extensive or patchy. (ii) Distortion of vessels – excessive straightening or bowing, and increased branching angles. (iii) A transradiant region (Fig. 14.5). The opacity of a lung depends on the degree of X-ray beam absorption and normally a reasonable assumption is that about half of the X-ray beam attenuation is by the soft tissues of the chest wall and the rest by the blood in the lungs. With the vascular loss of emphysema the lungs become more transradiant (darker) than usual. This may be a generalized change which makes it difficult to identify with certainty or it may be localized when increased transradiancy can be more reliably identified by comparison with normal areas.

A focal transradiancy that is approximately rounded and surrounded at least in part by a hairline wall is called a bulla [63]. Bullae may be seen as part of generalized emphysema or may be an isolated finding (Chapter 22).

A number of patients with emphysema demonstrate 'increased markings' rather than arterial deficiency and it has been shown that if this sign is disregarded on chest radiographs then cases of emphysema will be missed [64]. In one series of 73 patients with chronic airflow obstruction, a surprising number (63%) of those with severe emphysema assessed by macroscopic pathologic changes had this pattern [65]. 'Increased markings' is characterized by small peripheral vessels becoming more prominent, irregular and indistinct. Non-vascular linear opacities possibly due to scarring may also play a part. With this pattern of disease hyperinflation is absent or mild and there are usually signs of pulmonary arterial hypertension [64]. It is much more commonly seen with centriacinar than with panacinar emphysema [64]. The underlying functional or pathologic process is unclear. High resolution CT should go a long way to explaining these appearances but so far this study has not been performed.

The use of the above signs in diagnosing emphysema is based on a number of papers that appeared between 1962 and 1978 that correlated radiologic and pathologic findings in about 560 patients [60,61,64,66–69]. It is not easy to draw common conclusions from these papers as there is a great variation in the severity of disease, methods of pathologic assessment and the radiologic signs used. Some of the problems with these studies have been reviewed [70]. Nevertheless it is possible to draw the following conclusions:

1. The chest radiograph reliably detects severe generalized emphysema and can be used to exclude severe disease. It will also detect severe local disease.
2. The chest radiograph diagnoses about 50% of subjects with moderate disease but very few with mild disease.
3. In the various studies the accuracy of the chest radiograph has ranged between about 65 and 80% [71] with values for

sensitivities that are about the same except for a figure of 24% in one study [69]. This exceptionally low figure was due to the fact that most subjects only had mild/mild–moderate disease.
4. Specificity is good with low false positive rates in the order of 0–5% [70,71].
5. Some of the studies have recorded a sizeable inter- and intra-observer variation in relation to radiologic signs – 25% inter-observer and 12% intra-observer variation in one series [61]. Vascular signs were subject to more variation than those of hyperinflation, diminishing their usefulness [71].
6. The majority of studies indicate that the best predictor of generalized emphysema is overinflation as judged by the position of the diaphragm (in relation to anterior ribs) combined with flattening of the diaphragm [60,61,64,67,68]. Vascular criteria were in general less reliable apart from two studies [66,69].
7. A low, flat diaphragm as assessed by lung height and diaphragmatic angle has been shown to correlate strongly with static lung volumes in patients with clinical COPD [72]. More sophisticated studies have found a close correlation between measurements taken from the chest radiograph and total lung capacity in COPD [73]. With digitized chest radiography, measurements of radiologic TLC should become more widely available, at least for research studies.

14.6 AIRSPACES – COMPUTED TOMOGRAPHY

Computed tomography (CT) has high contrast resolution and being a tomographic technique, it allows direct visualization of emphysematous areas unobstructed by overlapping structures [74]. The first CT description of emphysema was as recent as 1982 [75] and since this time CT has been used to detect, grade as regards severity, and characterize emphysema. CT can detect all types of emphysema and is far better at identifying mild and moderate degrees of disease than the chest radiograph [74–78]. All modern scanners are capable of imaging emphysema and with exposure times of 2–3 seconds, breath-holding even in dyspneic patients is usually not a problem. CT studies are usually performed at TLC even though contrasts between normal and emphysematous lung may be greater at smaller lung volumes.

The signs of emphysema on CT are: (i) non-marginated, low attenuation areas (Fig. 14.6); (ii) vascular tree simplification due to pruning (Fig. 14.6); (iii) abnormal vascular con-

figurations (swept vessels, wide branching angles); and (iv) vascular attenuation [74,75,77,79]. In a study comparing various signs, non-peripheral, low attenuation areas on *in vivo* CT correlated best with emphysema assessed post-mortem [77]. It is sometimes possible to distinguish the various types of emphysema especially when changes are not severe [74,80]. Such distinctions involve assessing the distribution of lesions and their fine features, often best demonstrated with high resolution computed tomography (HRCT) [74,81–83]. Thus centriacinar emphysema (CAE) is characterized by a patchy, predominantly upper zone

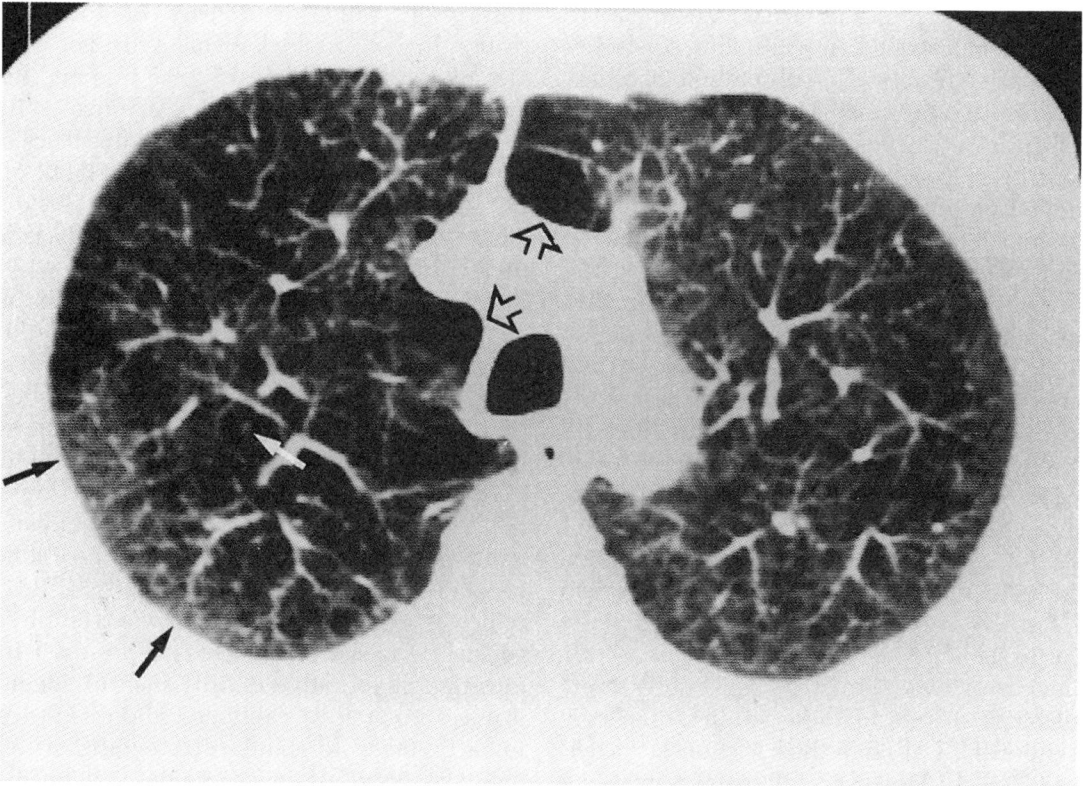

Fig. 14.6 CT taken just above carina in patient with generalized emphysema (centriacinar). On the right side there is a rim of lung with normal structure and density (black arrows). Deep to this zone there are numerous low density areas, some rounded and others with complex shapes. Some are poorly marginated, but others are in part well marginated by vessels or septa. In some areas preserved centrilobular arteries (white arrow) can be identified surrounded by low density, a typical appearance in centriacinar emphysema. Bullae are seen in one of their characteristic locations, against the mediastinum (open arrows).

distribution of centriacinar lucencies related to centrilobular arteries while in panacinar emphysema (PAE) there is uniform and often extensive lobular destruction with a lower zone predominance. Mild and sometimes even moderate PAE may be very difficult to detect because of its subtle widespread and even nature [84]. Paraseptal emphysema (PSE) is characterized by multiple, thin-walled air cysts that are often well marginated and which occur commonly along vessels and airways, lobular septa, or pleural surfaces (azygoesophageal recess, adjacent to the left ventricle, and anterior junctional region) [79].

CT can be used to quantify emphysema using visual assessment or density measurements. The accuracy of visual assessment has been demonstrated in a number of studies comparing *in vivo* CT with pathologic quantitation of emphysema post-mortem or on surgical specimens. In most studies only macroscopic emphysema has been quantitated pathologically using lesion counting (point counts or grids) or panel matching and similar techniques have been used to assess the CT scans. Recently a few studies have measured microscopic emphysema in pathologic specimens using airspace wall surface area per unit volume [85]. The earliest study of 25 post-mortem lungs and 10 mm thick CT sections in patients with CAE showed CT to be 87% sensitive and 80% accurate [77]. Other more recent studies using a variety of CT section thickness (1–10 mm) showed good correlations between pathology scores and CT scores with r values ranging from about 0.6 to 0.8 [79,83,84]. HRCT (1.5 mm section thickness) was shown to be slightly more sensitive in one of these studies than conventional CT (10 mm thick sections); $r = 0.85$ vs 0.81 [84]. However, CT usually missed a number of cases with mild disease in these studies, e.g. 6/33 [84], 2/6 [77] because CT and even HRCT could not reliably identify parenchymal holes smaller than 5 mm diameter. Most cases in the above studies had CAE and there is some evidence that the sensitivity

of CT is less with the more ill-defined and diffuse lesions of PAE – an 18% false negative rate in one study [84]. A low false positive rate of about 2.3% is also described for emphysema in general [70] possibly due to the misinterpretation of focal perivascular low densities produced as movement artefacts particularly near the diaphragm and left heart. The above studies have all been characterized by low inter- and intra-observer variation [79,84,86].

The other method for the quantitative assessment of emphysema depends on measuring CT density. A CT image is made up of a 512×512 matrix of picture-elements (pixels) each representing on a grey scale the X-ray absorption value or density of the corresponding volume-elements (voxels). The face of a voxel is about 0.5×0.5 mm and its depth depends on slice thickness (range 1–10 mm). CT density is expressed on a linear scale of Hounsfield units (water, 0; air, –1000) or rarely as EMI units (water, 0; air, –500). Surprisingly over this range CT density is a direct measure of physical density. CT density is determined by the relative mix of air, blood, interstitial fluid and tissue (walls of vessels, airways and alveoli) in a given voxel. The normal CT density characteristics of lung have been described [75,76,87–90]. In one study mean figures ranged from –770 to –875 (overall mean –817) Hounsfield units [90]. As might be expected there is a gradient from front to back in the supine position, range +20 to +68 Hounsfield units at TLC, which is increased in patients with emphysema [91]. If a CT scanner is to be used to generate quantitative density measurements it must be carefully calibrated and great care must be taken to standardize conditions as many factors affect density values [90]. In emphysema lung density is lower than normal and histograms can be constructed containing values for all the pixels in a CT lung section (Fig. 14.7(a)). Such histograms are skewed with a tail of high densities produced by large vessels and airways. Emphysematous lungs

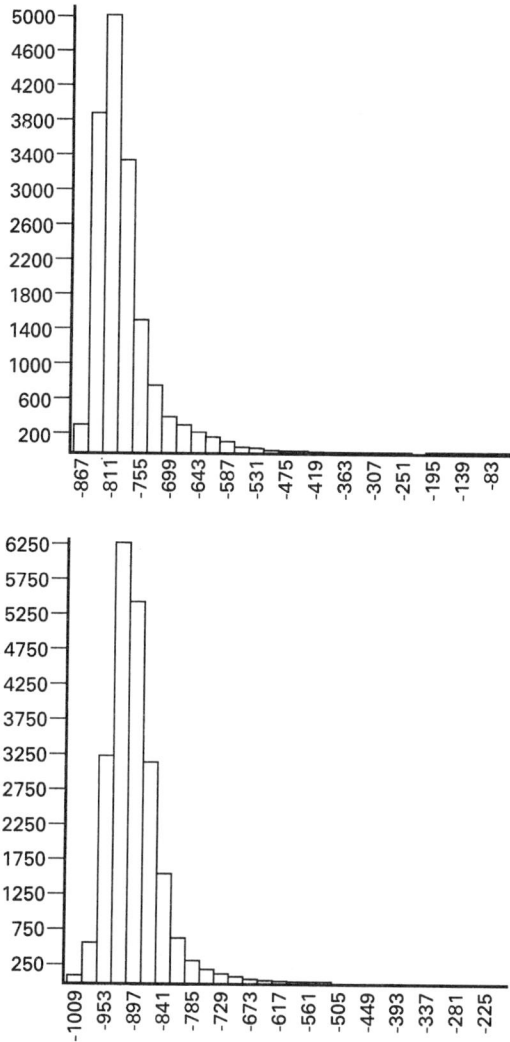

Fig. 14.7 Histogram of lung pixel values taken from a single CT section (X-axis, pixel density values in Hounsfield units; Y-axis, number of pixels). (a) normal lung. The modal value is about −820 Hounsfield units and the curve has a tail to the right mainly because of the higher density of vascular structures. (b) emphysema. The curve is left shifted and the modal value is about −920 Hounsfield units. Note different scales.

have an excess of low density pixels and the whole curve is left shifted (Fig. 14.7(b)) [76]. Pixels below a certain CT number can be

highlighted on the CT image (Fig. 14.8) and expressed as a percentage of total pixels in a given CT section permitting automated data collection. Using this 'density mask' method one group found that a CT density of −910 Hounsfield units gave the best cut-off point in assessing emphysema when compared with picture graded pathology scores at the same level ($r = 0.94$) [86]. In this study correlation was no better with a visual CT scoring system but the density mask was simpler, quicker and more reproducible. The optimum cut-off level must be expected to vary a little from machine to machine and ideally should be established by experiment for any given CT scanner. A study looking at microscopic emphysema assessed as airspace wall surface area per unit volume and comparing with the lowest fifth percentile of lung CT density measurements (this exaggerates density differences between normal and emphysematous lungs) found a correlation of 0.77 [85]. The use of a 'density mask' method and expiratory as well as inspiratory scans has been advocated to distinguish between areas of emphysema and simple hyperinflation without tissue destruction [92]. The degree of emphysema as determined by CT correlates well with carbon monoxide transfer coefficient but less well with airflow obstruction [93]. In other studies HRCT detected emphysema in symptomatic patients with reduced diffusion capacity but no evidence of airflow limitation [94] and in subjects with no defect of diffusion or airflow [95].

CT is currently the most sensitive and specific imaging technique for assessing emphysema *in vivo* with an accuracy commensurate with macroscopic visual assessment of excised lung slices.

14.6.1 ALPHA₁-ANTITRYPSIN DEFICIENCY

Emphysema that develops in α_1-antitrypsin deficiency (α_1-ATD) is panacinar with a strong basal predilection. In a study of 165 PiZ homozygous patients all but 2% had

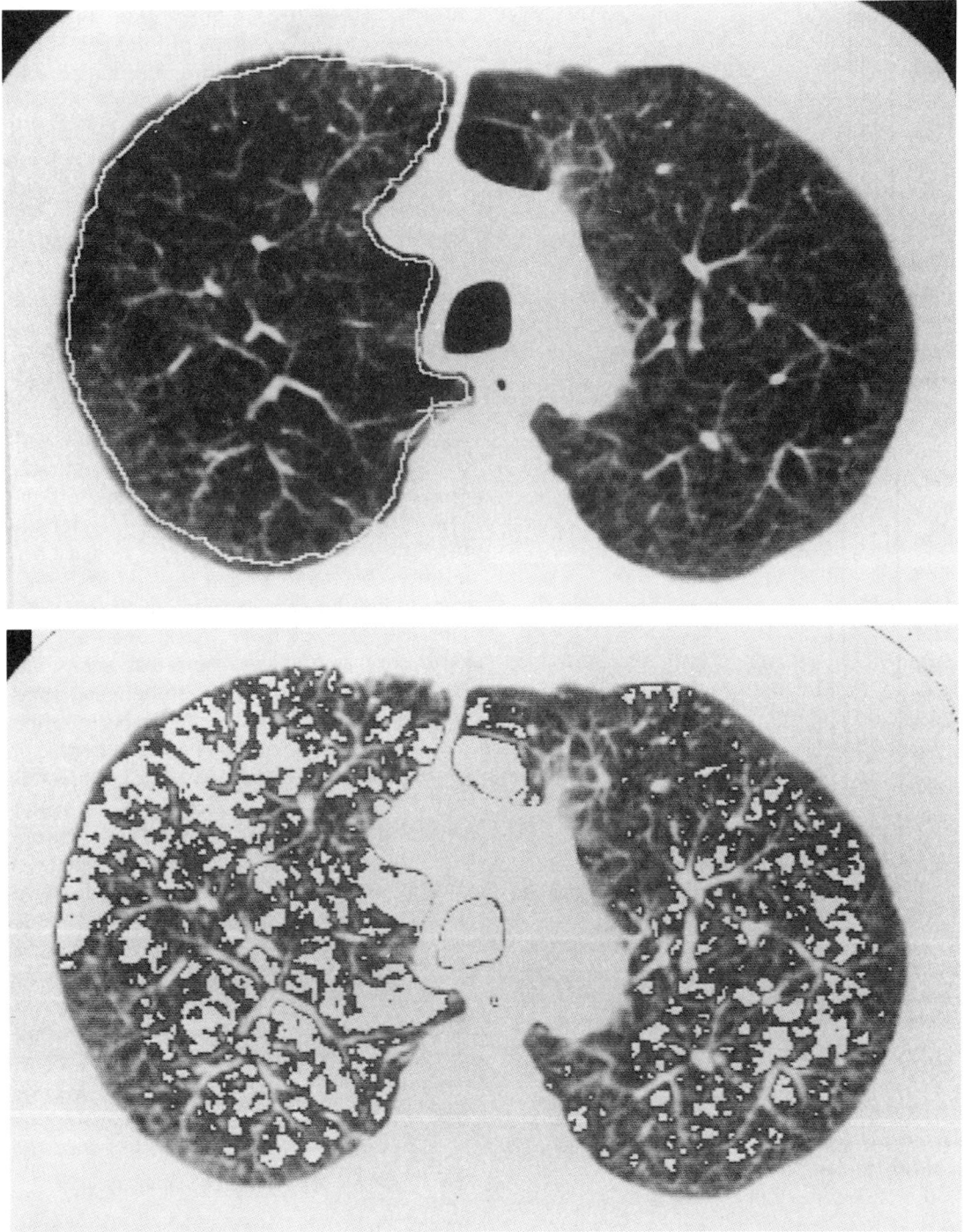

Fig. 14.8 'Density mask' assessment of generalized emphysema. (a) unmodified scan (apart from region of interest envelope). (b) All pixels with a CT number equal to or less than –910 Hounsfield units have been highlighted, indicating emphysematous areas.

radiologic lower zone involvement as judged by vascular changes. In a quarter the lower zone was the only zone affected [96]. This pattern of isolated lower zone change is only seen in about 8% of PiM patients with emphysema [97]. Bullae are not a major feature of α_1-ATD but they do occur [98]. When radiologic changes occur in heterozygotes they are similar. CT findings have recently been described in 17 homozygotes [99]. They confirm that in many patients changes are lower zone predominante but that upper zones are also regularly affected by emphysema; an unexpected finding was a 40% prevalence of bronchial wall thickening and/or dilatation.

14.7 BULLAE AND BULLOUS LUNG DISEASE

Bullae may occur in isolation or may be associated with generalized emphysema constituting one of its classic signs [100]. Pathologically, bullae are sharply demarcated regions of emphysema 1 cm or more in diameter.

On chest radiographs bullae appear as localized, avascular transradiancies usually separated from the rest of the lung at least in part by a curvilinear hairline wall (Fig. 14.9). Sometimes the wall is radiologically absent and in this situation bullae are very difficult to detect and it is well recognized that chest radiographs grossly underestimate the number of bullae [66]. The distinction between a bleb and bulla cannot be made radiographically. Bullae may be single or multiple and range in size from 1 cm to giant ones that occupy a whole hemithorax causing compensatory collapse of the adjacent lung. Isolated bullous disease is usually considered to be due to localized paraseptal emphysema and in this condition bullae show an upper zone predilection [101]. Bullae that are part of generalized emphysema tend to be distributed more evenly throughout the lung [102].

CT is much more sensitive than the chest radiograph in detecting bullae and is now the imaging investigation of choice (Fig. 14.10) when considering bullectomy [63,103–106].

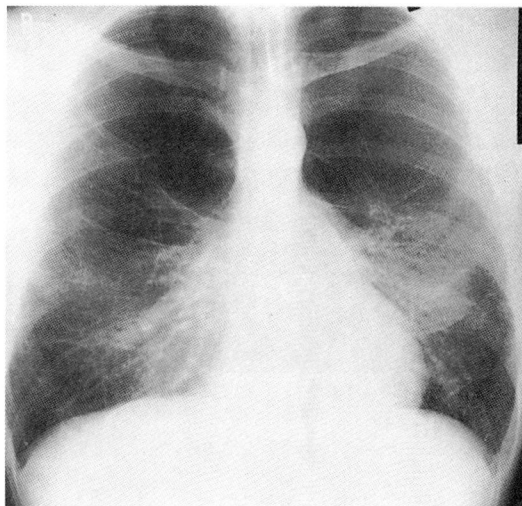

Fig. 14.9 Bullous disease. Gross bilateral mid/upper zone bullous disease. Affected zones are avascular and in part marginated by thin curvilinear structures. Note the preserved curvature of the hemidiaphragms suggesting the absence of generalized emphysema.

CT allows assessment of the number, size and position of bullae, can assess the ventilation of bullae (with inspiratory/expiratory images) and enables the state of the intervening lung to be evaluated (Fig. 14.10). Other techniques used in the past to assess patients before bullectomy such as bronchography and pulmonary angiography have been essentially replaced by CT.

The main complications of bullae are pneumothorax, infection or hemorrhage, all of which are detectable on imaging. With infection the wall of a bulla may thicken and an air–fluid level develops (Fig. 14.10) [107,108]. These changes often take a long time to clear [109] and may be followed by obliteration of the bulla. Hemorrhage is less common but radiologically similar.

14.8 COR PULMONALE

Cor pulmonale is a recognized complication of COPD and is seen almost exclusively with

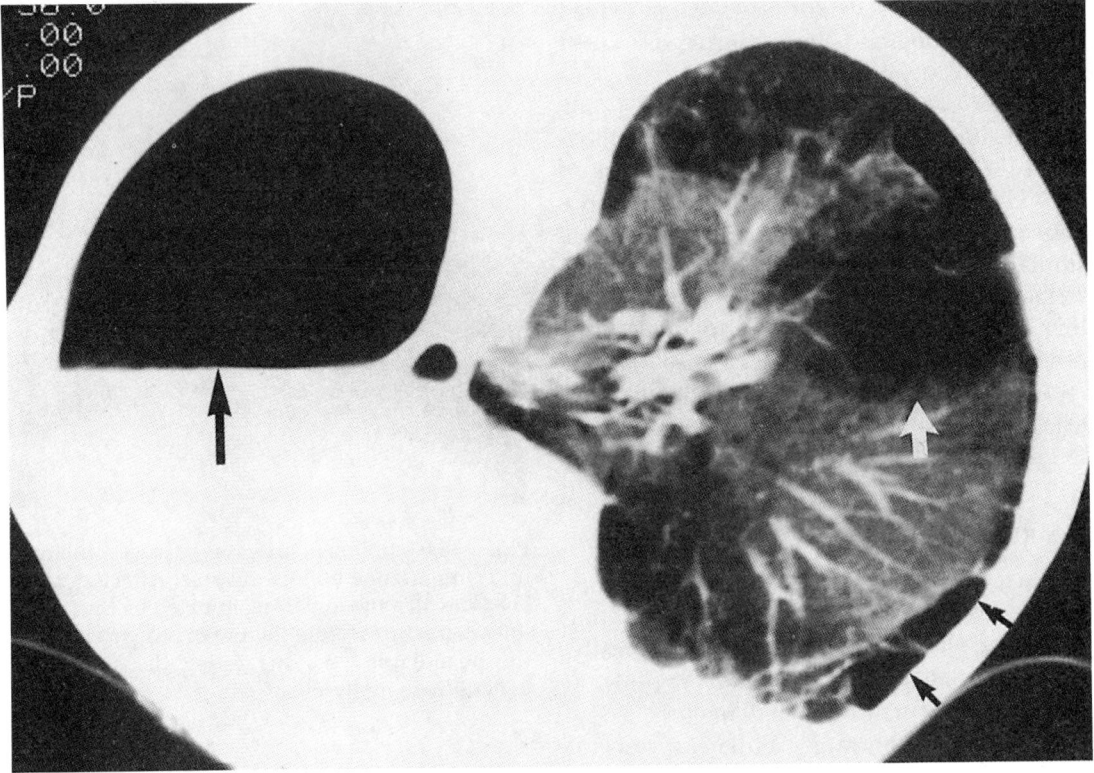

Fig. 14.10 Prone CT in bullous lung disease. There are large avascular areas, some poorly marginated, representing bullae (white arrow). Smaller subpleural bullae (small black arrows) have a configuration typical of paraseptal emphysema. Intervening lung between small black and white arrows looks essentially normal. On the left side an extremely large infected bulla displaces the rest of the lung and contains an air fluid level (large black arrow).

hypoxic patients at the chronic bronchitis end of the spectrum. With the onset of heart failure the heart silhouette increases in size and there is dilatation of proximal and mid-lung vessels. These signs subside after treatment but with repeated episodes radiologic evidence of pulmonary arterial hypertension becomes established. Cardiac enlargement in the acute phase is usually quite non-specific. However, vascular changes are often characteristic and relatively specific. They are like those seen in a left-to-right intracardiac shunt, all vessels between the main pulmonary artery (MPA) and a few divisions beyond the segmental vessels becoming dilated – the appearances of plethora (Fig. 14.11) [110].

The probable explanation of these changes is that hypoxic vasoconstriction occurs in vessels that are beyond the resolution of the chest radiograph and central blood volume is expanded.

There is a large literature correlating pulmonary artery (PA) size and pressure in diverse conditions. However, PA wall compliance varies among these disorders and extrapolations to cor pulmonale from, for instance, mitral value disease is quite likely to be invalid. Central arteries that lend themselves to measurement include the right PA, the left PA in lateral view, and combined measurements notably the transhilar width [111–113]. The most widely used measure-

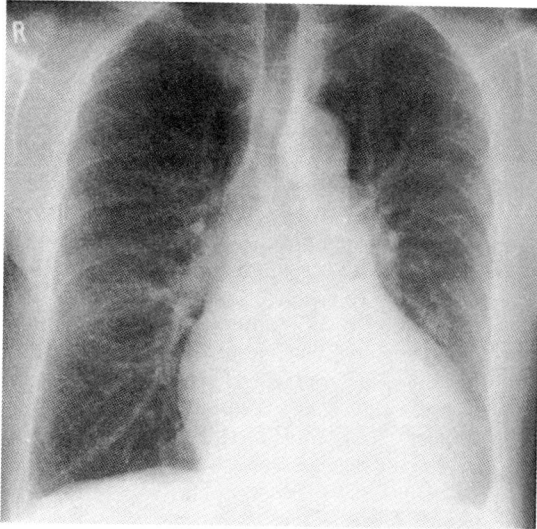

Fig. 14.11 Cor pulmonale. The chest radiographic appearance in an acute exacerbation of cor pulmonale closely resembles that of a left-to-right shunt. The radiograph shows a large heart, a big main pulmonary artery and generalized plethora of lung vessels which are equally big in all zones.

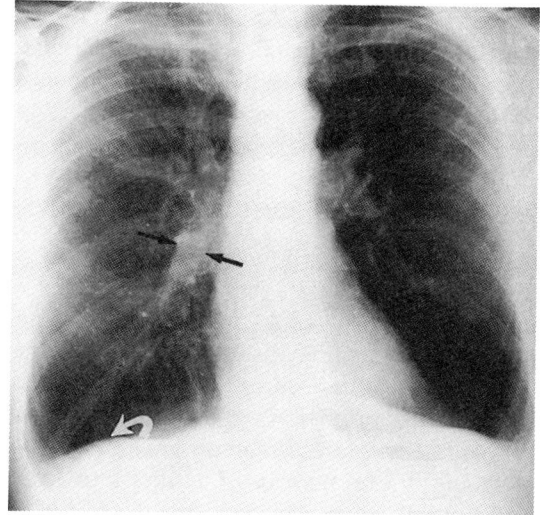

Fig 14.12 Generalized emphysema, pulmonary artery hypertension. The width of the descending right pulmonary artery (black arrows) is 18 mm indicating pulmonary arterial hypertension. The patient has generalized emphysema as indicated by low flat diaphragms (white arrow indicates anterior end of seventh rib).

ment is the width of the descending right pulmonary artery (RPA) taken about 1 cm below the Y point of the right hilum just before the artery gives off middle lobar branches (Fig. 14.12). The borders of the artery are well delineated against air in lung laterally and air in intermediate stem bronchus medially. The upper limit of normal range is taken as 16 mm in males and 15 mm in females based on a series of 1085 normal subjects (40% male, age range 18–72 years) [114]. Smaller series of normal patients give similar data with upper ranges of 17 mm (males) and 15 mm (females) [115] and 17.4 mm (male dominated series) [113]. When 'normal' data have been collected from subjects with chronic bronchitis but PA pressures less than 20 mmHg the upper limits as might be expected have been 1 or 2 mm greater [112,116–118]. For detecting pulmonary artery hypertension various series, using upper limits for the descending right pulmonary artery that range between 16 and 20 mm, have had sensitivities of 68% to 95% and specificities of 65% to 88% [112,115–117]. Reasonable RPA threshold measurements to diagnose pulmonary arterial hypertension, with a low false positive rate, would be diameters of 17 mm or more for females and 18 mm or more for males. Correlation coefficients in the above studies lie generally between 0.4 and 0.6 indicating that only about a third of the variation of PA diameter is due to PA pressure. Thus, while PA diameter can be used to detect the presence or absence of pulmonary artery hypertension it cannot be used to predict the level of PA pressure.

The main pulmonary artery segment, normally flat or slightly convex becomes more prominent and more convex with PA hypertension. The assessment of MPA prominence is usually made subjectively though successful measurements have been devised in patients with mitral valve disease [119]. Prominence of the MPA has not proved a very reliable way of assessing PA hypertension [116] possible because it is sensitive to patient rotation about both X- and Y-axes [116].

14.9 COPD AND OTHER CHEST DISORDERS

When COPD coexists with other pulmonary disorders radiologic signs are sometimes modified. This is well recognized in pneumonia where coexisting CAE commonly produce small (2–5 mm) rounded transradiancies within areas of infective consolidation. These transradiancies are frequently misinterpreted as being due to necrosis. The distribution of pulmonary edema in left heart failure is modified by emphysema, oligemic areas remaining edema free. An extreme example of this is unilateral edema in the Swyer–James syndrome [120]. At the same time left heart failure may modify the signs of emphysema with reduction or loss of the signs of hyperinflation ascribed to the reduced compliance of edematous lungs [100,121].

REFERENCES

1. Greene, R. and Lechner, G.L. (1975) 'Saber sheath' trachea: a clinical and functional study of marked coronal narrowing of the intrathoracic trachea. *Radiology*, **115**, 265–8.
2. Greene, R. (1978) 'Saber sheath' trachea: relation to chronic obstructive pulmonary disease. *Am. J. Roentgenol.*, **130**, 441–5.
3. Gamsu, G. and Webb, W.R. (1982) Computed tomography of the trachea: normal and abnormal. *Am. J. Roentgenol.*, **139**, 321–6.
4. Thurlbeck, W.M. (1990) Pathophysiology of chronic obstructive pulmonary disease. *Clinics Chest Med.*, **11**, 389–403.
5. Bates, D.V., Gordon, C.A., Paul, G.I., *et al.* (1966) Chronic bronchitis: report on the third and fourth stages of the co-ordinated study of chronic bronchitis in the Department of Veterans Affairs, Canada. *Med. Serv. J. Can.*, **22**, 1–59.
6. Simon, G. and Galbraith, H.J.B. (1953) Radiology of chronic bronchitis. *Lancet*, **2**, 850–2.

7. Simon, G. (1959) Chronic bronchitis and emphysema: a symposium: III. Pathological findings and radiological changes in chronic bronchitis and emphysema: B. Radiological changes in chronic bronchitis. *Br. J. Radiol.*, **32**, 292–4.
8. Fraser, R.G., Fraser, R.S., Renner, J.W. *et al.* (1976) The roentgenologic diagnosis of chronic bronchitis: a reassessment with emphasis on parahilar bronchi seen end-on. *Radiology*, **120**, 1–9.
9. Remy-Jardin, M., Remy, J., Gosselin, B. *et al.* (1993) Lung parenchymal changes secondary to cigarette smoking: pathologic–CT correlations. *Radiology*, **186**, 643–51.
10. Fraser, R.G. (1961) Measurements of the calibre of human bronchi in three phases of respiration by cinebronchography. *J. Can. Assoc. Radiol.*, **12**, 102–12.
11. Macklem, P.T. and Wilson, N.J. (1965) Measurement of intrabronchial pressure in man. *J. Appl. Physiol.*, **20**, 653–63.
12. Wright, J.L., Cagle, P., Churg, A. *et al.* (1992) Diseases of the small airways. *Am. Rev. Respir. Dis.*, **146**, 240–62.
13. Epler, G.R. (1992) Bronchiolitis obliterans organizing pneumonia: definition and clinical features: *Chest*, **102**, 2S–6S.
14. Theodore, J., Starnes, V.A. and Lewiston, N.J. (1990) Obliterative bronchiolitis. *Clinics Chest Med.*, **11**, 309–21.
15. Epler, G.R. (1988) Bronchiolitis obliterans and airways obstruction associated with graft-versus-host disease. *Clinics Chest Med.*, **9**, 551–6.
16. Gosink, B.B., Friedman, P.J. and Liebow, A.A. (1973) Bronchiolitis obliterans. Roentgenologic-pathologic correlation. *Am. J. Roentgenol.*, **117**, 816–32.
17. McLoud, T.C., Epler, G.R., Colby, T.V. *et al.* (1986) Bronchiolitis obliterans. *Radiology*, **159**, 1–8.
18. Breatnach, E. and Kerr, I (1982) The radiology of cryptogenic obliterative bronchiolitis. *Clin. Radiol.*, **33**, 657–61.
19. Turton, C.W., Williams, G. and Green, M. (1981) Cryptogenic obliterative bronchiolitis in adults. *Thorax*, **36**, 805–10.
20. Sweatman, M.C., Millar, A.B., Strickland, B. *et al.* (1990) Computed tomography in adult obliterative bronchiolitis. *Clin. Radiol.*, **41**, 116–9.
21. Geddes, D.M., Corrin, B., Brewerton, D.A. *et al.* (1977) Progressive airway obliteration in

adults and its association with rheumatoid disease. *Q. J. Med.*, **46**, 427–44.

22. Cornelius, E.A. and Betlach, E. H. (1960) Silo-filler's disease. *Radiology*, **74**, 232–8.

23. Lowry, T. and Schuman, L.M. (1956) 'Silo-filler's disease': a syndrome caused by nitrogen dioxide. *JAMA*, **162**, 153–60.

24. Charan, N.B., Myers, C.G., Lakshminarayan, S. *et al.* (1979) Pulmonary injuries associated with acute sulfur dioxide inhalation. *Am. Rev. Respir. Dis.*, **119**, 555–60.

25. Wyatt, S.E., Nunn, P. and Hows, J.M. (1984) Airways obstruction associated with graft versus host disease after bone marrow transplantation. *Thorax*, **39**, 887–94.

26. Ostrow, D., Buskard, N., Hill, R.S. *et al.* (1985) Bronchiolitis obliterans complicating bone marrow transplantation. *Chest*, **87**, 828–30.

27. Skeens, J.L., Fuhrman, C.R. and Yousem, S.A. (1989) Bronchiolitis obliterans in heart-lung transplantation patients: radiologic findings in 11 patients. *Am. J. Roentgenol.*, **153**, 253–6.

28. Morrish, W.F., Herman, S.J., Weisbrod, G.L. *et al.* (1991) Bronchiolitis obliterans after lung transplantation: findings at chest radiography and high-resolution CT. *Radiology*, **179**, 487–90.

29. Padley, S.P.G., Adler, B.D., Hansell, D.M. *et al.* (1993) Bronchiolitis obliterans: high resolution CT findings and correlation with pulmonary function tests. *Clin. Radiol.*, **47**, 236–40.

30. Swyer, P.R. and James, G.C.W. (1953) A case of unilateral pulmonary emphysema. *Thorax*, **8**, 133–6.

31. MacLeod, W.M. (1954) Abnormal trans-radiancy of one lung. *Thorax*, **9**, 147–53.

32. Reid, L. and Simon, G. (1962) Unilateral lung transradiancy. *Thorax*, **17**, 230–9.

33. O'Dell, C.W., Taylor, A., Higgins, C.B. *et al.* (1976) Ventilation-perfusion lung images in the Swyer–James syndrome. *Radiology*, **121**, 423–6.

34. McKenzie, S.A., Allison, D.J., Singh, M.P. *et al.* (1980) Unilateral hyperlucent lung: the case for investigation. *Thorax*, **35**, 745–50.

35. Moore, A.D.A., Godwin, J.D., Dietrich, P.A. *et al.* (1992) Swyer–James syndrome: CT findings in eight patients. *Am. J. Roentgenol.*, **158**, 1211–5.

36. Marti-Bonmati, L., Perales, F.R., Catala, F. *et al.* (1989) CT findings in Swyer–James syndrome. *Radiology*, **172**, 477–80.

37. Alderson, P.O. and Line, B.R. (1980) Scintigraphic evaluation of regional pul-monary ventilation. *Semin. Nucl. Med.*, **10**, 218–42.

38. Fazio, F., Lavender, J.P. and Steiner, R.E. (1978) 81mKr ventilation and 99mTc perfusion scans in chest disease: comparison with standard radiographs. *Am. J. Roentgenol.*, **130**, 421–8.

39. Cunningham, D.A. and Lavender, J.P. (1981) Krypton 81m ventilation scanning in chronic obstructive airways disease. *Br. J. Radiol.*, **54**, 110–16.

40. Welch, M.H., Richardson, R.H., Whitcomb, W.H. *et al.* (1969) The lung scan in α1-antitrypsin deficiency. *J. Nucl. Med.*, **10**, 687–90.

41. Ernst, H., Herxheimer, H., Koppenhagen, K. *et al.* (1970) Diagnosis of destructive emphysema by scintigraphy. *Am. Rev. Respir. Dis.*, **102**, 274–9.

42. Murata, K., Itoh, H., Senda, M. *et al.* (1986) Stripe sign in pulmonary perfusion scintigraphy: central pattern of pulmonary emphysema. *Radiology*, **160**, 337–40.

43. Alderson, P.O., Secker-Walker, R.H. and Forrest, J.V. (1974) The detection of obstructive pulmonary disease. *Radiology*, **112**, 643–8.

44. Wagner, P.D., Dantzker, D.R., Dueck, R. *et al.* (1977) Ventilation-perfusion inequality in chronic obstructive pulmonary disease. *J. Clin. Invest.*, **59**, 203–16.

45. Alderson, P.O., Lee, H. and Summer, W.R. (1979) Comparison of xenon-133 washout and single-breath imaging for the detection of ventilation abnormalities. *J. Nucl. Med.*, **20**, 917–22.

46. Krumholz, R.A., Burnham, G.M. and DeLong, J.F. (1972) Lung scan utilization in the diagnosis of pulmonary disease. *Chest*, **62**, 4–8.

47. Alderson, P.O., Biello, D.R., Sachariah, K.G. *et al.* (1981) Scintigraphic detection of pulmonary embolism in patients with obstructive pulmonary disease. *Radiology*, **138**, 661–6.

48. The PIOPED Investigators (1990) Value of ventilation/perfusion scan in acute pulmonary embolism. Results of the prospective investigation of pulmonary embolism diagnosis (PIOPED). *JAMA*, **263**, 2753–9.

49. James, J.M., Lloyd, J.J., Leahy, B.C. *et al.* (1992) 99TcM Technegas and krypton-81m ventilation scintigraphy: a comparison in known respiratory disease. *Br. J. Radiol.*, **65**, 1075–82.

50. Chamberlain, M.J., Morgan, W.K.C. and Vinitski, S. (1983) Factors influencing the

regional deposition of inhaled particles in man. *Clin. Sci.*, **64**, 69–78.

51. Lin, M.S. and Goodwin, D.A. (1976) Pulmonary distribution of an inhaled radio-aerosol in obstructive pulmonary disease. *Radiology*, **118**, 645–51.

52. Hayes, M. (1980) Lung imaging with radio-aerosols for the assessment of airway disease. *Sem. Nucl. Med.*, **10**, 243–51.

53. Isawa, T., Wasserman, K. and Taplin, G.V. (1970) Lung scintigraphy and pulmonary function studies in obstructive airways disease. *Am. Rev. Respir. Dis.*, **102**, 161–72.

54. Taplin, G.V., Poe, N.D. and Greenberg, A. (1966) Lung scanning following radioaerosol inhalation. *J. Nucl. Med.*, **7**, 77–87.

55. Hughes, J.M.B. (1990) Radionuclides and the lung: past, present, and future. *Am. J. Roentgenol.*, **155**, 455–63.

56. Schuster, D.P. (1989) Positron emission tomography: theory and its application to the study of lung disease. *Am. Rev. Respir. Dis.*, **139**, 818–40.

57. Brudin, L.H., Rhodes, C.G., Valind, S.O. *et al.* (1992) Regional structure-function correlations in chronic obstructive lung disease measured with positron emission tomography. *Thorax*, **47**, 914–21.

58. Fraser, R.G., Paré, J.A.P., Paré, P.D. *et al.* (1990) *Diagnosis of Diseases of the Chest*, 3rd edn, Vol. III. Saunders, Philadelphia.

59. Lennon, E.A. and Simon, G. (1965) The height of the diaphragm in the chest radiograph of normal adults. *Br. J. Radiol.*, **38**, 937–43.

60. Katsura, S. and Martin, C.J. (1967) The roentgenologic diagnosis of anatomic emphysema. *Am. Rev. Respir. Dis.*, **96**, 700–6.

61. Nicklaus, T.M., Stowell, D.W., Christiansen, W.R. *et al.* (1966) The accuracy of the roentgenologic diagnosis of chronic pulmonary emphysema. *Am. Rev. Respir. Dis.*, **93**, 889–99.

62. Simon, G., Pride, N.B., Jones, N.L. *et al.* (1973) Relation between abnormalities in the chest radiograph and changes in pulmonary function in chronic bronchitis and emphysema. *Thorax*, **28**, 15–23.

63. Morgan, M.D.L., Denison, D.M. and Strickland, B. (1986) Value of computed tomography for selecting patients with bullous lung disease for surgery. *Thorax*, **41**, 855–62.

64. Thurlbeck, W.M., Henderson, J.A., Fraser, R.G. *et al.* (1970) Chronic obstructive lung disease. A comparison between clinical, roentgeno-logic, functional and morphologic criteria in chronic bronchitis, emphysema, asthma and bronchiectasis. *Medicine*, **49**, 81–145.

65. Boushy, S.F., Aboumrad, M.H., North, L.B. *et al.* (1971) Lung recoil pressure, airway resistance and forced flows related to morphologic emphysema. *Am. Rev. Respir. Dis.*, **104**, 551–61.

66. Laws, J.W. and Heard, B.E. (1962) Emphysema and the chest film: a restrospective radiological and pathological study. *Br. J. Radiol.*, **35**, 750–61.

67. Reid, L. and Millard, F.J.C. (1964) Correlation between radiological diagnosis and structural lung changes in emphysema. *Clin. Radiol.*, **15**, 307–11.

68. Sutinen, S., Christoforidis, A.J., Klugh, G.A. *et al.* (1965) Roentgenologic criteria for the recognition of nonsymptomatic pulmonary emphysema. *Am. Rev. Respir. Dis.*, **91**, 69–76.

69. Thurlbeck, W.M. and Simon, G. (1978) Radiographic appearance of the chest in emphysema. *Am. J. Roentgenol.*, **130**, 429–40.

70. Pratt, P.C. (1987) Role of conventional chest radiography in diagnosis and exclusion of emphysema. *Am. J. Med.*, **82**, 998–1006.

71. Sanders, C. (1991) The radiographic diagnosis of emphysema. *Radiol. Clin. North. Am.*, **29**, 1019–29.

72. Rothpearl, A., Varma, A.O. and Goodman, K. (1988) Radiographic measures of hyperinflation in clinical emphysema. *Chest*, **94**, 907–13.

73. Loyd, H.M., String, S.T. and DuBois, A.B. (1966) Radiographic and plethysmographic determination of total lung capacity. *Radiology*, **86**, 7–14

74. Bergin, C., Müller, N.L. and Miller, R.R. (1986) CT in the qualitative assessment of emphysema. *J. Thorac. Imag.*, **1**, 94–103.

75. Goddard, P.R., Nicholson, E.M., Laszlo, G. *et al.* (1982) Computed tomography in pulmonary emphysema. *Clin. Radiol.*, **33**, 379–87.

76. Hayhurst, M.D., MacNee, W., Flenley, D.C. *et al.* (1984) Diagnosis of pulmonary emphysema by computerised tomography. *Lancet*, **ii**, 320–2.

77. Foster, W.L., Pratt, P.C., Roggli, V.L. *et al.* (1986) Centrilobular emphysema: CT-pathologic correlation. *Radiology*, **159**, 27–32.

78. Klein, J.S., Gamsu, G., Webb, W.R. *et al.* (1992) High-resolution CT diagnosis of emphysema in symptomatic patients with normal chest radiographs and isolated low diffusing capacity. *Radiology*, **182**, 817–21.

79. Bergin, C., Müller, N., Nichols, D.M. *et al.* (1986) The diagnosis of emphysema. A computed tomographic-pathologic correlation. *Am. Rev. Respir. Dis.*, **133**, 541–6.

80. Foster, W.L., Gimenez, E.I., Roubidoux, M.A. *et al.* (1993) The emphysemas: radiologic-pathologic correlations. *Radiographics*, **13**, 311–28.

81. Murata, K., Itoh, H., Todo, G. *et al.* (1986) Centrilobular lesions of the lung: demonstration by high-resolution CT and pathologic correlation. *Radiology*, **161**, 641–5.

82. Hruban, R.H., Meziane, M.A., Zerhouni, E.A. *et al.* (1987) High resolution computed tomography of inflation-fixed lungs. Pathologic-radiologic correlation of centrilobular emphysema. *Am. Rev. Respir. Dis.*, **136**, 935–40.

83. Kuwano, K., Matsuba, K., Ikeda, T. *et al.* (1990) The diagnosis of mild emphysema. Correlation of computed tomography and pathology scores. *Am. Rev. Respir. Dis.*, **141**, 169–78.

84. Miller, R.R., Müller, N.L., Vedal, E. *et al.* (1989) Limitations of computed tomography in the assessment of emphysema. *Am. Rev. Respir. Dis.*, **139**, 980–3.

85. Gould, G.A., MacNee, W., McLean, A. *et al.* (1988) CT measurements of lung density in life can quantitate distal airspace enlargement – an essential defining feature of human emphysema. *Am. Rev. Respir. Dis.*, **137**, 380–92.

86. Müller, N.L., Staples, C.A., Miller, R.R. *et al.* (1988) 'Density mask'. An objective method to quantitate emphysema using computed tomography. *Chest*, **94**, 782–7.

87. Fromson, B.H. and Denison, D.M. (1988) Quantitative features in the computed tomography of healthy lungs. *Thorax*, **43**, 120–6.

88. Wegener, O.H., Koeppe, P. and Oeser, H. (1978) Measurement of lung density by computed tomography. *J. Comp. Assist. Tomogr.*, **2**, 1251–6.

89. Rosenblum, L.J., Mauceri, R.A., Wellenstein, D.E. *et al.* (1980) Density patterns in the normal lung as determined by computed tomography. *Radiology*, **137**, 409–16.

90. Adams, H., Bernard, M.S. and McConnochie, K. (1991) An appraisal of CT pulmonary density mapping in normal subjects. *Clin. Radiol.*, **43**, 238–42.

91. Millar, A.B. and Denison, D.M. (1990) Vertical gradients of lung density in supine subjects with fibrosing alveolitis or pulmonary emphysema. *Thorax*, **45**, 602–5.

92. Knudson, R.J., Standen, J.R., Kaltenborn, W.T. *et al.* (1991) Expiratory computed tomography for assessment of suspected pulmonary emphysema. *Chest*, **99**, 1357–66.

93. Gould, G.A., Redpath, A.T. and Ryan, M (1991) Lung CT density correlates with measurements of airflow limitation and the diffusing capacity. *Eur. Respir. J.*, **4**, 141–6.

94. Klein, J.S., Gamsu, G., Webb, W.R. *et al.* (1992) High-resolution CT diagnosis of emphysema in symptomatic patients with normal chest radiographs and isolated low diffusing capacity. *Radiology*, **182**, 817–21.

95. Gurney, J.W., Jones, K.K., Robbins, R.A. *et al.* (1992) Regional distribution of emphysema: correlation of high-resolution CT with pulmonary function tests in unselected smokers. *Radiology*, **183**, 457–63.

96. Gishen, P., Saunders, A.J.S., Tobin, M.J. *et al.* (1982) Alpha 1-antitrypsin deficiency: the radiological features of pulmonary emphysema in subjects of Pi type Z and Pi type SZ: A survey by the British Thoracic Association. *Clin. Radiol.*, **33**, 371–7.

97. Hepper, N.G., Mulm, J.R., Sheehan, W.C. *et al.* (1978) Roentgenographic study of chronic obstructive pulmonary disease by alpha-1-antitrypsin phenotype. *Mayo Clin. Proc.*, **53**, 166–72.

98. Rosen, R.A., Dalinka, M.K., Gralino, B.J. *et al.* (1970) The roentgenographic findings in alpha-1-antitrypsin deficiency (AAD). *Radiology*, **95**, 25–8.

99. Guest, P.J. and Hansell, D.M. (1992) High resolution computed tomography (HRCT) in emphysema associated with alpha-1-antitrypsin deficiency. *Clin. Radiol.*, **45**, 260–6.

100. Simon, G. (1964) Radiology and emphysema. *Clin. Radiol.*, **15**, 293–306.

101. Boushy, S.F., Kohen, R., Billig, D.M. *et al.* (1968) Bullous emphysema: clinical, roentgenologic and physiologic study of 49 patients. *Dis. Chest*, **54**, 327–34.

102. Reid, L. (1967) *The Pathology of Emphysema*, Lloyd-Luke, London.

103. Fiore, D., Biondetti, P.R., Sartori, F. *et al.* (1982) The role of computed tomography in the evaluation of bullous lung disease. *J. Comp. Assist. Tomogr.*, **6**, 105–8.

104. Morgan, M.D.L. and Strickland, B. (1984) Computed tomography in the assessment of bullous lung disease. *Br. J. Dis. Chest*, **78**, 10–25.

105. Gaensler, E.A., Jederlinic, P.J. and Fitzgerald, M.X. (1986) Patient work up for bullectomy. *J. Thorac. Imaging*, **1**, 75–93.

106. Klingman, R.R., Angelillo, V.A. and DeMeester, T.R. (1991) Cystic and bullous lung disease. *Ann. Thorac. Surg.*, **52**, 576–80.

107. Mahler, D. and D'Esopo, N.O. (1981) Peri-emphysematous lung infection. *Clin. Chest Med.*, **1**, 51–7.

108. McCluskie, R.A. (1981) Unusual fate of emphysematous bullae. *Thorax*, **36**, 77.

109. Stark, P., Gadziala, N. and Greene, R. (1980) Fluid accumulation in pre-existing pulmonary air spaces. *Am. J. Roentgenol.*, **134**, 701–6.

110. Jefferson, K. and Rees, S. (1980) *Clinical Cardiac Radiology*, 2nd edn, Butterworths, London.

111. Hicken, P., Green, I.D. and Bishop, J.M. (1968) Relationship between transpulmonary artery distance and pulmonary arterial pressure in patients with chronic bronchitis. *Thorax*, **23**, 446–50.

112. Chetty, K.G., Brown, S.E. and Light, R.W. (1982) Identification of pulmonary hypertension in chronic obstructive pulmonary disease from routine chest radiographs. *Am. Rev. Respir. Dis.*, **126**, 338–41.

113. Bush, A., Gray, H. and Denison, D.M. (1988) Diagnosis of pulmonary hypertension from radiographic estimates of pulmonary arterial size. *Thorax*, **43**, 127–31.

114. Chang, C.H. (1962) The normal roentgenographic measurement of the right descending pulmonary artery in 1085 cases. *Am. J. Roentgenol.*, **87**, 929–35.

115. Teichmann, V., Jezek, V. and Herles, F. (1970) Relevance of the width of right descending branch of pulmonary artery as a radiological sign of pulmonary hypertension. *Thorax*, **25**, 91–6.

116. Matthay, R.A., Schwarz, M.I., Ellis, J.H. *et al.* (1981) Pulmonary artery hypertension in chronic obstructive pulmonary disease: determination by chest radiography. *Invest. Radiol.*, **16**, 95–100.

117. Keller, C.A., Shepard, J.W., Chun, D.S. *et al.* (1986) Pulmonary hypertension in chronic obstructive pulmonary disease. *Chest*, **90**, 185–92.

118. Bishop, J.M. and Csukas, M. (1989) Combined use of non-invasive techniques to predict pulmonary arterial pressure in chronic respiratory disease. *Thorax*, **44**, 85–96.

119. Milne, E.N.C. (1963) Physiological interpretation of the plain radiograph on mitral stenosis, including a review of criteria for the radiological estimation of pulmonary arterial and venous pressures. *Br. J. Radiol.*, **36**, 902–13.

120. Saleh, M., Miles, A.I. and Lasser, R.P. (1974) Unilateral pulmonary edema in Swyer–James syndrome. *Chest*, **66**, 594–7.

121. Milne, E.N. and Bass, H. (1969) Roentgenologic and functional analysis of combined chronic obstructive pulmonary disease and congestive cardiac failure. *Invest. Radiol.*, **4**, 129–47.

SMOKING CESSATION AND PREVENTION

15

J. Foulds and M. J. Jarvis

15.1 INTRODUCTION

Tobacco smoking is the major cause of chronic obstructive pulmonary disease (COPD), its contribution to COPD morbidity and mortality far outweighing all other factors [1]. The closeness of the association between smoking and lung disease was perhaps best shown in the study of Auerbach and colleagues [2] which found at autopsy that while almost all (94.5%) smokers of more than a pack per day had some degree of emphysema, almost all never-smokers (93.8%) had either no or minimal emphysema. Smoking cessation improves lung function by about 5% within a few months in patients *without* COPD and a number of studies have found that even amongst patients with advanced COPD, smoking cessation is followed by a reduction in the annual loss of lung function [3]. It is therefore clear that smoking prevention and cessation are central to prevention and treatment of COPD.

This chapter will briefly review some of the interventions which have been studied and suggest a general strategy for health care workers' interventions with smokers, which may be applied both in general medical practice and hospital outpatient departments.

First, however, a brief outline of the prevalence, natural history and reasons for difficulty stopping smoking is provided.

15.2 PREVALENCE AND NATURAL HISTORY

In the UK about 31% of men and 29% of women are current cigarette smokers [4], with an additional 9% of men being pipe or cigar smokers [5]. In the US the prevalence is similar, with 29% of the adult population being cigarette smokers. In both countries there is a strong relationship between social class and smoking, e.g. in UK men, the prevalence of cigarette smoking in unskilled manual workers (48%) is triple that in professionals (16%) [4].

Surveys suggest that currently about 40% of the UK population have never become daily smokers, 35% being never smokers and about 5% having a history of intermittent occasional smoking [6]. Of those who do become daily smokers about 60% will still be smoking at age 60 [5].

It has been estimated that at least 80–90% of COPD patients have been regular smokers at some time [7]. Studies of prevalence and natural history of smoking in patients after diagnosis of COPD have generally suffered from lack of reliability of patients' self-reports of their current smoking status. It has been found that even when patients are informed that their smoking status will remain confidential and not be passed on to their physician, around 20% of hospital outpatients who claim to be non-smokers show unambiguous evidence of tobacco smoke inhalation on sensitive biochemical tests [8].

Chronic Obstructive Pulmonary Disease. Edited by Dr P. Calverley and Professor N. Pride. Published in 1995 by Chapman & Hall, London. ISBN 0 412 46450 0

The vast majority of smokers start smoking before the age of 18. This typically begins with experimentation with a few cigarettes at around age 13, which quickly develops into daily smoking by the age of 16. It has been shown that these young smokers at the early stages of their smoking career are already inhaling significant quantities of nicotine, with concomitant pharmacologic effects (e.g. calming effect, dizziness), and experience craving and other withdrawal symptoms when attempting to stop smoking [9–11]. The majority of adult regular smokers smoke 10–20 cigarettes per day (average = 16), with fewer than 10% being content to consistently smoke 5 or less per day.

It is a consistent finding in large scale surveys that at least 90% of smokers believe that smoking is bad for one's health (e.g. that it causes lung cancer), 70% express a desire to stop smoking, and 60% have made at least one serious attempt to quit [6]. Fig. 15.1 gives an indication of the strength of motivation to quit in smokers attending their GP, and suggests that about 50% of such smokers have a strong desire to quit at any one time. Despite these facts it is unfortunately the case that less than 40% of regular smokers succeed in permanently quitting by their sixtieth birthday [5].

Thus the typical smoking COPD patient will probably have a history of smoking an average of one cigarette during every waking hour for the previous thirty or more years. They may not have experienced a day without tobacco in their adult life other than during brief periods of serious illness or brief attempts to quit which ended in failure.

15.3 NICOTINE ADDICTION

It has only recently become widely accepted that tobacco smoking is addictive in the same way as heroin and cocaine, and that nicotine is the drug in tobacco which produces the reinforcing psychoactive effects which result in compulsive use [1]. Some of the evidence producing this consensus is outlined below.

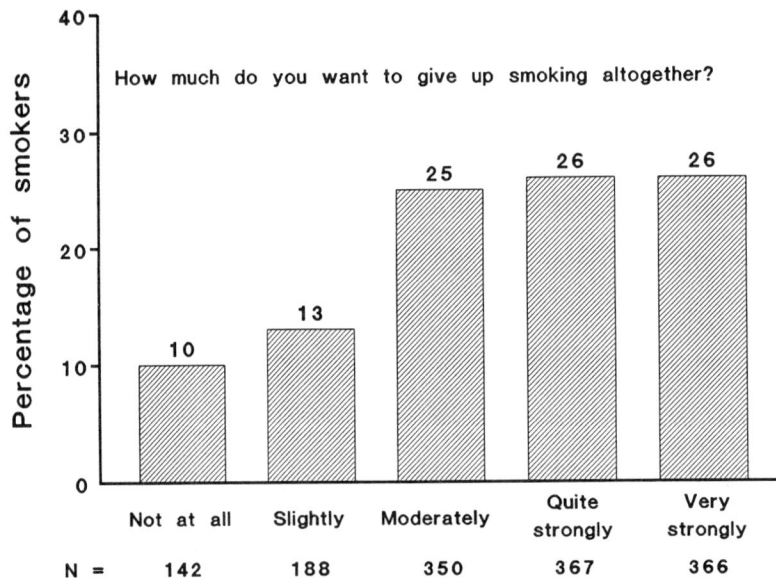

Fig. 15.1 Self-reported desire to give up smoking from a survey of smokers (n = 1413) in South London general practices.

(a) Tobacco has only ever been consumed by humans in ways which permit absorption of pharmacologically significant amounts of nicotine into the blood and brain. Cigarette smoking is a particularly efficient way of administering nicotine, which reaches the brain in a concentrated bolus within ten seconds of each puff, amounting to 70 000 nicotine 'hits' per year in a pack-a-day smoker [12].

(b) Nicotine acts as a primary reinforcer such that laboratory animals will work in order to receive intravenous injections of nicotine but not placebo [13], as do human smokers [14,15].

(c) Smokers smoke in a manner which enables them to regulate their plasma levels of nicotine, e.g. after cutting down the number of cigarettes smoked per day or switching to cigarettes providing a lower yield of nicotine they inhale more smoke from each cigarette in a manner which helps them achieve plasma nicotine levels closer to their usual levels [16,17]. Similarly when smokers are provided with extra nicotine from another source (e.g. transdermal nicotine) they inhale less smoke from their cigarettes, as indicated by lower levels of expired carbon monoxide [18].

(d) When regular smokers cease or cut down their nicotine intake they experience a withdrawal syndrome characterized by craving for nicotine, irritability, anxiety, difficulty concentrating, restlessness and increased appetite [19] as well as physical signs such as slowing of EEG, reduced heart rate and increased weight [20]. Studies have shown that these symptoms are relieved by nicotine replacement using nicotine chewing gum but not by placebo gum [21]. At least 68% of smokers who quit smoking for one week without nicotine replacement in a general practice study experienced symptoms fulfilling formal psychiatric criteria for the nicotine withdrawal syndrome [21].

(e) Numerous placebo-controlled smoking cessation trials have now shown that providing smokers with nicotine replacement (in the form of nicotine gum, skin patches or nasal spray) increases their chances of remaining abstinent from cigarettes for a year by between 50 and 100%. For example, a review of randomized trials in smoking cessation clinics [22] found mean one year sustained abstinence rates of 23% in subjects receiving nicotine gum and 13% in subjects receiving placebo gum.

(f) Surveys of patients (n=1000) attending drug treatment clinics seeking treatment for alcohol, cocaine or heroin dependence (about 90% of whom are cigarette smokers) have found that when asked, the majority (57%) said their cigarettes would be harder to quit than their problem substance [23].

15.4 INTERVENTIONS

15.4.1 PREVENTION

Given the evidence outlined above of rapid progression of nicotine intake and subsequent difficulty in quitting, the most attractive option would appear to be to take steps to prevent the current high initiation rate (450 children start smoking in Great Britain every day [24]). Such approaches have generally been conducted at two levels: (1) specific interventions at school or community level targeted at providing children with both information and skills which will make them less likely to begin smoking; (2) legislation designed to reduce children's exposure to cigarette advertising or availability of cigarettes to children.

A number of studies have found that intensive smoking prevention programmes initiated at school at age 11–14 can be effective in reducing the prevalence of smoking up to age 16 [25]. However, recent studies which have continued follow-up to age 18 have found that by this point there is no difference in smoking prevalence between children who received the intervention and those who did not [26–28]. This does not necessarily imply that such programmes are useless, but does indicate the great difficulty of preventing young people from initiating a behavior which is considered socially acceptable by adults, is carried out on a daily basis by their own adult family members, and indeed is strongly encouraged by intensive advertising.

A detailed analysis of the effects of availability and advertising of tobacco to children is beyond the scope of this chapter. A recent review commissioned by the UK Department of Health concluded that advertising does have a positive effect on consumption and that in each country in which advertising has been banned there was a reduction in tobacco consumption which cannot be attributed to other factors [29]. There is therefore little doubt that banning tobacco advertising would result in a reduction in tobacco-related death and illness. The other issue which can be expected to have an impact on tobacco consumption in both children and adults is that relating to the effects of passive smoking. There is now a consensus that passive smoking is a health hazard [30] and this will force employers to make the workplace a smoke-free zone or risk personal injury litigation. This advent of smoke-free work and leisure conditions will itself motivate more smokers to quit and reduce the availability of smoking role models for children. Two further points are perhaps worth making. First, despite voluntary agreements not to aim tobacco advertising at young people [31] it is clear that through sports sponsorship and other marketing methods children are exposed to and attracted by the industry's promotional activities [32]. Second, health professionals *can* make an impact in this area by lending their support to the various campaigns and pressure groups which attempt to achieve changes in the relevant legislation. An example of this was the recent tightening of the law and increases in fines for selling cigarettes to children under 16 in the UK [24], which followed pressure by the charity 'Parents Against Tobacco'. This charity was supported by many health professionals and by research reports on the availability of tobacco to young people [33].

Both controlled evaluations of interventions and recent data on prevalence of smoking in young people suggest that we do not yet have available effective methods of preventing the uptake of smoking in teenagers. It may be that health educational messages to young people would have more impact if they focused more on the immediate harm and imminent risk of becoming addicted to nicotine rather than on the distant risks to health which may mean little to teenagers. It may also be the case that in the long run one of the most effective methods of reducing uptake of smoking in young people will be to reduce the availability of adult smoking role models. This inevitably involves helping existing smokers to quit.

15.4.2 SMOKING CESSATION ADVICE AND TREATMENT

A vast number of products and techniques have been claimed to help smokers to quit. Most have not been evaluated properly and so their efficacy is dubious at best. Many are expensive and time-consuming as well and thus are clearly unacceptable to the majority of patients and physicians. Rather than describing all available methods, this section will try to highlight those methods which have been shown to be most helpful *and* cost effective, i.e. those which are likely to produce the largest number of long term ex-smokers.

(a) Gradual or immediate reduction?

One of the first choices to be faced when confronted by a smoking patient is whether to advise cutting down cigarette consumption gradually or to advise quitting abruptly. Given the evidence cited above about difficulty of quitting and the likely role of withdrawal symptoms in exacerbating this, it would seem plausible that (as is usually advised with cessation of benzodiazepines) gradual reduction would be easier and perhaps produce higher success rates. Indeed, methods of gradual reduction are commonly advocated in intensive behavioral smoking cessation programs [34]. These programs sometimes advocate 'nicotine fading' – gradual reduction of nicotine content of cigarettes smoked, followed by gradual reduction in number of cigarettes smoked per day. Experimental studies have confirmed that less severe withdrawal symptoms occur during partial reduction or reduction in nicotine yield per cigarette [35,36]. However, there is also considerable evidence that smokers who are apparently cutting down their smoking this way actually tend to increase their inhalation from each cigarette in a manner which seems to be designed to help them attain their usual blood nicotine levels [16,17]. One of the few studies which actually randomized smokers to either gradual reduction or abrupt quitting on a target date found the latter to produce a greater reduction in smoking [37]. It has also been found that smokers in cessation trials who do not succeed in quitting abruptly also show no signs of successfully cutting down their smoking in the long term [38,39]. It is clear, therefore, that there is little sense in trying to cut down and stay at a lower level as it seems that the chances of success are extremely low and that even if the patient did succeed then a likely consequence is an increase in inhalation of toxins per cigarette resulting in negligible overall health benefit. It has also been suggested that as the smoker cuts down the number of cigarettes per day each one becomes more reinforcing and hence the point of total abstinence becomes harder to reach [34].

In the absence of adequate randomized trials comparing gradual and immediate cessation, the weight of evidence suggests that smokers should be advised to quit abruptly on a target date, particularly when no ongoing treatment is provided to ensure that the smoker continues to cut down to zero cigarettes per day, and particularly when using concurrent nicotine replacement.

(b) Brief or intensive treatment?

Another difficult treatment option is the choice between offering a treatment which is relatively brief and simple (e.g. less than 30 minutes of advice), or one which is more intensive in terms of therapist time, and perhaps also in the demands made on the patient (e.g. keeping behavioral diaries, listening to relaxation tapes, etc.)

Although it is widely assumed that more intensive treatments will produce better results, very few studies have actually randomized patients to low and high intensity treatments in a manner which can provide clear evidence on this point. Those which have done this have generally found a small (non-significant) increment in success rates resulting from providing slightly more time-intensive advice and follow-up procedures [40–44]. One recent large study [45] randomized 647 motivated family practice patients to receive either a brief intervention comprising two appointments (17 minutes) or the same intervention plus the offer of four further supportive follow-up appointments (at quit-date and then 1, 4 and 16 weeks later). There was little difference in the 1-year abstinence rate between the two groups (10.2% vs 12.5%) and it was concluded that numerous long-term follow-up visits are of unproven value.

Despite this it is clear that patients who attend smokers' clinics providing intensive psychologic counselling have a better chance of long-term cessation than those receiving only a brief intervention by their GP. One factor which provides a likely explanation for this is *patient motivation*, i.e. the degree to which a patient wants to stop smoking and is therefore willing to put time and effort into it. By contacting a smokers' clinic and agreeing to attend numerous appointments for counselling a patient has demonstrated a considerable motivation to stop smoking. Results from a treatment trial based on this self-selected group will clearly not be applicable to an unselected group of smokers. For example, one study conducted in primary care offered some of the participants the opportunity to contact a Health Visitor for further advice and counselling [46]. Less than 2% of the patients took up this offer of further counselling (and only 13% claimed abstinence 1 year later). In another study patients were randomized to receive 15 minutes advice on self-quitting or 15 minutes advice *plus* encouragement to attend a free smoking cessation programme involving 9 group sessions [44]; 11% of those who were encouraged to, attended the intensive treatment (compared with less than 1% in the advice only group). Although the 3 month abstinence rate was higher in the 11% who actually *attended* the intensive treatment compared with the majority who chose not to (33% versus 10%), the cigarette abstinence rates were similar (12.9% and 14.1%) in the advice only and advice plus offer of treatment conditions as whole groups. It is therefore clear that trying to make unmotivated patients participate in time-intensive treatments will not have the desired effects. It is similarly obvious that comparison of 'success rates' found in different studies is meaningless in view of the great differences in motivation evident between unselected smokers in primary care and those few who elect to attend a smokers' clinic.

Another important factor which must be considered when choosing between low and high intensity treatments is their efficiency, both in terms of cost and time. Even assuming that it is the case that an intensive (5 hours per individual) treatment yields higher long term abstinence rates (e.g. 25%) than a minimal intervention (achieving only 4%)

success from 4 minutes of advice), if the therapist only has one hour per week to spend on smoking cessation, the intensive intervention can only be delivered to 10 individual patients per year (producing 2 or 3 ex-smokers) whereas the minimal intervention can be delivered to 800, producing 32 ex-smokers. It is clear that time-intensive treatments with individual smokers are not generally very efficient. A preferable format for delivering a more intensive treatment is in the context of a group. In 50 hours a therapist could run 10 groups (5 × 1 hour), seeing 160 patients and with a 25% success rate could produce 40 ex-smokers. As mentioned above, however, very few clinics have a large enough throughput of patients to be able to recruit 160 patients with high enough motivation to attend 5 1-hour treatment sessions.

(c) Non-pharmacologic aids to smoking cessation

The essential features common to most methods of helping smokers to quit are that they provide the smoker with a strategy and a rationale, i.e. a plan of what to do and a convincing reason for following that plan of action. It is likely that any intervention which provides these two components will be of some help in motivating an individual to progress from being someone with a vague intention of stopping smoking to someone who actually makes a real attempt. At the simplest level this can take the form of reminding a patient that the single best thing they can do for their health is to stop smoking, that it would be a good idea to flush all their remaining tobacco down the toilet on Sunday night, make Monday their 'quit day', and never smoke again.

A range of additional methods are commonly used to try to decrease the individual's desire for a cigarette (e.g. 'rapid smoking' to the point of nausea prior to quitting in behavioral treatments, or suggestions to this effect in hypnosis), to help the smoker cope with withdrawal symptoms (e.g. relaxation exercises) and to help maintain motivation (e.g. viewing a video of the health consequences of smoking and making a public promise to quit). Indeed there are so many proposed aids and methods that few have been properly evaluated in controlled studies and so it is impossible to say for certain whether they help or not.

Two aids do, however, deserve particular consideration. One of these is the use of a portable carbon-monoxide analyzer to measure end-expired carbon monoxide. Portable CO monitors provide an accurate quantitative guide to smoke inhalation (correlation with blood carboxyhemoglobin >0.95 [47]) which takes less than a minute to measure and can immediately be shown to the patient and lead to a discussion of the health effects of CO from cigarettes. They can also be informed that the high CO levels found in smokers (typically in the range 15 to 60 parts per million) return to those of non-smokers (less than 10 parts per million) within a matter of days and so this is a tangible and quick benefit of stopping smoking. Although the expired carbon monoxide measure is slightly less accurate in patients with COPD the error due to impairment of lung function is negligible for most purposes [48]. Some studies have shown that the measuring of expired carbon monoxide in this way can improve long-term cessation rates, particularly in the lower socioeconomic groups who now make-up the majority of smokers [46]. As the CO monitor is also 90% accurate in discriminating smokers from non-smokers it is useful tool in validating claims of abstinence, both on first contact and after a quit attempt [8]. These CO monitors are now readily available at a relatively low cost (around £400) and so should form part of the routine assessment procedure in any health setting which claims to have a serious interest in helping patients to stop smoking.

The other non-pharmacologic aid to smoking cessation which is appropriate when more intensive psychologic support is indicated is the use of group processes to help smokers quit. As well as the benefits in terms of cost efficiency mentioned above, there is now evidence that a particular type of smoking cessation group format may be particularly effective in helping smokers to quit [49,50]. This group format involves weekly group meetings over four weeks, with the general aim being for smokers to quit at the first group meeting and then support each other through the first few weeks in which nicotine withdrawal symptoms are at their worst. Rather than adopting a typical didactic teaching style the therapist concentrates on encouraging the cohesion of the group (by providing name-labels, asking group members to introduce themselves, encouraging contacts outside the group, encouraging group discussion, etc.) and enhancement of group pressure to maintain abstinence (by initiating publicly declared commitments to remain abstinent). It has been found that such 'group-oriented' groups produce higher end-of-treatment abstinence rates and better attendance than do traditional 'therapist-oriented' groups. This type of group treatment also has the advantage that as it is relatively simple (does not involve the therapist in teaching many techniques) it may be easily adopted by non-specialist therapists.

(d) Pharmacologic aids to stopping smoking

The possibility of an effective pharmacologic aid to smoking cessation has always been very attractive to smokers who are all too often looking for a magical wonder cure – something which when swallowed will effortlessly remove all withdrawal symptoms and desire for a cigarette. Physicians, too, are naturally attracted to the idea of an effective prescribable treatment. However, complex voluntary behavior such as puffing on a cigarette, or any other behavior which has become so compulsive as to be emitted seventy thousand times per year for years on end is unlikely ever to respond simply and completely to drug treatment.

There is an important difference between prescribing a medication to treat a physical illness (e.g. antibiotics for an infection) and prescribing medication to help promote a behavior change. It is therefore crucial that when a pharmacologic aid is prescribed for smoking cessation, it should be combined with a rationale and plan of how it is to be used and realistic expectations of both the effects of the medication and the role of the patient. Provision of such 'psychologic packaging' need not necessarily be very time-consuming (5–10 minutes) but may be essential for any pharmacologic adjunct to aid smoking cessation.

There has been considerable progress in the development and evaluation of pharmaceutic aids to smoking cessation in the past 15 years such that there are now a number of products which have been shown to help smokers stop and others which show some promise for the future. These are outlined below.

(i) Nicotine gum

Nicotine gum is the most thoroughly evaluated pharmacologic aid and has been shown to almost double long-term abstinence rates when compared with placebo in specialist smokers clinics providing intensive psychologic support [51]. The outcome of one such study [52] carried out at the Maudsley Hospital Smokers Clinic in London is shown in Fig. 15.2, suggesting a clear advantage of nicotine gum, even when using the strict criterion of one-year without a puff of tobacco smoke (biochemically validated).

A meta-analysis of randomized controlled trials of nicotine gum found a clear improvement in sustained abstinence rates at 1 year (23% vs 13%) in smokers' clinics but no effect in general medical practice (11% vs 12%) [22]. Since then further studies have confirmed this pattern – a family practice study in the United States found that 10% of those receiving nicotine gum and 7% of those receiving placebo reported (biochemically confirmed) continuous abstinence for 11 months [53] and a general hospital study in the UK reported 20% abstinence at 1 year in both nicotine and placebo gum groups [54]. Numerous reasons have been suggested for the poorer performance of nicotine gum in medical settings: patients in these settings may lack the motivation to quit, may not be dependent on nicotine, physicians may not give adequate instruction or enough support to encourage patients to persist with proper gum use. There does seem to be good evidence of poor compliance with gum use in medical settings, e.g. with only 45% collecting more than one box of gum (enough for one or two weeks) [53], and 60% rating the gum as unpleasant to use [55]. It is therefore clear that when nicotine gum is used by motivated nicotine-dependent patients given adequate instruction and follow-up it helps them to stop smoking, but under the conditions more normal in medical practice the beneficial effects are less apparent.

(ii) Nicotine skin patches

More recently nicotine skin patches have been developed which are capable of administering a slow infusion of nicotine and providing plasma nicotine levels of one-third to a half of smoking levels after four hours of wearing. A number of placebo-controlled trials of transdermal nicotine have been published and these have generally produced results similar to those of trials of nicotine gum [56]. Two early trials, however, have provided some indication that the patch may be more successful than the gum outside the smokers' clinic. One study, carried out in a chest clinic in Denmark (but mainly on healthy volunteers) found that 17% of the nicotine group and 4% of the placebo group achieved one year sustained abstinence when the patch was combined with relatively low intensity psychologic support [57]. Another study com-

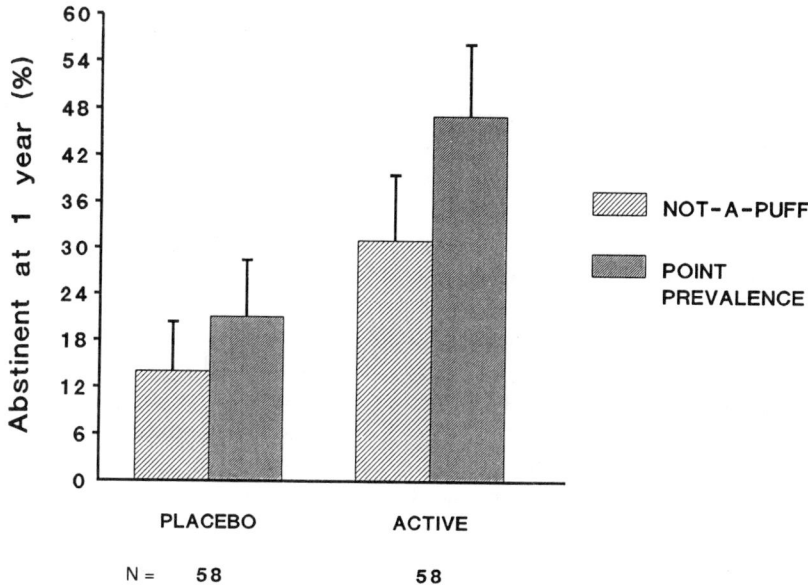

Fig. 15.2 Outcome of a randomized trial of nicotine gum combined with group support in a smokers' clinic [52]. Errors bars are 95% confidence intervals.

bining the patch with brief monthly appointments with the GP [58] found abstinence rates of 18% vs 12% at one year. These studies have prompted further evaluations of transdermal nicotine in general hospitals and primary care. Two recent studies carried out in hospital chest departments and targeting patients with smoking-related diseases [59,60] found an advantage of active over placebo patches in the early stages but by 12 weeks the advantage was relatively small. The two much larger trials in primary care both found a clear advantage of the nicotine patch over placebo at 12 weeks [61, 62], and the trial reported by Russell and colleagues [62] found that despite the expected high relapse rate over the year, there was still an advantage of active over placebo patches for 12 months' continuous abstinence (9% vs 5%). This result is particularly impressive as this study targeted heavy smokers (15 or more cigarettes per day) and the patients did not receive intensive counselling or group support. Taken together these trials of transdermal nicotine in medical pa-

tients suggest that nicotine patches are an effective smoking cessation aid when combined with the relatively brief advice and follow-up support which can be routinely provided by doctors and nurses in a National Health Service setting.

In the UK and some other countries the nicotine patch is available over the counter from pharmacies at full price to the customer (roughly equivalent to the costs of buying tobacco in a pack-a-day smoker). This has prompted a massive direct marketing campaign by the pharmaceutical companies. While some anti-smoking campaigners may feel uneasy about an anti-smoking campaign being associated with a particular product, there are potentially significant public health benefits of an anti-smoking advertising campaign far larger than those paid for by public funds. It is to be hoped that the widespread availability of the product does not detract from the important role of the doctor in providing appropriate advice on smoking and the use of nicotine replacement.

(iii) Nasal nicotine spray

Both nicotine gum and patches provide relatively slow absorption of nicotine. Consequently although they may provide some relief of nicotine withdrawal symptoms they do not provide a nicotine 'hit' in the form of a bolus which results from absorption via the pulmonary circulation. Perhaps the ideal nicotine replacement product would be an inhaler which is capable of delivering pure nicotine directly to the lungs and directly mimicking a cigarette (without the tar and carbon monoxide which cause most tobacco-related disease). Such a product has yet to be developed but perhaps the closest thing so far is nasal nicotine spray. This product has completed pilot testing [63] and initial results from a placebo-controlled trial suggest that, although there is no nicotine bolus, the fast absorption via the nasal cavity is able to reduce craving for a cigarette and produce a clear enhancement of placebo one-year continuous abstinence rates (26% vs 10%) in a smokers' clinic with intensive support [64]. It is likely that this product will be particularly suitable for more dependent smokers but may not be appropriate for brief interventions because the spray is initially perceived as quite aversive and requires encouragement to persist through the first week or so.

With all of the nicotine replacement products there is a risk of the nicotine addiction simply being transferred onto the new nicotine source. The size of this risk is thought to be related to the degree to which the nicotine replacement product mimics nicotine delivery from a cigarette. In smokers' clinics where use of nicotine replacement is encouraged, up to 6% of nicotine gum users continue using the gum for a least a year (25% of one year tobacco abstainers) [65] and the corresponding figure for nasal nicotine spray is 11% (43% of one year successes) [64]. Patch treatment generally has a weaning procedure built into the treatment programme (in the form of progressively smaller patches) and so tends to

avoid this problem. At the moment there are few data on health hazards from long-term nicotine replacement but there are good reasons for thinking that these will be minimal in comparison to the risks from continued smoking: there is a complete absence of tar and carbon monoxide, the quantities and speed of nicotine delivery are markedly lower than smoking, and finally there is evidence from studies of snuff users in Sweden that long-term nicotine exposure similar to that produced by nicotine replacement products results in lower risk of myocardial infarction than smoking and no increased risk compared with using no tobacco products at all [66].

(iv) Other pharmacologic treatments

A number of pharmacologic treatments other than nicotine replacement have begun to be evaluated. These include Buspirone, Clonidine, Doxepin, and lobeline-based products. Although some of these (e.g. Buspirone) have shown some promise in early studies it is frequently the case that when subject to more rigorous evaluation this early promise is not supported (as in the case of the lobeline-based products [67]). The use of these products for smoking cessation must therefore be considered as strictly experimental at this stage.

A summary of the key feature of effective smoking cessation treatment which have some support in the literature is presented in Table 15.1.

15.5 A SMOKING PREVENTION AND CESSATION STRATEGY

Thus far a number of different approaches to smoking cessation and prevention have been discussed. This section will attempt to describe how these different approaches may be effectively combined in a complementary manner as part of a coordinated smoking strategy.

Table 15.1 Aspects of smoking cessation treatment supported in the literature

Treatment variable	Method of choice
Speed of tobacco withdrawal	Abruptly on quit date
Intensity of treatment	Brief for all smokers, plus intensive for highly motivated moderate/heavy smokers
Timing of psychological support	Appointments concentrated in first 4 weeks when withdrawal symptoms are strong
Group or individual treatment	Group treatment whenever practical
Pharmacological aids	Nicotine replacement
Additional components	Measurement of expired carbon monoxide before and after cessation

The strategy for smoking prevention and cessation proposed here is largely based on data provided by a series of studies conducted by the smoking research team at the Institute of Psychiatry (directed by Professor Michael Russell). It is intended to be applicable to any healthcare setting dealing with a large number of outpatients (e.g. 3000 per year), such as General Practice or General Hospital outpatient clinics and assumes that only a limited amount of time (e.g. 100 hours per year) is available for smoking interventions.

The first step a healthcare worker needs to make to change smoking habits in patients is to find out whether they actually smoke. A doctor who does not even ask about this is implying that smoking is not relevant to health, whereas for many patients it will be the single most important determinant of their future health status. By asking whether they smoke and recording it in the notes (ideally using coloured labels on the outside of the notes) the doctor is showing both smokers and non-smokers that this is an important issue. This can of course be reinforced by informing the smokers just how important an issue it is and providing some brief advice on this together with a leaflet on how to go about it:

'The single best thing you can do for your health is to stop smoking. I advise you to stop smoking as soon as possible by selecting a quit date within the next week or so and stopping completely on that day. I'd like you to take this leaflet which provides some tips on stopping smoking.'

This type of brief intervention takes only one or two minutes per patient and has been shown to produce a small but very important effect. For example, one study [68] randomized all of the adult smokers attending five General Practices over a one month period to one of four groups: 1. No intervention. 2. Given a brief smoking questionnaire. 3. Given brief advice to stop smoking. 4. Advised to stop smoking, given an information leaflet and warned that they would be followed up. As shown in Fig. 15.3 there was a small but significant effect such that the proportions who stopped smoking during the first month and were still not smoking a year later were 0.3%, 1.6%, 3.3% and 5.1% in the four groups respectively.

This effect was achieved by motivating more people to try to stop smoking rather than increasing the success rate amongst those who did try. Successful quitting was also most apparent in the lighter smokers. When subjects were categorized as: (a) smokers (no quit attempt), (b) triers (made a quit attempt but didn't stop), (c) relapsers (abstained at one month but smoking at one year), and (d) quitters (abstinent at both one

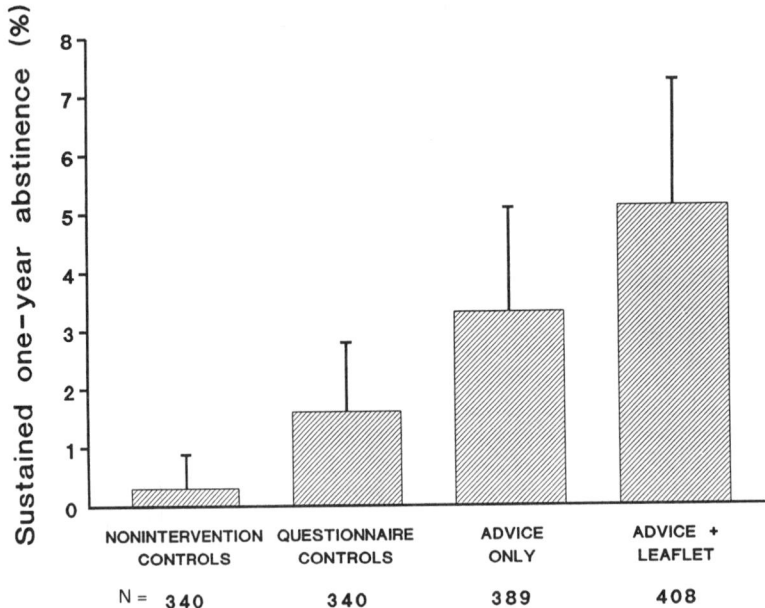

Fig. 15.3   Effect of GP advice on giving up smoking [68]. Error bars are 95% confidence intervals.

month and one year) there was a clear inverse relationship between the effects of GP advice and dependence, as measured at baseline by questionnaire ratings of severity of craving and perceived difficulty quitting [69]. This relationship is shown in Fig. 15.4.

As mentioned above, this effect of a brief intervention may be enhanced further by measurement of expired carbon monoxide in smokers, and indeed, given the frequency of inaccurate self-reports of smoking to doctors (around 20% of claimed non-smokers in general practice or hospitals have traces of recent smoking on sensitive biochemical measures [8, 46]) it may be worthwhile obtaining a measure of expired carbon monoxide as part of routine tests on *all* patients prior to asking about their smoking status.

In a subsequent study [70] with a similar design another group were offered a prescription of nicotine gum (provided free of charge), in addition to brief advice and a booklet. It was found that the offer of nicotine gum increased one year sustained abstinence rate from 4.1% in the advice plus booklet group to 8.8% in the group also offered nicotine gum. As before, these percentages are based on all cigarette smokers who attended the surgeries, including those who did not wish to stop and those in the gum group who did not even try the gum (47%). In addition to motivating more patients to try to stop smoking, the offer of gum increased the success rate amongst those who tried to quit (from 13.8% in the advice plus leaflet group to 19.5% in the gum group). In this study dependence, as measured at baseline, was negatively associated with subsequent 'success', and this relationship was attenuated in the gum group, i.e. highly dependent smokers were particularly helped by the offer of nicotine gum [71]. Similarly, motivation (as measured at baseline by questions about how much the person wants to quit) was positively related to success and this relationship was stronger in heavier smokers, i.e. heavier smokers need to have a particularly strong

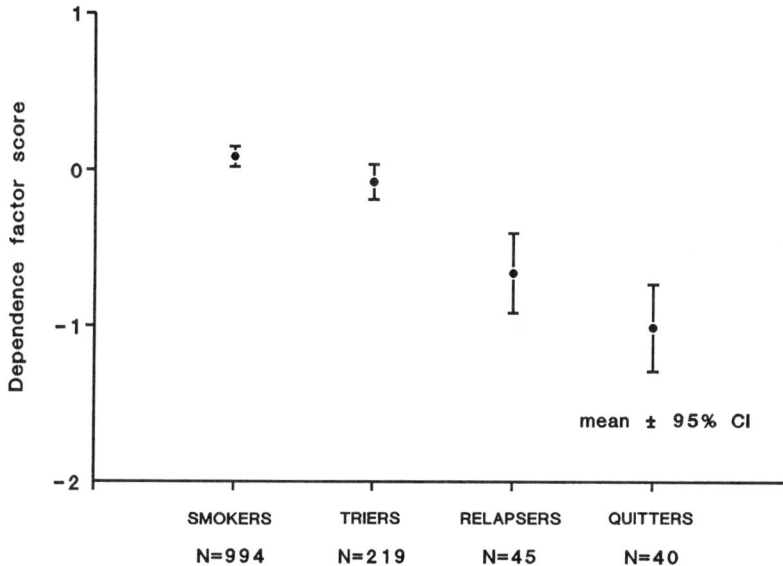

Fig. 15.4 Relationship of dependence to outcome in a GP intervention study [68]. Plotted values are scores from a factor analysis of questionnaire items completed before seeing the doctor [69].

desire to quit if they are to stand any chance of success.

A similar study carried out in a primary care setting in Canada also found a similar result, with 4.4% sustained abstinence at 1 year in those receiving usual care compared with 8.8% in patients of physicians who had been trained in the use of nicotine gum [72]. Interestingly this study found an intermediate (6.1%) success rate in patients who were offered the nicotine gum by physicians not trained in its use. Amongst other differences, these physicians were less likely to provide reading materials, ask for a quit date or offer a further appointment.

These studies suggest that doctors asking about patients' smoking and giving brief advice on quitting can have three important effects: (a) increasing smokers' motivation and intention to stop, (b) increasing the number who actually make a quit attempt, (c) increasing the number of their patients who become long term non-smokers, but this effect is mainly found in light (not heavily nicotine dependent) smokers. In addition, the

offer of nicotine gum as an aid to cessation motivates more smokers to try to quit but also increases the success rate. Nicotine replacement is of particular benefit to those heavier smokers who are less likely to succeed in quitting after brief advice alone.

The strategy suggested by these studies is one which attempts to reach as many patients as possible. The first step is to create an environment which makes it clear that smoking is not condoned and which offers both information and help for smokers considering quitting. Thus the hospital/practice should be clearly labelled as a non-smoking area and posters informing smokers of the health consequences of smoking and quitting should be clearly visible in waiting areas, as should posters and leaflets informing patients of what help is locally available (including an invitation to ask the doctor or nurse for help in quitting).

The next step is for clinicians to ask every single patient who attends whether or not they smoke, and to write the answer in the notes, ideally on a colour-coded label on the

Table 15.2 Overall smoking prevention and cessation strategy for outpatient medical settings

Intervention	Who to?	Time per patient	Total time	Success rate[a]	No. of successes
1. Ask about smoking, record on notes	All attenders (n = 3000)	10 seconds	8 hours	Prevention?	
2. Measure CO, give advice +leaflet	800 smokers (no extra help requested)	4 minutes	53 hours	4%	32
3. Prescribe nicotine replacement, arrange quit-date + follow-up	Those who ask for extra help (n = 160)	15 minutes	40 hours	10%	16
4. Group treatment with nicotine replacement (5 × 1 hour per group)	Those who ask for more support (n = 40, 13 or 14 per group)	22.5 minutes	15 hours	25%	10
Overall strategy	All patients	mean = 2.3 minutes per patient	116 hours	5.8% of smokers	58

[a]A 'success' is a patient who stops smoking immediately following the intervention and maintains abstinence for at least a year (and does not include those prevented from initiating smoking).

front. This simple behavior need take only 10 seconds, requiring a total of 8 hours of clinic time in a department seeing about 3000 patients per year. Table 15.2 summarizes the expected time required and outcome for various levels of intervention applied to the 1000 patients who are likely to admit they are smoking. In this example it is suggested that *all smokers* should be given the brief intervention, i.e. informed that they should stop smoking, have their expired carbon monoxide measured and explained, and given a leaflet on quitting. As discussed above, this simple intervention is likely to have a small but worthwhile effect, mainly on light smokers (those who consistently smoke less than ten cigarettes per day).

The clinician then has to decide on which of these smokers it would be worthwhile spending more time. The two important variables here are of course motivation and dependence on nicotine: clinic time is too precious to use trying to persuade those with little intention of quitting, and lighter

smokers may not require extra help (and will also have lower health risks). Until we have quick and valid measures of these variables a simple and pragmatic way of allocating further time is to only offer further help to patients who are motivated enough to actually request it (having already been informed that help is available by clinic posters). Those motivated patients who smoke at least 10 cigarettes per day may be offered a prescription for nicotine replacement (in the UK the patient will have to pay the full price less VAT), told how it works, asked to choose a quit date, and offered a follow-up appointment a week after their quit date. Those who are motivated enough to request more intensive treatment should have their name put on the waiting list for a stop-smoking group like the one described above (Section 15.4.2(c)).

The estimated numbers and results shown in Table 15.1 are based on the results of similar interventions reported in the scientific literature. This suggests that about 100 hours spent as described in the table will produce around 50 long-term ex-smokers, i.e. 2 hours per ex-smoker. This may not sound particularly impressive but it should be borne in mind that this two hours of work will have produced an additional life expectancy of between 1 and 6 years [73], or put another way, will (in an individual in their 40s) have reduced the quitter's risk of dying in the next 15 years by one-half (e.g. about 14% to 7%) compared with continuing smoking [3].

In addition to these cautious estimates of the number of long-term ex-smokers produced, this strategy will also have an important effect of provoking a general shift in attitudes to smoking such that intentions to abstain become stronger across the patient population as a whole [68]. This can be thought of as producing a shift to the right in Fig. 15.1 (Section 15.2), such that when the strategy is applied year on year more smokers become motivated to make a quit attempt and smoking prevalence continues to decline at a faster rate than if no organized intervention was being carried out [74].

The figures and suggestions given in Table 15.2 are mainly based on studies conducted in primary care, and of course things may be different in different situations, e.g. an outpatient hospital chest clinic. One recent study conducted in this setting [75] and focusing on patients with smoking-related diseases found that brief advice by the physician produced a long-term success rate of 5.1% which could be increased to 8.1% by also sending patients 6 brief letters from the doctor encouraging abstinence. These results are consistent with those presented in Table 15.2 and suggest one additional cost-effective method of helping patients to maintain their motivation in the months after their appointment at the hospital. The strategy proposed here can therefore be adjusted to meet the demands of different settings but it contains the main components which are supported in the scientific literature, namely (a) brief advice given to all smokers, (b) measurement of carbon monoxide as a method of validating smoking status and increasing cessation, (c) prescribing nicotine replacement with appropriate additional advice as an aid in motivated patients, and (d) use of a group format combined with nicotine replacement to administer more intensive treatment to dependent smokers with a strong desire to quit.

The main difficulty for clinicians is to maintain *their* efforts and motivation to keep these smoking cessation activities going. This is particularly the case with COPD patients – the hard cases who continue to smoke despite advice to the contrary and severe ill-health. The experience of advising large numbers of such patients against smoking and seeing the majority of them return to the clinic, continuing to smoke and with worsening symptoms can be a demoralizing one. However, the methods proposed above have been shown to help patients to stop smoking and are available now. Clinicians who carry out these procedures in a consistent manner can therefore do so in the knowledge that although the resulting overall annual smoking cessation rate will be low, it will be more than double that produced by 'usual care' procedures.

ACKNOWLEDGEMENTS

The financial support of the Medical Research Council and Imperial Cancer Research Fund is gratefully acknowledged.

REFERENCES

1. US Department of Health and Human Services (1988) *The Health Consequences of Smoking: Nicotine Addiction*. A report of the Surgeon General. US Government Printing Office, Washington D.C.
2. Auerbach, O., Hammond, E.C., Kirman, D. *et al.* (1972) Relation of smoking and age to emphysema: whole-lung section study. *N. Engl. J. Med.*, **286**, 853–7.
3. US Department of Health and Human Services (1990) *The Health Benefits of Smoking Cessation*.

A report of the Surgeon General. US Government Printing Office, Washington D.C.

4. Office of Population Censuses and Surveys (1992) *General Household Survey 1990.* HMSO, London.

5. Jarvis, M.J. and Jackson, P.H. (1988) Cigar and pipe smoking in Britain: implications for smoking prevalence and cessation. *Br. J. Addict.,* **83**, 323–30.

6. Cox, B.D., Blaxter, M, Buckle A.L.J. *et al.* (1987) *The Health and Lifestyle Survey.* Health Promotion Research Trust, London.

7. US Department of Health and Human Services. (1984) *The Health Consequences of Smoking: Chronic Obstructive Lung Disease.* A report of the Surgeon General. US Government Printing Office, Washington D.C.

8. Jarvis, M.J., Tunstall-Pedoe, H., Feyerabend, C. *et al.* (1987) Comparison of tests used to distinguish smokers from non-smokers. *Am. J. Public Health,* **77**, 1435–8.

9. McNeill, A.D., Jarvis, M.J., Stapleton, J.A. *et al.* (1989) Prospective study of factors predicting uptake of smoking in adolescents. *J. Epidem. Community Health,* **43**, 72–8.

10. McNeill, A.D., West, R.J., Jarvis, M.J. *et al.* (1986) Cigarette withdrawal symptoms in adolescent smokers. *Psychopharmacol.,* **90**, 533–6.

11. McNeill, A.D., Jarvis, M.J. and West, R.J. (1987) Subjective effects of cigarette smoking in adolescents. *Psychopharmacol.,* **92**, 115–7.

12. Russell, M.A.H. and Feyerabend, C. (1978) Cigarette smoking: a dependence on high-nicotine boli. *Drug Metab. Rev.,* **2**, 29–57.

13. Goldberg, S.R., Spealman, R.D., Risner, M.E. and Henningfield, J.E. (1983) Control of behaviour by intravenous nicotine injections in laboratory animals. *Pharmacology Biochem. Behav.,* **19**, 1011–20.

14. Henningfield, J.E. and Goldberg, S.R. (1983) Nicotine as a reinforcer in human subjects and laboratory animals. *Pharmacology Biochem. Behav.,* **19**, 989–92.

15. Henningfield, J.E., Miyasato, K. and Jasinski, D.R. (1983) Cigarette smokers self-administer intravenous nicotine. *Pharmacology Biochem. Behav.,* **19**, 887–90.

16. Benowitz, N.L., Hall, S.M., Herning, R.I. *et al.* (1983) Smokers of low-yield cigarettes do not consume less nicotine. *N. Engl. J. Med.,* **309**, 139–42.

17. Benowitz, N.L., Jacob, P III, Kozlowski, L.T. and Yu, L. (1986) Influence of smoking fewer cigarettes on exposure to tar, nicotine, and carbon monoxide. *N. Engl. J. Med.,* **315**, 1310–3.

18. Foulds, J., Stapleton, J., Feyerabend, C. *et al.* (1992) Effect of transdermal nicotine patches on cigarette smoking: a double blind crossover study. *Psychopharmacol.,* **106**, 421–7.

19. American Psychiatric Association (1987) *Diagnostic and Statistical Manual for Mental Disorders.* DSM-III-R (3rd edn revised), Washington D.C.

20. Hughes, J.R., Higgins, S.T and Hatsukami, D.K. (1990) Effects of abstinence from tobacco: a critical review, in *Research Advances in Alcohol and Drug Problems*, Vol. 10, (eds L.T. Koslowski, H. Annis, H.D Cappel *et al.*) Plenum Press, New York, pp. 317–98.

21. Hughes, J.R., Gust, S.W., Skoog, K. *et al.* (1991) Symptoms of tobacco withdrawal: a replication and extension. *Archives Gen. Psychiatry,* **48**, 52–9.

22. Lam, L., Sze, P.C., Sacks, H.S. *et al.* (1987) Meta-analysis of radomized controlled trials of nicotine chewing gum. *Lancet,* **ii**, 27–29.

23. Kozlowski, L.T., Wilkinson, D.A., Skinner, W. *et al.* (1989) Comparing tobacco cigarette dependence with other drug dependencies. *JAMA,* **261**, 898–901.

24. Royal College of Physicians (1992) *Smoking and the Young.* Lavenham Press, London.

25. Murray, D., Davis-Hearn, M., Goldman, A. *et al.* (1988) Four and five year follow-up results from four seventh grade smoking prevention strategies. *J. Behav. Med.,* **11**, 395–405.

26. Flay, B.R., Koeoke, D., Thomson, S.J. *et al.* (1989) Six year follow-up of the first Waterloo school smoking prevention trial. *Am. J. Public Health,* **79**, 1371–6.

27. Murray, D.M., Pirie, P., Luepker, R.V. *et al.* (1989) Five and six year follow-up results from four seventh grade smoking prevention strategies. *J. Behav. Med.,* **12**, 207–18.

28. Murray, D.M., Perry, C.L., Griffin, G. *et al.* (1992) Results from a statewide approach to adolescent tobacco use prevention. *Prev. Med.,* **21**, 449–72.

29. Smee, C. (1992) *Effect of Tobacco Advertising on Tobacco Consumption: a Discussion Document Reviewing the Evidence*, London, Economic and Operational Research Division, Department of Health.

30. Wald, N.J. (Chairman, Editorial Board) (1991) *Passive Smoking: a Health Hazard*, London,

Imperial Cancer Research Fund and Cancer Research Campaign.

31. Nelson, E.M. and Charlton, A. (1991) Children and advertising: does the voluntary agreement work? *Health Educ. J.*, **50**, 1.

32. Aitken, P.P., Leathar, D.S., O'Hagan, F.J. and Squair, S.I. (1987) Children's awareness of cigarette advertisements and brand imagery. *Br. J. Addict.* **82**, 615–22.

33. Jarvis, M.J. and McNeill, A.D. (1990) Children's purchases of single cigarettes: evidence for drug pushing? *Br. J. Addict.*, **85**, 1317–21.

34. Schwartz, J.L. (1987) *Review and Evaluation of Smoking Cessation Methods: the United States and Canada 1978–1985*, National Cancer Institute, Washington D.C.

35. Hatsukami, D.K., Dahlgren, L., Zimmerman, R. and Hughes, J.R. (1988) Symptoms of tobacco withdrawal from total cigarette cessation versus partial cigarette reduction. *Psychopharmacol.*, **94**, 242–7.

36. West, R.J., Russell, M.A.H., Jarvis, M.J. and Feyerabend, C. (1984) Does switching to an ultra-low nicotine cigarette induce nicotine withdrawal effects? *Psychopharmacol.*, **84**, 120–3.

37. Flaxman, J. (1978) Quitting smoking now or later: gradual, abrupt, immediate, and delayed quitting. *Behav. Ther.*, **9**, 260–70.

38. Hill, D., Weiss., Walker, D.L., and Jolley, D. (1988) Long-term evaluation of controlled smoking as a treatment outcome. *Br. J. Addict.*, **83**, 203–7.

39. Norregaard, J., Tonnesen, P., Somonsen, K. *et al.* (1992) Smoking habits in relapsed subjects from a smoking cessation trial after one year. *Br. J. Addict.*, **87**, 1189–94.

40. Slama, K., Redman, S., Perkins, J. *et al.* (1990) The effectiveness of two smoking cessation programmes for use in general practice: a randomised clinical trial. *Br. Med. J.*, **300**, 1707–9.

41. Marshall, A. and Raw, M. (1985) Nicotine chewing-gum in general practice: effect of follow-up appointments. *Br. Med. J.*, **290**, 1397–8.

42. Hall, S.M., Tunstall, C., Rugg, D. *et al.* (1985) Nicotine gum and behavioral treatment in smoking cessation. *J. Consult. Clin. Psychol.*, **53**, 256–8.

43. Fagerstrom, K. (1984) Effects of nicotine chewing-gum and follow-up appointments in physician-based smoking cessation. *Prev. Med.*, **13**, 517–27.

44. Hollis, J.F., Lichenstein, E., Mount, K. *et al.* (1991) Nurse-assisted smoking counseling in medical settings: minimizing demands on physicians. *Prev. Med.*, **20**, 497–500.

45. Gilbert, J.R., Wilson, D.M.C., Singer, J. *et al.* (1992) A family physician smoking cessation program: an evaluation of the role of follow-up visits. *Am. J. Prev. Med.*, **8**, 91–5.

46. Jamrozik, K., Vessey, M., Fowler, G. *et al.* (1984) Controlled trial of three different antismoking interventions in general practice. *Br. Med. J.*, **288**, 1499–503.

47. Jarvis, M.J., Belcher, M., Vesey, C. and Hutchison, D.C.S. (1986) Low cost carbon monoxide monitors in smoking assessment. *Thorax*, **41**, 886–7.

48. Jarvis, M.J., Russell, M.A.H. and Saloojee, Y. (1980) Expired air carbon monoxide: a simple breath test of tobacco smoke intake. *Br. Med. J.*, **281**, 484–5.

49. Hajek, P., Belcher, M. and Stapleton, J. (1985) Enhancing the impact of groups: an evaluation of two group formats for smokers. *Br. J. Clin. Psychol.*, **24**, 289–94.

50. Hajek, P. (1989) Withdrawal-oriented therapy for smokers. *Br. J. Addict.* **84**, 591–8.

51. Jarvis, M.J. and Russell, M.A.H. (1989) Treatment for the cigarette smoker. *Int. Rev. Psychiatry*, **1**, 139–47.

52. Jarvis, M.J., Raw, M., Russell, M.A.H. and Feyerabend, C. (1982) Randomised controlled trial of nicotine chewing gum. *Br. Med. J.*, **285**, 537–40.

53. Hughes, J.R., Gust, S.W., Keenan, R.M. *et al.* (1989) Nicotine vs placebo gum in general medical practice. *JAMA*, **261**, 1300–5.

54. Campbell, I.A., Prescott, R.J. and Tjeder-Burton, S.M. (1991) Smoking cessation in hospital patients given repeated advice plus nicotine or placebo chewing gum. *Respir. Med.*, **85**, 155–7.

55. British Thoracic Society (1983) Comparison of four methods of smoking withdrawal in patients with smoking related diseases. *Br. Med. J.*, **286**, 595–7.

56. Fiore, M.C., Jorenby, D.E., Baker, T.B. and Kenford, S.L. (1992) Tobacco dependence and the nicotine patch: clinical guidelines for effective use. *JAMA*, **286**, 2687–94.

57. Tonnesen, P., Norregaard, J., Simonsen, K. *et al.* (1991) A double-blind trial of a 16-h transdermal nicotine patch in smoking cessation. *N. Engl. J. Med.*, **325**, 311–15.

58. Abelin, T., Buehler, A., Muller, B. *et al.* (1989) Controlled trial of transdermal nicotine patch in tobacco withdrawal. *Lancet*, **i**, 7–10.

59. Campbell, I., Prescott, R.J. and Tjeder-Burton, S.M. (1992) Nicotine patches vs placebo in 234 hospital patients. *Thorax*, **47**, 886 (Abstract).

60. Foulds, J., Stapleton, T., Hayward, M. *et al.* (1993) Transdermal nicotine patches with low-intensity support to aid smoking cessation in outpatients in a general hospital: a placebo-controlled trial. *Arch. Fam. Med.*, **2**, 417–23.

61. Imperial Cancer Research Fund General Practice Research Group (1993) Effectiveness of a nicotine patch in helping people to stop smoking: results of a randomised trial in general practice. *Br. Med. J.*, **306**, 1304–8.

62. Russell, M.A.H., Stapleton, J.A., Feyerabend, C. *et al.* (1993) Targeting heavy smokers in general practice: randomised controlled trial of transdermal nicotine patches. *Br. Med. J.*, **306**, 1308–12.

63. Jarvis, M.J., Hajek, P., Russell, M.A.H. *et al.* (1987) Nasal nicotine solution as an aid to cigarette withdrawal: a pilot clinical trial. *Br. J. Addict.*, **82**, 983–8.

64. Sutherland, G., Stapleton, J.A., Russell, M.A.H. *et al.* (1992) Randomised controlled trial of nasal nicotine spray in smoking cessation. *Lancet*, **340**, 324–9.

65. Hajek, P., Jackson, P. and Belcher, M. (1988) Long term use of nicotine chewing gum: outcome, determinants and effect on weight gain. *JAMA*, **260**, 1593–6.

66. Huhtasaari, F., Asplund, K., Lundberg, V. *et al.* (1992) Tobacco and myocardial infarction: is snuff less dangerous than cigarettes? *Br. Med. J.*, **305**, 1252–6.

67. Sachs, D.P.L. and Leischow, J. (1991) Pharmacologic approaches to smoking cessation. *Clinics Chest Med.*, **12**, 769–91.

68. Russell, M.A.H., Wilson, C., Taylor, C. *et al.* (1979) Effect of general practitioners' advice against smoking. *Br. Med. J.*, **2**, 231–5.

69. Jarvis, M.J. (1994) Change in the addictions: does treatment make a difference? in *Addictions: Processes of Change*, (eds M. Lader and G. Edwards), Oxford University Press.

70. Russell, M.A.H., Merriman, R., Stapleton, J.A. *et al.* (1983) Effect of nicotine chewing gum as an adjunct to general practitioners' advice against smoking. *Br. Med. J.*, **287**, 1782–5.

71. Jackson, P.H., Stapleton, J.A., Russell, M.A.H. *et al.* (1986) Predictors of outcome in a General Practitioner intervention against smoking. *Prev. Med.*, **15**, 244–53.

72. Wilson, D.M.C., Taylor, D.W., Gilbert, J.R. *et al.* (1988) A randomized trial of a family physician intervention for smoking cessation. *JAMA*, **260**, 1570–4.

73. D'Agostino, R.B., Kannel, W.B., Belanger, A.J. *et al.* (1989) Trends in CHD risk factors at age 55–64 in the Framingham Study. *Int. J. Epidemiol.*, **18** (3, Suppl. 1) s67–s72.

74. Russell, M.A.H., Stapleton, J.A., Hajek, P. *et al.* (1988) District programme to reduce smoking: can sustained intervention by general practitioners affect prevalence? *J. Epidemiol. Community Health*, **42**, 111–5.

75. British Thoracic Society (1990) Smoking cessation in patients: Two further studies by the BTS. *Thorax*, **45**, 835–40.

BRONCHODILATORS: BASIC PHARMACOLOGY

P.J. Barnes

16.1 INTRODUCTION

Bronchodilators are widely used in the therapy of COPD and provide modest relief of symptoms and increase the exercise tolerance. The pharmacology of bronchodilators is largely concerned with the relaxation of airway smooth muscle, although it is increasingly recognized that bronchodilators may also affect other cell types. This chapter discusses the molecular, biochemical and clinical pharmacology of bronchodilators currently used in the treatment of COPD and also describes some novel bronchodilators under development.

Bronchodilator drugs have an 'anti-bronchoconstrictor' effect, which may be demonstrated directly *in vitro* by a relaxant effect on precontracted airway preparations. Bronchodilators cause immediate reversal of airway obstruction *in vivo*, and this is believed to be due to a direct effect on airway smooth muscle, although additional indirect effects on other airway cells (such as reduced microvascular leakage, reduced release of bronchoconstrictor mediators from inflammatory cells and reduced neurotransmitter release) may contribute to the reduction in airway narrowing. In COPD the most important spasmogen is likely to be acetylcholine released from cholinergic nerves in the airway, although it is possible that other spasmogens such as neuropeptides, certain inflammatory mediators and peptides such as endothelin may also be contributory.

Only three types of bronchodilator are in current clinical use:

β-adrenoceptor agonists (sympathomimetics)
Methylxanthines (theophylline)
Anticholinergic drugs

Drugs such as sodium cromoglycate, which prevent bronchoconstriction in some patients with mild asthma, have no direct bronchodilator action and are ineffective once bronchoconstriction has occurred. Corticosteroids, while gradually improving airway obstruction in asthmatic patients, have no direct effect on contraction of airway smooth muscle and are not therefore considered to be bronchodilators. The potential role of anti-inflammatory treatments in COPD is currently under investigation and is discussed in Chapter 18.

16.2 β-ADRENOCEPTOR AGONISTS

β-Adrenoceptor agonists are the most widely used bronchodilator agents for the relief of airway obstruction. While in asthma they are clearly the most effective agents available, in COPD they are often similar in efficacy to anticholinergics.

Chronic Obstructive Pulmonary Disease. Edited by Dr P. Calverley and Professor N. Pride. Published in 1995 by Chapman & Hall, London. ISBN 0 412 46450 0

16.2.1 CHEMISTRY

The development of β_2-agonists was a logical development of substitutions in the catecholamine structure. The catechol ring consists of hydroxyl groups in the 3 and 4 positions of the benzene ring (Fig. 16.1). Noradrenaline differs from adrenaline only in the terminal amine group, which therefore indicates that modification at this site confers β-receptor selectivity. Further substitution of the terminal amine resulted in β_2-receptor selectivity, as in salbutamol and terbutaline.

Endogenous catecholamines are rapidly removed by two active uptake processes.

1. *Uptake*$_1$ is localized to sympathetic nerve terminals and noradrenaline is rapidly returned to storage vesicles.
2. *Uptake*$_2$ facilitates uptake into non-neural tissue, such as smooth muscle cells, where enzymatic degradation occurs.

Isoprenaline is not a substrate for uptake$_1$, but is avidly taken up by uptake$_2$, whereas non-catecholamine β-agonists (such as salbutamol) are not taken up by either process.

Catecholamines are rapidly metabolized by the enzyme catechol-o-methyl transferase (COMT), which methylates in the 3-hydroxyl position, and accounts for the short duration of action of catecholamines. Modification of the catechol ring, as in salbutamol and terbutaline, prevents this degradation and therefore prolongs their effect. Catecholamines are also broken down by monoamine oxidase (MAO) in sympathetic nerve terminals and in the gastrointestinal tract which cleaves the side chain. Isoprenaline, which is a substrate for MAO, is therefore metabolized in the gut, making absorption variable. Substitution in the amine group confers resistance to MAO and ensures reliable absorption. Many other β_2-selective agonists have now been introduced and, while there may be differences in potency, there are no clinically significant differences in selectivity. Inhaled β_2-selective drugs in current clinical use (apart from rimiterol which is broken down by COMT) have a similar duration of action.

Recently, inhaled β_2-selective drugs which have a much longer duration of effect (over 12 hours), such as salmeterol and formoterol,

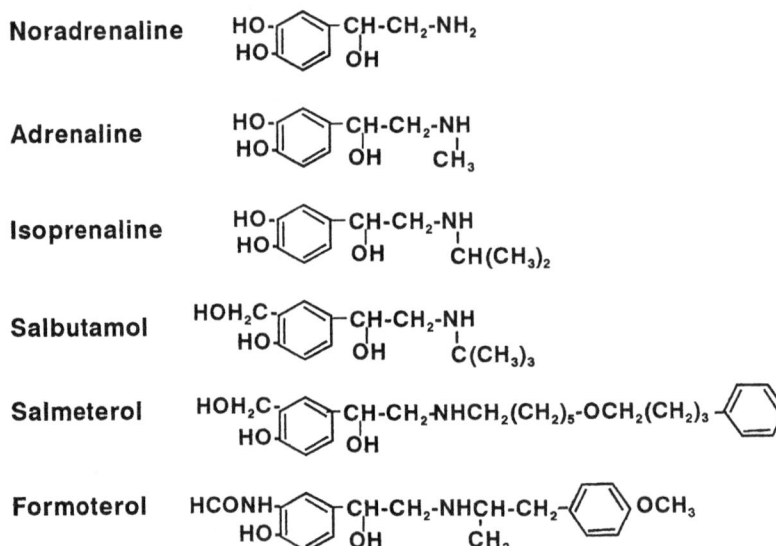

Fig. 16.1 Chemical structure of some adrenergic agonists showing development from catecholamines.

have been developed and are now available in several countries [1]. The mechanism for their long duration of action may be related to a high lipophilicity, which may keep the molecule in the vicinity of the receptor.

16.2.2 MECHANISM OF ACTION

$β$-Agonists produce all their effects via the activation of surface $β$-receptors. Their major target is airway smooth muscle, although it is now recognized that they may have additional therapeutic effects on other cell types [2].

(a) Airway smooth muscle

Autoradiographic studies have demonstrated the presence of $β$-receptors in airway smooth muscle of animal and human airways from the trachea down to terminal bronchioles [3,4]. In some species both $β_1$ and $β_2$-receptors have been demonstrated functionally in airway smooth muscle; the presence of $β_1$-receptors is related to the presence of sympathetic innervation of airway smooth muscle [5]. Human airway smooth muscle lacks a functional sympathetic innervation and this is consistent with the autoradiographic evidence that in humans only $β_2$-receptors are expressed in smooth muscle at all airway levels [6]. Recent studies have demonstrated the expression of the $β_2$-receptor gene in cultured human airway smooth muscle cells using Northern blotting and in airway smooth muscle by *in situ hybridization* [7]. The amount of $β_2$-receptor mRNA in airway smooth muscle is high relative to the low receptor density; this may indicate a rapid turnover of $β_2$-receptors and may account for the relative resistance of airway smooth muscle to desensitization (or tolerance). Functional studies also demonstrate that relaxation of both central and peripheral human airways is mediated solely via $β_2$-receptors [8]. $β$-Agonists act as functional antagonists and inhibit or reverse the con-

tractile response irrespective of the constricting stimulus.

The intracellular mechanisms involved in mediating the relaxant effect of $β$-agonists in airway smooth muscle have recently been elucidated (Fig. 16.2). $β$-Receptor stimulation increases intracellular cyclic AMP which activates protein kinase A (PKA). PKA phosphorylates several proteins in the cell resulting in relaxation [9]. In airway smooth muscle PKA directly inhibits myosin light chain phosphorylation [10], inhibits phosphoinositide hydrolysis and thereby reduces intracellular Ca^{2+} release [11], promotes Ca^{2+}/Na^+ exchange [12], thus resulting in a fall in intracellular Ca^{2+}, and stimulates Na^+/K^+ ATPase [13]. These effects are observed at relatively high concentrations of $β$-agonist when maximal relaxation responses have been exceeded. An important effect of $β$-agonists is the opening of membrane potassium (K^+) channels. Charybdotoxin and iberiotoxin, which are selective blockers of large conductance Ca^{2+}-activated K^+ channels (maxi-K channels) inhibit the bronchodilator responses to $β$-agonists and to other agents which elevate cyclic AMP [14,15]. These effects are observed at low concentrations of $β$-agonists in human airways *in vitro*, suggesting that this is a major mechanism of airway smooth muscle response to $β$-agonists [16]. Patch clamp studies have confirmed that elevation of cyclic AMP opens a maxi-K channel in airway smooth muscle cells [17]. More recently evidence has been obtained that $β$-receptors may activate the maxi-K channel in airway smooth muscle cells directly via the $α$-subunit of G_s [18]. This suggests that relaxation of airway smooth muscle may occur independently of a rise in intracellular cyclic AMP and explains why there is a discrepancy between the low concentration of $β$-agonists needed to relax airway smooth muscle and the relatively high concentrations needed to elevate cyclic AMP concentrations. Furthermore it explains why forskolin, which causes a large increase in intracellular cyclic AMP

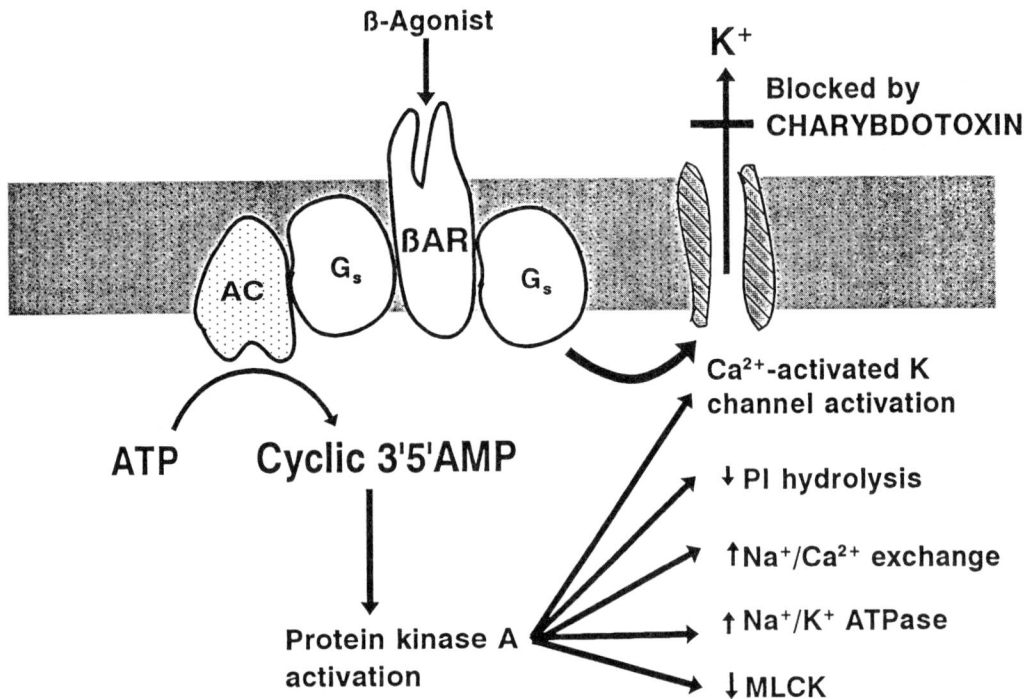

Fig. 16.2 Molecular mechanisms of action of β-agonists on airway smooth muscle cells. β-Agonists activate surface β-receptors which are coupled to adenylyl cyclase (AC) via a coupling protein (G_s). This causes an increase in cyclic AMP which activates protein kinase A (PKA) which then phosphorylates several substrates leading to molecular events that result in relaxation. β-Receptors may also directly be coupled via G_s to a large conductance potassium channel (K_{Ca}).

concentration in airway smooth muscle, is a relatively poor bronchodilator [19].

(b) Effects on nerves

β-Agonists may also modulate neurotransmission in airways via prejunctional receptors on airway nerves [20]. In canine and feline airways exogenous noradrenaline and endogenously-released catecholamines inhibit cholinergic nerve-induced bronchoconstriction to a greater extent than an equivalent contraction induced by acetylcholine, indicating a pre-junctional effect. This effect in dogs is mediated via pre-junctional β_1-receptors localized to postganglionic cholinergic nerves [21], although other studies suggest that β_2-receptors are also involved

[22]. β-Agonists may also modulate neurotransmission in parasympathetic ganglia via an effect on preganglionic nerve endings [23]. In human airways β-agonists modulate cholinergic neurotransmission *in vitro* via prejunctional β_2-receptors on postganglionic cholinergic nerves [24,25]. Although there are close anatomic associations between adrenergic and cholinergic nerves in human airways [26], stimulation of endogenous noradrenaline release from sympathetic nerves by tyramine has no modulatory effect [24]. It is more likely that circulating adrenaline regulates prejunctional β_2-receptors in human airways.

β-Agonists may also have effects on sensory nerves. β-Agonists inhibit excitatory non-adrenergic non-cholinergic (NANC) bronchoconstrictor responses in guinea-pig bronchi *in vitro* at concentrations which do not block equivalent tachykinin-induced responses [27]. This modulatory effect is mediated via a β_2-receptor on capsaicin-sensitive sensory nerves in the airways [27], although recently some evidence has suggested that an atypical β-receptor (β_3) may be involved [28]. Whether β-receptors modulate sensory nerves in human airways is not certain. Some evidence which suggests that β_2-receptors may be modulatory is provided by the inhibitory action of salbutamol on cough responses [29]. However an inhaled β_2-agonist, even in a high dose, has no additional protective effect on inhaled metabisulphite (which is believed to act on airway sensory nerves) than on methacholine challenge [30].

(c) Effects on vessels

β-Agonists are vasodilators and their vasodilator action within the pulmonary circulation may have a potentially deleterious effect in patients with COPD, particularly during exacerbations, since the reversal of hypoxic vasoconstriction in poorly ventilated areas may result in increased shunting of blood and increased hypoxemia. In practice the effect of high dose nebulized β-agonists in decreasing PaO_2 is usually small (<5 mmHg), although in occasional patients greater falls are observed [31]. Any fall in PaO_2 can be reversed by increasing the inspired oxygen concentration [31].

β-Agonists are also vasodilators in the bronchial circulation. This may be a potential disadvantage since theoretically this might increase plasma exudation by increased delivery of blood to leaky postcapillary venules and increase the thickness of airway tissue by increasing the blood volume. In fact β-agonists have been found to reduce plasma exudation in rodent airways after inhalation, probably due to a direct effect on postcapillary venular endothelial cells [32,33].

(d) Effects on inflammatory cells

The effect of β-agonists on airway inflammation is a controversial area [34], partly because of the differing understanding of what inflammation involves. The role of inflammation in COPD is less well defined than in asthma. Since β-agonists are clearly capable of inhibiting plasma exudation in the airways in response to inflammatory mediators they must be considered to be anti-inflammatory. β-Agonists also inhibit mast cells which participate in the acute allergic inflammatory response. However, β-agonists have little or no effect on the chronic inflammatory response which underlies airway hyperresponsiveness and chronic asthma. This is most clearly demonstrated by biopsy studies which show that regular treatment with β-agonists, including salmeterol, fails to resolve the inflammatory process as judged by the presence of activated mast cells, eosinophils and macrophages [35,36].

β-Agonists inhibit the release of histamine from chopped human lung and dispersed human lung mast cells via β_2-receptors [37]. Whether these *in vitro* studies are relevant to *in vivo* use of β-agonists is less certain. Inhaled salbutamol inhibits the increase in plasma histamine induced by allergen exposure in asthmatic patients [38], but there are some doubts about the interpretation of plasma histamine measurements. Urinary leukotriene E_4 excretion may be a more accurate reflection of airway mediator release after allergen exposure, but the effects of inhaled β-agonists are relatively small [39]. Functional evidence suggests that inhaled β-agonists may have an effect on mast cells *in vivo* since a nebulized β-agonist has a significantly greater effect on adenosine 5'-monophosphate- (AMP) induced bronchoconstriction than on histamine- or methacholine-induced bronchoconstriction [30]. This increased protective effect is also seen after the normal therapeutic dose of β-agonist from a metered dose inhaler [30]. The increased protection against AMP challenge compared with the directly acting constrictors may reflect an additional effect on airway mast cells, since adenosine and AMP cause bronchoconstriction indirectly via the release of histamine from mast cells.

β-Agonists also have inhibitory effects on eosinophils [40] and lymphocytes [41], but these effects are small and usually rapidly desensitized. β-Agonists do not inhibit alveolar macrophages [42]. These findings are consistent with the view that β-agonists do not have a useful therapeutic effect on chronic inflammation of the airways.

(e) Airway secretions

β-Agonists increase mucus secretion from submucosal glands in human airways [43] and ion transport across airway epithelium [44]. In addition β-agonists may increase ciliary beat frequency in cultured human airway epithelial cells [45]. These effects may enhance mucociliary clearance, and therefore reverse any defect in clearance found in COPD. However, β-agonists appear to selectively stimulate mucous rather than serous cells, which may result in a more viscous mucus secretion [46].

16.2.3 SAFETY OF β-AGONISTS

Because of a possible relationship between adrenergic drug therapy and the rise in asthma deaths in several countries during the early 1960s, doubts have been cast on the safety of β-agonists in patients with airway obstruction. A causal relationship between β-agonists use and mortality has never been established, although in retrospective studies this would not be possible. More recently, these doubts have been revived and the use of high doses of β-agonists given by nebulizers at home was linked to the increase in asthma deaths in New Zealand. However, there is no convincing evidence that nebulized β-agonists directly contribute to

asthma deaths, which can usually be ascribed to underestimation and under-treatment of the disease. There has never been any convincing evidence that β-agonists cause death by inducing cardiac arrhythmias, and in asthma patients who had near-death episodes there was no evidence for dangerous arrhythmias [47].

A particular β2-agonist, fenoterol, has been linked to the recent rise in asthma deaths in New Zealand since significantly more of the fatal cases were prescribed fenoterol than the case-matched control patients [48,49]. However, the evidence is controversial and it is likely that any increased risk in mortality may be explained by the fact that fenoterol, as a more potent bronchodilator, was used in more severe asthmatics who are at higher risk. A recent study based in Saskatchewan, Canada, examined the links between drugs dispensed for asthma and death or near-death from asthma attacks, based on computerized records of prescriptions. There was a marked increase in the risk of death with high doses of all inhaled β-agonists [50]. The risk was greater with fenoterol, but when the dose was adjusted to the equivalent dose for salbutamol there was no significant difference in the risk for these two drugs. The link between high β-agonist usage and increased asthma mortality does not prove a causal association, since patients with more severe and poorly controlled asthma, and who are therefore more likely to have an increased risk of fatal attacks, are more likely to be using higher doses of β-agonist inhalers and less likely to be using effective anti-inflammatory treatment. Indeed in the patients who used regular inhaled steroids there was a significant reduction in risk of death.

Recent evidence suggests that the regular use of inhaled β-agonists may increase asthma morbidity. In a study carried out in New Zealand the regular use of fenoterol was associated with poorer control and a small increase in airway hyperresponsiveness compared with patients using fenoterol 'on demand' for symptom control [51]. Another study showed that regular salbutamol was associated with a more rapid decline in lung function over a period of two years compared with use of salbutamol 'on demand' in both COPD and asthma patients [52]. A similar finding was obtained with an anticholinergic bronchodilator. Other studies have shown that regular inhaled β-agonists (salbutamol or terbutaline) are associated with a rebound increase in airway responsiveness [53–55], although the magnitude of the changes described is small and of doubtful clinical significance.

These concerns about inhaled β-agonists indicate that further research is needed with carefully controlled trials in large numbers of patients [34]. It is now clear that inhaled β_2-agonists of short or long duration do not suppress the underlying inflammation of asthma in the way steroids do [35,36], and yet they may control the symptoms of asthma. The position of β-agonists in patients with COPD is even less clear as no significant studies have addressed the issue.

16.2.4 TOLERANCE

Continuous treatment with an agonist often leads to tolerance or subsensitivity, which may be due to down-regulation of the receptor. For this reason there have been many studies of bronchial β-receptor function after prolonged therapy with β-agonists [56]. Tolerance of non-airway β-receptor responses, such as tremor and cardiovascular and metabolic responses, is readily induced in normal and asthmatic subjects. But whether tolerance of airway β-receptors occurs is debatable. Tolerance of human airway smooth muscle to β-agonists *in vitro* has been demonstrated, although the concentration of agonist necessary is high and the degree of desensitization is variable [57,58]. Animal studies suggest that airway β-receptors may be more resistant to desensitization than β-receptors elsewhere [59].

In normal subjects bronchodilator tolerance has been demonstrated in some studies after high dose inhaled salbutamol, but not in others. In asthmatic patients tolerance to the bronchodilator effects of β-agonists has not usually been found. However, even when tolerance has been demonstrated, the effect is very small and probably clinically insignificant; the more readily demonstrable tolerance of extrapulmonary effects has the benefit that side-effects tend to disappear with continued use. Recent evidence suggests that tolerance develops to the mast cell stabilizing effect of β-agonists, but not to the bronchodilator effect [60]; this might explain why intermittent use of β-agonists may be more effective than regular use in asthma. The relative resistance of airway smooth muscle β-receptors to desensitization may reflect the high level of β_2-receptor gene expression in airway smooth muscle cells [7].

Although tolerance to the bronchodilator effects of long-acting β_2-agonists has not been reported [61,62], the protective effect of salmeterol against methacholine challenge appears to be reduced after 4 weeks of administration [63].

The mechanisms of tolerance have been investigated at a molecular level. Short-term desensitization involves uncoupling of the β-receptor via phosphorylation of the receptor and its G-protein through the activation of specific kinases [64], but longer exposure to β-agonists results in reduced messenger RNA levels due to reduced stability [65]. Even more prolonged exposure to β-agonists results in down-regulation of β-receptors in lung with reduced gene transcription [59].

Experimental studies have shown that corticosteroids prevent the development of tolerance in airway smooth muscle, and prevent and reverse the fall in pulmonary β-receptor density [66,67]. Thus, any tendency for tolerance to develop with high dose inhaled β-agonists should be prevented by concomitant administration of corticosteroids.

16.3 ANTICHOLINERGICS

Anticholinergic drugs are useful broncho-dilators in patients with COPD and may be as effective as β-agonists.

16.3.1 CHOLINERGIC MECHANISMS

Cholinergic nerves are the dominant neural bronchoconstrictor pathway in animal and human airways [68], and there has been considerable interest in why airway cholinergic mechanisms are exaggerated in COPD. Many triggers which induce bronchospasm (such as sulfur dioxide, prostaglandins, histamine and cold air) also stimulate sensory receptors in the airways and may therefore lead to reflex cholinergic bronchoconstriction [69].

(a) Neural pathways

Cholinergic motor nerves arise in the nucleus ambiguus of the brain stem and travel down the vagus nerve to relay in parasympathetic ganglia which are situated within the airways. From these intrinsic ganglia short postganglionic fibres innervate the target cells, such as airway smooth muscle, bronchial vessels and submucosal glands (Fig. 16.3). In animals and normal human subjects there is a certain degree of resting cholinergic tone which may be demonstrated by vagus nerve section or by administration of atropine which blocks the effect of endo-genously released acetylcholine on mus-carinic receptors.

Cholinergic innervation is greatest in large airways and diminishes peripherally [68]. Studies in animals have demonstrated that cholinergic nerve effects are greatest in large airways and minimal in small airways. Receptor mapping studies have demonstrated a high density of muscarinic receptors in smooth muscle of large airways, but few in peripheral airways of ferrets [70], although in human airways muscarinic receptors are also seen in peripheral airways [71]. In humans, studies which have tried to distinguish large and small airway effects have shown that cholinergic bronchoconstriction predomi-nantly involves larger airways, whereas β-ag-onists are equally effective in large and small airways [72]. This relative diminution of cholinergic control in small airways may have important clinical implications, since anti-cholinergic drugs should be less useful than β-agonists when bronchoconstriction in-volves small airways, as seems likely in COPD.

(b) Reflex bronchoconstriction

Cholinergic efferent pathways may be activated reflexly via stimulation of afferent nerves both within and outside the airways. There may be increased cholinergic reflex bronchoconstriction due to stimulation of sensory receptors in the airways. A wide variety of stimuli are able to elicit reflex cholinergic bronchoconstriction [73]. Sensory afferent endings, which include irritant receptors and unmyelinated nerve endings (C-fibers), are found in airway epithelium, larynx and nasopharynx [74]. Sensory receptors may be triggered by many stimuli, including dust, cigarette smoke, mechanical stimulation and mediators such as histamine, prostaglandins and bradykinin, which will lead to reflex bronchoconstriction. Reflex bronchoconstriction may be inhibited by anti-cholinergic drugs, which may therefore have a variable effect on airway obstruction which will be dependent on the degree of chol-inergic reflex bronchoconstriction. Recent neurophysiologic studies with single fiber recording suggest that bradykinin may be the most important activator of C-fibers in the airways [75]. The role of inflammatory media-tors in COPD is less certain, but it is possible that bradykinin may be formed from exuded plasma, or may be secreted from mucus-secreting glands.

Reflex bronchoconstriction may also be initiated from sensory receptors in the larynx,

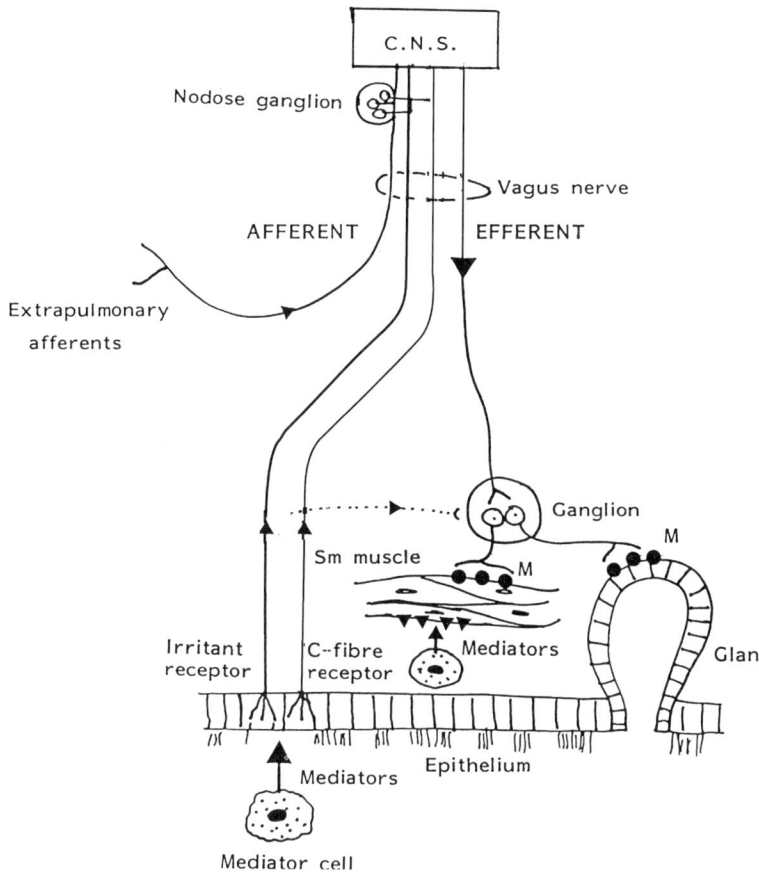

Fig. 16.3 Cholinergic neural pathways arise in the brain stem, travel down the vagus nerve and relay in parasympathetic ganglia within the airway wall. Short postganglionic fibers innervate target organs such as airway smooth muscle and submucosal glands. Cholinergic pathways may be activated reflexly via afferent receptors in the airways. (M = muscarinic receptors.)

nose and esophagus. Rhinitis may exacerbate airway obstruction through enhanced cholinergic reflex bronchoconstriction. There is evidence that esophageal acid reflux may exacerbate asthma through cholinergic mechanisms, since anticholinergic drugs inhibit the bronchoconstriction associated with reflux ('the reflux reflex') [76].

(c) Acetylcholine release

Acetylcholine is released from airway sensory nerves and acts on muscarinic receptors on target cells. The release of acetylcholine may be modulated via a number of prejunctional receptors [20]. Inflammatory mediators and neuropeptides released from airway nerves may either increase or decrease acetylcholine release.

16.3.2 CHOLINERGIC MECHANISMS IN COPD

Since cholinergic nerves are the predominant neural bronchoconstrictor mechanism it is not surprising that they are involved in obstructive diseases of the airways. In COPD there is

structural narrowing of airways which is irreversible. This appears to be a combination
of fibrosis, particularly in peripheral airways,
and muscle hyperplasia, whereas in emphysema it is due to narrowing of peripheral
airways due to loss of elastic recoil provided
by the alveolar wall attachments. In addition,
there is a degree of vagal bronchomotor tone.
While, in normal airways, this tone has little
effect on airway caliber, when the airways are
narrowed the same degree of tone will have a
much more marked effect on airway resistance (which is inversely proportional to the
fourth power of the radius) (Fig. 16.4).
Reversing this tone by anticholinergic drugs
will, therefore, have a significant beneficial
effect. The relative benefit of anticholinergic
drugs versus β-agonists is likely to be greater
in COPD than in asthma, in which additional
factors (such as direct effects of mediators
such as leukotriene D_4 on airway smooth
muscle) are likely to be operative. There is
some day-to-day variability in airway function in patients with COPD and evidence that
anticholinergics reduce this variability which
may suggest that changes in vagal cholinergic
tone are the major determinant of this variability [77]. Anticholinergics are as effective
as β_2-agonists in exacerbations of COPD indicating that, as in asthmatic patients, the major
component of increased airway obstruction is
due to an increase in cholinergic tone [78].

Anticholinergic drugs usually cause bronchodilatation in normal subjects and patients
with asthma and COPD. The extent of bronchodilatation is variable between individuals,
which presumably reflects the degree of vagal
tone. Anticholinergic drugs are competitive
antagonists of acetylcholine, so the bronchodilator effect is related to the dose given
until maximal blockade of endogenous acetylcholine is obtained. In asthmatic patients the
degree of bronchodilatation seen with anticholinergic drugs is less marked than with β-
agonists (which will relax airway smooth
muscle irrespective of the constrictor stimuli).
This may demonstrate that airway narrowing

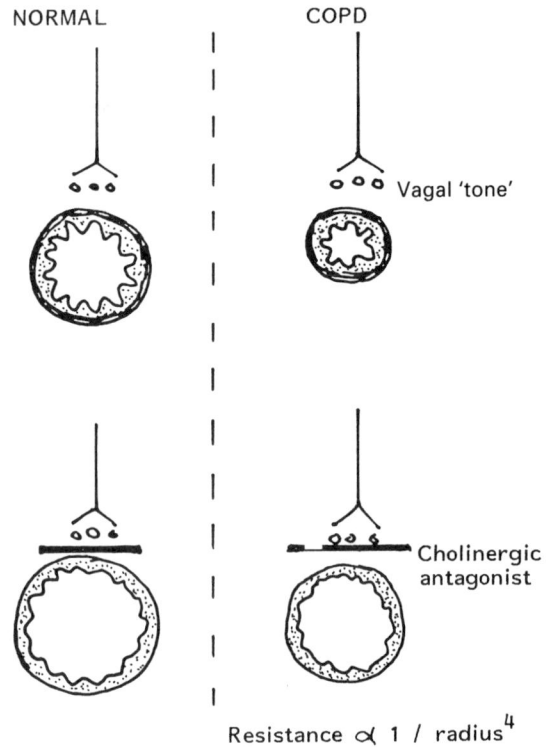

$$\text{Resistance} \propto 1 \: / \: \text{radius}^4$$

Fig. 16.4 Normal airways have a certain amount
of cholinergic tone, resulting in a small degree of
airway narrowing which is revealed by a small
bronchodilator response to anticholinergics. In
COPD, in which there is fixed narrowing of the
airways, the same amount of cholinergic tone will
have a greater effect on airway resistance for geometric reasons. Conversely anticholinergics will
have a relatively greater bronchodilator effect. In
COPD cholinergic tone may be the only reversible
component of airway narrowing.

in asthma is due to more factors than vagal
tone alone. In COPD, however, anticholinergics may produce equivalent or even greater
bronchodilatation than β-agonists since vagal
tone is the major reversible element in such
patients [79]. Anticholinergics often appear to
be of similar efficacy to β-agonists in COPD
patients [80,81], and sometimes an even
greater improvement has been reported with
anticholinergics [82,83], although very few
studies have investigated dose–response relationships (Chapter 17).

The reason why anticholinergics sometimes have a greater effect on airway function in COPD is uncertain, since if cholinergic tone were the only reversible component it may be predicted that β_2-agonists would be equally effective in inhibiting cholinergic tone. Perhaps anticholinergics might have a greater effect than β-agonists in COPD because of some additional effect on mucus secretion. Cholinergic agonists are potent stimulants of mucus secretion in human airways *in vitro* [80,84], and act predominantly on submucosal glands which are the major source of mucus in proximal airways. In more peripheral airways the only source of airway mucus is epithelial goblet cells, and there is evidence in animals that these are under cholinergic control [85]. In addition cigarette smoke is a potent stimulus to goblet cell discharge in animals and the effects of the particulate phase are mediated by a cholinergic reflex [86]. If the same applies to human airways, it is possible that inhaled anticholinergics reduce goblet cell secretions and thereby improve the airway obstruction in peripheral airways.

Although the onset of bronchodilatation after anticholinergic drugs may be slower than after a β-agonist, the duration of bronchodilatation may be greater than 8 hours and therefore significantly longer than conventional inhaled β_2-agonists such as salbutamol [80]. This may be used to advantage when the two drugs are used in combination. The prolonged duration of bronchodilatation compared with β-agonists may be of advantage in these patients. It is likely that the fall in lung function which occurs at night in patients with COPD [87] may also benefit from high-dose anticholinergic drugs given at night, since an increase in vagal tone is the most likely mechanism for the increased nocturnal bronchoconstriction [88,89].

16.3.3 MUSCARINIC RECEPTOR SUBTYPES

Cholinergic effects on the airways are mediated by muscarinic receptors on target cells in the airways [90,91]. More is now known about muscarinic receptor structure, and muscarinic receptors have now been cloned [92]. Recently, several different subtypes of muscarinic receptor have been distinguished, raising the possibility of developing more selective anticholinergic agents. In the airways, smooth muscle muscarinic receptor activation results in rapid phosphoinositide hydrolysis [93–95] and the formation of inositol (1,4,5) trisphosphate which releases calcium ions from intracellular stores. Muscarinic receptor activation also inhibits adenylyl cyclase and therefore reduces cyclic AMP in airway smooth muscle [96], which may counteract the bronchodilator effects of β-agonists (Fig. 16.5). These two biochemical events are mediated by different receptor subtypes in airway smooth muscle.

Muscarinic receptors mediate the mucus secretory response to vagus nerve stimulation. Cholinergic agonists are potent secretagogues and stimulate mucus secretion from submucosal glands [97] and also from goblet cells in the epithelium, which are the major source of mucus in peripheral airways [85].

With the development of selective drugs, subclasses of muscarinic receptors have now been demonstrated in many tissues [92]. Receptor subtypes have been cloned and expressed, and at least 5 distinct receptor proteins have now been recognized in animal and human tissues [92]. Three distinct subtypes of receptor have been recognized pharmacologically in humans. M_1-receptors are pirenzepine-sensitive and are usually localized to neuronal structures. M_2-receptors are present in atrium and mediate the heart rate slowing with cholinergic stimulation. M_2-receptors are selectively blocked by AF-DX 116, methoctramine or gallamine and are different from muscarinic receptors on smooth muscle (M_3-receptors) which are sensitive to 4-diphenylocetoxy-N-methyl-piperidine methiodide (4-DAMP) and hexahydro-siladifenidol. All three muscarinic

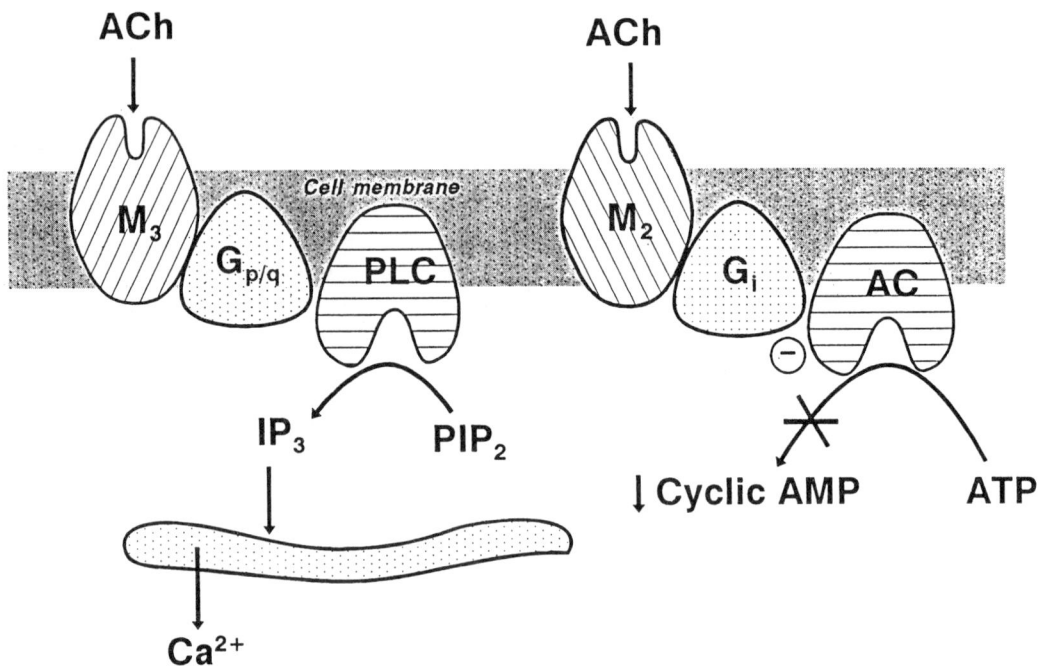

Fig. 16.5 Coupling of muscarinic receptors in airway smooth muscle cells. Muscarinic receptors (M_3-receptors) may be coupled via G-proteins to phospholipase C (PLC), leading to formation of inositol 1,4,5 triphosophate (IP_3) and release of intracellular calcium ions. M_2-receptors are coupled via G_i to inhibition of adenylyl cyclase (AC), resulting in a fall in cyclic AMP which may increase contractile responses.

receptor subtypes have now been described in airways [91,98], but their precise relevance to airway disease and therapy is not yet certain.

(a) M_1-receptors

The discovery that the muscarinic antagonist pirenzepine was able to discriminate between high and low affinity muscarinic receptor binding sites [99] supported previous suggestions that subtypes of muscarinic receptor might exist. Receptors with a high affinity for pirenzepine, which are designated M_1-receptors, are found in cerebral cortex and autonomic ganglia, in contrast to lower affinity receptors which predominate in heart and smooth muscle (which were therefore all classified by exclusion as M_2-receptors). M_1-receptors are usually localized to neurones

and in the peripheral nervous system have been demonstrated in autonomic ganglia. There is evidence for facilitatory M_1-receptors on parasympathetic ganglia in rabbit bronchi [100]. M_1-receptors may also be present in human airway ganglia, since inhaled pirenzepine has a much greater inhibitory effect on reflex bronchoconstriction (triggered by SO_2 inhalation) than on bronchoconstriction due to the direct effect of inhaled methacholine, whereas the non-selective ipratropium bromide is equally effective on both challenges [101].

The physiologic role of the M_1-receptors in ganglia is still not certain. Classically, ganglionic transmission is via nicotinic cholinergic receptors which are blocked by hexamethonium. It is possible that excitatory M_1-receptors are facilitatory to nicotinic receptors and may be involved in 'setting' the

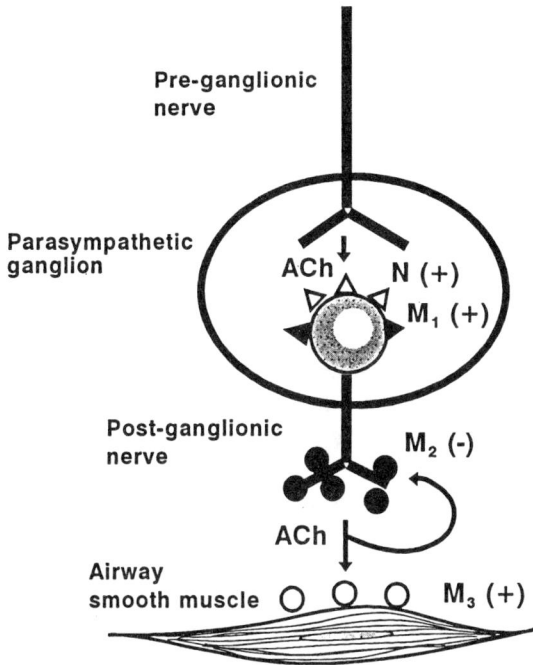

Fig. 16.6 Muscarinic receptor subtypes in airways. Ganglionic transmission is mediated via nicotinic receptors (N), but M_1-receptors may play a facilitatory role. M_2-receptors at the postganglionic terminal may inhibit the release of acetylcholine (ACh), which acts on M_3-receptors on airway smooth muscle.

efficacy of ganglionic transmission. Activation of these receptors probably closes K^+ channels, resulting in a slow depolarization of the ganglion cell [102]. Perhaps they might be involved in the chronic regulation of cholinergic tone, whereas nicotinic receptors (which act as 'fast' receptors and open ion channels) are more important in rapid signalling, such as occurs during reflex activation of the cholinergic pathway (Fig. 16.6). If so, then M_1-antagonists such as pirenzepine and telenzepine might have a useful therapeutic role in asthma and COPD, since they may reduce vagal tone. Since increased vagal tone may be important in COPD, M_1-selective antagonists might prove to be efficacious. A recent study has found

that telenzepine had no significant beneficial effect on airway function in patients with COPD however [103].

The results of binding studies in lung are unexpected. Binding of the non-selective muscarinic antagonist [³H]quinuclidinyl benzilate in human peripheral lung membranes is displaced by pirenzepine with a shallow inhibitory curve, suggesting the presence of high and low affinity sites [104]. The high affinity binding site has the characteristic expected of an M_1-receptor and this is confirmed by the use of [³H]pirenzepine to label the receptors. M_1-receptors make up more than half of the binding sites in lung of both species which cannot be accounted for by receptors on airway ganglia or nerves, which would make up only a small fraction of the membranes. Autoradiographic mapping studies suggest that M_1-receptors in human airways are present on submucosal glands, and are also seen in alveolar walls [71]. These autoradiographic studies have recently been supported by *in situ* hybridization studies using cDNA and oligonucleotide probes, which hybridize to the specific messenger RNA encoded by the genes for the different muscarinic receptor subtypes [105]. In human lung M_1-receptor mRNA is localized to submucosal glands and to alveolar walls, whereas in rabbit lung the muscarinic receptors localized to the peripheral lung appear to belong to the M_4-receptor subtype (Mak and Barnes, unpublished), which corresponds with recent functional data in this species [106].

(b) M_2-receptors

Muscarinic receptors which inhibit the release of acetylcholine from cholinergic nerves have been described in the gut [107]. Such muscarinic autoreceptors have also been described in the airways, and have been characterized as M_2-receptors, thus differing from the muscarinic receptor subtypes on airway smooth muscle which are classified as M_3-

receptors [20]. These muscarinic receptors appear to be located prejunctionally on post-ganglionic parasympathetic nerves and have a powerful inhibitory influence on acetylcholine release (Fig. 16.6). Muscarinic autoreceptors have been demonstrated in guinea pig [108–110], cat [111], rat [112] and dog [22,113]. The presence of prejunctional M_2-receptors on airway cholinergic nerves has recently been confirmed in guinea-pig trachea by direct measurement of acetylcholine release [114,115].

Similar feedback inhibitory receptors have also been localized to postganglionic cholinergic nerves in human airways *in vitro* [109]. In normal subjects pilocarpine, which selectively stimulates the prejunctional receptors, has an inhibitory effect on cholinergic reflex bronchoconstriction induced by SO_2, suggesting that these inhibitory receptors are present *in vivo*, and presumably serve to limit cholinergic bronchoconstriction [116]. Other evidence now also supports this observation [117]. In asthmatic patients pilocarpine has no such inhibitory action, indicating that there might be some dysfunction of the autoreceptor, which would result in exaggerated cholinergic reflex bronchoconstriction [116, 118]. A functional defect in muscarinic autoreceptors may also explain why β-blockers produce such marked bronchoconstriction in asthmatic patients, since any increase in cholinergic tone due to blockade of inhibitory β-receptors on cholinergic nerves would normally be switched off by M_2-receptors in the nerves, and a lack of such receptors may lead to increased acetylcholine release, resulting in exaggerated bronchoconstriction [119]. Support for this idea is provided by the protective effect of oxitropium bromide against propranolol-induced bronchoconstriction in asthmatic patients [120]. Whether there may be a similar defect in muscarinic autoreceptors in patients with COPD has not yet been determined.

The mechanism by which M_2-autoreceptors on cholinergic nerves may become dysfunc-

tional is not certain. It is possible that chronic inflammation in airways may lead to down-regulation of M_2-receptors which may have an important functional effect if the density of prejunctional muscarinic receptors is relatively low. Recently experimental studies have demonstrated that influenza virus may inactivate M_2 rather than M_3-receptors [121]. This may be related to the action of viral neuraminidase on sialic acid residues of M_2-receptors [122]. This provides a possible explanation for increased airway reactivity after influenza infections. There is also evidence that the eosinophil cationic protein major basic protein may selectively impair M_2-receptor function through an allosteric effect [123]. Reactive oxygen species released in the acute inflammatory reaction may also result in impaired M_2-receptor function, and this could be important in acute exacerbations of asthma, when cholinergic bronchoconstriction apparently increases. It is possible that oxidants in cigarette smoke may also have an inhibitory effect on M_2-receptors and this could be relevant in COPD.

Although the bronchoconstrictor responses to cholinergic agonists appear to involve the activation of M_3-receptors leading to phosphoinositide hydrolysis, binding studies have indicated a high proportion of M_2-receptors in airway smooth muscle [124]. This has been confirmed in cultured human airway smooth muscle cells using cDNA probes to the human M_2-receptor [105]. Recently it has been established that these M_2-receptors have a functional role in counteracting the bronchodilator response to β-agonists, both *in vitro* [125] and *in vivo* [126] (Fig.16.5).

(c) M_3-receptors

Muscarinic receptors on airway smooth muscle are sensitive to 4-DAMP and hexahydrosiladifenidol and are therefore classified as M_3-receptors. Binding studies in guinea-pig and human lung membranes indicate the presence of M_3-receptors [104]. Autoradio-

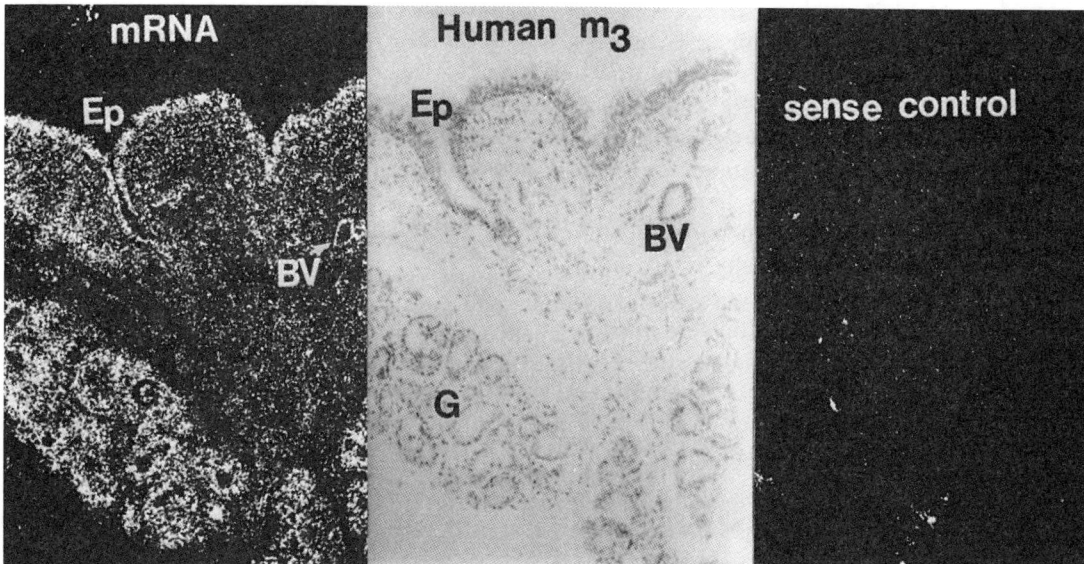

Fig. 16.7 *In situ* hybridization using a cDNA probe to the human M$_3$-receptor, showing the expression of the M$_3$-receptor gene in human airways.

graphic studies have demonstrated M$_3$-receptors in airway smooth muscle of large and small human airways [71], and this has been confirmed by *in situ* hybridization studies with M$_3$-selective cDNA probes [105] (Fig. 16.7).

M$_3$-receptors are also localized to submucosal glands in human airways, which appear to have mixed population of M$_1$- and M$_3$-receptors in a proportion of 1:2 [71]. This is consistent with functional studies which have demonstrated a secretory response to cholinergic agonists that is intermediate between an M$_1$- and M$_3$-receptor mediated response [127,128].

(d) M$_4$- and M$_5$-receptors

In rabbit lung there is evidence from binding studies for the existence of an M$_4$-receptor and this has been confirmed by the presence of M$_4$-receptor mRNA on Northern blotting [106]. *In situ* hybridization has demonstrated that this M$_4$-receptor mRNA is localized to alveolar walls, and vascular and airway smooth muscle (Mak and Barnes, unpublished observations). In human lung Northern analysis has not revealed any evidence of either M$_4$ or M$_5$-receptor mRNA and *in situ* hybridization has not revealed any evidence for expression of these receptor subtypes [105].

(e) Clinical relevance of muscarinic receptor subtypes

The discovery of at least three muscarinic subtypes in lung has important clinical implications, since it raises the possibility of more selective anticholinergic therapy in the future. Atropine, ipratropium bromide and oxitropium bromide are non-selective as anticholinergic drugs and therefore block prejunctional (M$_2$) and postjunctional (M$_3$) receptors. Inhibition of the autoreceptor means that more acetylcholine will be released during cholinergic nerve stimulation and this may overcome postjunctional blockade, thus making these non-selective antagonists less efficient than a selective antagonist of M_3-receptors. Direct evidence for this is the increase in acetylcholine release on nerve stimulation which occurs in the presence of atropine [114,129], and the fact that ipratropium bromide in low doses causes an increase in vagally mediated bronchoconstriction [108]. A similar analogy exists with α-adrenoceptors and the non-selective antagonist phentolamine which, by acting on a prejunctional α_2-receptor, increases noradrenaline release and is thus far less effective in the treatment of high blood pressure than a selective α_1-antagonist such as prazosin, which acts only on the postjunctional receptor. Unfortunately, muscarinic drugs with the high selectivity shown by prazosin for postjunctional receptors are not yet available for clinical use.

Blockade of muscarinic autoreceptors by drugs such as ipratropium bromide might account for some of the cases of paradoxical bronchoconstriction after inhaled anticholinergic drugs in patients with COPD [130]. Presumably anticholinergic drugs selective for M_3-receptors may be more effective and should not have the same risk of precipitating paradoxical bronchoconstriction.

The demonstration of different muscarinic receptor subtypes in airways may have important clinical implications. Further elucidation of the physiologic role for these receptor subtypes will depend on the development of more selective antagonists. Drugs such as methoctramine, which have a high degree of selectivity for M_2-receptors, are promising tools for elucidation of the role of muscarinic receptor subtypes, but drugs with a higher selectivity for M_3-receptors are likely to be most useful clinically in airway disease. Active efforts are underway to develop such selective drugs, but it has proved difficult to develop highly selective drugs and this may be related to the fact that the binding site for acetylcholine is highly conserved between the different subtypes of muscarinic receptor [131]. The most selective muscarinic antagonists, such as gallamine and methoctramine

appear to interact non-competitively and this may be due to interaction with an allosteric site. Recently a long-acting muscarinic antagonist, tiotropium (Ba679) that has selectivity for M_1 and M_3 receptors has been developed for use in COPD and clinical trials are now underway [132].

16.4 THEOPHYLLINE

Although theophylline has been in clinical use for more than 50 years its mechanism of action is still uncertain. Several modes of action have been proposed. Theophylline is widely used in the treatment of COPD and is still regarded as a bronchodilator. Theophylline increases exercise tolerance even when there is no improvement in spirometry [133,134]: it may reduce trapped gas volume, suggesting an effect on peripheral airways, and this may explain why some patients obtain considerable symptomatic improvement [135]. Theophylline is a poor relaxant of human airway smooth muscle at concentrations that are achieved therapeutically and this has suggested that it may have a nonbronchodilator action in airway obstruction, either by modulation of the inflammatory or immune response in the airways or by affecting respiratory muscles.

16.4.1 PHOSPHODIESTERASE INHIBITION

It is widely held that the bronchodilator effect of theophylline is due to inhibition of phosphodiesterase (PDE), which breaks down cyclic AMP in the cell, thereby leading to an increase in intracellular cyclic AMP concentrations. Theophylline is a non-selective PDE inhibitor, but the degree of inhibition is small at concentrations of theophylline which are therapeutically relevant, and there is no evidence that airway smooth muscle cells concentrate theophylline to achieve higher intracellular than circulating concentrations. Furthermore, inhibition of PDE should lead to synergistic interaction with β-agonists, but this has not been convincingly demonstrated *in vivo*. Several isoenzyme families of PDE have now been recognized [136,137] and some are more important in smooth muscle relaxation [138,139] (see below). There is some evidence that PDE activity may be increased in inflammatory cells of asthmatic patients [140] and this could theoretically increase the effectiveness of theophylline as a PDE inhibitor as a greater degree of inhibition may be achieved.

16.4.2 ADENOSINE RECEPTOR ANTAGONISM

Theophylline is a potent inhibitor of adenosine receptors at therapeutic concentrations, suggesting that this could be the basis for its bronchodilator effects. Although adenosine has little effect on human airway smooth muscle *in vitro*, it causes bronchoconstriction in asthmatic subjects when given by inhalation, by releasing histamine from airway mast cells, which is prevented by therapeutic concentrations of theophylline [141]. However, this only confirms that theophylline is capable of antagonizing the effects of adenosine at therapeutic concentrations. Enprofylline, which is more potent than theophylline as a bronchodilator, has little inhibitory effect on adenosine receptors at therapeutic concentrations, suggesting that adenosine antagonism is an unlikely explanation for the bronchodilator effect of theophylline [142]. However, adenosine antagonism may account for some of the side-effects of theophylline, such as central nervous system stimulation, cardiac arrhythmias and diuresis.

16.4.3 OTHER MECHANISMS

Several other actions of theophylline have been claimed to account for its anti-asthma effect. These include increased secretion of adrenaline from the adrenal medulla, inhibition of prostaglandin effects and inhibition of intracellular calcium ion release. None of these effects is convincing at therapeutically

relevant concentrations of theophylline, however. Despite extensive study, it has been difficult to elucidate the molecular mechanism for the bronchodilator or other anti-asthma actions of theophylline. It is possible that any beneficial effect in asthma is related to its action on other cells (such as platelets, T-lymphocytes or macrophages) or on airway microvascular leak and edema in addition to airway smooth muscle relaxation. Indeed theophylline is a rather ineffective bronchodilator and its anti-asthma effect is more likely to be explained by some other effect. It may be relevant that theophylline is ineffective when given by inhalation, but is effective when a critical plasma concentrations is reached [143]. This may indicate that it is having important effects on cells other than those in the airway. It is possible that theophylline acts as an immunomodulater and has effects on T-lymphocyte (CD8+) function [144], and it has some effect in suppressing graft rejection [145].

16.4.4 ACTIONS OF THEOPHYLLINE

The primary effect of theophylline is assumed to be relaxation of airway smooth muscle and *in vitro* studies have shown that it is equally effective in large or small airways. However, theophylline is a very weak bronchodilator at therapeutically relevant concentrations, suggesting that some other target cell may be more relevant. Theophylline inhibits mast cell mediator release, increases mucociliary clearance and prevents the development of microvascular leakiness and therefore has been considered 'anti-inflammatory' [146]. Theophylline inhibits the late response to allergen challenge more effectively than the early response, which may also indicate an anti-inflammatory effect [147]. Theophylline has a stimulatory effect on suppressor T-lymphocytes (CD8+) which may be relevant to the control of chronic airway inflammation [144,148], but has no effect on eosinophil degranulation at clinically relevant concentrations [149], which is in agreement with its lack of effect in reducing airway hyper-responsiveness [150,151].

In addition, aminophylline apparently increases the contractility of the fatigued diaphragm in man [152], although this has not been confirmed in other studies [153]. Whether this action of theophylline is relevant clinically in respiratory failure is uncertain.

16.4.5 PHARMACOKINETICS

There is a close relationship between improvement in airway function and serum theophylline concentration. Below 10 mg/l therapeutic effects (at least in terms of rapid improvement in airway function) are small and above 25 mg/l additional benefits are outweighed by side effects, so that the thera-peutic range is usually taken as 10–20 mg/l [154]. The dose of theophylline required to give these therapeutic concentrations varies between subjects, largely because of dif-ferences in clearance. In addition, there may be differences in bronchodilator response to theophylline and, with acute broncho-constriction, higher concentrations may be required to produce bronchodilatation.

Theophylline is rapidly and completely absorbed, but there are large inter-individual variations in clearance, due to differences in hepatic metabolism. Theophylline is metab-olized in the liver by the cytochrome P450/P448 microsomal enzyme system, and a large number of factors may influence hepatic metabolism.

(a) Increased clearance

Increased clearance is seen in children (1–16 years), and in cigarette and marijuana smokers. Concurrent administration of phenytoin and phenobarbitone increases ac-tivity of P450, resulting in increased meta-bolic breakdown, so that higher doses may be required.

(b) Reduced clearance

Reduced clearance is found in liver disease, pneumonia and heart failure and doses need to be reduced to half and plasma levels moni-tored carefully. Increased clearance is also seen with certain drugs, including ery-thromycin, certain quinolone antibiotics (ciprofloxacin, but not ofloxacin), allopurinol and cimetidine (but not ranitidine) which interfere with cytochrome P450 function. Thus, if a patient on maintenance theo-phylline requires a course of erythromycin, the dose of theophylline should be halved. Viral infections and vaccination may also reduce clearance, and this may be particularly important in children. Because of these vari-ations in clearance individualization of theo-phylline dosage is required and plasma concentrations should be measured 4 h after the last dose with slow-release preparations when steady state has usually been achieved. There is no significant circadian variation in theophylline metabolism.

16.5 NEW BRONCHODILATORS

Several new classes of bronchodilator are cur-rently under development, but it is difficult to envisage more effective bronchodilators than inhaled β_2-agonists and anticholinergic drugs in COPD. Novel bronchodilators may result from improvements in existing classes of bronchodilator, or by adopting novel approaches. The most significant advance has been the development of inhaled long-acting β_2-agonists such as salmeterol and for-moterol, which have already been discussed. Theophylline may be improved by sub-stitutions in the methylxanthine ring which retain the anti-asthma effect but reduce side effects. One such example is enprofylline which is five-fold more potent than theo-phylline as a bronchodilator and is effective as an anti-asthma drug [142]. Side effects are fewer, since enprofylline is not an effective adenosine receptor antagonist at therapeutic concentrations, as discussed above. Enprofylline is not being developed as there are toxicologic problems, but other novel xanthines are currently under development. Anticholinergics in current clinical use (ipratropium and oxitropium bromide) are nonselective muscarinic antagonists. Selective antagonists are under development [119]. Antagonism of M_1- and particularly M_3-receptors should be beneficial, but inhibition of prejunctional M_2-receptors on cholinergic nerves may increase acetylcholine release and therefore reduce the efficacy of muscarinic blockade at airway smooth muscle and may even exacerbate bronchoconstriction [119]. M_3- and combined M_1/M_3-selective antagonists are currently under development.

16.5.1 K+ CHANNEL OPENERS

Potassium (K+) channels are involved in recovery of excitable cells after depolarization and therefore are important in stabilization of cells. K+ channel openers such as cromakalim or lemakalim (the *levo*-isomer of cromakalim) open K+ channels in smooth muscle and therefore relax airway smooth muscle [155]. This has suggested that K+ channel activators may be a novel class of bronchodilator [156]. Preliminary clinical studies suggest that cromakalim, given in a single oral dose at night, has a useful protective effect against nocturnal asthma [157], although when taken by the same route there is no protection against bronchoconstrictor challenges in asthmatic patients [158]. The cardiovascular side effects of these drugs (postural hypotension, flushing) limit the oral dose, however. Perhaps inhaled K+ channel openers may be more useful in the future but it is difficult to see how they would be an improvement on β-agonists, unless there are additional beneficial properties.

The K+ channel that is most important in airway smooth muscle relaxation and which is involved in the bronchodilator responses to β-agonists and theophylline is the maxi-K channel which is blocked by charybdotoxin [15,16]. An agonist for this channel would be of potential benefit since these channels are relatively less important in vascular smooth muscle [159], so that vasodilator side effects may be less of problem.

16.5.2 SELECTIVE PHOSPHODIESTERASE INHIBITORS

Phosphodiesterase (PDE) breaks down cyclic AMP and, if inhibited, causes cyclic AMP to increase, leading to bronchodilatation. It is now recognized that there are at least five isoenzyme families of PDE which may be selectively inhibited [136,137]. In human airway smooth muscle PDE III and IV isoenzymes are important in relaxation [160], and thus selective inhibitors may be useful bronchodilators [138,139]. Since PDE IV is also important in inhibition of inflammatory cells [161], such as eosinophils, mast cells and lymphocytes, these drugs may have additional anti-inflammatory effects (Fig. 16.8). In animal studies PDE III/IV inhibitors are very effective in reducing airway inflammation and airway hyperresponsiveness after allergen [162].

16.5.3 NITROVASODILATORS

In vitro nitrovasodilators such as glyceryl trinitrate and nitroprusside are effective relaxants of airway smooth muscle [163,164] and nitric oxide is the endogenous neural bronchodilator in human airways [164]. These agents relax airway smooth muscle by activating soluble guanylyl cyclase and thereby increasing cyclic GMP. Such agents may therefore form the basis for novel bronchodilators, although cyclic GMP is the major intracellular mechanism mediating vasodilatation so that side effects might be a problem.

Atrial natriuretic peptide has bronchodilator actions mediated via activation of particulate guanylyl cyclase, thus increasing

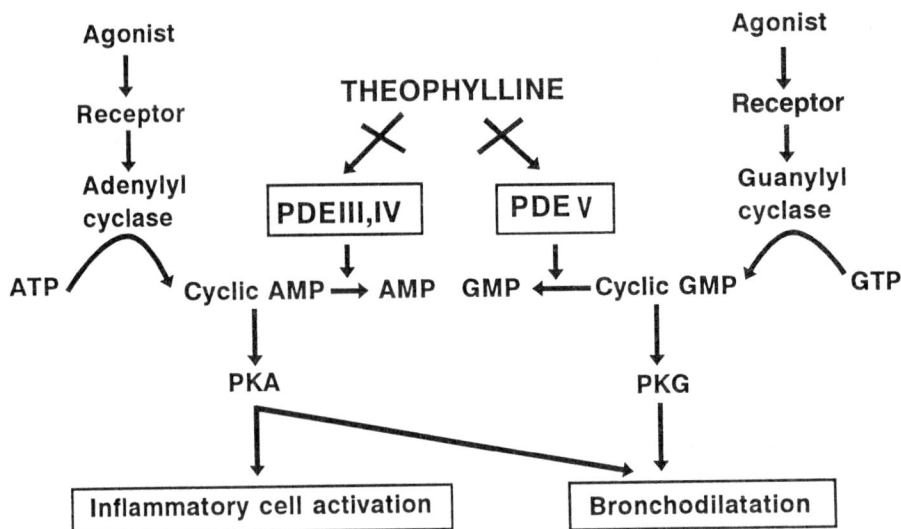

Fig. 16.8 Several types of phosphodiesterase are now recognized in airway cells. PDE III and IV are involved in metabolism of cyclic AMP and selective inhibitors may have bronchodilator and anti-inflammatory effects. PDE V is involved in metabolism of cyclic GMP and may also be involved in bronchodilator effects.

intracellular cyclic GMP and has been found to have a bronchodilator action in man [165].

[169] and it is possible that these drugs may have a role in the treatment of COPD in the future.

16.5.4 MEDIATOR ANTAGONISTS

Anticholinergic drugs cause bronchodilatation in COPD by blocking the constrictor action of endogenously released acetylcholine. It is possible that other spasmogens may be contributing to the airway narrowing in COPD and that other receptor antagonists may therefore be useful. In asthma both antihistamines [166] and a leukotriene D_4 antagonist [167] have some bronchodilator effect, but it is unlikely that these mediators are important in COPD. There has been considerable interest in the possibility that tachykinins released from sensory nerves in the airways may contribute to the bronchoconstriction and inflammation of asthma [168], but it is possible that tachykinins released by the action of irritant cigarette smoke might also be involved in COPD. Potent selective non-peptide tachykinin antagonists have now been developed

REFERENCES

1. Löfdahl, C.G. and Chung, K.F. (1991) Long-acting β_2-adrenoceptor agonists: a new perspective in the treatment of asthma. *Eur. Resp. J.*, **4**, 218–26.
2. Barnes, P.J. (1992) β-Receptors on airway smooth muscle, nerves and inflammatory cells. *Life Sci.*, **52**, 2101–9.
3. Barnes, P.J., Basbaum, C.B., Nadel, J.A. and Roberts, J.M. (1982) Localization of β-adrenoceptors in mammalian lung by light microscopic autoradiography. *Nature*, **299**, 444–7.
4. Carstairs, J.R., Nimmo, A.J. and Barnes, P.J. (1984) Autoradiographic localisation of beta-adrenoceptors in human lung. *Eur. J. Pharmacol.*, **103**, 189–90.
5. Barnes, P.J., Nadel, J.A., Skoogh, B-E. and Roberts, J.M. (1983) Characterization of beta-adrenoceptor subtypes in canine airway smooth muscle by radioligand binding and physiological responses. *J. Pharmacol. Exp. Ther.*, **225**, 456–61.

6. Carstairs, J.R., Nimmo, A.J. and Barnes, P.J. (1985) Autoradiographic visualization of β-adrenoceptor subtypes in human lung. *Am. Rev. Respir. Dis.*, **132**, 541–7.

7. Hamid, Q.A., Mak, J.C., Sheppard, M.N. *et al.* (1991) Localization of β₂-adrenoceptor messenger RNA in human and rat lung using *in situ* hybridization: correlation with receptor autoradiography. *Eur. J. Pharmacol.*, **206**, 133–8.

8. Nijkamp, F.P., Engels, F., Henricks, P.A.J. and van Oosterhout, A.J.M. (1992) Mechanisms of β-adrenergic receptor regulation in lung and its implication for physiological responses. *Physiol. Rev.*, **72**, 323–67.

9. Giembycz, M.A. and Raeburn, D. (1991) Putative substrates for cyclic nucleotide-dependent protein kinases and the control of airway smooth muscle tone. *J. Autonomic Pharmacol.*, **166**, 365–98.

10. Gerthoffer, U.T. (1986) Calcium dependence of myosin phosphorylation and airway smooth muscle contraction and relaxation. *Am. J. Physiol.*, **250**, C597–604.

11 Hall, I.P. and Hill, S.J. (1988) Beta₂-adrenoceptor stimulation inhibits histamine stimulated inositol phospholipid hydrolysis in bovine tracheal smooth muscle. *Br. J. Pharmacol.*, **95**, 1204–12.

12. Twort, C.A.C. and van Breemen, C. (1989) Human airway smooth muscle in cell culture: control of the intracellular calcium store. *Pulm. Pharmacol.*, **2**, 45–53.

13 Gunst, S.J. and Stropp, J.Q. (1988) Effect of Na-K adenosine triphosphatase activity on relaxation of canine tracheal smooth muscle. *J. Appl. Physiol.*, **64**, 635–41.

14. Jones, T.R., Charette, L., Garcia, M.L. and Kaczorowski, G.J. (1990) Selective inhibition of relaxation of guinea-pig trachea by charybdotoxin, a potent Ca⁺⁺-activated K⁺ channel inhibitor. *J. Pharmacol. Exp. Ther*, **225**, 697–706.

15. Jones, T.R., Charette, L., Garcia, M.L. and Kaczorowski, G.J. (1993) Interaction of iberiotoxin with β-adrenoceptor agonists and sodium nitroprosside on guinea pig trachea. *J. Appl. Physiol.*, **74**, 1879–84.

16. Miura, M., Belvisi, M.G., Stretton, C.D. *et al.* (1992) Role of potassium channels in bronchodilator responses in human airways. *Am. Rev. Respir. Dis.*, **146**, 132–6.

17. Kume, H., Takai, A., Tokuno, H., and Tomita, T. (1989) Regulation of Ca²⁺-dependent K⁺-channel activity in tracheal myocytes by phosphorylation. *Nature*, **341**, 152–4.

18. Kume, H., Hall, I.P., Washabau, R.J. *et at.* (1994) β-Adrenergic agents regulate K_{Ca} channels in airway smooth muscle by CAMP-dependent and -independent mechanisms. *J. Clin. Invest.*, **93**, 371–9.

19. Waldeck, B. and Widmark, E. (1985) Comparison of the effects of forskolin and isoprenaline on tracheal, cardiac and skeletal muscles from guinea-pig. *Eur. J. Pharmacol.*, **112**, 349–53.

20. Barnes, P.J. (1992) Modulation of neurotransmission in airways. *Physiol. Rev.*, **72**, 699–729.

21. Danser, A.H.J., van den Ende, R., Lorenz, R.R. *et al.* (1987) Prejunctional β₁-adrenoceptors inhibit cholinergic neurotransmission in canine bronchi. *J. Appl. Physiol.*, **62**, 785–90.

22. Janssen, L.J. and Daniel, E.E. (1991) Characterization of the prejunctional β-adrenoceptors in canine bronchial smooth muscle. *J. Pharmacol. Exp. Ther.*, **254**, 741–9.

23. Skoogh, B-E. and Svedmyr, N. (1989) β₂-Adrenoceptor stimulation inhibits ganglionic transmission in ferret trachea. *Pulm. Pharmacol.*, **1**, 167–72.

24. Rhoden, K.J., Meldrum, L.A. and Barnes, P.J. (1988) Inhibition of cholinergic neurotransmission in human airways by β₂-adrenoceptors. *J. Appl. Physiol.*, **26**, 65–72.

25. Aizawa, H., Inoue, H., Miyazaki, N. *et al.* (1991) Effects of procaterol, a beta₂-adrenoceptor stimulant, on neuroeffector transmission in human bronchial tissue. *Respiration*, **58**, 163–6.

26. Daniel, E.E., Kannan, M., Davis, C. and Posey-Daniel, V. (1986) Ultrastructural studies on the neuromuscular control of human tracheal and bronchial muscle. *Respir. Physiol.*, **63**, 109–28.

27. Verleden, G.M., Belvisi, M.G., Rabe, K.F. *et al.* (1993) β₂-Adrenoceptors inhibit NANC neural bronchoconstrictor responses *in vitro*. *J. Appl. Physiol.*, **74**, 1195–9.

28. Itabashi, S., Aikawa, T., Sekizawa, K. *et al.* (1992). Evidence that an atypical β-adrenoceptor mediates the prejunctional inhibition of non-adrenergic non-cholinergic contraction in guinea pig bronchi. *Eur. J. Pharmacol.*, **218**, 187–90.

29. Nichol, G., Nix, A., Barnes, P.J. and Chung, K.F. (1990) Prostaglandin F_{2α} enhancement of capsaicin induced cough in man: modulation

by β_2-adrenergic and anticholinergic drugs. *Thorax*, **45**, 694–8.

30. O'Connor, B.J., Ridge, S.M., Barnes, P.J. and Fuller, R.W. (1992) Comparative effect of terbutaline on mast cell and neurally mediated bronchoconstriction in asthma. *Thorax*, **46**, 745P.

31. Maguire, W.C. and Nair, S. (1978) Ventilation and perfusion effects of inhaled alpha and beta agonists in asthma patients. *Chest*, **73** (Suppl), 983–5.

32. Erjefält, I. and Persson, C.G.A. (1986) Anti-asthma drugs attenuate inflammatory leakage into airway lumen. *Acta Physiol. Scand.*, **128**, 653–5.

33. Tokuyama, K., Lötvall, J.O., Löfdahl, C.-G. *et al.* (1991) Inhaled formoterol inhibits histamine induced airflow obstruction and airway microvascular leakage. *Eur. J. Pharmacol. Sci.*, **193**, 35–40.

34. Barnes, P.J. and Chung, K.F. (1992) Questions about inhaled β_2-agonists in asthma. *Trends Pharmacol. Sci*, **13**, 20–3.

35. Laitinen, L.A., Laitinen, A., and Haahtela, T. (1992) A comparative study of the effects of an inhaled corticosteroid, budesonide, and of a β_2-agonist, terbutaline, on airway inflammation in newly diagnosed asthma. *J. Allergy Clin. Immunol.*, **90**, 32–42.

36. Roberts, J.A., Bradding, P., Wallis, A.F. *et al.* (1992) The influence of salmeterol xinafoate on mucosal inflammation in asthma. *Am. Rev. Respir. Dis.*, **145**, A418.

37. Church, M.K. and Hiroi, J. (1987) Inhibition of IgE-dependent histamine release from human dispersed lung mast cells by anti-allergic drugs and salbutamol. *Br. J. Pharmacol.*, **90**, 421–9.

38. Howarth, P.H., Durham, S.R., Lee, T.K. *et al.* (1985) Influence of albuterol, cromolyn sodium and ipratropium bromide on the airway and circulating mediator responses to allergen bronchial provocation in asthma. *Am. Rev. Respir. Dis.*, **132**, 986–92.

39. Taylor, I.K., O'Shaughnessy, K.M., Choudry, N.B. *et al.* (1992) A comparative study in atopic subjects with asthma of the effects of salmeterol and salbutamol on allergen-induced bronchoconstriction, increase in airway reactivity and increase in urinary leukotriene E_4 excretion. *J. Allergy Clin. Immunol.*, **89**, 575–83.

40. Yukawa, T., Ukena, D., Chanez, P. *et al.* (1990) Beta-adrenergic receptors on eosinophils: binding and functional studies. *Am. Rev. Respir. Dis.*, **141**, 1446–552.

41. Didier, M., Aussel, C., Ferrua, B. and Fehlman, M. (1987) Regulation of interleukin 2 synthesis by cAMP in human T cells. *J. Immunol.*, **139**, 1179–84.

42. Fuller, R.W. O'Malley, G., Baker, A.J. and MacDermot, J. (1988) Human alveolar macrophage activation: inhibition by forskolin but not β-adrenoceptor stimulation or phosphodiesterase inhibition. *Pulm. Pharmacol.*, **1**, 101–6.

43. Phipps, R.J., Williams, I.P., Richardson, P.S. *et al.* (1982) Sympathetic drugs stimulate the output of secretory glycoprotein from human bronchi *in vitro*. *Clin. Sci.*, **63**, 23–8.

44. Knowles, M., Murray, G., Shallal, J. *et al.* (1984) Bioelectric properties and ion flow across excised human bronchi. *J. Appl. Physiol.*, **56**, 868–77.

45. Devalia, J.L., Sapsford, R.J., Rusznak, C. *et al.* (1992) The effects of salmeterol and salbutamol on ciliary beat frequency of cultured human bronchial epithelial cells *in vitro*. *Pulm. Pharmacol.*, **5**, 257–63.

46. Leikhauf, G.D., Ueki, I.F. and Nadel, J.A. (1984) Selective autonomic regulation of the viscoelastic properties of submucosal gland secretions from cat trachea. *J. Appl. Physiol.*, **56**, 426–30.

47. Molfino, N.A., Nannini, L.J., Martelli, A.N. and Slutsky, A.S. (1991) Respiratory arrest in near-fatal asthma. *N. Engl. J. Med.*, **324**, 285–8.

48. Crane, J., Pearce, N., Flatt, A. *et al.* (1989) Prescribed fenoterol and death from asthma in New Zealand 1981–83: case-control study. *Lancet*, **i**, 917–22.

49. Grainger, J., Woodsman, K., Pearce, N. *et al.* (1991) Prescribed fenoterol and death from asthma in New Zealand 1981–7: a further case control study. *Thorax*, **46**, 105–11.

50. Spitzer, W.O., Suissa, S., Ernst, P. *et al.* (1992) The use of β-agonists and the role of death and near-death from asthma. *N. Engl. J. Med.*, **326**, 503–6.

51. Sears, M.R., Taylor, D.R., Print, C.G. *et al.* (1992) Regular inhaled beta-agonist treatment in bronchial asthma. *Lancet*, **336**, 1391–6.

52. Van Schayck, C.P., Dompeling, E., van Herwaarden, C.L.A. *et al.* (1991) Bronchodilator treatment in moderate asthma or chronic bronchitis: continuous or on demand? A randomised controlled study. *Br. Med. J.*, **303**, 1426–31.

53. Kraan, J., Koeter, G.H., Van der Mark, T.W. *et al.* (1985) Changes in bronchial hyperactivity induced by 4 weeks of treatment with antiasthmatic drugs in patients with allergic asthma: a comparison between budesonide and terbutaline. *J. Allergy Clin. Immunol.*, **76**, 628–36.

54. Kerrebijn, K.F., Von Essen-Zandvliet, E.E.M. and Neijens, H.J. (1987) Effect of long-term treatment with inhaled corticosteroids and beta-agonists on bronchial responsiveness in asthmatic children. *J. Allergy Clin. Immunol.*, **79**, 653–9.

55. Van Schayck, C.P., Graafsma, S.J., Visch, M.B. *et al.* (1990) Increased bronchial hyper-responsiveness after inhaling salbutamol during 1 year is not caused by subsensitization to salbuterol. *J. Allergy Clin. Immunol.*, **86**, 793–800.

56. Tattersfield, A.E. (1985) Tolerance to beta-agonists. *Clin. Resp. Physiol.*, **21**, 1–5S.

57. Hasegawa, M. and Townley, R.G. (1984) Differences between lung and spleen susceptibility to desensitization to terbutaline. *J. Allergy Clin. Immunol.*, **71**, 230–8.

58. Guillot, C., Fornaris, M., Badger, M. and Orehek, J. (1984) Spontaneous and provoked resistance to isoproterenol in isolated human bronchi. *J. Allergy Clin. Immunol.*, **74**, 713–8.

59. Nishikawa, M., Mak, J.C.W., Shirasaki, H. *et al.* (1994) Long-term exposure to norepinephrine results in down-regulation and reduced mRNA expression of pulmonary β-adrenergic receptors in guinea pigs. *Am. J. Respir. Cell. Mol. Biol.*, **10**, 91–9.

60. O'Connor, B.J., Aikman, S.L. and Barnes, P.J. (1992) Tolerance to the non-bronchodilator effects of inhaled β_2-agonists. *N. Engl. J. Med.*, **327**, 1204–8.

61. Ullman, A., Hedner, J. and Svedmyr, N. (1990) Inhaled salmeterol and salbutamol in asthmatic patients. An evaluation of asthma symptoms and the possible development of tachyphylaxis. *Am. Rev. Respir. Dis.*, **142**, 571–5.

62. Kesten, S., Chapman, K.R., Broder, I. *et al.* (1991) A 3 month comparison of twice daily inhaled formoterol versus four times daily inhaled albuterol in the management of stable asthma. *Am. Rev. Respir. Dis.*, **144**, 622–5.

63. Cheung, D., Timmers, M.C., Zwinderman, A.H. *et al.* (1992) The prolonged effects of salmeterol on airway hyperresponsiveness in asthma. *N. Engl. J. Med.*, **327**, 1198–1203.

64. Collins, S., Caron, M.G. and Lefkowitz, R.J. (1992) From ligand binding to gene expression: new insights into the regulation of G-protein-coupled receptors. *Trends Pharmacol. Sci.*, **17**, 37–9.

65. Hadcock, J.R., Wang, H.Y. and Malbon, C.C. (1989) Agonist-induced destabilization of β-adrenergic receptor mRNA: attenuation of glucocorticoid-induced up-regulation of β-adrenergic receptors. *J. Biol. Chem.*, **264**, 19928–33.

66. Davis, A.O. and Lefkowitz, R.J. (1984) Regulation of beta adrenergic receptors by steroid hormones, *Ann. Rev. Physiol.*, **46**, 119–30.

67. Mak, J.C.W., Adcock, I. and Barnes, P.J. (1992) Dexamethasone increases β_2-adrenoceptor gene expression in human lung. *Am. Rev. Respir. Dis.*, **145**, A834.

68. Barnes, P.J. (1987) Cholinergic control of airway smooth muscle. *Am. Rev. Respir. Dis.*, **136**, S42–S45.

69. Widdicombe, J.G., Karlsson, J-A. and Barnes, P.J. 1991. Cholinergic mechanisms in bronchial hyperresponsiveness and asthma, in *Asthma: Its Pathology and Treatment*, (eds. Kaliner, M.A., Barnes, P.J. and Persson, C.G.A.), Marcel Dekker, New York, pp. 327–56.

70. Barnes, P.J., Basbaum, C.B. and Nadel, J.A. (1983) Autoradiographic localization of autonomic receptors in airway smooth muscle: marked differences between large and small airways. *Am. Rev. Respir. Dis.*, **127**, 758–62.

71. Mak, J.C.W. and Barnes, P.J. (1990) Autoradiographic visualization of muscarinic receptor subtypes in human and guinea pig lung. *Am. Rev. Respir. Dis.*, **141**, 1559–68.

72. Ingram, R.H. Jr, Wellman, J.J., McFadden, E.R. Jr *et al.* (1977) Relative contribution of large and small airways to flow limitation in normal subjects before and after atropine and isoproterenol. *J. Clin. Invest.*, **59**, 696–703.

73. Nadel, J.A. and Barnes, P.J. (1984) Autonomic regulation of the airways. *Ann. Rev. Med.*, **35**, 451–67.

74. Karlsson, J-A., Sant'Ambrogio, G. and Widdicombe, J.G. (1988) Afferent neural pathways in cough and reflex broncho-constriction. *J. Appl. Physiol.*, **65**, 1007–23.

75. Fox, A.J., Barnes, P.J., Urban, L. and Dray, A. (1993) An *in vitro* study of the properties of single vagal afferents innervating guinea-pig airways. *J. Physiol. (Land.)*, **469**, 21–35.

76. Herve, P., Denjean, A., Jian, R. *et al.* (1986) Intraesophageal perfusion of acid increases the bronchomotor response to methacholine and to isocapnic hyperventilation in asthmatic subjects. *Am. Rev. Respir. Dis.*, **139**, 986–9.

77. Gross, N.J., Co, E. and Skorodin, M.S. (1989) Cholinergic bronchomotor tone in COPD: estimates of its amount in comparison with that in normal subjects. *Chest*, **96**, 984–7.

78. Patrick, D.M., Dales, R.E., Stark, R.M. *et al.* (1990) Severe exacerbations of COPD and asthma: incremental benefit of adding ipratropium to usual therapy. *Chest*, **98**, 295–7.

79. Lefcoe, N.M., Toogood, J.H., Blennerhassett, G. *et al.* (1982) The addition of an aerosol anticholinergic to an oral beta agonist plus theophylline in asthma and bronchitis. *Chest*, **82**, 300–5.

80. Gross, N.J. and Skorodin, M.S. (1984) Anticholinergic, antimuscarinic bronchodilators. *Am. Rev. Respir. Dis.*, **129**, 856–70.

81. Chapman, K.R. (1990) The role of anticholinergic bronchodilators in adult asthma and COPD. *Lung*, **168** (Suppl.), 295–303.

82. Gross, N.J. and Skorodin, M.S. (1984) Role of the parasympathetic system in airway obstruction due to emphysema. *N. Engl. J. Med.*, **311**, 321–5.

83. Braun, S.R., McKenzie, W.N. Copeland, C. *et al.* (1989) A comparison of the effect of ipratropium and albuterol in the treatment of chronic obstructive airway disease. *Arch. Intern. Med.*, **149**, 544–7.

84. Rogers, D.F., Aursudkij, B., and Barnes, P.J. (1989) Effects of tachykinins on mucus secretion on human bronchi *in vitro*. *Eur. J. Pharmacol.*, **174**, 283–6.

85. Tokuyama, K., Kuo, H-P., Rohde, J.A.L. *et al.* (1990) Neural control of goblet cell secretion in guinea pig airways. *Am. J. Physiol.*, **259**, L108–L115.

86. Kuo, H-P., Barnes, P.J. and Rogers, D.F. (1992) Cigarette smoke induced goblet cell secretion: dose-dependent differential nerve activation. *Am. J. Physiol.*, **7**, L161–L167.

87. Connolly, C.K. (1979) Diurnal rhythms in airway obstruction. *Br. J. Dis. Chest*, **73**, 357–66.

88. Coe, C.I. and Barnes, P.J. (1986) Reduction of nocturnal asthma by an inhaled anticholinergic drug. *Chest*, **90**, 485–8.

89. Morrison, J.F.J., Pearson, S.B. and Dean, H.G. (1988) Parasympathetic nervous system in nocturnal asthma. *Br. Med. J.*, **296**, 1427–9.

90. Barnes, P.J. (1987) Muscarinic receptors in lung. *Postgrad. Med. J.*, **63** (Suppl.), 13–19.

91. Barnes, P.J. (1990) Muscarinic receptors in airways: recent developments. *J. Appl. Physiol.*, **68**, 1777–85.

92. Hulme, E.C., Birdsall, N.J.M. and Buckley, N.J. (1990) Muscarinic receptor subtypes. *Ann. Rev. Pharmacol.*, **30**, 633–73.

93. Chilvers, E.R., Challiss, R.A.J., Barnes P.J. and Nahorski S.R. (1989) Mass changes of inositol (1,4,5)trisphosphate in trachealis muscle following agonist stimulation. *Eur. J. Pharmacol.*, **164**, 587–90.

94. Chilvers, E.R., Batty, I.H., Challiss, R.A.J. *et al.* (1990) Formation of inositol polyphosphates in airway smooth muscle after muscarinic receptor stimulation. *J. Pharmacol. Exp. Ther.*, **252**, 786–91.

95. Roffel, A.F., Elzinga, C.R.S. and Zaagsma, J. (1990) Muscarinic M_3-receptors mediate contraction of human central and peripheral airway smooth muscle. *Pulm. Pharmacol.*, **3**, 47–51.

96. Jones, C.A., Madison, J.M., Tom-Moy, M. and Brown, J.K. (1987) Muscarinic cholinergic inhibition of adenylate cyclase in airway smooth muscle. *Am. J. Physiol.*, **253**, C90–C104.

97. Ueki, I., German, V. and Nadel, J. (1980) Micropipette measurement of airway submucosal gland secretion: autonomic effects. *Am. Rev. Respir. Dis.*, **121**, 351–7.

98. Minette, P.A. and Barnes, P.J. (1990) Muscarinic receptor subtypes in airways: function and clinical significance. *Am. Rev. Respir. Dis.*, **141**, S162–S165.

99. Hammer, R., Berrie, C.P., Birdsall, N.J.M. *et al.* (1980) Pirenzepine distinguishes between different subclasses of muscarinic receptors. *Nature*, **283**, 90–2.

100. Bloom, J.W., Baumgartener-Folkerts, C., Palmer, J.D. *et al.* (1988) A muscarinic receptor subtype modulates vagally stimulated bronchial contraction. *J. Appl. Physiol.*, **65**, 2144–50.

101. Lammers, J.-W.J., Minette, P., McCusker, M. and Barnes, P.J. (1989) The role of pirenzepine-sensitive (M_1) muscarinic receptors in vagally mediated bronchoconstriction in humans. *Am. Rev. Respir. Dis.*, **139**, 446–9.

102. Ashe, J.H. and Yarosh, C.A. (1984) Differential and selective antagonism of the slow-inhibitory postsynaptic potential and slow-excitatory postsynaptic potential by gallanin and pirenzepine in the superior cervical ganglion of the rabbit. *Neuropharmacology*, **23**, 1321–9.

103. Ukena, D., Wehinger, C., Engelstatter, R. *et al.* (1993) The muscarinic M_1-receptor selective antagonist telenzepine has no bronchodilator effects in patients with chronic obstructive airways disease. *Eur. Resp. J.*, **6**, 378–82.

104. Mak, J.C.W. and Barnes P.J. (1989) Muscarinic receptor subtypes in human and guinea pig lung. *Eur. J. Pharmacol.*, **164**, 223–30.

105. Mak, J.C.W., Baraniuk J.N. and Barnes P.J. (1992) Localization of muscarinic receptor subtype messenger RNAs in human lung. *Am. J. Resp. Cell. Mol. Biol.*, **7**, 344–8.

106. Lazareno, S., Buckley, N.J. and Roberts, F.F. (1990) Characterization of muscarinic M_4 binding sites in rabbit lung, chicken heart and NG 108–15 cells. *Mol. Pharmacol.*, **38**, 805–15.

107. Kilbinger, H. and Wessler, T. (1980) Inhibition by acetylcholine of the stimulation-evoked release of [^{3}H]acetylcholine from guinea-pig myenteric plexus. *Neurosci.*, **5**, 1331–40.

108. Fryer, A.D. and Maclagan, J. (1984) Muscarinic inhibitory receptors in pulmonary parasympathetic nerves in the guinea-pig. *Br. J. Pharmacol.*, **83**, 973–8.

109. Minette, P.A. and Barnes, P.J. (1988) Prejunctional inhibitory muscarinic receptors on cholinergic nerves in human and guinea-pig airways. *J. Appl. Physiol.*, **64**, 2532–7.

110. Watson, N., Barnes, P.J. and Maclagan, J. (1992) Action of methoctramine, a muscarinic M_2-receptor antagonist, on muscarinic and nicotine cholinoceptors in guinea pig airways *in vivo* and *in vitro*. *Br. J. Pharmacol.*, **105**, 107–12.

111. Blaber, L.C., Fryer, A.D. and Maclagan, J. (1985) Neuronal muscarinic receptors attenuate vagally-induced contraction of feline bronchial smooth muscle. *Br. J. Pharmacol.*, **86**, 723–8.

112. Aas, P. and Maclagan, J. (1990) Evidence for prejunctional M_2 muscarinic receptors in pulmonary cholinergic nerves in the rat. *Br. J. Pharmacol.*, **101**, 73–6.

113. Ito, Y. and Yoshitomi, T. (1988) Autoregulation of acetylcholine release from vagus nerve terminals through activation of muscarinic receptors in the dog trachea. *Br. J. Pharmacol.*, **93**, 636–46.

114. Kilbinger, H., Schoreider, R., Siefken, H. *et al.* (1991) Characterization of prejunctional muscarinic autoreceptors in guinea pig trachea. *Br. J. Pharmacol.*, **103**, 1757–63.

115. Del Monte, M., Omini, C. and Subissi, A. (1990) Mechanism of the potentiation of neurally-induced bronchoconstriction by gallamine in the guinea pig. *Br. J. Pharmacol.*, **99**, 582–8.

116. Minette, P.A.H., Lammers, J., Dixon, C.M.S. *et al.* (1989). A muscarinic agonist inhibits reflex bronchoconstriction in normal but not in asthmatic subjects. *J. Appl. Physiol.*, **67**, 2461–5.

117. Ayala, L.E. and Ahmed, T. (1991) Is there a loss of a protective muscarinic receptor mechanism in asthma? *Chest*, **96**, 1285–91.

118. Barnes, P.J. (1989) Muscarinic autoreceptors in airways: their possible role in airway disease. *Chest*, **96**, 1220–1.

119. Barnes, P.J. (1989) Muscarinic receptor subtypes: implications for lung disease. *Thorax*, **44**, 161–7.

120. Ind, P.W., Dixon, C.M.S., Fuller, R.W. and Barnes, P.J. (1989) Anticholinergic blockade of beta-blocker induced bronchoconstriction. *Am. Rev. Respir. Dis.*, **139**, 1390–4.

121. Fryer, A.D. and Jacoby, D.B. (1991) Parainfluenza virus infection damages inhibitory M_2-muscarinic receptors on pulmonary parasympathetic nerves in the guinea pig. *Br. J. Pharmacol.*, **102**, 267–71.

122. Gies, J-P. and Landry, Y. (1988) Sialic acid is selectively involved in the interaction of agonists at M_2 muscarinic acetylcholine receptors. *Biochem. Biophys. Res. Commun.*, **150**, 673–80.

123. Jacoby, D.B., Gleich, G.J. and Fryer, A.D. (1992) Human eosinophil major basic protein is an endogenous allosteric antagonist at the inhibitory muscarinic M_2 receptor. *Am. Rev. Respir. Dis.*, **145**, A436.

124. Roffel, A.F., Elzinga, C.R.S., van Amsterdam, R.G.M. *et al.* (1988) Muscarinic M_2-receptors in bovine tracheal smooth muscle: discrepancies between binding and function. *Eur. J. Pharmacol.*, **153**, 73–82.

125. Yang, C.M., Chow, S-P. and Sung, T-C. (1991) Muscarinic receptor subtypes coupled to generation of different second messengers in isolated tracheal smooth muscle cells. *Br. J. Pharmacol.*, **104**, 613–8.

126. Fernandes, L.B., Fryer, A.D. and Hirschman, C.A. (1992) M_2 muscarinic receptors inhibit isoproterenol-induced relaxation of canine airway smooth muscle. *J. Pharmacol. Exp. Ther.*, **262**, 119–26.

127. Gater, P., Alabaster, V.A. and Piper, I. (1989) Characterisation of the muscarinic receptor subtype mediating mucus secretion in the cat trachea *in vitro. Pulm. Pharmacol.*, **2**, 87–92.

128. Yang, C.M., Farley, J.M. and Dwyer, T.M. (1988) Muscarinic stimulation of submucosal glands in swine trachea. *J. Appl. Physiol.*, **64**, 200–9.

129. D'Agostino, G., Chiari, M.C., Grana, E. and Kilbinger, H. (1990) Muscarinic inhibition of acetylcholine release from a novel *in vitro* preparation of the guinea pig trachea. *Naunyn-Schmiedeberg's Arch. Pharmacol.*, **342**, 141–5.

130. Connolly, C.K. (1982) Adverse reaction to ipratropium bromide. *Br. Med. J.*, **285**, 934–5.

131. Kurtenbach, E., Curtis, C.A.M., Pedder, E.K. *et al.* (1990) Muscarinic acetylcholine receptors. *J. Biol. Chem.*, **265**, 13702–8.

132. Maesen, F.P.V., Smeets, J.J., Costongs, M.A.L. *et al.* (1992) B679 BR. A new long-acting antimuscarinic bronchodilator. *Eur. Resp. J.*, **5** (Suppl. 15), 211S.

133. Taylor, D.R., Buick, B., Kinney, C. *et al.* (1985) The efficacy of orally administered theophylline, inhaled salbutamol, and a combination of the two as chronic therapy in the management of chronic bronchitis with reversible airflow obstruction. *Am. Rev. Respir. Dis.*, **131**, 747–51.

134. Murciano, D., Avclair, M-H., Pariente, R. and Aubier, M. (1989) a randomized controlled trial of theophylline in patients with severe chronic obstructive pulmonary disease. *N. Engl. J. Med.*, **320**, 1521–5.

135. Chrystyn, H., Mulley, B.A. and Peake, M.D. (1988) Dose response relation to oral theophylline in severe chronic obstructive airway disease. *Br. Med. J.*, **297**, 1506–10.

136. Beavo, J.A. and Reifsnyder, D.H. (1990) Primary sequence of cyclic nucleotide phosphodiesterase isoenzymes and the design of selective inhibitors. *Trends Pharmacol. Sci.*, **11**, 150–5.

137. Nicholson, C.D., Challiss, R.A.J. and Shahid, M. (1991) Differential modulation of tissue function and therapeutic potential of selective inhibitors of cyclic nucleotide phosphodiesterase isoenzymes. *Trends Pharmacol. Sci.*, **12**, 19–27.

138. Torphy, T.J. and Undem., R.J. (1991) Phosphodiesterase inhibitors: new opportunities for the treatment of asthma. *Thorax*, **46**, 499–503.

139. Giembycz, M.A. (1992) Could selective cyclic nucleotide phosphodiesterase inhibitors render bronchodilator therapy redundant in the treatment of bronchial asthma? *Biochem. Pharmacol.*, **43**, 2041–51.

140. Bachelet, M., Vincent, D., Havet, N. *et al.* (1991) Reduced responsiveness of adenylate cyclase in alveolar macrophages from patients with asthma. *J. Allergy Clin. Immunol.*, **88**, 322–8.

141. Cushley, M.J., Tattersfield, A.E. and Holgate, S.T. (1984) Adenosine-induced bronchoconstriction in asthma: antagonism by inhaled theophylline. *Am. Rev. Respir. Dis.*, **129**, 380–4.

142. Persson, C.G.A. (1986) Development of safer xanthine drugs for the treatment of obstructive airways disease. *J. Allergy Clin. Immunol.*, **78**, 817–24.

143. Cushley, M.J. and Holgate, S.T. (1985) Bronchodilator actions of xanthine derivatives administered by inhalation in asthma. *Thorax*, **40**, 176–9.

144. Shohat, B., Volovitz, B. and Varsano, I. (1983) Induction of suppressor T cells in asthmatic children by theophylline treatment. *Clin. Allergy*, **13**, 487–93.

145. Guillou, P.J., Ramsden, C., Kerr, M. *et al.* (1984) A prospective controlled clinical trial of aminophylline as an adjunct immunosuppressive agent. *Transpl. Proc.*, **16**, 1218–20.

146. Persson, C.G.A. (1988) Xanthines as airway anti-inflammatory drugs. *J. Allergy Clin. Immunol.*, **81**, 615–7.

147. Pauwels, R., van Revterghem, D., van der Straeten, M. *et al.* (1985) The effect of theophylline and enprophylline on allergen-induced bronchoconstriction. *J. Allergy Clin. Immunol.*, **76**, 583–90.

148. Fink, G., Mittelman, M., Shohat, B. and Spitzer, S.A. (1987) Theophylline-induced alterations in cellular immunity in asthmatic patients. *Clin. Allergy*, **17**, 313–6.

149. Yukawa, T., Kroegel, C., Dent, G. *et al.* (1989) Effect of theophylline and adenosine on eosinophil function. *Am. Rev. Respir. Dis.*, **140**, 327–33.

150. Cockcroft, D.W., Murdock, K.Y., Gore, B.P. *et al.* (1991) Theophylline does not inhibit allergen-induced increase in airway respons-

iveness to methacholine. *J. Allergy Clin. Immunol.*, **83**, 913–20.

151. Dutoit, J.I., Salome, C.M. and Woolcock, A.J. (1987) Inhaled corticosteroids reduce the severity of bronchial hyperresponsiveness in asthma, but oral theophylline does not. *Am. Rev. Respir. Dis.*, **136**, 1174–8.

152. Aubus, P., Cosso, B., Godard, P. *et al.* (1984) Decreased suppressor cell activity of alveolar macrophages in bronchial asthma. *Am. Rev. Respir. Dis.*, **130**, 875–8.

153. Moxham, J. (1988) Aminophylline and the respiratory muscles: an alternative view. *Clin. Chest Med.*, **2**, 325–40.

154. Weinburger, M. (1984) The pharmacology and therapeutic use of theophylline. *J. Allergy Clin. Immunol.*, **73**, 525–40.

155. Black, J.L., Armour, C.L., Johnson, P.R.A. *et al.* (1990) The action of a potassium channel activator BRL 38227 (lemakalim) on human airway smooth muscle. *Am. Rev. Respir. Dis.*, **142**, 1384–9.

156. Black, J.L. and Barnes, P.J. (1990) Potassium channels and airway function: new therapeutic approaches. *Thorax*, **45**, 213–8.

157. Williams, A.J., Lee, T.H., Cochrane, G.M. *et al.* (1990) Attenuation of nocturnal asthma by cromakalim. *Lancet*, **336**, 334–6.

158. Kidney, J.C., Fuller, R.W., Wordsell, Y.M. *et al.* (1993) Effect of oral potassium channel activator BFL 38227 on airway function and responsiveness in asthmatic patients: comparison with salbutamol. *Thorax*, **48**, 130–4.

159. Crawley, D., Liu, S.F., Evans, T.W. *et al.* (1992) Role of potassium channels in relaxations of human small pulmonary arteries. *Am. Rev. Respir. Dis.*, **145**, A228.

160. Belvisi, M.G., Miura, M., Peters, M.J. *et al.* (1992) Effect of isoenzyme-selective cyclic nucleotide phosphodiesterase inhibitors on human tracheal smooth muscle tone. *Br. J. Pharmacol.*, **107**, 53P.

161. Dent, G., Giembycz, M.A., Rabe, K.F. and Barnes, P.J. (1991) Inhibition of eosinophil cyclic nucleotide PDF activity and opsonized zymosan-stimulated respiratory burst by 'type IV' PDE inhibitors. *Br. J. Pharmacol.*, **103**, 1339–46.

162. Sanjar, S., Aoki, S., Kristersson, A. *et al.* (1990) Antigen challenge induces pulmonary eosinophil accumulation and airway hyperreactivity in sensitized guinea pigs: the effect of anti-asthma drugs. *Br. J. Pharmacol.*, **99**, 679–86.

163. Gruetter, C.A., Childers, C.C., Bosserman, M.K. *et al.* (1989) Comparison of relaxation induced by glyceryl trinitrate, isosorbide dinitrate and sodium nitroprusside in bovine airways. *Am. Rev. Respir. Dis.*, **139**, 1192–7.

164. Belvisi, M.G., Stretton, C.D. and Barnes, P.J. (1992) Nitric oxide is the endogenous neurotransmitter of bronchodilator nerves in human airways. *Eur. J. Pharmacol.*, **210**, 221–2.

165. Hulks, G., Jardine, A.G., Connell, J.M.C. and Thomson, N.C. (1989) Bronchodilator effect of atrial natriuretic peptide in asthma. *Br. Med. J.*, **292**, 1081–2.

166. Cookson, W.O.C.M. (1987) Bronchodilator action of the antihistamine terfenadine. *Br. J. Clin. Pharmacol.*, **24**, 120–1.

167. Hui, K.P. and Barnes, N.C. (1991) Lung function improvement in asthma with a cysteinyl-leukotriene receptor antagonist. *Lancet*, **337**, 1062–3.

168. Barnes, P.J., Baraniuk, J. and Belvisi, M.G. (1991) Neuropeptides in the respiratory tract. *Am. Rev. Respir. Dis.*, **144**, 1187–98, 1391–9.

169. Watling, K.J. (1992) Non peptide antagonists herald a new era in tachykinin research. *Trends Pharmacol. Sci.*, **13**, 266–9.

SYMPTOMATIC BRONCHODILAT TREATMENT

P.M.A. Calverley

17.1 INTRODUCTION

The use of bronchodilator drugs to reduce the symptoms and increase the exercise tolerance of patients with chronic obstructive pulmonary disease (COPD) is a cornerstone of management in these patients. The basic pharmacology of these drugs has already been reviewed (Chapter 16) and this chapter focuses on the physiologic consequences of bronchodilator action as well as considering the evidence for their efficacy and the problems of treatment selection. Although 'functional' end points such as reductions in breathlessness and increases in self-paced waking distances are important to patients, it is only relatively recently that simpler and reliable methods of assessing these variables have been developed. Surrogate end points such as changes in FEV_1 or PEF after active bronchodilator have been reported in most clinical trials, usually over quite short periods of time and these may underestimate the potential benefit of treatment. Unlike bronchial asthma where drug treatment can restore normal pulmonary function in most mild to moderate cases, the structural changes in COPD (Chapter 2) preclude this and few studies have considered how effective a dose of bronchodilator is in relation to the maximum attainable bronchodilation for that subject [1,2]. Moreover, clinically relevant changes in FEV_1 may be so small in severe COPD patients that they fall within the day-to-day reproducibility of the measurement

(Chapter 13). Problems such as these hampei interpretation of clinical studies of bronchodilator action and lead to an unduly pessimistic view of the benefit of treatment [3].

Before considering the three principal groups of symptomatic bronchodilator: β-agonist, anticholinergic and theophylline derivatives, it is useful to review how they might modify the pathophysiology of the COPD patient.

17.2 PHYSIOLOGIC BASIS OF BRONCHODILATOR ACTION

Although the most important effects of bronchodilators appear to be related to relaxation of the airway smooth muscle, a range of other actions with potential or actual clinical benefit have been reported (Table 17.1).

17.2.1 CHANGES IN AIRWAY CALIBER

Central and peripheral airways resistance is increased in stable COPD at rest and falls after bronchodilator treatment [4,5], presumably due to airway smooth muscle relaxation. The consequences of this are discussed below.

17.2.2 A REDUCTION IN PULMONARY HYPERINFLATION

This has been documented in several studies [6–8] and is likely to reflect changes in

Chronic Obstructive Pulmonary Disease. Edited by Dr P. Calverley and Professor N. Pride. Published in 1995 by Chapman & Hall, London. ISBN 0 412 46450 0

...otential beneficial effects of bronchodilator drugs in COPD

...e in airway caliber		Central and/or peripheral
		Reduces inspiratory/expiratory airways resistance
		Reduces respiratory system time constants
		Mainly 'neural' i.e. abolishes ASM tone
2.	Reduction of pulmonary hyperinflation	Reduce the work of breathing
		Reduces passive and dynamic FRC
		Reduces threshold due to PEEP
		Parallels the change in FEV1 but not proportionately
		Changes in PIF may be a useful guide
3.	Changes in mucociliary clearance	A long-term benefit
		Clinical significance unclear
4.	Improved respiratory muscle strength/endurance	Shown in animal studies with several drugs
		Hard to separate from changes in 1 and 2
5.	Anti-inflammatory activity	Of speculative importance only as yet

dynamic expiratory flow patterns which permit more complete lung emptying. Pulmonary elastic recoil is an important determinant of airway caliber but is unlikely to be directly affected by bronchodilator drugs.

17.2.3 CHANGES IN MUCOCILIARY CLEARANCE

This is impaired in most forms of COPD [9] reflecting structural damage to the cilia and the ciliotoxic effects of cigarette smoke [10,11]. β-Agonists can increase ciliary beat frequency and accelerate mucociliary clearance whilst anticholinergic drugs might impair this although clinical studies suggest this is not the case (see below). There are no good clinical studies of the effects of long-term bronchodilators on mucociliary clearance which control for the effects of changes in cigarette smoking or of cough. This latter is a major mechanism of particulate clearance and is reduced by bronchodilator drugs. Clinically these effects appear to be insignificant.

17.2.4 IMPROVING RESPIRATORY MUSCLE FUNCTION

The debate about the ability of theophyllines to increase respiratory muscle endurance and strength grumbles on with evidence for [12] and against [13]. It is difficult to believe that there is a significant effect in spontaneously breathing patients at the accepted therapeutic levels of theophylline since the respiratory muscles appear to cope surprisingly well with their increased loading given their geometric disadvantage [14] (Chapter 9).

17.2.5 ANTI-INFLAMMATORY ACTIONS

Both β-agonists and theophyllines have some anti-inflammatory actions [15] but the significance of these effects remains debatable. There is increasing evidence that long-term corticosteroid therapy can influence the natural history of COPD and produce at least short-term bronchodilation in some patients [16]. This is reviewed in Chapter 18. Pathologic inflammation has been seen in both large and small airways [17,18] and is associated with airway wall thickening which might be modified by long-term symptomatic bronchodilator treatment. Unfortunately, the current NIHLBI lung health study has selected only an anticholinergic bronchodilator, ipratropium bromide, as its interventional drug. This drug is almost certainly devoid of any anti-inflammatory action and the question of the beneficial effects or otherwise of beta agonists in COPD is likely to remain open.

Of these various actions the major effects can be explained by changes in airway caliber secondary to smooth muscle relaxation. This can be achieved by abolition of the normal resting cholinergically mediated smooth muscle tone, a reduction in pathologically increased smooth muscle tone or a decrease in airway wall thickness either from anti-inflammatory or vascular effects. There is evidence for tonic ASM contraction as a minor degree of bronchodilatation occurs after inhaled atropine and ipratropium [19]. Studies in normal subjects and COPD suggest that day-to-day variations in airway caliber are due to fluctuations in this smooth muscle tone [20,21] (Fig. 17.1). Whether the degree of cholinergic tone is truly 'pathologic' or simply reflects normal fluctuations in smooth muscle activity in an airway of reduced baseline caliber, is much more debatable. In contrast thickening of the airway wall appears to be most marked in the 'peripheral', i.e. <2 mm airways in COPD patients and is less likely to contribute to resting airway resistance than it is in asthmatics [18].

Non-specific bronchial reactivity in response to either histamine or methacholine, is increased in COPD [22] but this is usually attributed to geometric factors since even a small change in airway caliber will increase resistance dramatically when the resting airway diameter is reduced [23]. A more elaborate analysis has been reported by Wiggs *et al.* [24]. Using data derived from directly measured airway wall thickness in asthmatic and COPD patients and applying a series of

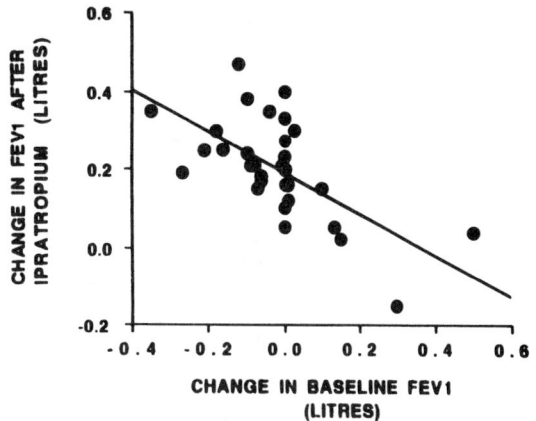

Fig. 17.1 Relationship between the change in airway caliber and the response to 500 μg nebulized ipratropium bromide in 33 stable COPD patients. Patients attended on two days and received ipratropium or salbutamol in randomized order. On days when airway caliber had increased, there was little or no further bronchodilatation with ipratropium and vice versa. This suggests that airway tone may be cholinergically mediated since anticholinergic blockade on days when airway tone was relatively low, i.e. FEV_1 had risen, was ineffective. (Reproduced with permission from reference [21].)

reasonable physiologic assumptions, they have developed a model for bronchial reactivity which emphasizes the role of airway wall thickness as the cause of increases in reactivity in both conditions. Moreover, these effects are greatly exaggerated by even modest changes in pulmonary elastic recoil (Fig. 17.2). Although they now believe that much of these results in asthmatics can be explained by smooth muscle hypertrophy, a comparable analysis for reactivity in COPD has not yet been developed. It is tempting but probably over-optimistic to hope that the apparently more favourable prognosis seen in the IPPB patients with the greatest degree of bronchodilator responsiveness [25] will relate to an increased airway wall thickening which itself will be amenable to treatment by either bronchodilator or anti-inflammatory therapy.

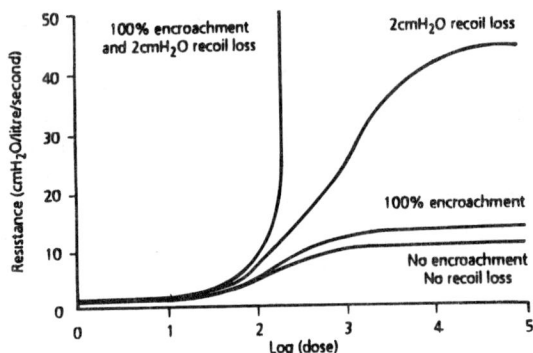

Fig. 17.2 Theoretical model predictions of changes in resistance with increasing dose of an agonist drug derived using actual measurements of airway wall thickness [18]. When there is no encroachment on the lumen and no loss of recoil a plateau of increasing resistance is reached after 3 log doses. With the addition of a 2 cm loss of elastic recoil, the airway resistance for a given change in agonist increases dramatically even with normal wall thickness. The *in vivo* situation is likely to lie between this relationship and that where there is 100% encroachment and a loss of recoil. This model takes no account of dynamic compensatory responses which might modify the behavior of the respiratory system *in vivo*. (Reproduced with permission from reference [24].)

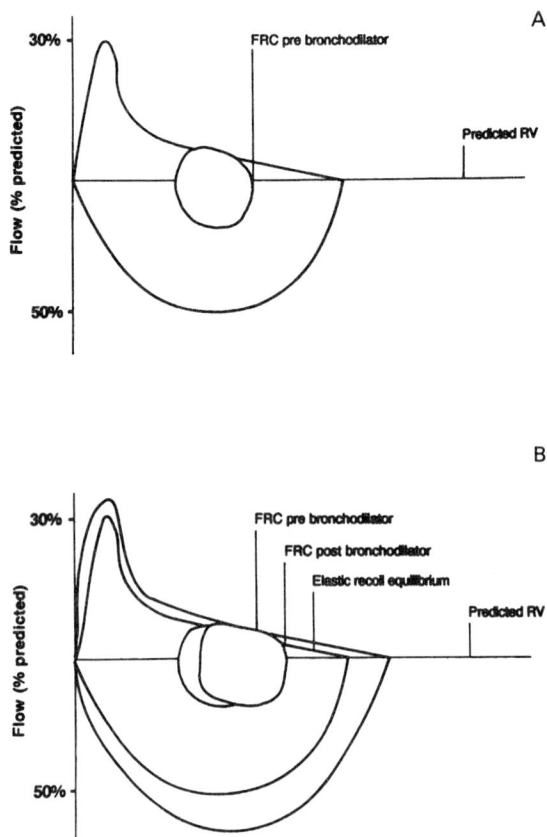

Fig. 17.3 Schematic flow volume loop before (panel A) and after an active bronchodilator drug. In panel B the changes are superimposed upon the baseline results for comparison. Inspiratory flows are downwards and expiratory flows upwards. In panel A residual volume is increased and there is an additional increase in dynamic FRC due to the breathing pattern adopted. Forced expiratory flow is flow limited at most lung volumes including those during tidal breathing. Expiratory flows can only be increased by a further increase in dynamic FRC. After the bronchodilator there is a fall in the dynamic FRC as well as in the residual volume. There are modest increases in mid and late expiratory flows (FEF_{50} and FEF_{75}) as well as an increase in peak expiratory and peak inspiratory flows. Tidal expiratory flows are still flow limited but the increase in peak inspiratory flow means it is possible to increase tidal inspiratory flows at the same lung volume without the same cost in terms of respiratory muscle energetics.

The consequences of bronchodilatation are complex. As well as improving the FEV_1 and peak expiratory flow, bronchodilators can promote a slower, deeper breathing pattern which favors more complete lung emptying. Whether this is due to some local reflex action or, as is more likely, simply to the reduction in inspiratory impedance associated with changes in airway caliber, is not yet clear. Not only do these changes reduce the work of breathing due to hyperinflation but they reduce the hidden threshold load of intrinsic PEEP (Chapter 7) and increase the previously diminished inspiratory force reserve [26]. A fall in airways resistance shortens the time constants of the respiratory system. These show marked frequency dependence in COPD (Chapter 7) and by reducing this effect, the bronchodilator not only increases maximum ventilation but allows this to be reached with a smaller degree of pulmonary hyperinflation. The relationships between tidal and maximum flows and the influence of resting lung volume are shown schematically in Fig. 17.3. A further result is a transient mismatch in ventilation and perfusion which can lead to a fall in PaO_2 at rest [27] (Chapter 8), although whether this is significant during exercise remains more questionable [28].

From this it is clear that relatively modest changes in airway dimension can have major effects on respiratory mechanics and hence symptoms as well as on maximum exercise capacity and perhaps more relevantly, the amount of exercise that can be undertaken before further dynamic hyperinflation occurs. This analysis suggests a number of end points, e.g. FEV_1, FVC, PEF, lung volume, symptoms and exercise tolerance that might demonstrate the benefits of a bronchodilator drug. However, not all of these variables will change to the same degree at the same time. In general, the effectiveness of a bronchodilator in COPD will depend upon:

1. Its potency and the dose used.
2. Its duration of action which itself can be influenced by (1) above.
3. Speed of onset of action – generally anti-inflammatory effects take weeks to months to be apparent whilst bronchodilators change airway caliber in minutes.
4. The clinical state of the patient – especially baseline FEV_1 which remains the simplest global measure of severity.

These features taken together with the side-effect profile and the simplicity of use of the drug itself, determine the acceptability of treatment to these patients.

17.3 BETA-AGONISTS

These are available in a range of formulations and dosage schedules, representative examples of which are given in Table 17.2. Oral β-agonists can be effective bronchodilators [29,30] but have lost favor even in older COPD patients as their simplicity of administration is marred by their higher side-effect profile and slow onset of bronchodilatation. This is clearly demonstrated in an acute study of 17 patients where conventional doses of 5 mg oral terbutaline and 400 mg theophylline were compared with 270 μg of inhaled salbutamol given from a metered dose inhaler (MDI). Oral therapy was marginally less effective (mean change in FEV_1 post-salbutamol 0.3 l vs 0.21 l after oral therapy). Tremor, anxiety and nausea were reported by 9 patients after oral treatment but by none after the inhaled drug [31].

Oral and intravenous β-agonists can act as pulmonary vasodilators at rest and may further reduce pulmonary artery pressure by lowering airways resistance [32,33]. The clinical significance of these effects remain dubious (Chapter 9).

Episodic reports of bronchodilatation after β-agonist inhalation in patients with 'emphysema' have been published for several years [7] but the IPPB Trial group were the first to study this systematically. They examined the response to 250 μg of inhaled isoprenaline in 965 COPD patients repeatedly over three years [34]. The majority showed a significant degree of bronchodilatation to β-agonists, however expressed, at one or more visits in this trial. Responders were more likely to complain of wheezing or reduced exercise capacity or to have shown a fall in baseline FEV_1 during the trial. There is an impression that conventional doses of salbutamol are more effective than orciprenaline (metaproterenol). Direct comparisons are lacking in COPD patients but data for each drug compared against the same dose of iptratropium supports this view [35]. Three useful dose response studies have examined the effects of salbutamol on spirometry in incompletely reversible or 'irreversible' COPD patients [36–38]. There appears to be a shallow but definite dose response relationship best seen with FEV_1. The timed peak response may be

Table 17.2 Commonly used formulations of bronchodilator drugs

Drug	Parenteral	Metered dose inhaled (μg)	Nebulizer (mg)	Oral (mg)	Duration of action (h)
Isoprenaline sulphate[a] (isoproterenol)	– –	200–400	0.8–4.0	–	1–2
Orciprenaline (metaproterenol)		750–1500	–	20	3–4
Salbutamol (albuterol)	3–20 μg/min	100–200	2.5–5.0	4	4–6
Terbutaline	1.5–5 μg/min iv	250–500	5–10	5	4–6
Fenoterol[b]	–	100–200	–	–	4–6
Salmeterol	–	50–100	–	–	12+
Ipratropium bromide	–	40–80	0.25–0.5	–	6–8
Oxitropium[c] bromide	–	200	–	–	7–9
Theophylline (SR)	–	–	–	100–400	Variable, up to 12
Aminophylline	500 μg/kg/h	–	–	225–450	Variable, up to 12

Data derived from ATS: Standards for the diagnosis and care of patients with chronic obstructive pulmonary disease (COPD) and asthma. *Am. Rev. Respir. Dis.* **136.** 225–44 and from the British National Formulary, 1993; 25.
Names in parentheses refer to North American generic terms where different from the UK.
Doses of β-agonists refer to average dose given up to 4 times daily whilst anticholinergic doses are bd or tds therapy depending on the drug used.
Theophyllines require dose titration depending on side effects and plasma theophylline (see text).
[a]Seldom used now as non-selective and potentially hazardous.
[b]Not available in USA – caution re dosage in view of concerns raised in asthmatic patients.
[c]Not available in USA.

slower than that reported in asthmatics but the time to 80% of the peak value is quite rapid. The duration of bronchodilatation and incidence of cardiac and metabolic side effects increases with the dose used [36,37] (Fig. 17.4) and there seems to be little benefit in giving more than 1 mg salbutamol. Whether this bronchodilatation is associated with broncho-protection and how it is influenced by base-line airway reactivity has not been assessed in COPD, although recent data in asthmatic patients suggest that broncho-protection is more short term [39]. Those patients who subsequently respond to corticosteroids often have the largest bronchodilator responses to β-agonists [16,40]. However, there is still evidence of dose response effect with inhaled β-agonists even in patients with a previously negative corticosteroid trial [38].

Patients who do not show 'significant' spirometric improvement can still benefit from β-agonist treatment (Table 17.3). Changes in 12-minute corridor walking distance do not relate well to changes in simple spirometry after β-agonists [41] (Chapter 12) but 12 minute walking distance increased by 62 (15 meters) after 200 μg of inhaled salbutamol in one study of 24 severe COPD patients (mean FEV_1 0.83 l). Even patients who show 'no bronchodilator response' can still have significantly improved treadmill and corridor walking times 112 (56 meters)

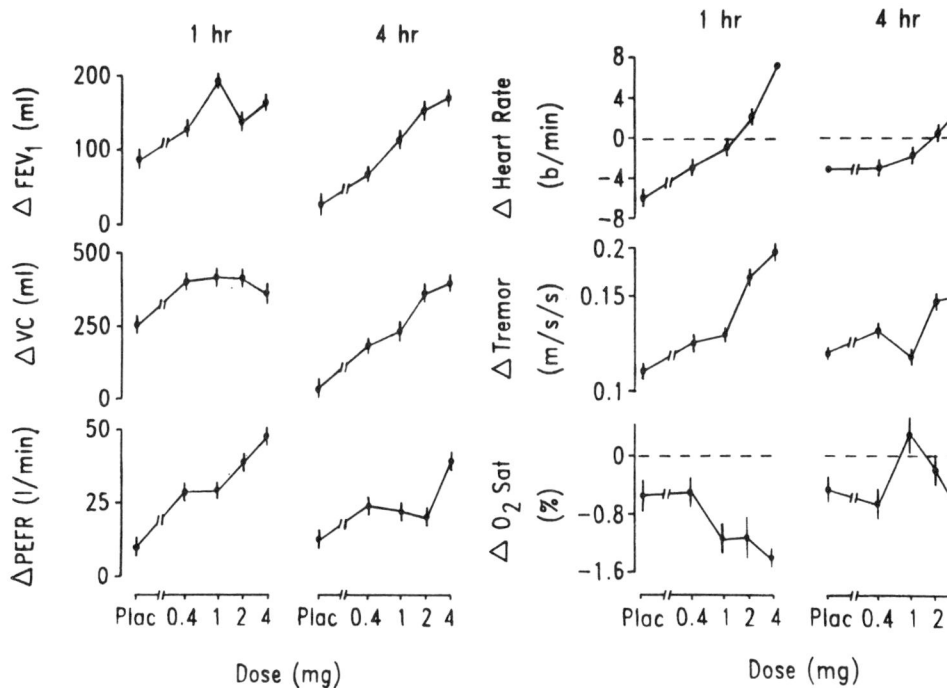

Fig. 17.4 Composite figure derived from those in reference [37], reproduced with permission. The two left-hand panels show the changes in FEV$_1$ vital capacity and peak expiratory flow after placebo and increasing doses of inhaled salbutamol given on different days in a group of 30 COPD patients, (mean FEV$_1$ 0.9 (0.26 l)). This demonstrates the dose response relationships with β-agonists and the preservation of the bronchodilator effect over a 4-hour period. The two right-hand panels refer to side effects noted at each dose increment. There was, again, a dose-related increase in heart rate, tremor and fall in oxygen saturation with the cardiovascular effects persisting more clearly at 4 hours than is the case with a change in saturation. The clinical significance of these effects for the group as a whole is likely to be small although individuals show marked idiosyncratic responses at least in terms of tremor and heart rate.

and 82 (46 meters) respectively after supranormal doses of orciprenaline [42].

As shown by the IPPB study [34] the response to β-agonist does not appear to reduce with time. Some workers have suggested that older COPD patients are less likely to respond to β-agonists [43,44] perhaps due to a loss of β receptors [45] but this view has been challenged [21]. Likewise concerns about the safety of regular β-agonists in patients with bronchial asthma [46] have been extended to COPD patients where maintenance bronchodilatation has always played a larger role. In a community-based study of the effects of medication and

dosage regimen on the decline in FEV$_1$, 144 patients completed the two-year protocol of whom 93 had 'chronic bronchitis'. In the whole group the FEV$_1$ declined more rapidly in those patients with continuous β-agonist (or anticholinergic) treatment than those where therapy was on demand, differences between the groups amounting to 52 ml/year of FEV$_1$ [47]. These findings are worrying but like the data on age and bronchodilator responses from the same group [44] the constitution of the study population is rather unusual. Thus, 86% of the chronic bronchitis were ex-smokers, their mean pack years of smoking not differing from the asthmatic

Table 17.3 Effect of beta-agonists on exercise capacity in COPD

Study	no	Dose	Baseline FEV(l)	FEV (l)	FVC (l)	Δ6MD (m)	Comment
Mohammed [30]	30	8 mg oral salb	1.03	0.09	0.17	30	6 weeks treatment n.s. compared to placebo
Evald	18	1.0 mg inh terb	0.92	0.08	0.24	11	ns compared to placebo
Corris [38]	8	400 μg 1600 μg inh salb	0.72 0.71	0.07 0.13	0.20 0.44	35[a] 38 [a]	Patients corticosteroid irreversible; change in PIF useful predictor
Vathenen [37]	30	400 μg 4 mg inh salb	0.09 0.9	0.12 0.16	0.36 0.42	20[a] 16[a]	Randomized study of multiple doses; no close related walking effect
Berger [42]	10	5 puffs orciprenaline	1.48	0.11	0.14	42[a]	Patients chosen to be 'irreversible'
Leitch [41]	24	200 μg inh salb	0.82	0.15	0.41	31[a]	Combination with anticholinergic beneficial

Δ6MD, change in six-minute walking distance in metres – data converted to this from 12 minute walks by simple division. FEV, forced expiratory volume in litres/sec; FVC, forced vital capacity in litres; inh, inhaled; terb, terbutaline; salb, salbutamol.
[a]Significantly better than placebo.

patients, whilst the patients on continuous therapy started from a slightly lower baseline FEV_1 and may have been subject to the 'horse race effect' of already having more progressive disease. Further studies in more typical COPD patients will be needed to clarify this potentially important effect especially as the authors claim for the loss of FEV_1 in this study is equivalent to that seen in patients who continue to smoke.

17.4 ANTICHOLINERGICS

Although smoking the leaves of *Datura stramonium* was one of the earliest herbal remedies for airflow limitation of all kinds [48], treatment with anticholinergic drugs fell from favor due to their systemic atropine-like effects. Therapeutic interest revived in the 1970s with the development of the poorly absorbed inhaled quaternary ammonium compound, ipratropium bromide. More recently a closely related derivative, oxitropium bromide has been investigated but this is currently available only in Europe and Japan but not North America. Detailed reviews of the clinical pharmacology of both are available [49,50]. Inhaled ipratropium affects both central and peripheral airways [5] and produces significant falls in resting FRC [6,7] (Fig. 17.5). When compared to β-agonists, anticholinergics have a somewhat slower time to peak effect, usually between 30 and 60 minutes in most COPD patients but are effective for rather longer than simple bronchodilators (approx. 6–10 hours) [49]. Dose response studies have been conducted with both ipratropium and oxitropium [51–56] and optimal bronchodilatation from a metered dose inhaler usually occurs with either 80 μg ipratropium or 200 μg oxitroprium. Direct comparisons of ipratropium and oxitropium are reported in two

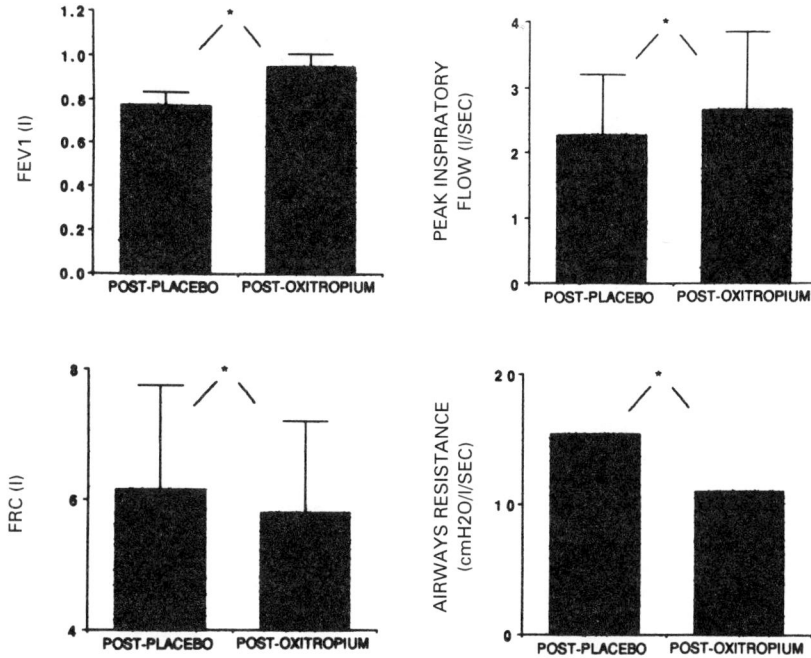

Fig. 17.5 Lung mechanics, corridor walking distance and breathlessness scores in a group of 32 stable COPD patients (mean FEV_1 0.8 l) recorded after 200 μg oxitropium bromide via an MDI or after an identical placebo. There are significant increases in FEV_1, peak inspiratory flow and falls in both functional and residual capacity in airways resistance. These are paralleled by small but significant increases in corridor walking distance and reductions in perceived breathlessness at the end of exercise. Changes in FEV_1 were not proportional to changes in either walking distance or perceived breathlessness. Changes in intensity of breathlessness at the end of exercise were best related to changes in PIF ($r = -0.57$).

studies. In one 200 μg oxitropium was compared to 40 μg ipratropium and a greater peak bronchodilatation and longer duration of action was seen with the latter [5], whilst the second study found no difference in the extent or duration of bronchodilatation when 80 μg ipratropium was compared with 200 μg oxitropium [57]. A more unfortunate problem is that the customary dose of ipratropium is 40 μg which is not optimally chosen given this dose response data for COPD patients. A better profile of bronchodilatation is achieved in COPD using 80 μg ipratropium [58] and this may explain the disparities between the direct comparisons with other drugs.

The same problem has afflicted the few studies that have examined functional variables (Table 17.4). Inhaled atropine produced small increases in maximum exercise ventilation in 18 COPD patient studied during cycle ergometry and also reduced their oxygen consumption at any given workload [59], a finding now replicated using oxitropium bromide [60]. However, Leitch and colleagues failed to find a significant improvement n corridor walking distance in 24 stable COPD patients one hour after conventional doses of ipratropium [41]. In contrast, Hay *et al.* reported significant (12%) improvement in walking distance 45 minutes after 200 μg oxitropium in 32 similar COPD patients [61]. These are similar to changes seen after orciprenaline [42] and salbutamol [41] and were accompanied by significant falls in resting and end exercise dyspnea scores. These studies have been extended to a

Table 17.4 Effects of inhaled anticholinergic and oral theophllines on exercise capacity in COPD

Study	No.	Dose	Baseline FEV	FEV	FVC	6MD (m)	Comment
Leitch et al. [41]	24	40 µg ipra	0.85	0.15	0.44	22	?Type II error or dose effect
Hay et al. [61]	32	200 µg oxi	0.70	0.18	0.41	27*	Spirometic reversibility did not predict improvement in breathless scores following active drug
Spence et al. [60]	32	200 µg oxi	0.77	0.18	0.42	20*	All patients unresponsive to a corticosteroid trial
Mahler et al. [75]	12	15 µg/ml theo	1.36	0.11	0.14	9.2	Improved overall dyspnea rating over 4 weeks therapy
Chrystyn et al. [8]	33	12.0 µg/ml 18.3 µg/nl theo	1.00 1.00	0.08 0.13	0.19 0.32	26* 56*	Dose-related reductions in 'trapped gas volume'; 8 weeks therapy
Mckay et al. [79]	15	9.1 µg/ml 16.8 µg/ml theo	0.92 0.92	0.10 0.13	0.11 0.17	65 80*	Not a true 6MD but a treadmill walk; improved quality of life scores on active drug; ? selection bias; 7 weeks therapy
Guyatt et al. [77]	19	10 µg/ml theo	N/A	N/A	N/A	40*	Changes equivalent to inhaled salbutamol; 2 weeks therapy

Symbols as for Table 17.3.
Ipra, ipratropium bromide; oxi, oxitropium bromide; theo, theophylline expressed as mean serum theophylline concentration.
Note the variable confidence intervals for significant change in the longer term oral theophylline studies reflecting the wider between day coefficient of variation in walking distance.

further group of similar patients by the same workers who showed that this dose of anticholinergic produces variable falls in FRC and more consistent reductions in airways resistance and increases in peak inspiratory flow, the latter two being the better predictors of subsequent functional improvement (Fig. 17.5).

Large studies of both ipratropium (n = 261) and oxitropium (n = 125) found no evidence of tachyphylaxis in their bronchodilator effect over 90 days [35,50] and the same was seen over six months in a cross-over Dutch general practice study [62]. The problems of accelerated loss of lung function with continuous treatment appear to extend to the anticholinergic agents but the same methodologic concerns remain [47] (see above). Unlike β-agonists there is no suggestion of a loss or responsiveness to inhaled anticholinergics with age [21,44].

17.5 THEOPHYLLINE

Despite the drawbacks of a substantial and erratic side-effect profile and limited efficacy as a bronchodilator, theophylline preparations are still widely prescribed among COPD patients although their popularity may be declining [63]. Theophyllines are only available orally which limits their role as acute symptom relievers and explains their propensity for systemic side-effects, particularly CNS and gastrointestinal ones. On the positive side they can potentially achieve similar concentrations throughout the airways, which may not be true of inhaled therapy. Earlier preparations were bedeviled by erratic absorption which may explain their lack of clinical effectiveness [64,65]. These problems have now been overcome aided by the development of simpler readily available laboratory theophylline assays and more reliable long acting formulations with a half-life of 12–18 hours are available [66,67]. Even when care is taken to ensure a stable plasma concentration, the bronchodilator action is limited in stable COPD patients (Table 17.5), changes in FEV_1 ranging from 0 to 20% [8,64,65,67–80]. There is evidence of a modest dose response effect [8] but the confidence intervals of these changes are wide and like many other studies this report does not indicate how many patients had to enter the study to achieve the study population reported.

Some patients do report subjective improvement after theophylline in the face of trivial spirometric changes and this may explain why formal assessments of breathlessness and exercise tolerance have been performed more often with this drug than with any other. Representative clinical trials data are summarized in Table 17.5. There are at least 11 reports of the effects of theophylline on the exercise capacity in COPD, although this has not been measured in any standardized way. Two of these found no change in corridor walking distance [72,75] and two further reports showed no improvement in the duration of cycle exercise [81]. However, each report may have been subject to Type II errors of varying severity. Three further studies report equivocal findings with responses in one variable but not another, e.g. improvement in walking distance after β-agonist and theophylline combined but not either alone [76]. In the remaining studies there is a small but clear improvement in corridor and treadmill walking after theophylline, although whether this differs from β-agonists is less clear [8,77,79,82]. There appears to be a dose response relationship in both studies [8,79] with clinically significant benefits only being seen at the higher dose levels. A similar pattern emerges in studies where dyspnea has been assessed (Table 17.5) with significant reduction in end exercise and resting levels of breathlessness when on active treatment. Quality of life assessments made after longer periods of treatment showed improvements in breathlessness during every day activities and reductions in perceived fatigue on higher (i.e. >17 μg/ml) doses of theophylline but whether these changes are greater than those seen after salbutamol is debatable [77,79].

The slow onset of action and the difficulties in achieving stable plasma levels mean that most studies occur after 2–6 weeks rather than a few hours as is the case with inhaled therapy. In these periods tachyphylaxis to theophyllines is not apparent but extended

Table 17.5   Effect of bronchodilator agents on spirometry and lung volumes in stable COPD

Study	Gross and Skorodin [1]	Easton et al. [85]	Spence [60]	Chrystyn et al. [8]	Murciano [78]	Taylor [86]
No	10	11	32	33	60	12
Drug	salb atr meth	salb ipra	oxi	theo	theo	theo
Dose	720 μg 3.0 mg	800 μg 120 μg	200 μg	12.1 μg/ml 18.3 μg/ml	14.8 μg/ml	12.0 μg/ml
FEV$_1$						
Baseline	1.12 1.19	0.95 1.02	0.77	1.00 1.00	31.5%p	1.14
Post-drug	1.42 1.51	1.34 1.31	0.95	1.08 1.13	35.7%p	1.27
% change	27 27	41 28	24	8 13	13	11
FVC						
Baseline	– –	– –	1.91	2.46 2.46	60.1 %p	2.55
Post-drug	– –	– –	2.33	2.65 2.78	63.2%p	2.69
% change	– –	– –	22	8 13	5	5
FRC						
Baseline	217%p 220%p	169%p 169%p	5.28	6.76 6.76	161%p	5.01
Post-drug	195%p 188%p	153%p 153%p	4.93	6.28 6.24	157%p	4.9
% change	10 14.5	9.4 9.4	7	7 7	2	2
RV						
Baseline	242%p 247%p	– –	4.24	4.23 4.23	– –	4.12
Post-drug	197%p 180%p	– –	3.93	3.32 3.06	– –	3.8
% Change	18.6 27	– –	7	22 28	–	8

Symbols as text.
FRC, functional residual capacity; RV, residual volume.
Data expressed absolute volumes (litres) or as % predicted (% p) depending on the paper.
Drug abbreviations as Tables 17.2 and 17.3.
atr meth, atropine methonitrite.

follow-up beyond 12 weeks in COPD patients has not been reported, at least for the functional end points which seem to be clinically most important.

The reasons for this functional improvement are still being investigated. *In vitro* studies and observations in normal volunteers led to the suggestion that theophyllines protected against respiratory muscle fatigue and increased respiratory muscle strength. In one particularly impressive placebo-controlled study in 60 patients with severe COPD there was a fall in FRC, an increase in inspiratory muscle strength and a lower ratio of Ppl/Ppl max after active therapy [78]. This group has argued that theophylline protects against inspiratory muscle fatigue [12]. However, there are substantial doubts about the applicability of their methodologies to the clinical situation, let alone whether they produce these effects at acceptable plasma levels. The lack of evidence of low frequency fatigue has already been noted (Chapter 5). Even during acute fatiguing inspiratory loads, oral theophylline did not reduce dyspnea in COPD patients [81]. Methodologic problems made reports of significant falls in trapped gas volume hard to interpret, although three studies have reported these [8,79,80] and attribute increases in exercise tolerance to them. Decreases in dynamic hyperinflation after theophylline may explain improvements seen in both symptoms and exercise tolerance. Thus Jenne and colleagues

found that the work of breathing was reduced in 10 patients at modest theophylline levels (mean 10.3 μg/ml) whilst maximum exercise ventilation increased [73] (Fig. 17.6). This is similar to data after an inhaled anticholinergic drug during cycle exercise where exercise desaturation and dyspnea were also reduced [60]. These findings make it unlikely that the beneficial effects of theophylline are occurring for reasons other than simple bronchodilatation.

17.6 SINGLE AGENT OR COMBINATION THERAPY

The problem of suboptimal dosing in different routes of administration make interpretation of the comparisons between agents very difficult.

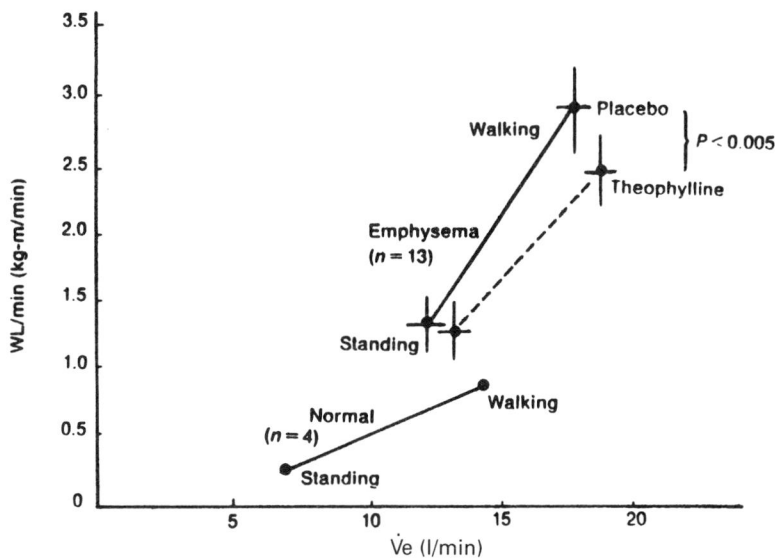

Fig. 17.6 Mechanical work on the lung (WL/min) plotted against minute ventilation ($\dot{V}E$ l/min) in 4 normal subjects and 13 patients with severe COPD before (solid lines) and after (dotted lines) treatment with oral theophylline for several days. (Reproduced from reference [73] with permission.)

Work performed on the lung is significantly increased in the COPD patient exceeding that achieved during the modest treadmill walking (1.2 mph) used as the exercise stimulus in this study. After theophylline there is a reduction in WL which is most marked during exercise and amounts to some 16% of peak level attained previously. This is very similar to the 15% change in FEV_1 and 16% change in FVC noted after theophylline treatment and suggests any effects of theophylline are related to its action as a bronchodilator drug rather than more subtle actions on the respiratory muscles.

Most data rely on spirometric end points and rather surprisingly there are no functional comparisons between high doses of β-agonists and high doses of inhaled anticholinergic in COPD. Such a trial would have to use nebulized drugs as dry powder anticholinergics have only just been developed. The problems of the existing data are illustrated by the one study to compare walking distance after both drugs in the same patients [41]. As already noted, salbutamol but not 40 μg ipratropium improved exercise performance in these patients. However, combining the two drugs did produce a further significant functional improvement (change in 12 MD post-salbutamol 62(15) meters; post-ipratropium 43(15) meters, post-combination 72(15) meters) suggesting that one or both of the other drugs were being given in suboptimal doses.

There is convincing evidence that β-agonists are more effective bronchodilators in asthmatics than are anticholinergics [83] but this is not true in COPD. Thus one reviewer found that 36 of 38 studies reported that anticholinergics were equivalent with or superior to β-agonists in COPD patients [84]. An earlier well-conducted dose response study suggested that inhaled atropine methonitrate could achieve more of the potentially available bronchodilatation than could salbutamol [1]. However, this finding is not universal [85]. Among milder COPD patients assessed by short-term responses to 80 μg ipratropium and 400 μg salbutamol respectively, more patients responded to the former and achieved most of their maximal bronchodilatation with ipratropium alone, a reverse of the situation in a parallel group of asthmatics [44]. Single agent studies over three months of regular use suggest that the initial benefit with ipratropium is maintained compared to orciprenaline [35] and salbutamol.

Comparative studies with oral theophyllines are more demanding and hence less numerous. Variations in the bio-availability of the preparation as well as the need to keep at the higher end of the therapeutic window to demonstrate significant functional benefit, make interpretation especially difficult. Using a spirometric end point Filuk *et al.* studied 16 COPD patients (11 men) comparing effects of either 800 μg salbutamol or sufficient intravenous theophylline to raise the serum theophylline level to 24 μg/ml [74]. The principal results are summarized in Fig. 17.7. When they categorized their patients retrospectively into responders (i.e. change in FEV_1 >200 ml and >10% baseline) and non-responders the same pattern emerged with theophylline producing significantly less complete bronchodilatation than salbutamol alone or the combination, whatever the order of administration. Similar findings have been reported by others [69,73].

A more complex study design was reported by Guyatt and co-workers who compared 200 μg q.d.s. salbutamol and aminophylline in high doses singly and in combination [77]. They included a placebo and each treatment period lasted four weeks. Although 612 COPD patients were screened, only 29 entered and 19 completed the study. Both bronchodilators produced similar significant improvements in PEF and patients walked further for less breathlessness on active treatment. The combination produced further improvements and the clinical symptoms of fatigue and emotional function assessed in the quality of life questionnaire improved on active treatment. The study highlights the selective nature of the population reported in clinical trials as well as the problem of choosing appropriate doses of drug to make comparisons. It is doubtful whether the benefits of combination treatment would be seen if a higher dose of salbutamol, e.g. 1 mg were used, at least extrapolating from earlier functional studies [37] which showed a clear superiority of these higher doses of β-agonists compared with those used in this study. Comparisons of theophylline with anticholinergic are less frequent, the most widely quoted study being that of Lefcoe *et al.* [83]. They compared ipratropium alone to

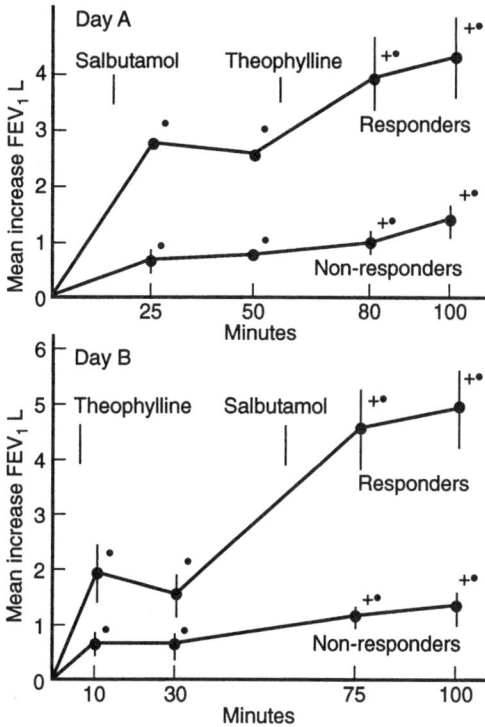

Fig. 17.7 Changes in FEV$_1$ in 16 COPD patients (mean baseline FEV$_1$ 0.73 l) given 800 μg salbutamol or sufficient theophylline to achieve a plasma level of approximately 24 μg/ml. Significance levels for increases in FEV$_1$L compared to baseline (•)0<0.05(+•) and after first drug to <0.015(+•). Patients received either salbutamol first then theophylline or the reverse order (days A and B respectively). They were divided into 8 individuals who showed a bronchodilator response, i.e. >200 ml change from baseline and 8 who did not. Salbutamol produced a larger bronchodilator response in this dose than did theophylline irrespective of the order of administration. However, the two drugs were synergistic although the extent of these changes was quite modest in the non-responder group. Whether these changes would still be present had a larger dose of salbutamol been used, is less clear – see Fig. 17.4 for possible additional effects of increasing the dose of salbutamol. Likewise, whether equivalent effects would be obtained with a longer acting drug such as salmeterol remains to be determined. (Reproduced from reference [74] with permission.)

theophylline and the β-agonist, fenoterol, in combination and found that the anticholinergic was marginally superior but the combination was, once more, additive. No comparative studies of functional end points have been reported with theophylline and anticholinergics.

17.7 REVERSIBILITY

The problems of defining a significant spirometric response to bronchodilator drugs have already been considered (Chapter 13) and are particularly important in COPD where baseline FEV$_1$ is often less than one liter. This has not deterred investigators from using short-term changes in spirometry after inhaled bronchodilators as an entry criterion for clinical studies or as a means of selecting patients for one or other form of treatment [87]. The limitations of this approach have already been stressed and the problems of differing baseline FEV$_1$, day-to-day variations in airway tone, variations in reversibility criteria and the uncertain relevance of all these to functional improvements, make it difficult to interpret much of the clinical data in COPD suggesting that bronchodilator reversibility should be used to select patient treatment. This does not mean that such tests are without value but emphasizes the need for a better understanding of the useful information they can give us such as the maximum degree of bronchodilatation that the patient can achieve, at least in the short term rather than the response to a specific drug or drug combination.

17.8 SIDE EFFECTS

Each of the three major bronchodilator groups exhibits dose-dependent side effects which limit their usefulness but vary widely in severity between different patients. Although current β-agonist drugs are relatively cardioselective, oral therapy increases heart rate probably by peripheral vasodilatation, and promotes muscle tremor irrespective of the drug chosen [65,88]. Larger doses given by MDI, i.e. above 1 mg, increase the heart rate and objectively reported somatic tremor as well as the patient's perception of side effects [36,37] (Fig. 17.4). Despite these changes in resting heart rate, there is no excess of arrhythmia in COPD patients without coexisting cardiac disease [89] but patients with ischemic heart disease do have more ventricular ectopic beats, the clinical significance of which remains unclear [90]. Detailed hemodynamic studies show that oral β-agonists can reduce pulmonary vascular resistance and increase cardiac output which may explain the patient's complaint of a more forceful heartbeat [32]. However, these favorable effects on tissue oxygen delivery are offset by falls in arterial saturation due to worsening ventilation perfusion mismatching and the overall benefit or improvement in these hemodynamic variables is very difficult to predict (Chapter 11).

Similar falls in oxygen saturation have been reported after high-dose inhaled β-agonists but these may not be relevant to everyday exercise as studies during self-paced corridor walking for 15 minutes and 2 hours after nebulized salbutamol show that exercise-induced desaturations which normally occur in these patients, are not worsened by pretreatment with a β-agonist but their exercise tolerance is increased [28]. Like all sympathomimetic drugs, β-agonists produce hypokalemia at least transiently, after their administration. Some have suggested that this may explain the excess of asthma deaths seen in New Zealand in the last decade [91] although it seems more likely that regular β-agonist use is a mark of disease severity rather than a cause in itself. In contrast, COPD patients are older, may have occult ischemic disease and are often transiently or permanently hypoxemic as well as receiving other treatment, e.g. thiazide diuretics which worsen β-agonist-induced hypokalemia [92].

Again, the lack of evidence of significant rhythm disturbances in these patients is reassuring, probably reflecting tachyphylaxis of these metabolic effects [93]. None the less, it is worth monitoring serum potassium during high-dose nebulizer treatment of an acute exacerbation (Chapter 19).

Inhaled anticholinergic drugs are relatively free from side effects although many patients complain of a slightly metallic taste which they dislike. The lack of systemic absorption even at high doses protects against GI and urinary problems although the occasional patient can develop acute glaucoma if they inadvertently allow the nebulized aerosol to enter their eyes [94,95]. Earlier reports of paradoxical bronchoconstriction were confined to asthmatic patients [96] and seem to have resolved after the benzalkonium chloride preservative was removed from the nebulizer formulation. Likewise, concerns about reduced mucociliary clearance have proven unfounded [97]. Unlike β-agonists anticholinergics do not affect resting oxygen tensions [27] and appear to improve exercise performance without changing the degree of exercise-induced desaturations [60].

Theophylline therapy has a deservedly bad reputation for side effects among COPD patients. In one large study of patients attending an emergency department 10% of 5557 patients in whom theophylline levels were measured had values >20 μg/ml and 116 cases exceeded 30 μg/ml [98]. Most of this toxicity was chronic and 6% of this group died of drug-related effects. Relatively minor problems include insomnia, headaches, nausea and gastrointestinal reflux symptoms (reflecting increased gastric acid production). However, serious cardiac rhythm disturbances can occur especially multifocal, atrial tachycardia and ventricular tachyarrhythmias [99]. Some patients present with grand mal epilepsy as a result of theophylline toxicity which can induce significant falls in cerebral blood flow [100] and increase brain hypoxia [101]. It is tempting to suggest that the ventilatory stimulant effects of theophylline, if they exist [102], are due to these mechanisms rather than its impact on CNS adenosine concentrations [103]. COPD patients often have coexisting vascular disease and acid reflux disorders due to their smoking which may explain why side-effects seem to occur at levels within the therapeutic range. Moreover, additional intravenous theophylline on a background of high–normal theophylline levels during an exacerbation is particularly hazardous and requires careful monitoring (Chapter 19).

Unlike other symptomatic treatments, oral theophylline needs considerable attention to detail if the modest benefits in terms of symptoms reduction and improved exercise tolerance (which require the highest tolerable theophylline levels) are not to provoke significant side effects (which requires the lowest practical serum levels). Theophylline is metabolized by the cytochrome P450 mixed function oxidase system and metabolizers may be fast or slow [104]. Theophylline clearance decreases with age [105] and is influenced by a host of other variables (Table 17.6).

Long-acting, readily absorbed theophylline preparations have greatly improved the pharamacokinetic profile of these drugs which may account for the success in treating overnight peak flow changes in asthmatics [66]. However, the once or twice daily recom-mended dose may be insufficient to give therapeutic serum theophylline levels in rapid metabolizers [106]. Slow-release theophyllines are still affected by the timing of the dose in relation to meals. When taken after a meal, absorption is slow and fluctuations in theophylline level reduced but if taken with food, especially if the fat content is high, then 'dose dumping' occurs and potentially toxic levels can developed due to enhanced absorption [107]. Given this multiplicity of problems, it is not surprising that routine theophylline treatment is so difficult, even when monitoring of serum levels is readily available.

17.9 DELIVERY DEVICES

Whatever its other problems oral therapy has the advantage of simplicity in use which is not shared by inhaled bronchodilators. Studies of patients' compliance with inhaled treatment in the Lung Health Study make depressing reading with an overall compliance with prescribed therapy of 65% and significant over reporting of inhaler use by patients keen to please their physician [108]. Recent data in asthmatic patients suggests that combinations of prophylactic and symptomatic therapy are no more likely to be taken than either alone. The reasons for poor patient compliance are in need of urgent exploration.

Table 17.6 Theophylline metabolism in COPD

Increased	Decreased
Cigarette smoking**	Arterial hypoxemia (<6.0 kPa) **
Anticonvulsant drugs	Respiratory acidosis *
Rifampicin	Congestive cardiac failure *
	Liver cirrhosis
	Erythromycin **
	Ciprofloxacin (not ofloxacin)
	Cimetidine (not ranitidine)
	Viral infections
	Old age *

Many factors influence theophylline metabolism and those posing particular problems in COPD are indicated by asterisks, the number depending upon the likely hazards.

Conventional MDIs pose particular problems especially for elderly patients [109]. The physics of aerosol generation and its deposition within the lungs have been studied in detail [110]. Key factors are the particle size, usually expressed as the mass median diameter, the hygroscopicity of the drug and the inspiratory flow rate. In general, particles between 2 and 5 MMDs are deposited in the airway rather than the alveoli or mouth. Particles tend to absorb moisture and increase their MMD the further along the airway they travel. High initial inspiratory flows promote impaction in the pharynx and increase the dose swallowed. An ideal MDI technique has been suggested [111], the principal features of which are summarized in Table 17.7 together with the particular problems for the older COPD patient. Incoordination of inspiratory effort and activation and breath-holding due to the 'cold freon' effect when the aerosol vaporizes appear to be particularly common [108].

Many attempts have been made to overcome this. Dry powder formulations need less patient cooperation and will undoubtedly replace current MDI use in the next 5–10 years as chlorofluorocarbons are withdrawn for environmental reasons. Unlike the MDI, dry powder inhalers need high inspiratory flow rates to ensure optimal lung deposition. Devices based on dry powder capsules (Rotacaps, Glaxo), foil disks (Rotadisk, Glaxo) or micronized pure drug (Turbohaler, Astra) are competing for this lucrative market, although the simplicity of use of the latter is particularly attractive in COPD. Radio-active tracer studies suggest that most of the inhaled drug from an MDI activation ends up in the stomach with only 10% reaching the lungs [110]. By introducing a space between the inhaler and the oropharynx, the aerosol forms a cloud which can be inhaled. Large volume 'spacer' devices (Nebuhaler, Volumatic in Europe; InspirEase in North America) utilize these effects. They involve less coordination and the larger particles deposit in the spacer before inhalation reducing the total drug dosage, although the amount reaching the lung is probably not very different. Although hard to assess directly at present with short-term bronchodilators drugs, studies with high-dose inhaled corticosteroids suggest that less drug is absorbed when spacers are used [112]. However, COPD patients may only be able to achieve low inspiratory flow rates. Usually the one-way plastic valve used in these devices opens even at flow rates of 40 l/min or less but it may stick if the spacer is not kept clean. Tube spacers represent an attempt to make these devices more portable but are generally less effective, at least in drug deposition terms [113].

Table 17.7 Inhaler technique in COPD

Ideal method	Difficulties in COPD
1. Remove cap	Occasionally forgotten
2. Shake inhaler	Occasionally forgotten
3. Hold inhaler upright	Often forgotten
4. Tilt head back 10–15°	Often forgotten
5. Hold inhaler in front of open mouth	Advice often confused about this
6. Begin to inspire and active inhaler	Co-ordination problems
7. Breathe in slowly and deeply	Difficult if hyperinflated already
8. Breath-hold for 10–15 s	Breath-hold time reduced
9. Breathe out slowly through the nose	High respiratory rate makes this harder
10. Use one puff at a time – wait 3–5 min between puffs	Often use multiple puffs in a single inspiration

The deposition patterns of nebulized drugs are similar to those of the spacer, larger particles being deposited within the face mask and tubing. They involve even less patient cooperation and yield a higher absolute dosage of the drug which may explain some of their popularity with patients (see below).

Despite the enthusiasm for better devices, there are surprisingly few data about the benefits of improved delivery systems or even modifications of inhaler technique in COPD patients. Most deposition studies examine whole lung deposition making it difficult to assess subtle differences resulting from change in delivery. Indeed, the poor 'clinical signal:noise ratio' in COPD makes practical clinical trials extremely difficult. However, change in airway caliber will influence the deposition pattern [114] and it seems likely that regular inhaled treatment will allow drug deposition more distally in the airways at doses that are associated with less systemic upset.

17.10 DOMICILIARY NEBULIZER THERAPY

The continuing debate about the efficacy and appropriateness of domiciliary nebulized bronchodilators in COPD illustrates many of the problems inherent in studies of bronchodilator action in these patients. There is a genuine concern that in some countries at least, the prescription of nebulizer solutions of bronchodilators from a portable compressor, has increased unnecessarily [115]. The initial belief that a complex IPPB machine is better than a compressor has not been borne out [116] although it would be interesting to know what effect IPPB and bronchodilator together have on intrinsic PEEP as either CPAP or IPAP can reduce this in some circumstances [117,118].

Using spirometric end points and corridor walking exercise, nebulized salbutamol seems to be no more effective than lower doses of the same drug given through a spacer device [36]. However, these comparisons were relatively brief and studies of up to one year suggest that most (27 of 32) of a group of predominant COPD patients found nebulized treatment better than their previous inhaled therapy and also demonstrated an increase in home PEF of 40 l/min [119]. Several factors may explain these changes.

First, the total dose of drug delivered to the airways is large and although the dose response effects of β-agonists and anticholinergics are not impressive, a small change in FEV_1 is likely to produce a disproportionately large improvement in effort tolerance (see above). Second, the higher the initial FEV_1 the longer is the duration of action. This is clearly seen in a multidose study of ipratropium where the mean FEV_1 after 0.6 mg was significantly higher than that after 40 μg through a metered dose inhaler and remained 33% higher at 8 hours [54]. Finally, facial cooling that occurs when the nebulizer solution condenses within the mask can, itself, reduce dyspnea independent of any effect on airway caliber [120].

Attempts at evaluating successful treatment have been restricted by the lack of suitable end points although a mixture of patient preference, home PEF and symptom scoring has been used [119,121,122]. Routine bronchodilator testing can separate relatively good responders [123] but was less useful in long-term studies [119,121,122]. In this last report changes in specific airways conductance in the laboratory did seem a promising means of selecting 'good responders'. At present prescribing nebulizer treatment is more likely to be influenced by the enthusiasm (or lack of it) of the physician together with the anxiety of both patient and family that every form of treatment should be used to reduce distress. There is obviously a need for further large-scale systematic investigation to provide clearer guidelines about the cost benefits of this treatment and its scientific basis.

17.11 NON-BRONCHODILATOR SYMPTOMATIC TREATMENT

Several alternatives to bronchodilator treatment are used with varying degrees of success to provide short and long-term symptomatic benefit in COPD patients. Some of these are considered in detail in other chapters (Chapters 10, 16, 20). None of the remaining therapies offer general help although some can be useful in specific circumstances.

17.11.1 MUCOLYTIC THERAPY

The classic epidemiologic definition of chronic bronchitis emphasizes the role of sputum production as a cardinal feature of the disease (Chapter 1) and this fact appears deeply embedded in the subconscious of physician and patient alike even when the utility of this definition has passed (Chapter 1). The best way to reduce mucus production is to stop smoking and avoid atmospheric pollutants. Increasing oral water intake had no effect on mucociliary clearance in elderly chronic bronchitic patients [124] whilst aerosolized hypertonic saline is as likely to provoke bronchoconstriction as it is a productive cough. Oral expectorants like guanifeniesin or iodides do not improve mucociliary clearance in COPD [125] nor do newer agents such as Ambroxol appear to be much better. However, β-agonists [126] and theophylline both increase mucociliary clearance although how much this contributes to their overall efficacy is unclear.

17.11.2 CARDIAC THERAPY

Digoxin continues to have its advocates as an inotropic drug in COPD although there is little evidence of any beneficial effect beyond its actions on the conducting system. One report has suggested that it can improve diaphragmatic contractility [127] but the relevance of this finding to clinical medicine remains obscure. Diuretics remain valuable as first-line treatment for peripheral edema but do not appear to influence mucociliary clearance. Both β-agonists and theophylline have favorable pulmonary vasodilator effects (see above and Chapter 11). However, anticholinergic drugs which have negligible systemic side effects produce equivalent improvements in exercise performance and symptoms suggesting that bronchodilatation is a principal action of all these agents.

17.11.3 INFECTION CONTROL

There is no evidence that prophylactic antibiotic treatment reduces the incidence of severity of infective exacerbations in COPD. However, antibiotics are beneficial during exacerbations where bacterial infection is present [128]. Prophylactic use of influenza vaccination and, more recently, pneumococcal vaccination, seems appropriate in COPD patients although the magnitude and consistency of this benefit is hard to evaluate.

17.12 CLINICAL STRATEGIES OF BRONCHODILATOR USE

Whilst there is a large body of data about specific actions for bronchodilator drugs in COPD, there is less agreement about the optimum way of using them singly or in combination. General guidance has been offered by the American Thoracic Society [87] and more specific guidelines have been developed by the Canadian Thoracic Society [129]. Much depends upon the clinical setting in which the patient presents, local availability of pharmaceuticals and, more particular, the health care system in which the physician operates. Thus, in the United Kingdom for patients attending their family physicians with early symptoms suggestive of COPD, then establishing the diagnosis firmly making some form of assessment of its severity, e.g. by PEF or spirometric measurements and encouraging the patients to stop smoking, should be the primary goals. Monotherapy with either β-agonists or anticholinergics to provide adequate symptom control particularly during exacerbations is often all that is required. Anticholinergics offer a marginal advantage if maintenance treatment is thought to be necessary. Time spent explaining inhaler technique and the purpose of treatment will be amply repaid.

In a patient presenting to a hospital out-patient clinic with persistent or worsening symptoms or one who needs increasing doses of symptomatic therapy, then additional assessments, including some measure of bronchodilator reversibility to determine the potential for improvement, is worthwhile. Ideally, this should consist of a combination of nebulized β-agonists and anticholinergic to ensure a maximum benefit. In this group regular inhaled ipratropium bromide 80 μg t.d.s. or oxitropium 200 μg t.d.s. stands the best chance of reducing cholinergic tone with the minimum of side effects. I normally couple this with advice to use β-agonists as relieving therapy on an as required basis. In many patients the dose of β-agonists used is influenced by the onset of tremor or tachycardia which is relatively idiosyncratic. If a patient remains symptomatic despite these measures which I usually couple with an assessment of the need for long-term inhaled corticosteroids (Chapter 13), then introduction of a carefully monitored dose of theophylline is worthwhile starting with a low dose, e.g. uniphyllin 100 mg b.d.s. and slowly building up to a dose at the upper limit of the therapeutic range over the next 2–4 weeks. Assessment of inhaler technique and an early change to simpler delivery systems such as spacers or dry powder devices, would give the patient more confidence and save time in the long run. A realistic explanation of the potential benefits and possible side effects particularly when taking theophyllines will help the patient to cope with their disability better. Whether such simple, traditional, medical attention is more effective than active bronchodilator therapy alone, has not been assessed. I reserve nebulized bronchodilator

treatment assessments for patients with very severe symptoms where all other therapies including a range of pulmonary rehabilitation measures, have failed and especially for patients who appear to be in the 'revolving door' situation with increasing frequent hospitalizations despite maximal home support. In these circumstances nebulizer therapy is likely to have a powerful placebo effect which may none the less be worthwhile for the patient.

17.13 FUTURE PROSPECTS

Several new developments are like to affect the symptomatic bronchodilator treatment of COPD patients. Long-acting β-agonists treatment with drugs like salmeterol and formoterol, have already established a place in asthma management and the first studies are appearing in COPD patients. which unsurprisingly confirm their extended bronchodilator action when compared with saline [130]. More detailed information about the functional consequences of these drugs, their impact on sleep quality, symptoms, exercise performance and quality of life is now needed but they may offer an attractive alternative to theophylline treatment. Studies in asthmatic patients suggest that 50 μg salmeterol b.d.s. is equivalent to 500 μg salbutamol q.d.s. [131] although whether the same equivalence exists in the COPD group is currently not known. However, increasing the dose of salmeterol to 100 μg per day produces a similar side effect profile to that of high-dose β-agonists. There is scope for a more potent and long-acting anticholinergic drug in COPD, the best candidate for which is a new agent currently designated as tiotropium bromide. This is believed to show differential receptor binding kinetics such that it blocks M_3-receptors longer than the M_2-receptors which may produce more prolonged and possibly more potent bronchodilatation. Preliminary data in 6 partially reversible COPD patients suggests that bronchodilatation lasting for more than 15 hours can be achieved with 80–160 μg given once daily [132]. Whether more specific M_1 and M_3 blocking drugs would offer clinical advantages is also a topic for further research. Attempts at modifying theophylline pharmacokinetics to produce a safer agent appear to have stalled for the time being whilst newer theophylline derivatives such as enprofylline have proved to be as toxic as their predecessors.

Whatever the category all inhaled drugs will have to move to CFC-free dry powder or wet nebulizer formulations giving further scope for innovative design solutions for the many patients who have difficulties using existing MDIs. However, the best hope for the immediate future lies in the development and testing of anti-inflammatory drugs such as the inhaled corticosteroids which may influence the rate of decline in lung function in COPD. This is the topic of the next chapter.

REFERENCES

1. Gross, N.J. and Skorodin, M.S. (1984) Role of the parasympathetic system in airway obstruction due to emphysema. *N. Engl. J. Med.*, **311**, 421–5.
2. Chaib, J., Belcher, N. and Rees, P.J. (1989) Maximum achievable bronchodilation in asthma. *Resp. Med.*, **83**, 497–502.
3. Rebuck, A.S. and Galko, B.M. (1991) Bronchodilators in the treatment of bronchitis and emphysema, in: *Chronic Obstructive Pulmonary Disease*, ed. N.S. Cherniack, Saunders, Philadelphia, pp. 487–9.
4. Yanni, M., Sekizawa, K., Ohrui, T. *et al.* (1992) Site of airways obstruction in pulmonary disease: direct measurement of intrabronchial pressure. *J. Appl. Physiol.*, **72**, 1016–23.
5. Takishima, T., Sekizawa, K., Tamura, G. and Inoue, H. (1990) Anticholinergics in treatment of COPD – site of bronchodilatation. *Res. Clin. Forums*, **13**, (Pt 2), 49–59.
6. Poppius, H. and Salorinne, Y. (1973) Comparative trial of a new anticholinergic bronchodilator Sch 1000 and salbutamol in chronic bronchitis. *Br. Med. J.*, **4**, 134–6.
7. Hughes, J.A., Tobin, M.J., Bellamy, D. and Hutchison, D.C.S. (1982) Effects of ipratropium bromide and fenoterol aerosols in pulmonary emphysema. *Thorax*, **37**, 667–70.
8. Chrystyn, H., Mulley, B.A. and Peake, M.D. (1988) Dose response relation to oral theophylline in severe chronic obstructive airways disease. *Br. Med. J.*, **297**, 1506–10.
9. Puchelle, E., Zahn, J.M., Girard, R. *et al.* (1980) Mucociliary transport *in vivo* and *in vitro*. Relations to sputum properties in chronic bronchitis. *Eur. J. Respir. Dis.*, **61**, 254–64.
10. Barton, A.D., Weiss, S.G.T., Lourenco, R.V. *et al.* (1977) Mucous glycoprotein content of chronic bronchitis sputum. *Proc. Soc. Exp. Biol. Med.*, **156**, 8–13.
11. Lourenco, R.V., Klimek, M.F. and Borouski, C.J. (1971) Deposition and clearance of 2 mcm particles in the tracheobronchial tree of normal subjects-smokers and non-smokers. *J. Clin. Invest.*, **50**, 1411–20.
12. Aubier, M. (1988) Pharmacology of respiratory muscles. *Clin. Chest. Med.*, **9**, 311–4.
13. Moxham, J. (1988) Aminophylline and the respiratory muscles. *Clin. Chest Med.*, **9**, 325–36.
14. Similowski, T., Yan, S., Gauthier, A.P. *et al.* (1991) Contractile properties of the human diaphragm during chronic hyperinflation. *N. Engl. J. Med.*, **325**, 917–23.
15. Howarth, P.H., Durham, S.R., Lee, T.H. *et al.* (1985) Influence of albuterol, cromolyn sodium and ipratropium bromide on the airway and circulating mediator responses to allergen bronchial provocation in asthma. *Am. Rev. Respir. Dis.*, **132**, 986–92.
16. Nisar, M., Walshaw, M., Earis, J.E. *et al.* (1990) Assessment of reversibility of airway obstruction in patients with chronic obstructive airways disease. *Thorax*, **45**, 190–4.
17. Ollerenshaw, S.L. and Woolcock, A.J. (1992) Characteristics of the inflammation in biopsies from large airways of subjects with asthma and subjects with chronic airflow limitation. *Am. Rev. Respir. Dis.*, **145**, 922–7.
18. Bosken, C.H., Wiggs, B.R., Paré, P.D. and Hogg, J.C. (1990) Small airway dimensions in smokers with obstruction of airflow. *Am. Rev. Respir. Dis.*, **142**, 563–70.
19. De Troyer, A., Yernault, J-C. and Rodenstein, D. (1979) Effects of vagal blockade on lung mechanics in normal man. *J. Appl. Physiol.*, **46**, 217–26.
20. Gross, N.J., Coe, E. and Skorodin, M.S. (1989) Cholinergic bronchomotor tone in COPD. *Chest*, **96**, 984–7.
21. Nisar, M., Earis, J.E., Pearson, M.G. and Calverley, P.M.A. (1992) Acute bronchodilator

trials in chronic obstructive pulmonary disease. *Am. Rev. Respir. Dis.*, **146**, 555–9.

22. Ramsdell, J.W., Nachtway, F.J. and Moser, K.M. (1982) Bronchial hyperreactivity in chronic obstructive bronchitis. *Am. Rev. Respir. Dis.*, **126**, 829–32.

23. Benson, M.K. (1975) Bronchial reactivity. *Br. J. Dis. Chest*, **69**, 227–39.

24. Wiggs, B.R., Bosken, C.H., Paré, P.D. *et al.* (1992) A model of airway narrowing in asthma and in chronic obstructive pulmonary disease. *Am. Rev. Respir. Dis.*, **145**, 1251–8.

25. Anthonisen, N.R., Wright, E.C., Hodgkin, J.E. and the IPPB Trial Group (1983) Prognosis in chronic obstructive pulmonary disease. *Am. Rev. Respir. Dis.*, **136**, 14–20.

26. Bellemare, F. and Grassino, A. (1983) Force reserve of the diaphragm in patients with chronic obstructive pulmonary disease. *J. Appl. Physiol.*, **55**, 8–15.

27. Gross, N.J. and Bankwala, Z. (1987) Effects of an anticholinergic bronchodilator on arterial blood gases of hypoxemic patients with chronic obstructive pulmonary disease: comparison with an adrenergic agent. *Am. Rev. Respir. Dis.*, **136**, 1091–4.

28. Spence, D.P.S., Pearson, M.G. and Calverley, P.M.A. (1992) Effect of oxitropium bromide and salbutamol on oxygen desaturation and breathlessness during six minute walking tests in chronic obstructive pulmonary disease. *Thorax*, **47**, 211P (abstract).

29. Marvin, P.M., Baker, B.J., Dutt, A.K. *et al.* (1983) Physiologic effects of oral bronchodilators during rest and exercise in chronic obstructive pulmonary disease. *Chest*, **84**, 684–9.

30. Mohammed, A.F., Anderson, K., Matusiewicz, S.P. *et al.* (1991) Effect of controlled-release salbutamol in predominantly non-reversible chronic airflow obstruction. *Resp. Med.*, **85**, 495–500.

31. Shim, C.S. and Williams, M.H. (1983) Bronchodilator response to oral aminophylline and terbutaline versus aerosol albuterol in patients with chronic obstructive pulmonary disease. *Am. J. Med.*, **75**, 697–701.

32. Teule, G.J.J. and Majid, P.A. (1980) Haemodynamic effects of terbutaline in chronic obstructive airways disease. *Thorax*, **35**, 536–42.

33. Peacock, A., Busst, C., Dawkins, K. and Denison, D.M. (1983) Response of pulmonary circulation to oral pirbuterol in chonic airflow obstruction. *Br. Med. J.*, **287**, 1178–80.

34. Anthonisen, N.R., Wright, E.C. and the IPPB Trial Group (1986) Bronchodilator response in chronic obstructive pulmonary disease. *Am. Rev. Respir. Dis.*, **133**, 814–9.

35. Tashkin, D.P., Ashutosh, K., Bleecker, E.R. *et al.* (1986) Comparison of the anticholinergic bronchodilator ipratropium bromide with metaproterenol in chronic obstructive pulmonary disease: a 90 day multi-center study. *Am. J. Med.*, **81** (suppl. 5A), 81–90.

36. Jenkins, S.C. and Moxham, J. (1987) High dose salbutamol in chronic bronchitis: comparison of 400 mcg, 1 mg, 1.6 mg, 2 mg and placebo delivered by rotahaler. *Br. J. Dis. Chest*, **81**, 242–7.

37. Vathenen, A.S., Britton, J.R., Ebden, P. *et al.* High-dose inhaled albuterol in severe chronic airflow limitation. *Am. Rev. Respir. Dis.*, **138**, 850–5.

38. Corris, P.A., Neville, E., Nariman, S. and Gibson G.J. (1983) Dose-response study of inhaled salbutamol powder in chronic airflow obstruction. *Thorax*, **38**, 292–6.

39. Cheung, D., Timmers, M.C., Zwinderman, A.H. *et al.* (1992) Long term effects of a long acting beta-2-adrenoreceptor agonist, salmeterol, on airway hyper-responsiveness in patients with mild asthma. *N. Engl. J. Med.*, **327**, 1198–203.

40. Mendella, L.A., Manfreda, J., Warren, C.P.W. and Anthonisen, N.R. (1982) Steroid response in the stable chronic obstructive pulmonary disease. *Ann. Intern. Med.*, **96**, 17–21.

41. Leitch, A.G., Hopkin, J.M., Ellis, D.A. *et al.* (1978) The effect of aerosol ipratropium bromide and salbutamol on exercise tolerance in chronic bronchitis. *Thorax*, **33**, 711–3.

42. Berger, R. and Smith, D. (1988) Effect of inhaled metaproterenol on exercise performance in patients with stable 'fixed' airway obstruction. *Am. Rev. Respir. Dis.*, **138**, 624–9.

43. Barros, M.J. and Rees, P.J. (1990) Bronchodilator responses to salbutamol followed by ipratropium bromide in partially reversible airflow obstruction. *Resp. Med.*, **84**, 371–5.

44. van Schayck, C.P., Folgering, H., Harbers, H. *et al.* (1991) Effects of allergy and age on response to salbutamol and ipratropium bromide in moderate asthma and chronic bronchitis. *Thorax*, **46**, 355–9.

45. Ziegler, M.G., Lake, C.R. and Kopin, I.J. (1979) Plasma noradrenaline increases with age. *Nature*, **261**, 33–5.

46. Sears, M.R., Taylor, D.R., Print, C.G. *et al.* (1990) Regular inhaled beta-agonist treatment in bronchial asthma. *Lancet*, **336**, 1391–6.

47. van Schayck, C.P., Dompeling, E., van Herwaarden, C.L.A. *et al.* (1991) Bronchodilator treatment in moderate asthma or chronic bronchitis: continuous or on demand? A randomised controlled study. *Br. Med. J.*, **303**, 1426–31.

48. Gandevia, B. (1975) Historical view of the use of parasympatholytic agents in the treatment of respiratory disorders. *Postgrad. Med. J.*, S1 (suppl. 7), 13–20.

49. Gross, N.J. (1988) Ipratropium bromide. *N. Engl. J. Med.*, **319**, 486–94.

50. Calverley, P.M.A. (1992) The clinical efficacy of oxitropium bromide. *Rev. Contemp. Pharmacother*, **3**, 189–96.

51. Lulling, J., Delwiche, J.P., Ledent, C. and Prignot, J. (1980) Controlled trial of the effect of repeated administration of ipratropium bromide on ventilatory function of patients with severe chronic airways obstruction. *Br. J. Dis. Chest.*, **74**, 135–41.

52. Gomm, S.A., Keaney, N.P., Hunt, L.P. *et al.* (1983) Dose-response comparison of ipratropium bromide from a metered dose inhaler and by jet nebulisation. *Thorax*, **38**, 297–301.

53. Allen, C.J. and Campbell, A.H. (1980) Dose response of ipratropium bromide assessed by two methods. *Thorax*, **35**, 137–9.

54. Gross, N.J., Petty, T.L., Freidman, M. *et al.* (1989) Dose response to ipratropium as a nebulized solution in patients with chronic obstructive pulmonary disease. *Am. Rev. Respir. Dis.*, **139**, 1188–91.

55. Peel, E.T. and Anderson, G. (1984) A dose response study of oxitropium bromide in chronic bronchitis. *Thorax*, **39**, 453–6.

56. Frith, P.A., Jenner, B., Dangerfield, R.N. *et al.* (1986) Oxitropium bromide. Dose response and time response study of a new anticholinergic bronchodilator drug. *Chest*, **89**, 249–53.

57. Peel, E.T., Anderson, G., Cheong, B. and Broderick, N. (1984) A comparison of oxitropium bromide and ipratropium bromide in asthma. *Eur. J. Respir. Dis.*, **65**, 106–8.

58. Burge, P.S., Harries, M.G. and I'Anson, E. (1984) Comparison of atropine with ipratropium bromide in patients with reversible airways obstruction unresponsive to salbutamol. *Br. J. Dis. Chest*, **74**, 259–62.

59. Brown, S.E., Pragen, R.S., Shinto, R.A. *et al.* (1986) Cardiopulmonary responses to exercise in chronic airflow obstruction. Effects of inhaled atropine sulphate. *Chest*, **89**, 7–11.

60. Spence, D.P.S., Hay, J.G., Carter, J. *et al.* (1993) Oxygen desaturation and breathlessness during corridor walking in chronic obstructive pulmonary disease: effect of oxitropium bromide. *Thorax*, **48**, 1145–50.

61. Hay, J.G., Stone, P., Carter, J. *et al.* (1992) Bronchodilator reversibility, exercise performance and breathlessness in stable chronic obstructive pulmonary disease. *Eur. Respir. J.*, **5**, 659–64.

62. van Schayck, C.P., Graafsma, S.J., Visch, M.B. *et al.* (1990) Increased bronchial hyperresponsiveness after inhaling salbutamol during 1 year is not caused by subsensitization to salbutamol. *J. Allergy Clin. Immunol.*, **86**, 793–800.

63. Rogers, R.M., Owens, G.R. and Pennock, B.E. (1985) The pendulum swings again toward a rationale use of theophylline. *Chest*, **87**, 280–2.

64. Alexander, M.R., Dull, W.L. and Kasik, J.E. (1980) Treatment of chronic obstructive pulmonary disease with orally administered theophylline. *JAMA*, **244**, 2286–90.

65. Jenkins, P.F., White, J.P., Jariwalla, A.J. *et al.* (1982) A controlled study of slow-release theophylline and aminophylline in patients with chronic bronchitis. *Br. J. Dis. Chest*, **76**, 57–60.

66. Busse, W.W. and Bush, R.K. (1985) Comparison of morning and evening dosing with a 24 hour sustained release theophylline, Uniphyl, for nocturnal asthma. *Am. J. Med.*, **79**, (Suppl. 6A) 62–6.

67. Greening, A.P., Baillie, E., Gribben, H.R. and Pride, N.B. (1981) Sustained release oral aminophylline in patients with airflow obstruction. *Thorax*, **36**, 303–7.

68. Eaton, M.L., Green, B.A, Church, T.R. *et al.* (1980) Efficacy of theophylline in 'irreversible' airflow obstruction. *Ann. Intern. Med.*, **92**, 758–61.

69. Barclay, J., Whiting, B., Meridith, P.A. and Addis, G.J. (1981) Theophylline-salbutamol interaction: bronchodilator response to salbutamol at maximally effective plasma theophylline concentrations. *Br. J. Clin. Pharmacol.*, **11**, 203–8.

70. Leitch, A.G., Morgan, A., Ellis, D.A. *et al.* (1981) Effect of oral salbutamol and slow release theophylline on exercise tolerance in chronic bronchitis. *Thorax*, **36**, 787–9.

71. Eaton, M. MacDonald, F., Church, T. and Niewohner, D.E. (1982) Effects of theophylline on breathlessness and exercise tolerance in patients with chronic airflow obstruction. *Chest*, **82**, 538–42.

72. Evans, W.V. (1984) Plasma theophylline concentrations, six minute walking distances and breathlessness in patients with chronic airflow obstruction. *Br. Med. J.*, **289**, 1649–51.

73. Jenne, J.W., Siever, J.R., Druz, W.S. *et al.* (1984) The effect of maintenance theophylline therapy on lung work in severe chronic obstructive pulmonary disease while standing and walking. *Am. Rev. Respir. Dis.*, **130**, 600–5.

74. Filuk, R.B., Easton, P.A. and Anthonisen, N.R. (1985) Responses to large doses of salbutamol and theophylline in patients with chronic obstructive pulmonary disease. *Am. Rev. Respir. Dis.*, **132**, 871–4.

75. Mahler, D.A., Matthay, R.A., Snyder, P.E. *et al.* (185) Sustained release theophylline reduces dyspnea in non-reversible obstructive airways disease. *Am. Rev. Respir. Dis.*, **131**, 22–5.

76. Dullinger, D., Kronenberg, R. and Niewohner, D.E. (1986) Efficacy of inhaled metaproterenol and orally administered theophylline in patients with chronic airflow obstruction. *Chest*, **89**, 171–3.

77. Guyatt, G.H., Townsend, M., Pugsley, S.O. *et al.* (1987) Bronchodilators in chronic airflow limitation. Effects on airway function, exercise capacity and quality of life. *Am. Rev. Respir. Dis.*, **135**, 1069–74.

78. Murciano, D., Auclair, M-H., Pariente, R. and Aubier, M. (1989) A randomized controlled trial of theophylline in patients with severe chronic obstructive pulmonary disease. *N. Engl. J. Med.*, **320**, 1521–5.

79. McKay, S.E., Howie, C.A., Thomson, A.H. *et al.* (1993) The value of theophylline treatment in patients severely handicapped by chronic obstructive pulmonary disease. *Thorax*, **48**, 227–32.

80. Mulloy, E. and McNicholas, W.T. (1993) Theophylline improves gas exchange during rest, exercise and sleep in severe chronic obstructive pulmonary disease. *Am. Rev. Respir. Dis.*, **148**, 1030–6.

81. Kongragunta, W.R., Druz, W.S. and Sharp, J.L. (1988) Dyspnea and diaphragmatic fatigue in patients with chronic obstructive pulmonary disease. *Am. Rev. Respir. Dis.*, **137**, 662–7.

82. Leitch, A.G., Morgan, A., Ellis, D.A. *et al.* (1981) Effect of oral salbutamol and slow-release theophylline on exercise tolerance in chronic bronchitis. *Thorax*, **36**, 787–9.

83. Lefcoe, N.M., Toogood, J.H., Blenner Lassett, G. *et al.* (1982) The addition of an aerosol anticholinergic to an oral beta agonist plus theophylline in asthma and bronchitis. *Chest*, **82**, 300–5.

84. Chapman, K.R. (1990) The role of anticholinergic bronchodilators in adult asthma and COPD. *Lung*, **168** (Suppl.), 295–303.

85. Easton, P.A., Jadue, C., Dhingra, S. and Anthonisen, N.R. (1986) A comparison of the bronchodilating effects of a beta-2 adrenergic agent (albuterol) and an anticholinergic agent (ipratropium bromide) given by aerosol alone or in sequence. *N. Engl. J. Med.*, **315**, 735–9.

86. Taylor, D.R., *et al.* (1985) The efficacy of orally administered theophylline, inhaled salbutamol and a combination of the two as chronic therapy in the management of chronic bronchitis with reversible air flow obstruction. *Am. Rev. Respir. Dis.*, **131**, 747–51.

87. American Thoracic Society (1987) Standards for the diagnosis and care of patients with chronic obstructive pulmonary disease (COPD) and asthma. *Am. Rev. Respir. Dis.*, **136**, 225–44.

88. Marvin, P.M., Baker, B.J., Dutt, A.K. *et al.* (1983) Physiologic effects of oral bronchodilators during rest and exercise in chronic obstructive pulmonary disease. *Chest*, **84**, 684–9.

89. Conradson, T.B., Eklundh, G., Olofsson, B. *et al.* (1985) Cardiac arrhythmias in patients with mild to moderate obstructive lung disease. *Chest*, **88**, 537–42.

90. Conradson, T.B., Eklundh, G., Olofsson, B. *et al.* (1987) Arrhythmogenicity from combined bronchodilator therapy in patients with obstructive lung disease and concomitant ischaemic heart disease. *Chest*, **91**, 5–9.

91. Pearce, N., Crane, J., Burgess, C. *et al.* (1991) Beta-agonists and asthma mortality: déjà vu. *Clin. Exp., Allergy*, **21**, 401–10.

92. Lipworth, B.J., McDevitt, D.G. and Strathers, A.D. (1990) Electrocardiographic changes induced by inhaled salbutamol after treatment with bendrofluazide: effects of replacement therapy with potassium, magnesium, and triamterene. *Clin. Sci.*, **78**, 255–9.

93. O'Connor, B.J., Aikman, S.L. and Barnes, P.J. (1992) Tolerance to the nonbronchodilator effects of beta-2-agonists in asthma. *N. Engl. J. Med.*, **327**, 1204–8.

94. Kalra, L. and Bone, M. (1988) The effect of nebulized bronchodilator therapy on intraocular pressure in patients with glaucoma. *Chest*, **93**, 739–41.

95. Shah, P., Dhurjon, L., Metacalfe, T. and Gibson, J.M. (1992) Acute angle closure glaucoma associated with nebulised ipratropium bromide and salbutamol. *Br. Med. J.*, **304**, 40–1.

96. Patel, K.R. and Tullett, W.M. (1983) Bronchoconstriction in response to ipratropium bromide (letter). *Br. Med. J.*, **286**, 1318.

97. Pavia, D., Bateman, J.R.M., Sheahan, N.F. and Clarke, S.W. (1979) Effect of ipratropium bromide on mucociliary clearance and pulmonary function in reversible airways obstruction. *Thorax*, **34**, 501–7.

98. Sessler, C.N. (1990) Theophylline toxicity: clinical features of 116 consecutive cases. *Am. J. Med.*, **88**, 567–76.

99. Levine, J.H., Michael, J.R. and Guarnien, T. (1985) Multifocal atrial tachycardia: A toxic effect of theophylline. *Lancet*, **i**, 12–14.

100. Bowton, D.L., Alford, P.T., McLees, B.D. *et al.* (1987) The effects of aminophylline on cerebral blood flow in patients with chronic obstructive pulmonary disease. *Chest*, **91**, 874–7.

101. Nishimura, N., Suzuki, A., Yoshioka, A. *et al.* (1992) Effect of aminophylline on brain tissue oxygen tension in patients with chronic obstructive lung disease. *Thorax*, **47**, 1025-9.

102. Swaminathan, S., Paton, J.Y., Davidson-Ward, S.L. *et al.* (1992) Theophylline does not increase ventilatory responses to hypercapnia or hypoxia. *Am. Rev. Respir. Dis.*, **146**, 1398–1401.

103. Parsons, S.T., Griffiths, T.L., Christie, J.M.L. and Holgate, S.T. (1991) Effect of theophylline and dipyridamole on the respiratory response to isocapnic hypoxia in normal human subjects. *Clin. Sci.*, **80**, 107–12.

104. Miller, C.A., Shisher, L.B. and Vesell, E.S. (1985) Polymorphism of theophylline metabolism in man. *J. Clin. Invest.*, **75**, 1415–25.

105. Randolph, W.C., Seaman, J.J., Dickson, B. *et al.* (1986) The effect of age on theophylline clearance in normal subjects. *Br. J. Clin. Pharmacol.*, **22**, 603–5.

106. Weinberger, M. and Hendeles, L. (1983) Slow-release theophylline: Rationale and basis for product selection. *N. Engl. J. Med.*, **308**, 760–4.

107. Hendeles, L., Weinberger, M., Milavetz, G. *et al.* (1985) Food-induced 'dose dumping' from a once-a-day theophylline product as a cause of theophylline toxicity. *Chest*, **87**, 758–65.

108. Rand, C.S., Wise, R.A., Nides, M. *et al.* (1992) Metered-dose inhaler adherence in a clinical trial. *Am. Rev. Respir. Dis.*, **146**, 1559–64.

109. Crompton, G.K. (1982) Problems patients have using pressurised aerosol inhalers. *Eur. J. Respir. Dis.*, **63**, (Suppl. 119), 101–4.

110. Newman, S.P., Pavia, D., Moren, F. *et al.* (1981) Deposition of pressurized aerosols in the human respiratory tract. *Thorax*, **36**, 52–5.

111. Dolovich, M.B., Ruffin, R.E., Roberts, R. and Newhouse, M.T. (1981) Optimal delivery of aerosols from metered-dose inhalers. *Chest*, **80**, (Suppl.), 911- 5.

112. Brown, P.H., Greening, A.P. and Crompton, G.K. (1993) Large volume spacer devices and the influence of high dose beclomethasone dipropionate on hypothalamo-pituitary-adrenal axis function. *Thorax*, **48**, 233–8.

113. Godden, D.J. and Crompton, G.K. (1981) An objective assessment of the tube spacer in patients unable to use a conventional pressurized aerosol effectively. *Br. J. Dis. Chest*, **75**, 165–8.

114. Pavia, D., Thomson, M.L., Clarke, S.W. and Shannon, H.S. (1977) Effect of lung function and mode of inhalation on penetration of aerosol into the human lung. *Thorax*, **32**, 194–7.

115. Editorial (1984) The nebulizer epidemic. *Lancet*, **ii**, 789–90.

116. Intermittent Positive Pressure Breathing Trial Group (1983) Intermittent positive pressure breathing therapy of chronic obstructive pulmonary disease: A clinical trial. *Ann. Intern. Med.*, **99**, 612–20.

117. Petrof, B.J., Calderini, E. and Gottfried, S.B. (1990) Effect of CPAP on respiratory effort and dyspnea during exercise in severe COPD. *J. Appl. Physiol.*, **69**, 179–88.

118. O'Donnell, D.E., Sanii, R., Gresbrecht, G. and Younes, M. (1988) Effect of continuous positive airway pressure on respiratory sensation in patients with chronic obstructive pulmonary disease during submaximal exercise. *Am. Rev. Respir., Dis.*, **138**, 1185–91.

119. O'Driscoll, B.R., Kay, E.A., Taylor, R.J. *et al.* (1992) A long-term prospective assessment of home nebulizer treatment. *Resp. Med.*, **86**, 317–25.

120. Spence, D.P.S., Graham, D.R., Ahmed, J. *et al.* (1993) Does cold air affect exercise capacity and dyspnea in stable chronic obstructive pulmonary disease? *Chest*, **103**, 693–6.

121. Teale, C., Morrison, J.F.J., Jones, P.C. and Muers, MF. (1991) Reversibility tests in chronic

obstructive airways disease: their predictive value with reference to benefit from domiciliary nebulizer therapy. *Resp. Med.*, **85**, 281–4.

122. Goldman, J.M., Teale, C. and Muers, M.F. (1992) Simplifying the assessment of patients with chronic airflow limitation for home nebulizer therapy. *Resp. Med.*, **86**, 33–8.

123. Allen, M.B., Pugh, J. and Wilson, R.S.E. (1988) Nebuhaler or nebulizer for high dose bronchodilator therapy in chronic bronchitis: a comparison. *Br. J. Dis. Chest*, **82**, 368–73.

124. Shim, C.S. and Williams, M.H. (1987) Lack of effect of hydration on sputum production in chronic bronchitis. *Chest*, **92**, 679–82.

125. Hirsch, S.R, Viernes, P.F. and Korg, K.C. (1973) The expectorant effect of glyceryl guiacolate in patients with chronic bronchitis. A controlled *in vitro* and *in vivo* study. *Chest*, **63**, 9–14.

126. Fazio, F. and Lafortuna, C. (1981) Effect of inhaled salbutamol on mucociliary clearance in patients with chronic bronchitis. *Chest*, **80**, 827–30.

127. Aubier, M., Murciano, D., Viires, N. *et al.* (1987) Effect of digoxin on diaphragm strength generation in patients with chronic obstructive pulmonary disease during acute respiratory failure. *Am. Rev. Respir. Dis.*, **135**, 544–8.

128. Anthonisen, N.R., Manfreda, J., Warren, C.P.W. *et al.* (1987) Antibiotic therapy in exacerbations of chronic obstructive pulmonary disease. *Ann. Intern. Med.*, **106**, 196–204.

129. Chapman, K.R., Bowie, D.M., Goldstein, R.S. *et al.* (1992) COPD Assessment and Management Guidelines: Consensus Statement of a Canadian Thoracic Society Workshop. *Can. Med. J.*, **147**, 420–8.

130. Palmer, J.B.D., Stuart, A.M., Shepherd, G.L. and Viskum, K. (1992) Inhaled salmeterol in the treatment of patients with moderate to severe reversible obstructive airways-disease – a 3-month comparison of the efficacy and safety of twice-daily salmeterol (100 mcg) with salmeterol (50 mcg). *Resp. Med.*, **86**, 409–17.

131. Smyth, E.T., Pavord, I.D., Wong, C.S. *et al.* (1993) Interaction and dose equivalence of salbutamol and salmeterol in patients with asthma. *Br. Med. J.*, **306**, 543–5.

132. Maesen, F.P.V., Smeets, J.J., Costongs, M.A.L. *et al.* (1993) Ba 679, a new long acting antimuscarinic bronchodilator: a pilot dose escalation study in COPD. *Eur. Respir. J.*, **6**, 1031–6.

CORTICOSTEROID TREATMENT 18

D.S. Postma and T.E.J. Renkema

18.1 INTRODUCTION

Pathophysiologic studies in patients with COPD show that there is a chronic inflammatory process in the wall and the lumen of the peripheral airways and a loss of elastic recoil in the supporting alveolar structure of the outer wall of the small airways. The inflammatory process in the small airways, being important both during the initial stage in the development of COPD [1,2] and in established COPD, consists of an increased number of lymphocytes, mononuclear cells, and neutrophils, increased connective tissue deposition and epithelial metaplasia and ulceration in the airway walls [3–6]. Bronchoalveolar lavage in smokers with or without airflow limitation shows that there is an increased percentage of neutrophils, patients with airflow limitation having higher numbers than the smokers without airflow limitation [3]. Moreover, macrophages of smoking patients with COPD show a higher activation level. Cigarettes may therefore be regarded as inflammatory agents.

These inflammatory processes in the airways may serve as an opening for institution of anti-inflammatory therapy in patients with COPD. This may circumstantially be supported by the observation that quitting smoking of cigarettes results in a significant slowing down in the deterioration of lung function [7,8]. The most potent anti-inflammatory therapeutic agents that are available are without any doubt glucocortico-steroids. In this chapter results of studies on the application of oral and topical corticosteroids in patients with established COPD with moderate to severe airways obstruction will be described.

18.2 ORAL CORTICOSTEROIDS

18.2.1 SHORT-TERM STUDIES

Corticosteroids have been used in the treatment of airways obstruction since 1950, when the first preparations of biosynthetically derived analogs of the adrenal cortical hormones became available. Today some 40 years later their role in COPD is still controversial, whereas they have a central place in everyday practice for the treatment of asthma. Several studies have investigated the effects of oral corticosteroids on the level of airways obstruction in patients with COPD [9–11], some of them having a controlled double-blind design [12–19]. But results from the latter type of studies are also conflicting. They at best show some beneficial effect in a subset of patients, even after extension of the duration of oral corticosteroid intake beyond the most commonly used 14 days. The latter seems to be important as Weir *et al.* found that FEV_1 continued to improve after 14 days of corticosteroid treatment in some subjects with COPD [20].

Characterization of the individuals who effectively will benefit from oral corticosteroids

Chronic Obstructive Pulmonary Disease. Edited by Dr P. Calverley and Professor N. Pride. Published in 1995 by Chapman & Hall, London. ISBN 0 412 46450 0

is, however, very difficult. No consistent pattern emerged from the above mentioned studies: greater reversibility and sputum and blood eosinophilia have been found to be weak predictors of improvement by some authors but not by others. One study stated that a response to oral prednisolone occurred as frequently in patients with physiologic features of emphysema as in those without [21].

Oral corticosteroids are capable of reducing the severity of hyper-responsiveness in asthmatic individuals even after short-term use [22]. One study investigated this effect in non-allergic patients with COPD and showed that oral corticosteroids do not change the level of hyper-responsiveness in these patients [22]. Furthermore Wempe *et al.* demonstrated that they also do not change the bronchodilator response to cumulatively applied doses of a β-agonist or anticholinergic [Fig. 18.1], nor alter the protection provided by either drug against histamine [23]. As only a small group of non-allergic COPD patients was investigated in this study, generalization to all patients is not suitable.

It is not yet clear whether beneficial effects of high-dose oral glucocorticosteroids on FEV_1, when they occur, are maintained when the doses are tapered off to clinically acceptable doses or when oral corticosteroids are supplemented by or replaced with inhaled corticosteroids. Only a small percentage of responders in two available studies [15,17] could maintain their response on low doses of inhaled corticosteroids. Harding and Freedman [12] showed that 4 of their responders (22% of the population) had a comparable improvement of ventilatory capacity when on single-blind therapy with 800 μg/day of beclomethasone valerate for 10 days, compared with 30 mg of prednisone daily for the same period. Another double-blind study in 18 patients with COPD [24] showed that addition of either 400 μg or 1600 μg of inhaled budesonide daily could comparably reduce the oral dose of corticosteroids by approximately 6.5 mg/day without changing the level of FEV_1 or hyper-responsiveness [Fig. 18.2]. In the group treated with 400 μg budesonide, prednisone was reduced from 8.1 to 1.4 mg, and in the group

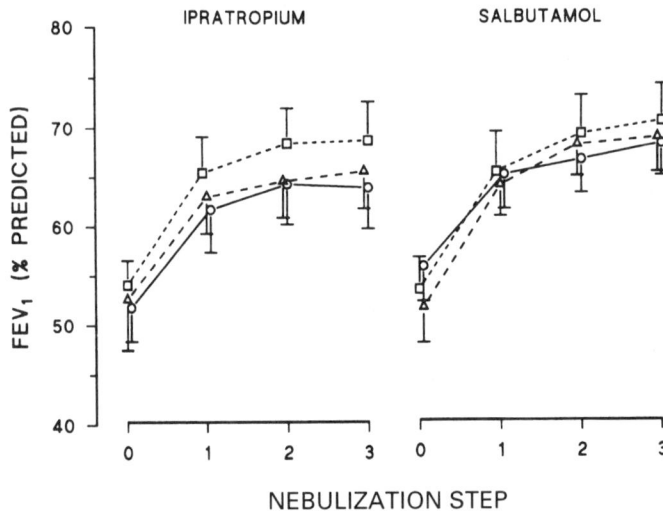

Fig. 18.1 Cumulative dose–response curves with nebulization of either ipratropium bromide (left panel) or salbutamol (right panel) after 3 weeks treatment with placebo (circle), budesonide (triangle) and prednisone (square). No significant differences in final FEV_1 existed between the treatments. (Reprinted with permission from [23].)

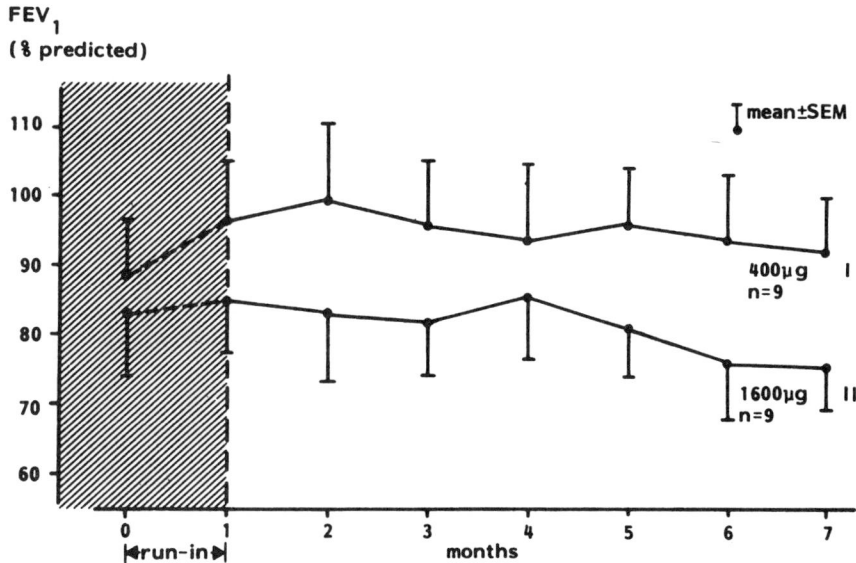

Fig. 18.2 Course of FEV_1 in 18 patients with COPD during reduction of prednisone (see text), while patients were on either 400 μg or 1600 μg daily of inhaled budesonide. (Reprinted with permission from [24].)

receiving 1600 μg budesonide, prednisone was reduced from 9.7 to 3.1 mg/day. This suggests that 400 μg/day of an inhaled corticosteroid may be sufficient. This is especially important since with this dose plasma cortisol values (after a Synacthen test) improved to normal levels. However, duration of follow-up was short, and results may be different at a later time. The same applies to the above mentioned studies investigating whether inhaled corticosteroids maintain the effect of oral corticosteroids.

Finally, little information is available on the role of oral corticosteroids in patients with an acute exacerbation [25–27]. Emerman found no effect of 100 mg methylprednisolone i.v. in addition to standard bronchodilator therapy. In contrast, Albert *et al.* found significant improvement with methylprednisolone (0.5 mg/kg i.v. every 6 hours over 72 hours) with regard to pre- and postbronchodilator FEV_1. The differences might be explained by the observation that the study of Albert showed significant effects after 6 hours, while Emerman investigated the patients for only up to 7 hours (see Chapter 19).

The most common side-effects are presented in Table 18.1. Though a short course of corticosteroids may result in only a few side-effects, long-term use even at lower dosages, is frequently associated with adverse reactions. In the 20 years' follow-up study on COPD patients treated with oral corticosteroids [28, 29] many patients had to stop therapy due to side-effects. The main reasons for stopping were: 20% due to hypertension, 20% with recurrent gastrointestinal ulcers, 40% with far advanced osteoporosis or fractures, 10% due to diabetes mellitus, and 10% miscellaneous (compliance, glaucoma, mood disorders). Thus severe osteoporosis with or without fractures is the most common side-effect. The advantage of using inhaled corticosteroids is that side-effects are reduced for the equivalent therapeutic effect, because of their low systemic effects. Nevertheless local side-effects are known, i.e. dysphonia, hoarseness, sore throat and oropharyngeal candida infection. The most important clinical side-effect of adrenocortical suppression is thought to occur with doses above 1500 μg/day [30,31], although some studies suggest an effect on bone

Table 18.1 Side-effects of oral corticosteroids

Short term, high dose
diabetes mellitus
hypertension
sodium and water retention
mood disorders
glaucoma
pancreatitis
peptic ulceration
Long term
hypothalamic–adrenal axis suppression
cushingoid features (e.g. striae, acne, skin atrophy, easy bruising, centripetal obesity)
osteoporosis
aseptic bone necrosis
posterior subcapsular cataract
hyperlipidemia
growth failure
impaired wound healing
proximal myopathy
suppression of immune response
oral candidiasis

turnover at lower dosages [32,33]. It has to be kept in mind, however, that the latter results pertain to healthy volunteers, treated for a very short time. Results may be different at longer time of follow-up. A recent report [34] does suggest that easy bruising is also a frequent side-effect, increasing in frequency with increasing age, dosage and duration of use. Future studies have yet to determine whether bone turnover is also affected by inhaled corticosteroids when given over longer periods of follow-up and with advanced age.

18.2.2 LONG-TERM STUDIES

Only two long-term intervention studies with oral glucocorticosteroids are available, both retrospective in nature [28,29]. These studies in patients with COPD show a favorable effect of prednisolone on the course of the FEV_1 over 20 years of follow-up. A close association existed between the pattern of change in FEV_1 over time and the intake and dosage of prednisolone [Fig. 18.3]. When 10 mg/day or more

was taken FEV_1 remained stable or even increased over the many years of follow-up. Improvement in FEV_1 as shown in the first study [28] was thought to be quite remarkable. Patients in this study were initially investigated because of a low FEV_1 (below 1 liter) and less than 15% improvement (from baseline prebronchodilator FEV_1) over the first year of follow-up in order to try to exclude patients with asthmatic features. In this study allergic patients were not systematically excluded, and this might have influenced the results. Therefore a similar study was started in patients without any sign of allergy. Comparable results were obtained [29].

Both studies showed that reduction below 10 mg/day or cessation of prednisolone resulted in further decline of FEV_1. The studies were retrospective in nature, but patients who were given or withheld prednisolone in a later stage of their follow-up could be regarded as their own control (CON+ and CON– in Fig. 18.3). One of the clinically important findings is that a change in FEV_1

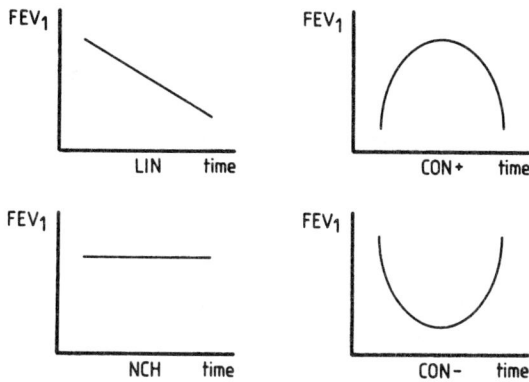

Fig. 18.3 Patterns of the course in FEV_1 over 20 years of follow-up in patients with COPD: LIN = linear, CON+ = convex, CON– = concave, NCH = no change. The course appeared to be related to institution or withdrawal of oral corticosteroids. (Reprinted with permission from [29].)

could only be observed after 6–24 months of therapy. This is in striking contrast with asthma, where glucocorticosteroids have an almost instantaneous effect. As COPD is slowly progressive disease this delay in effect may just reflect the difference in the etiology of airways obstruction. It may also underline the importance of long-term follow-up to detect any change in lung function when in-

tervention studies are undertaken in COPD and may explain the lack of effect observed in many short-term studies.

18.3 INHALED CORTICOSTEROIDS

There is little doubt that inhaled corticosteroids are an effective treatment for asthma, resulting in improvement of symptoms, number of exacerbations, lung function and hyper-responsiveness, both in short-term [35–39] and long-term studies [40–43]. It is only recently that inhaled corticosteroids have also drawn attention of researchers to application in patients with COPD.

18.3.1 SHORT-TERM STUDIES

There have been some 7 studies [23, 44–49] showing that inhaled corticosteroids administered over a period of 3–12 weeks generally do not change the level of airways obstruction, as assessed by FEV_1 and PEF, or airways hyper-responsiveness to histamine in patients with COPD. Baseline characteristics of these studies are presented in Table 18.2.

In the studies of Engel *et al.* [44] and Wesseling *et al.* [45] one could expect that no

Table 18.2 Baseline characteristics and change in FEV_1 in 7 short-term studies with inhaled corticosteroids in COPD

Reference	Engel [44]	Wesseling [45]	Watson [46]	Thompson [47]	Wempe [23]	Auffarth [48]	Weir [49]
No.	18	35	14	30	10	24	107
Age (years)	50	52	60	50	57	57	63
Smoking (no.)	18	16	14	30	6	24	41
Atopy (no.)	0	–	3	–	0	0	46
FEV_1 (% pred)	97	96	80	72	59	53	44
ΔFEV_1 (%) in	–	–	11	8	10	7	11
PC_{20} (mg/ml)	0.61	–	2.8	–	0.52	0.96	0.81
Dose (μg/day)	800	1600	1200	1000	1600	1600	1500
Duration (wk)	12	6	12	6	3	8	2
Improvement in FEV_1	none	none	none	10%[a]	7.5%[a]	none	[b]

–, not determined.
ΔFEV_1, % in, improvement with bronchodilator expressed as increase in % above baseline; PC_{20}, concentration of inhaled histamine provoking a fall in FEV_1 of 20% or more; % pred, percentage predicted value.
[a] improvement in FEV_1 with inhaled corticosteroids.
[b] > 20% improvement in FEV_1 in 8/34 with inhaled corticosteroids and 3/35 with placebo (not significant).

change in FEV_1 would occur after therapy with inhaled corticosteroids, as the patients all had near-normal lung function ('chronic bronchitis'). The same is true, although to a lesser extent, for the study of Watson *et al.* [46]. Although in the other studies a certain improvement should be detectable, it could not be demonstrated in most patients even at reasonably high doses of inhaled corticosteroids up to 1600 μg/day. There are nevertheless two studies showing some or even a significant response of FEV_1 to inhaled corticosteroids compared with placebo. The first one [49] shows that 12 out of 34 patients responded with a $\geq 10\%$ increase in FEV_1, FVC

and PEF, but many of these patients had an allergic background. The other one [47], shows in smokers with mild airways obstruction an improvement of 10% in predicted FEV_1 in the beclomethasone group and a 3% improvement in the placebo group, the difference being statistically significant (Fig. 18.4). These patients appeared to be hardly reversible on a bronchodilator, while hyperresponsiveness was not tested. Atopy was also not tested and this may have influenced the results, as it has been shown in a mixed population with airways obstruction that more allergic individuals are more likely to respond to inhaled corticosteroids [43]. An interesting observation in the study of Thompson and co-workers [47] was that not only FEV_1 but also the parameters in the bronchoalveolar lavage fluid reflecting epithelial permeability and cellularity improved in the beclomethasone-treated group (Fig. 18.5). Therefore, asthma and COPD might have some expressions of airways inflammation in common. However, the significant difference between the two groups was largely due to increased leakage over the

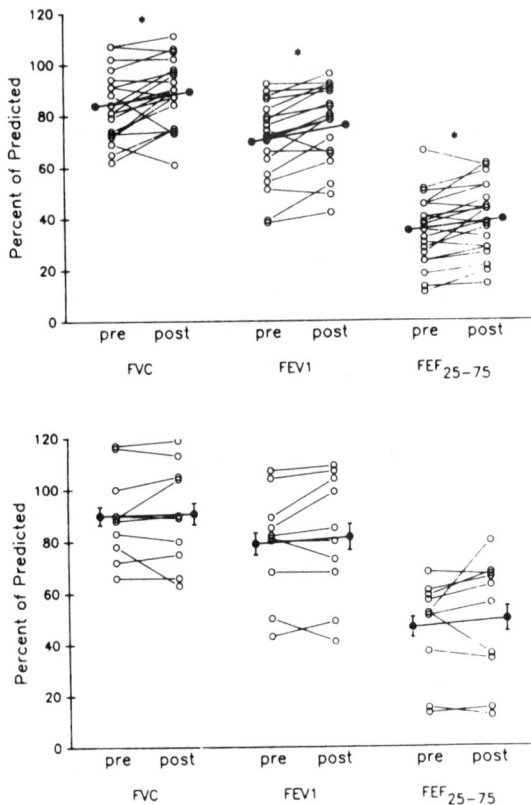

Fig. 18.4 Spirometric changes after 6 weeks of treatment with beclomethasone (top) or placebo (bottom). FEF_{25-75} forced expiratory flow between 25% and 75% of vital capacity. (Reprinted with permission from [47].)

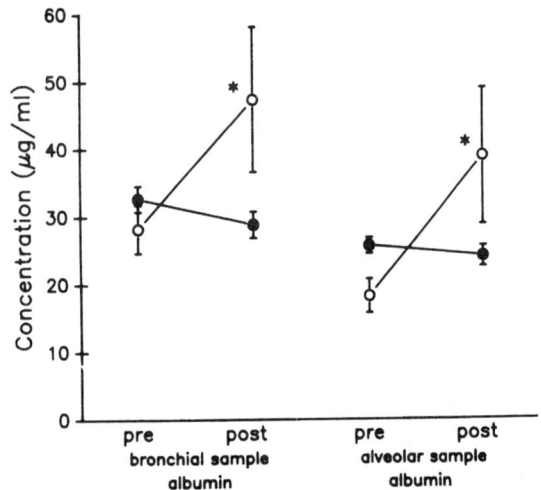

Fig. 18.5 Changes in estimated epithelial lining fluid albumin concentrations after treatment with beclomethasone (closed circles) or placebo (open circles). (Reprinted with permission from [47].)

6 weeks of follow-up in the placebo-treated group. This increase was so big that one wonders what would happen if this were continued over many years. Therefore, further results on anti-inflammatory effects of corticosteroids in patients with COPD have to be awaited.

Next to objective functional criteria, subjective improvement may be an important measure of treatment effect. It is for instance well known that patients who hardly improve or even show deterioration in lung function after inhaling a bronchodilator may have symptomatic benefit. It is as yet not certain what should be tested to assess treatment effects best. Yet it is certain that in the future quality of life will be one of the issues. In the available studies on short-term therapy of inhaled corticosteroids in patients with COPD there are some positive effects in subjective symptoms, like cough [44], sputum production [47], and dyspnea [48]. When other parameters were assessed in the former studies, they all showed a trend for improvement in the corticosteroid group.

Based on these short-term effects one could only hypothesize that longer duration of treatment might perhaps show larger effects. As there is no clearcut dose–effect relationship of inhaled corticosteroids in the above mentioned short-term studies, a more pronounced effect with higher doses could not be expected. Moreover, higher doses of inhaled corticosteroids are not warranted considering the current knowledge on side-effects.

18.3.2 LONG-TERM STUDIES

Only one recently published article has studied the effect of inhaled corticosteroids in patients with COPD after one year of therapy [50]. Patients in this study were selected from a former study [51] based on their rapid decline in lung function over the previous 2 years when they did not use any inhaled corticosteroids. They served as their own controls when 800 μg/day of inhaled

Table 18.3 Patient characteristics in the study of Dompeling *et al.* [50]

	Asthma	*COPD*
No.	28	28
Age (yrs)	49 (12)	54 (12)
Gender, male	12	16
Pack-years	13 (14)	23 (3)[a]
Smokers (no.)	14	17
Allergy (no.)	14	2
FEV_1 (% pred)	67 (17)	70 (16)
ΔFEV_1 (% pred)	14 (9)	7 (4)[a]
PC_{20} (mg/ml)	0.8	6.2[a]

[a] significant difference.
% pred = percentage predicted; ΔFEV_1 (% pred), bronchodilator response expressed as % predicted value of FEV1.

beclomethasone was instituted after the first two years. The patients in this study were categorized as either 'asthma' or 'COPD', but overlap in clinical features between the two groups was considerable (Table 18.3). Atopy appeared to be more prominent in asthmatics, as expected. However, level of FEV_1 and smoking was not that different between those with asthma and with COPD.

Both groups showed a mean fall in FEV_1 in the first 2 years of about 160 ml/year, which is unusually high, especially in patients with asthma. After institution of beclomethasone, patients with COPD improved their prebronchodilator FEV_1 significantly by 160 ml in the first 6 months of treatment, but the fall in FEV_1 continued in the next 6 months by 70 ml (Fig. 18.6). Therefore the authors suggest that longer follow-up is necessary to establish whether this is due to chance variation or real decline. Hyper-responsiveness deteriorated by 1.8 doubling dose ($P = 0.07$) during the year of beclomethasone treatment. Exacerbations were the same in the first 2 years without inhaled corticosteroids and the third year with inhaled corticosteroids (mean 1.8 exacerbations per year in both periods). Exacerbations were less frequent in the asthma group (mean 1.3/year in the first 2 years, and significantly lower in the third year: 0.6 per year). As the study did

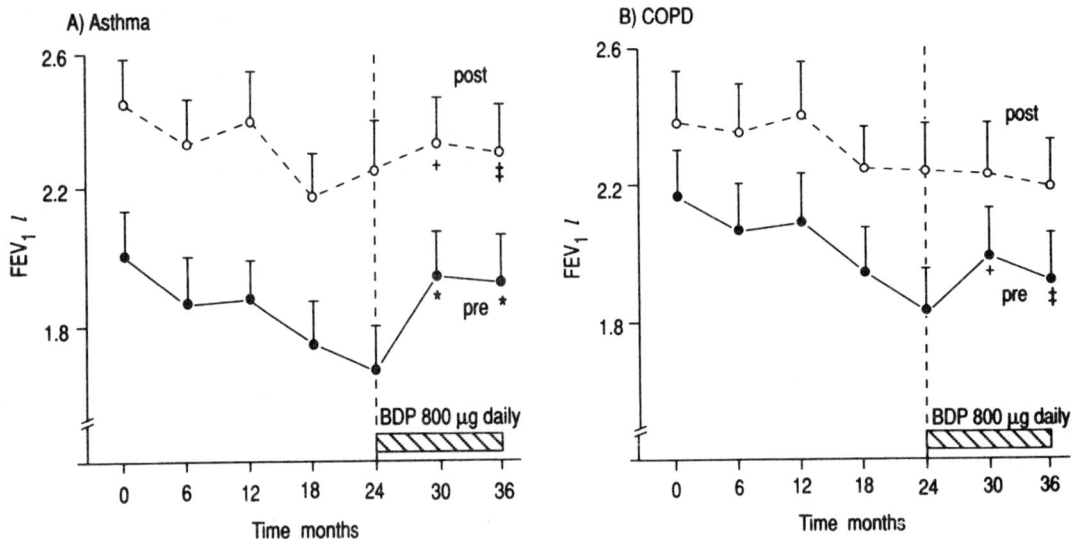

Fig. 18.6 The course of prebronchodilator (closed circles) and postbronchodilator (open circles) FEV_1 after three years treatment with bronchodilators alone (0–24 months) and beclomethsasone (24–36 months). Left panel shows results of asthmatics, right panel of patients with COPD. Values were compared with 24 months' values. Asthma: *: $P = 0.001$; +: $P = 0.07$; ++: $P = 0.32$; COPD: +: $P = 0.09$; ++: $P = 0.29$. (Reprinted with permission from [50].)

not have a control group on placebo, it is possibly only justified to compare the 'asthma' with the 'COPD' group. This shows that the improvement in FEV_1 and PEF in the latter group is smaller than in the former. Moreover, exacerbations were less frequent in the asthma group.

The last observations of the study of Dompeling *et al.* [50] are compatible with the findings of another long-term study, where patients with both asthma and COPD were included, not on the basis of a clinical diagnosis, but on objective criteria, i.e. the presence of airways obstruction and hyper-responsiveness [43]. In this study with 2.5 years follow-up all patients received an inhaled β-agonist, 500 μg q.i.d. with addition of either (a) placebo 2 puffs q.i.d., (b) ipratropium bromide, 40 μg q.i.d., or (c) inhaled beclomethasone, 200 μg q.i.d. Patients with a symptom-based diagnosis of asthma responded more favorably with their FEV_1 than those with COPD. This study also showed a beneficial effect on the number of ex-

acerbations at follow-up [43] in both groups (Fig. 18.7).

The study was not designed to investigate differences between asthma and COPD, and questionnaire-based diagnoses were made after inclusion of the patients. It showed that a subgroup of patients could not be classified as either asthmatic or COPD as they had features of both (called 'asthmatic bronchitis'). This group had a somewhat less positive response to inhaled corticosteroids. Thus, it seems worthwhile to investigate a COPD-group with or without allergic and hyper-responsiveness features and with or without chronic cough and sputum, to determine who will benefit from long-term inhaled corticosteroids.

Finally, there is one abstract [52] of a study of 58 non-allergic individuals with irreversible airways obstruction, who were all hyper-responsive. In this study patients were treated with either (a) placebo, (b) 1600 μg budesonide or (c) 1600 μg budesonide and 5 mg pred-

no. exacerbations/
patient-year

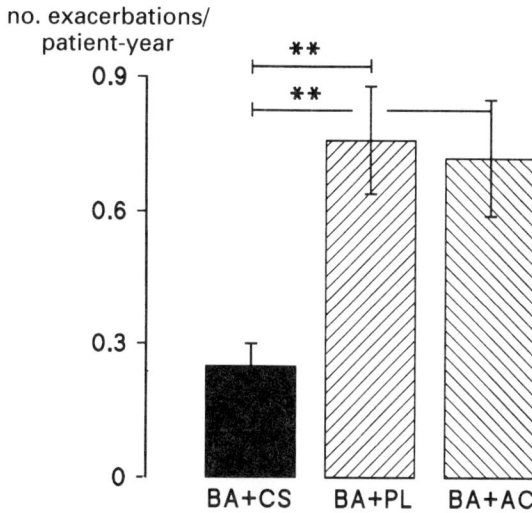

Fig. 18.7 Number of exacerbations per year that the patient is in the study in a symptom-based subgroup of patients with COPD. BA = β-agonist; CS = inhaled corticosteroids; PL = placebo; AC = anti-cholinergic. ** = significant difference. (Data of Dutch CNSLD Study Group [43].)

therapy. Over the 2 years of follow-up, there appeared to be a positive effect of inhaled corticosteroids on decline in FEV_1. These effects were small and only reached significance in the group that was treated with inhaled corticosteroids alone. The duration of exacerbations tended to decrease and symptoms improved in the two groups treated with corticosteroids.

Although the numbers of patients in the above mentioned studies are small, and some of these studies have not been designed for testing the effects of inhaled corticosteroids in COPD, the results of the three studies point in the same direction. Inhaled corticosteroids might thus reduce exacerbations in the long run and improve symptoms. Possibly, decline of lung function is also reduced (Table 18.4). The latter appears to be true for prebronchodilator FEV_1. Whether the same is true for postbronchodilator FEV_1 is not yet clear.

18.4 INTERACTION OF CORTICOSTEROIDS WITH BRONCHODILATORS

nisolone orally daily. In addition to this double-blind treatment, patients continued their regular use of inhaled and oral bronchodilators. The three small groups were comparable at the start of the study with regard to smoking habits, airways obstruction and hyper-responsiveness and bronchodilator

Corticosteroids are known to restore β-adrenergic responsiveness of the smooth muscle in previously non-responsive asthmatics [53] and in normal subjects [54]. Moreover, *in vitro* studies have shown an increase in β-receptors after corticosteroids [55]. At this moment there is one investigation in patients with

Table 18.4 Baseline characteristics and results from long-term studies with inhaled corticosteroids in COPD

	Dompeling et al. [50]	*Dutch SGO [43]*	*Renkema et al. [52]*
No.	28	33	58
FEV_1 (% pred)	63	62	63
Δ FEV_1 (% baseline)	12	6	10
PC_{20} (mg/ml)	8.4	0.44	1.3
Duration (years)	1	2.5	2
Dose (μg/24 h)	800	800	1600
Reduction exa[a]	–	+	+
Improvement FEV_1	+	+	±
Improvement PC_{20}	–	+	–

[a] reduction of days or number of exacerbations by inhaled corticosteroids.
% pred = % predicted

COPD studying an interactive effect of inhaled and oral corticosteroids with bronchodilators, i.e. the anticholinergic drug ipratropium bromide and the β-adrenergic drug salbutamol [23]. There was no modifying effect of corticosteroids on bronchodilator action, though only a small group of patients was studied for a relatively short period. Nevertheless a higher, though non-significant, post-ipratropium FEV_1 was found after treatment with prednisone compared with placebo treatment (Fig. 18.1). The latter occurred without an effect of prednisone on prebronchodilator FEV_1. This may suggest some synergistic effect, and more studies are warranted in this field.

18.5 CONCLUSIONS

Results of the few published studies show some circumstantial evidence for a beneficial effect of corticosteroids in COPD. It is astonishing how much is known of their effects in asthma, and how relatively little in COPD. Some important points emerge from the available data.

First, several studies have pointed to the fact that corticosteroids have a much slower onset of action in COPD than in asthma. As a consequence trials of both oral and inhaled corticosteroids in COPD – in larger groups, but in individual patients as well – should proceed for longer time periods than we have become used to in asthma.

The use of oral corticosteroids is clearly limited by their serious side-effects. However, as with any pharmaceutical intervention, side-effects of oral corticosteroids in patients with COPD should be carefully weighed against their benefits. Dosages should be reduced to the lowest possible level, and perhaps supplemented with inhaled corticosteroids.

The role of inhaled corticosteroids in clinical practice as opposed to oral corticosteroids is even less clear. Short-term studies do not show a large beneficial effect in ventilatory capacity or hyper-responsiveness, although there appears to be some subjective improvement in symptoms. There is as yet only one abstract showing that inhaled corticosteroids prevent accelerated decline at 2 years' follow-up. As with oral corticosteroids, there seems to be a subgroup of patients that responds favorably. It is as yet, however, unclear which patient characteristics separate 'responders' from 'non-responders'. Clearly this has to be established in further long-term studies before all patients with COPD, regardless of age, smoking habits, atopy, reversibility, and hyper-responsiveness are given inhaled corticosteroids life-long. More research needs to be directed at distinguishing subgroups in order to be able to predict corticosteroid sensitivity. Large scale long-term studies such as the Euroscop study currently in progress [57] should give the answers.

Finally, it is an unresolved problem which parameters should be assessed to determine corticosteroid sensitivity: exacerbation rates and measures of quality of life are increasingly being recognized as important parameters. Taking improvements in FEV_1 as the only measure may well lead to insufficient patient care.

REFERENCES

1. Hogg, J.C., Macklem, P.T. and Thurlbeck, W.M. (1968). Site and nature of airway obstruction in chronic obstructive lung disease. *N. Engl. J. Med.*, **278**, 1355–60.
2. Niewoehner, D.E., Kleinerman, J. and Rice, D.B. (1974) Pathologic changes in the peripheral airways of young cigarette smokers. *N. Engl. J. Med.*, **291**, 755–8.
3. Thompson, A.B., Draughton, D. Robbins, R.A. *et al.* (1989) Intraluminal airway inflammation in chronic bronchitis. Characterization and correlation with clinical parameters. *Am. Rev. Respir. Dis.*, **140**, 1527–37.
4. Martin, T.R., Raghu, G., Maunder, R.J. and Springmeyer, S.C. (1985) The effects of chronic bronchitis and chronic air-flow obstruction on lung cell populations recovered by bron-

choalveolar lavage. *Am. Rev. Respir. Dis.*, **132**, 254–60.

5. Ollerenshaw, S.L. and Woolcock, A.J. (1992) Characteristics of the inflammation in biopsies form large airways of subjects with asthma and subjects with chronic airflow limitation. *Am. Rev. Respir. Dis.*, **145**, 922–7.

6. Bosken, C.H., Hards, J., Gatter, K. and Hogg, J.C. (1992) Characterization of the inflammatory reaction in the peripheral airways of cigarette smokers using immunocytochemistry. *Am. Rev. Respir. Dis.*, **145**, 911–17.

7. Fletcher, C., Peto, R., Tinker, C. and Speizer, F.E. (1976). *The Natural History of Chronic Bronchitis and Emphysema. An Eight Year Study of Early Chronic Obstructive Lung Disease in Working Men in London.* Oxford University Press, Oxford.

8. Postma, D.S. and Sluiter, H.J. (1989) Prognosis of chronic obstructive pulmonary disease: the Dutch experience. *Am. Rev. Respir. Dis.*, **140**, S100–S105.

9. Eliasson, O., Hoffman, J., Trueb, D. *et al.* (1986) Corticosteroids in COPD. A clinical trial and reassessment of the literature. *Chest*, **89**, 484–90.

10. Postma, D.S., Renkema, T.E.J. and Koëter, G.H. (1990) Effects of corticosteroids in 'chronic bronchitis' and 'chronic obstructive airway disease'. *Agents Actions*, **30** suppl. 41–67.

11. Callahan, C.M., Dittus, R.S. and Katz, B.P. (1991) Oral corticosteroid therapy for patients with stable chronic obstructive pulmonary disease. A meta-analysis. *Ann. Intern. Med.*, **114**, 216–23.

12. Harding, S.M. and Freedman, S. (1978) A comparison of oral and inhaled corticosteroids in patients with chronic airways obstruction: features determining response. *Thorax*, **33**, 214–8.

13. Evans, J.A., Morrison, I.M. and Saunders, K.B. (1974) A controlled trial of prednisone, in low dosage, in patients with chronic airways obstruction. *Thorax*, **29**, 401–6.

14. Lam, W.K., So, S.Y. and Yu, D.Y.C. (1983) Response to oral corticosteroids in chronic airflow obstruction. *Br. J. Dis. Chest*, **77**, 189–98.

15. Mendella, L.A., Manfreda, J., Warren, C.P.W. and Anthonisen, N.R. (1982) Steroid response in stable chronic obstructive pulmonary disease. *Ann. Intern. Med.*, **96**, 17–21.

16. Mitchell, D.M., Gildeh, P., Rehahn, M. *et al.* (1984) Effects of prednisolone in chronic airflow limitation. *Lancet*, **ii**, 193–5.

17. Shim, C., Stover, D.E. and Williams, M.H. Jr. (1978) Response to corticosteroids in chronic bronchitis. *J. Allergy Clin. Immunol.*, **62**, 363–7.

18. Sahn, S.A. (1978) Corticosteroids in chronic bronchitis and pulmonary emphysema. *Chest*, **73**, 389–96.

19. Stokes, T.C., O'Reilly, J.F., Shaylor, J.M. and Harrison, B.D.W. (1982) Assessment of steroid responsiveness in patients with chronic airflow obstruction. *Lancet*, **ii**, 345–8.

20. Weir, D.C., Robertson, A.S., Gove, R.I. and Burge, P.S. (1990) Time course of response to oral and inhaled corticosteroids in non-asthmatic chronic airflow obstruction. *Thorax*, **45**, 118–21.

21. Weir, D.C., Gove, R.I., Robertson, A.S. *et al.* (1991). Response to corticosteroids in chronic airflow obstruction: relationship to emphysema and airways collapse. *Eur. Respir. J.*, **4**, 1185–90.

22. Wempe, J.B., Postma, D.S., Breederveld, N. *et al.* (1992) Separate and combined effects of corticosteroids and bronchodilators on airflow obstruction and airway hyperresponsiveness in asthma. *J. Allergy Clin. Immunol.*, **89**, 679–87.

23. Wempe, J.B., Postma, D.S., Breederveld, N. *et al.* (1992) Effects of corticosteroids on brochodilator action in chronic obstructive pulmonary disease. *Thorax*, **47**, 616–21.

24. Overbeek, S.E., Hilvering, C., Bogaard, J.M. *et al.* (1986) A comparison of the efficacy of high dose and normal dose budosonide in prednisone dependent patients with chronic obstructive lung disease (COLD). *Eur. J. Respir. Dis.*, **69**, Suppl. 146, 581–7.

25. Emerman, C.L., Connors, A.E., Lukens, T.W. *et al.* (1989) A randomized clinical trial of methylprednisolone in the emergency treatment of acute exacerbations in COPD. *Chest*, **95**, 563–7.

26. Albert, R.K., Martin, T.R. and Lewis, S.W. (1980) Controlled clinical trial of methylprednisolone in patients with chronic bronchitis and acute repiratory insufficiency. *Ann. Intern. Med.*, **92**, 753–8.

27. Glenny, R.W. (1987) Steroids in COPD: the scripture according to Albert. *Chest*, **91**, 289–90.

28. Postma, D.S., Steenhuis, E.J., Weele, van der LTh. and Sluiter, H.J. (1985) Severe chronic airflow obstruction: can corticosteroids slow down progression? *Eur. J. Respir. Dis.*, **67**, 56–64.

29. Postma, D.S., Peters, I., Steenhuis, E.J. and Sluiter, H.J. (1988) Moderately severe chronic airflow obstruction. Can corticosteroids slow down progression? *Eur. Respir. J.*, **1**, 22–6.

458   *Corticosteroid treatment*

30. Smith, M.J. and Hodson, M.E. (1983) Effects of long term inhaled high dose beclomethasone dipropionate on adrenal function. *Thorax*, **38**, 676–81.
31. Gordon, A.C.H., McDonald, C.F., Thomson, S.A. *et al.* (1987) Dose of inhaled budesonide required to produce clinical suppression of plasma cortisol. *Eur. J. Respir. Dis.*, **71**, 10–14.
32. Ali, N.J., Capewell, S. and Ward, M.J. (1991) Bone turnover during high dose inhaled corticosteroid activity. *Thorax*, **46**, 160–5.
33. Pouw, E.M., Prummel, M.F., Oosting, H. *et al.* (1991) Beclomethasone inhalation decreases serum osteocalcin concentration. *Br. Med. J.*, **302**, 627–8.
34. Mak, V.H.F., Melchor, R. and Spiro, S.G. (1992) Easy bruising as a side-effect of inhaled corticosteroids. *Eur. Respir. J.*, **5**, 1068–74.
35. Kraan, J., Köeter, G.H., Mark, van der ThW. *et al.* (1988) Dosage and time effects of inhaled budesonide on bronchial hyperreactivity. *Am. Rev. Respir. Dis.*, **137**, 44–8.
36. Kraan, J., Köeter, G.H., Mark, van der ThW. *et al.* (1985) Changes in bronchial hyperreactivity induced by 4 weeks of treatment with anti-asthmatic drugs in patients with allergic asthma: a comparison between budeesonide and terbutaline. *J. Allergy Clin. Immunol.*, **76**, 628–36.
37. Kerrebijn, K.F., Van Essen-Zandvliet, E.E.M. and Neijens, H.J. (1987) Effect of long-term treatment with inhaled corticosteroids and beta-agonists on the bronchial responsiveness in children with asthma. *J. Allergy Clin. Immunol.*, **79**, 653–9.
38. Svendsen, U.G., Frolund, L., Madsen, F. and Nielsen, N.H. (1989). A comparison of the effects of nedocromil sodium and beclomethasone diproprionate on pulmonary function, symptoms, and bronchial responsiveness in patients with asthma. *J. Allergy Clin. Immunol.*, **84**, 224–31.
39. Baets, de F.M., Goetheyn, M. and Kerrebijn, K.F. (1990) The effect of two months of treatment with inhaled budesonide on bronchial responsiveness to histamine and house dust mite antigen in asthmatic children. *Am. Rev. Respir. Dis.*, **142**, 581–6.
40. Juniper, E.F., Kline, P.A., Vanzieleghem, M.A. *et al.* (1990) Long-term effects of budesonide on airway responsiveness and clinical asthma severity in inhaled steroid-dependent asthmatics. *Eur. Respir. J.*, **3**, 1122–7.
41. Juniper, E.F., Kline, P.A., Vanzieleghem, M.A. *et al.* (1990) Effect of long-term treatment with an inhaled corticosteroid (budesonide) on airway hyperresponsiveness and clinical asthma in nonsteroid-dependent asthmatics. *Am. Rev. Respir. Dis.*, **142**, 832–6.
42. Haahtela, T., Järvinen, M., Kava, T. *et al.* (1991) Comparison of a beta-agonist, terbutaline, with an inhaled corticosteroid, budesonide, in newly detected asthma. *N. Engl. J. Med.*, **325**, 388–92.
43. Kerstjens, H.A.M., Brand, P.L.P., Hughes, M.D. and the Dutch CNSLD Group (1992) A comparison of bronchodilator therapy with or without inhaled corticosteroid therapy in obstructive airways disease. *N. Engl. J. Med.*, **327**, 1413–19.
44. Engel, T., Heinig, J.H., Madsen, O. *et al.* (1989) A trial of inhaled budesonide on airway hyperresponsiveness in smokers with chronic bronchitis. *Eur. Respir. J.*, **2**, 935–9.
45. Wesseling, G.J., Quaedvlieg, M. and Wouters, E.F.M. (1991) Inhaled budesonide in chronic bronchitis. Effects on respiratory impedance. *Eur. Respir. J.*, **4**, 1101–5.
46. Watson, A., Lim, T.K., Joyce, H. and Pride, N.B. (1992) Failure of inhaled corticosteroids to modify bronchoconstrictor or bronchodilator responsiveness in middle-aged smokers with mild airflow obstruction. *Chest*, **101**, 350–5.
47. Thompson, A.B., Mueller, M.B., Heires, A.J. *et al.* (1992) Aerosolized beclomethasone in chronic bronchitis. Improved pulmonary function and diminished airway inflammation. *Am. Rev. Respir. Dis.*, **146**, 389–95.
48. Auffarth, B., Postma, D.S., de Monchy, J.G.R. *et al.* (1991) Effects of inhaled budesonide on spirometry, reversibility, airway responsiveness and cough threshold in smokers with COPD. *Thorax*, **46**, 327–33.
49. Weir, D.C., Gove, R.I., Robertson, A.S. *et al.* (1990) Corticosteroid trials in non-asthmatic chronic airflow obstruction: a comparison of oral prednisolone and inhaled beclomethasone dipropionate. *Thorax*, **45**, 112–7.
50. Dompeling, E. van Schayck, C.P., Folgering, H. *et al.* (1992) Inhaled beclomethasone improves the course of asthma and COPD. *Eur. Respir. J.* **5**, 945–52.
51. van Schayck, C.P., Dompeling, E., van Herwaarden, C. *et al.* (1991) Bronchodilator treatment in moderate asthma or chronic bronchitis: continuous or on demand? A randomised controlled study. *Br. Med. J.*, **303**, 1426–31.

52. Renkema, T.E.J., Sluiter, H.J., Koëter, G.H. and Postma, D.S. (1990) A two-year prospective study on the effect of inhaled and inhaled plus oral corticosteroids in chronic airflow obstruction. *Am. Rev. Respir. Dis.*, **141**, A504.

53. Ellul-Micallef, R. and Fenech, F.F. (1975) Effects of intravenous prednisolone in asthmatics with diminished adrenergic responses. *Lancet*, **ii**, 375–7.

54. Holgate, S.T., Baldwin, C.J. and Tattersfield, A.E. (1977) β-Adrenergic agonist resistance in normal human airways. *Lancet*, **ii**, 375

55. Fraser, C.M. and Venter, J.C. (1980) The synthesis of beta-adrenergic receptors in cultured human lung cells: induction by glucocorticosteroids. *Biochem. Biphys. Res. Commun.*, **94**, 390–7.

56. Hui, K.P., Conolly, M.E. and Tashkin, D.P. (1982) Reversal of human lymphocyte beta-adrenergic receptor desensitization by glucocorticoids. *Clin. Pharmacol. Ther.*, **32**, 566–71.

57. Pauwels, R.A., Löfdahl, C-G., Pride, N.B. *et al.* (1992) European Respiratory Society Study on chronic obstructive pulmonary disease (EUROSCOP): hypothesis and design. *Eur. Respir. J.*, **5**, 1254–61.

ACUTE RESPIRATORY FAILURE

M.J. Mador and M.J. Tobin

19.1 INTRODUCTION

Chronic obstructive pulmonary disease (COPD) is an extremely common disorder in industrialized countries. In 1986, approximately 11.4 and 2 million Americans were estimated to have chronic bronchitis and emphysema, respectively [1]. Almost 2 million hospitalizations were due to COPD. COPD was the fifth leading cause of death (3.6% of all deaths) [2]. Morbidity and mortality rates are even higher in the UK. These patients are extremely vulnerable to a wide variety of insults. Thus, a bronchial infection which would have only minor effects in a healthy individual can tip the COPD patient into frank respiratory failure. In this chapter we will review the clinical presentation and treatment of acute respiratory failure in patients with COPD.

19.2 CLINICAL MANIFESTATIONS

Patients with acute respiratory failure and COPD may present with features of the precipitating illness, worsening of the underlying obstructive lung disease, carbon dioxide (CO_2) narcosis, or complications arising from acute respiratory failure. The symptoms of the precipitating illness can obviously be quite variable. Worsening of the underlying COPD usually results in increasing dyspnea and the typical patient with acute respiratory failure is in obvious respiratory distress. Tachypnea and prominent accessory muscle recruitment are generally present. Sputum production may increase or the patient may complain of difficulty in expectorating sputum. There is often a recent history of upper respiratory tract infection and/or the production of purulent yellow-green sputum. Peripheral edema and weight gain may be present suggesting a worsening of right heart failure. Wheezing may be heard and breath sounds are usually diminished.

When considering the effects of carbon dioxide retention on gas exchange, it is useful to examine the carbon dioxide–oxygen diagram of Rahn and Fenn (Fig. 19.1) [3]. This diagram shows that a rise in the arterial carbon dioxide (Pa_{CO_2}) is always accompanied by a fall in the arterial oxygen tension (Pa_{O_2}). The slope of the alveolar line relating oxygen tension (P_{O_2}) to carbon dioxide tension (P_{CO_2}) depends on the respiratory exchange ratio, which is usually 0.8. Thus, an increase in Pa_{CO_2} of 10 mmHg will result in a 12.5 mmHg fall in Pa_{O_2}. Studies in patients with COPD and acute respiratory failure have shown that the lowest Pa_{O_2} level compatible with life is approximately 20 mmHg [4,5]. Therefore, the highest tolerable Pa_{CO_2} while breathing room air is approximately 80–90 mmHg. Since patients with COPD have an increased

Chronic Obstructive Pulmonary Disease. Edited by Dr P. Calverley and Professor N. Pride. Published in 1995 by Chapman & Hall, London. ISBN 0 412 46450 0

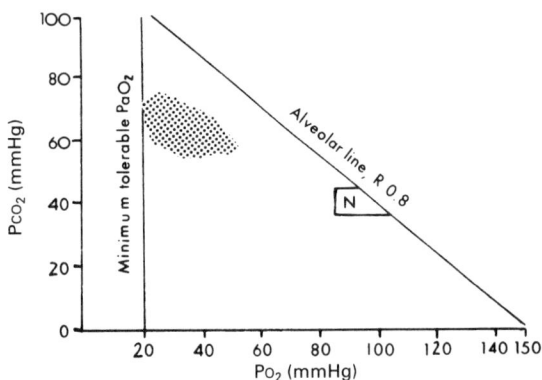

Fig. 19.1 The relationship between oxygen tension (P_{O_2}) and carbon dioxide tension (P_{CO_2}) in patients breathing room air is depicted in this oxygen–carbon dioxide diagram. The slope of the alveolar line depends on the respiratory exchange ratio (R), which is assumed to be 0.8. The boxed area (N) represents the range of arterial blood gas values in normal persons. The horizontal distance of PaO_2 value from the alveolar line represents the alveolar–arterial oxygen gradient.

Studies of patients with chronic obstructive pulmonary disease in acute respiratory failure reveal that a PaO_2 of 20 mmHg is the lowest PaO_2 value compatible with life while breathing room air. The stippled area represents the usual range of $PaCO_2$ values in patients with acute respiratory failure who are breathing room air. (Reproduced from reference [4].)

alveolar–arterial oxygen gradient, $PaCO_2$ rarely exceeds 80 mmHg while breathing room air [5].

The major clinical features of hypercapnia are those that affect the central nervous system and to a lesser degree the cardiovascular system. The central nervous system findings range from irritability to coma and include disorientation, confusion, somnolence and combativeness [6,7]. Coma is uncommon in patients who are breathing room air, since the level of $PaCO_2$ necessary to cause coma is usually associated with a PaO_2 that is incompatible with life [8]. Motor findings include tremor, myoclonic jerks, asterixis and seizures [6]. The vasodilator action of CO_2 may raise intracranial pressure causing

headache or papilledema [7–9]. Focal signs mimicking a cerebrovascular accident may rarely occur.

The level of consciousness correlates reasonably well with cerebrospinal fluid pH, which, in turn, is usually decreased in proportion to blood pH in patients with respiratory acidosis [10]. The rapidity of the increase in $PaCO_2$ and the severity of the accompanying hypoxemia are also important factors [11]. In a study of patients receiving long-term oxygen therapy no evidence of obvious central nervous system dysfunction was noted at $PaCO_2$ levels ranging from 75 to 110 mmHg [12]. The fact that these patients had a normal or only mildly depressed arterial pH and PaO_2 suggests that acidosis and hypoxemia are probably the major factors that account for the clinical manifestations of CO_2 narcosis.

The cardiovascular features of hypercapnia are caused by the vasodilator and sympathetic stimulant effects of carbon dioxide [11]. These effects include warm flushed skin, diaphoresis and a bounding pulse [13].

19.3 DIAGNOSIS

Obtaining an arterial blood gas is imperative in assessing the patient with acute respiratory failure. The PaO_2 reveals the patient's state of oxygenation. The conventional criterion for the diagnosis of respiratory failure due to failure of oxygenation is a PaO_2 of less than 55 mmHg. The $PaCO_2$ measures the adequacy of alveolar ventilation.

$$PaCO_2 = (\dot{V}CO_2 / \dot{V}A) \times k$$

where $\dot{V}CO_2$ = CO_2 production, $\dot{V}A$ = alveolar ventilation, and k = constant. An elevated $PaCO_2$ value due to a decrease in $\dot{V}A$ may in turn be due to a decrease in minute ventilation or an increase in dead space. An increase in CO_2 production is normally compensated for by an increase in minute ventilation, and, thus, it is never solely responsible for an increase in $PaCO_2$. The patient's acid–base status should be evaluated as it is important to remember that an increase in $PaCO_2$ is a normal compensatory response to metabolic alkalosis [14]. A $PaCO_2$ of 86 mmHg has been reported in a patient with metabolic alkalosis who had no evidence of lung disease [15]. Thus, it is crucial to check the pH to determine the primary acid–base disturbance. In the absence of metabolic alkalosis, a diagnosis of hypercapnic respiratory failure is generally made when the $PaCO_2$ is greater than 45 mmHg. The chronicity of the respiratory failure can be determined by evaluating the pH and serum bicarbonate. As a rule of thumb, an acute increase in $PaCO_2$ of 10 mmHg is associated with a decrease in pH of 0.08 units and a decrease in serum bicarbonate of 1 mEq/l [16]. A chronic increase in $PaCO_2$ of 10 mmHg is associated with a decrease in pH of 0.03 units and an increase in bicarbonate of 3.5 mEq/l [16].

19.4 THERAPY

19.4.1 IMPROVEMENT IN OXYGENATION

Hypoxemia is the most immediate life-threatening abnormality, and, thus, improving oxygenation should be the first priority of treatment. The physiologic mechanisms primarily responsible for hypoxemia in these patients are hypoventilation and ventilation–perfusion mismatch (provided severe pneumonia or pulmonary edema is not present, as either condition typically produces a shunt). As a result, a relatively modest increase in FIO_2 will usually provide adequate oxygenation. However, when supplemental oxygen is given to patients with COPD who are in acute respiratory failure, $PaCO_2$ usually increases [5]. In most cases, this increase is quite modest, 1 to 5 mmHg for a 10 mmHg increase in PaO_2 [5]. Occasionally, a greater increase in $PaCO_2$ occurs, and uncontrolled oxygen therapy can cause severe CO_2 retention [4].

In the past, it was considered that patients with COPD depended primarily on their hypoxic drive to breathe since their responsiveness to CO_2 was believed to be impaired [4]. According to this theory, correction of hypoxemia with supplemental oxygen removed the hypoxic drive to breathe, leading to a fall in minute ventilation and a rise in $PaCO_2$. The lack of CO_2 responsiveness prevented the respiratory system from compensating for the fall in minute ventilation. Recent studies have challenged this view. Aubier and colleagues administered 100% oxygen for 15 minutes to 22 COPD patients with acute respiratory failure [17]. PaO_2 increased from 38 ± 2 to 225 ± 23 mmHg. $PaCO_2$ increased from 65 ± 3 to 88 ± 5 mmHg. However, minute ventilation fell by only 7% and could not account for the increase in $PaCO_2$. The authors attributed the increase in $PaCO_2$ primarily to an increase in VD/VT although this interpretation has been disputed [18]. In another study, the same authors found that mouth occlusion pressure $(P_{0.1})$, an index of central respiratory drive, was markedly increased in COPD patients in acute respiratory failure [19]. While supplemental oxygen resulted in a significant reduction in $P_{0.1}$, the values still remained higher than those obtained in the chronic state (i.e. the drive to breathe remained high). More recently, Dunn and colleagues examined 13 ventilator dependent patients with COPD [20]. They found that hyperoxia produced both a breathing pattern independent increase in VD/VT and a decrease in respiratory drive. Correction of hypoxemia also shifts the hemoglobin–CO_2 binding curve (Haldane effect) which will increase $PaCO_2$ for a given CO_2 content. Thus, the mechanism by which oxygen supplementation worsens hypercapnia is multifactorial. However, the relative importance of the various mechanisms remains controversial and some investigators believe that removal of the hypoxic stimulus to breathe is still the most important factor [18]. In the vast majority of patients, careful administration of oxygen achieves adequate oxygenation with only modest increases in $Paco_2$ that are without any significant clinical sequelae.

Supplemental oxygen should be administered either by nasal cannula at 1 to 2 l/min [21,22] or via a Venturi mask set at 24–28% oxygen [21,22]. The flow rate (nasal cannula) or oxygen concentration (Venturi mask) is then adjusted according to the resultant arterial blood gases. On average, the arterial Po_2 increases by 10 mmHg when the Fio_2 is increased from room air (21%) to 24% in patients with COPD and acute respiratory failure and by 20 mmHg when the Fio_2 is increased to 28% [22].

The inspired concentration of oxygen (Fio_2) delivered by nasal cannula can vary considerably between patients depending on the patient's ventilatory pattern. Bazuaye and colleagues estimated the Fio_2 in seven patients with stable COPD receiving oxygen via nasal cannula [23]. At a flow rate of 2 l/min, the Fio_2 ranged from 23.7 to 34.9%. The variability in Fio_2 is likely to be even greater in patients who are clinically unstable. Clearly more precise control of the inspired oxygen concentration can be achieved by Venturi masks which may reduce the incidence of severe CO_2 retention during oxygen therapy. However, nasal cannuls are often better tolerated than a facemask in acutely dyspneic patients. In addition, nasal cannula do not have to be removed for expectoration, suctioning or eating. Regardless of the method of oxygen delivery, the goal of therapy is to achieve a Pao_2 of about 60–70 mmHg. Following a change in supplemental oxygen therapy, it is important to obtain an arterial blood gas approximately 15 min later to ensure that the desired effect has been achieved.

Pulse oximeters have become ubiquitous in many intensive care units. Because of their non-invasive nature, it would be desirable if oximetry could be used to guide supplemental oxygen therapy. However, oximetry provides no information on arterial Pco_2. Furthermore, the 95% confidence limits for pulse oximetry are ± 4% [24]. Thus, an oximeter reading of 95% could represent an oxygen saturation between 91% (arterial Po_2 60 mmHg) and 99% (arterial Po_2 160 mmHg). From this discussion, it is clear that tight control of arterial Po_2 cannot be achieved with pulse oximetry and arterial blood gas measurements are required. Pulse oximetry is still very important for patient monitoring since it can alert the clinician that the patient is deteriorating during therapy (as evidenced by a fall in oxygen saturation).

(a) Respiratory stimulants

Respiratory stimulants have been employed in an attempt to prevent or delay life-threatening respiratory acidosis allowing definitive therapy (bronchodilators, steroids, etc.) adequate time to take effect, and, thus, potentially avoid intubation and mechanical ventilation. Conceptually, the use of respiratory stimulants is based on the notion that respiratory drive in patients with COPD and acute respiratory failure is insufficient. Studies clearly demonstrate that central respiratory drive is very high in such patients [19,25,26]. Furthermore, these patients may be quite susceptible to the development of inspiratory muscle fatigue. Indeed, small changes in breathing pattern can produce electromyographic changes consistent with incipient diaphragmatic fatigue in patients with stable but severe COPD [27]. Thus, pharmacologic increases in central respiratory drive in an unstable critically ill patient with COPD could be enough to produce frank inspiratory muscle fatigue. There have been no studies in the literature that conclusively show clear benefit from the administration of respiratory stimulants. In an early, prospective double-blind comparison of doxapram (a commonly used respiratory stimulant) and placebo, patients who received doxapram had better blood gas values after 2 hours of administration compared with patients who received placebo [28]. However, the number of patients ultimately requiring mechanical ventilation was similar in the two groups, 15 of 40 in the doxapram group and 12 of 38 in the placebo group.

More recently, Jeffrey and colleagues examined the effect of a continuous infusion of doxapram to patients with COPD who developed respiratory acidosis (pH <7.26) during controlled oxygen therapy [29]. In this study, 17 deaths occurred during 139 episodes of acute respiratory failure in 95 patients with COPD. Doxapram was administered during 39 episodes while mechanical ventilation was employed in only 4 episodes. The investigators raised the possibility that the low incidence of mechanical ventilation in this study could be related to employment of doxapram therapy; however, it more likely reflects their conservative approach to initiation of mechanical ventilation. It is important to note that the overall mortality rate in this study was quite acceptable (12%) compared to other studies in which mechanical ventilation was more frequently employed. Given the lack of data demonstrating benfit from respiratory stimulants, their potential toxicity [30], and the questionable conceptual basis for their administration, we do not routinely use these agents.

19.4.2 RELIEF OF AIRWAY OBSTRUCTION

In the past, patients with COPD were considered to have 'irreversible' or 'fixed' airway obstruction. However, recent studies have shown that airflow increases substantially following bronchodilator administration in many patients with COPD [31,32]. Furthermore, patients with features typical of emphysema have similar bronchodilator responsiveness [31,33]. Accordingly, COPD patients with acute respiratory failure should receive bronchodilator therapy.

(a) Sympathomimetic agents

β_2-Agonists play a central role as bronchodilating agents in patients with COPD and acute respiratory failure. Parenteral, oral and inhalational forms of these agents are available. The inhalational route is preferred since its use results in greater bronchodilatation and fewer side effects at comparable doses [34–36]. β_2-Agonists can be inhaled via a jet nebulizer or metered-dose inhaler.

In the acutely ill patient, it has been traditional to administer β_2-agonists via a hand-held jet nebulizer. The jet nebulizer uses compressed air to create an aerosol of the medication which the patient breathes until the desired dose has been delivered. A dose of 15 mg of metaproterenol or 2.5 mg of albuterol can be administered every 3–4 hours. Nebulization rate and particle size distribution are affected by the flow rate of compressed air, initial solution volume, solution composition, the plumbing used to connect the nebulizer to the patient, and the structural design of the nebulizer [37,38]. Recent work has also demonstrated a disturbingly high degree of variability between units for many common brands of hand-held nebulizers [38]. Accordingly, the rate of nebulization should be periodically assessed as a quality control measure. It has been suggested that nebulization rate should be at least 0.2 ml/min and unit-to-unit variability in nebulization rate should be < 75%.

Recently, a number of investigators have attempted to determine whether jet nebulization offers any therapeutic advantages over metered-dose inhalers. In several carefully controlled studies, the cumulative dose of β_2-agonist required to produce maximal bronchodilatation was established for the jet nebulizer and metered-dose inhaler. When this dosage was administered chronically, there was no difference in the degree of bronchodilatation achieved by the two delivery systems [39,40]. Thus, optimal therapy is determined by the dose delivered to the lower respiratory tract rather than the mode of delivery. Unfortunately, the optimal dosage varies from patient to patient, and it may increase during acute exacerbations; it is usually greater than the recommended dosage via metered-dose inhaler (2 puffs) [41]. A number of investigators have compared administration of 2–4 puffs of β_2-agonist via a metered-dose inhaler (with or without a spacer device) with the administration of much larger dosages of β_2-agonists via a jet nebulizer. In the majority of studies, there have been no discernible differences in the degree of bronchodilatation achieved by the two delivery systems. These studies have been performed both in patients with stable disease and in patients with acute exacerbations [42–44], although patients with acute respiratory failure have been specifically excluded. Thus, at the present time β_2-agonists should probably be administered by jet nebulization to COPD patients with acute respiratory failure (who are not being mechanically ventilated). However, it appears that therapy can be switched to metered-dose inhaler with or without a spacer device, much earlier in the course of hospitalization than was customary in the past. This approach can result in considerable cost savings [42,45].

In addition, a recent study of mechanically-ventilated patients found similar improvements in passive expiratory flow when β_2-agonists were administered by metered-dose inhaler compared with jet nebulizer [46]. In another study of mechanically-ventilated patients, lung deposition of β_2-agonists was $5.7 \pm 1.1\%$ when administered via metered-dose inhaler and only $1.2 \pm 0.4\%$ when administered by jet nebulizer [47]. These findings require confirmation but it is clear that jet nebulizer therapy is undergoing a period of intense scrutiny and it is likely that indications for nebulizer therapy in the future will be considerably more restricted than they are at the present time. When therapy is switched from nebulizer to metered-dose inhaler, it is essential that the patients receive adequate instruction and training to ensure that the metered-dose inhaler is used appropriately. This task can be performed by the allied health staff during the time that they would otherwise have allotted to administration of nebulizer therapy.

(b) Anticholinergic agents

Ipratropium bromide is a synthetic congener of atropine that is at least as potent as the β_2-agonists in patients with stable COPD [48]. In fact, when administered in currently recommended dosages (2 puffs), ipratropium bromide almost always produces greater bronchodilatation than β_2-agonists [49–51]. However, dose response curves clearly demonstrate that two puffs of ipratropium or β_2-agonist usually do not provide maximal bronchodilatation [52,53]. When sequential doses of β_2-agonists are administered until maximal bronchodilatation is achieved, administration of ipratropium either augments bronchodilatation slightly [52] or has no effect [53].

Ipratropium bromide is not yet available as a nebulized solution in the United States, although it is available in many other countries. In a double-blind randomized Canadian study involving 51 patients with an acute exacerbation of COPD (mean FEV_1 0.7 ± 0.29 l), the effects of 0.5 mg of nebulized ipratropium bromide, 1.25 mg of nebulized fenoterol hydrobromide, or a combination of the two agents were compared [54]. All three regimens resulted in improved spirometric function at 45 and 90 min post treatment but there were no detectable differences between the three regimens (Fig. 19.2). In particular, no benefit could be demonstrated for combination therapy. In another study, patients with an acute exacerbation of COPD were treated for seven days with either nebulized ipratropium or fenoterol [55]. There were no differences in the degree of improvement in FEV_1 from baseline, arterial blood gases or duration of hospitalization between the two regimens. Thus β_2-agonist and anticholinergic agents (ipratropium) appear to be equally effective in the treatment of acute exacerbations of COPD. At the present time, there are no

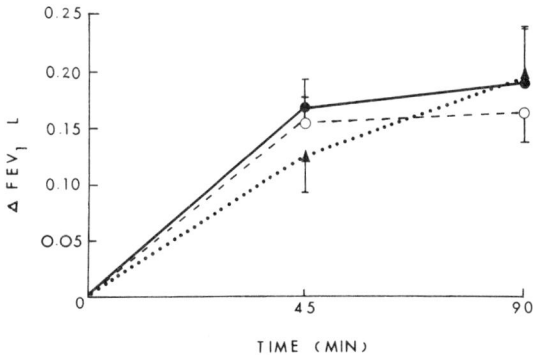

Fig. 19.2 Mean increases in 1-sec forced expiratory volume (FEV$_1$) above baseline after inhalation of ipratropium (triangles), fenoterol (open circles), or the combination (solid circles), in 51 patients with chronic obstructive pulmonary disease. There was no significant difference between the three treatment regimens. Bars represent ± standard error. (Reproduced from reference [54].)

data to suggest that combination therapy is of additional benefit during acute COPD exacerbations and such therapy is not recommended.

(c) Methylxanthines

The role of methylxanthines in obstructive lung disease is undergoing a period of reassessment [56]. In patients with stable COPD, theophylline produces modest bronchodilatation with mean changes in the FEV$_1$ in the range of 10–15% [57,58]. Since methylxanthines have multiple side effects with considerable potential for serious toxicity, whereas inhaled bronchodilators are generally safe, a more relevant question is whether theophylline provides any additional benefit in patients already receiving inhaled bronchodilators at optimal dosage. Studies have shown that some patients (40–50%) [59,60] display additional bronchodilatation (increase in FEV$_1$ of 32% or 0.22 l) [59] when theophylline is added to large doses of inhaled bronchodilator. Whether this additional bronchodilatation translates into improved exercise performance or symptomatic benefit remains to be determined.

The role of theophylline in acute exacerbations of COPD is very poorly defined. Rice and colleagues studied 28 patients who received either intravenous aminophylline or placebo in a randomized double-blind trial [61]. Patients received an otherwise standard treatment regimen consisting of nebulized β_2-agonist, intravenous steroids, antibiotics and oxygen. Over the first 72 hours of hospitalization, there were no significant differences in the degree of improvement in spirometry, arterial blood gases or sensation of dyspnea between the aminophylline and placebo groups.

Given the limitations of the data base, no firm recommendations can be made concerning the role of methylxanthines in acute exacerbations of COPD and the clinician must use his/her own clinical judgement. If one elects to administer methylxanthines, the dose must be carefully individualized since the therapeutic range is narrow (10–20 mg/l) and clearance rates can differ markedly and unpredictably between patients, particularly those that are critically ill [62]. For initiation of intravenous therapy in patients not already receiving the drug, the recommended loading dose of aminophylline (equivalent to 80% anhydrous theophylline) is 6 mg/kg. In patients already receiving oral theophylline, a theophylline level should be obtained prior to initiation of intravenous therapy. The intravenous maintenance dosage is 0.5 mg/kg/h in a healthy non-smoking adult. Factors that alter theophylline clearance requiring adjustment of the maintenance dose are listed in Table 19.1. In addition, large interindividual variations in theophylline clearance exist between patients so that serum levels should be monitored daily until the patient's condition stabilizes.

In addition to their bronchodilator effects, methylxanthines have been shown to improve cardiac and diaphragmatic performance in some studies. Matthay and

Table 19.1   Adjustment of theophylline dosage with various underlying conditions

Condition	Correction factor
Patient characteristics	
Normal adult non-smoker <60 years	1.0
Age >60 years	0.6
Adult smoker <40 years	1.6
Disease state	
Congestive heart failure	0.4
Pneumonia	0.4
Liver failure	0.2–0.4
Severe airway obstruction	0.8
Drugs	
Erythromycin	0.7
Troleandomycin	0.5
Cimetidine	0.7
Oral contraceptives	0.7
Phenytoin	1.5
Phenobarbital	1.2
Carbamazepine	>1.0
Rifampin	>1.0

Caution should be exercised when correction factors exceed one or when multiple correction factors apply.

colleagues found that acute infusion of aminophylline improved right and left ventricular function (in both normal subjects and COPD patients), at least as assessed by the ejection fraction [63]. However, the increases in ejection fraction were very modest (45–52% for the right ventricle and 60–67% for the left ventricle). In a follow-up study, oral theophylline produced similar results which were sustained at 16 weeks [64]. The clinical significance of these very modest changes in ejection fraction remains to be determined. However, it is of interest that subcutaneous administration of 0.25 mg of terbutaline has been reported to produce more pronounced effects on cardiac function in COPD patients [65]. Theophylline has been shown to improve diaphragmatic contractility and fatiguability in animals [66], normal volunteers [67] and patients with COPD [68]. However, other investigators have been unable to replicate these findings [69–71], so that it seems unlikely that theophylline in therapeutic dosages has a clinically significant effect on diaphragmatic function. This topic has been reviewed previously [72].

(d) Corticosteroids

While the benefits of chronic administration of steroids in patients with COPD remains unclear, a single randomized double-blind placebo controlled study supports the use of methylprednisolone during acute exacerbations [73]. In this study of 44 patients, they received either methylprednisolone, 0.5 mg/kg every 6 hours, or placebo for 3 days. Spirometric improvement was greater in the methylprednisolone group (Fig. 19.3). Furthermore, a 40% or greater increase in the FEV_1 at 72 hours was observed in 12 of 22 patients receiving methylprednisolone but in only 3 of 21 patients receiving placebo. In this study, results were analyzed as the percent change from baseline and absolute values were neither presented nor analyzed. This approach has been subsequently criticized [74].

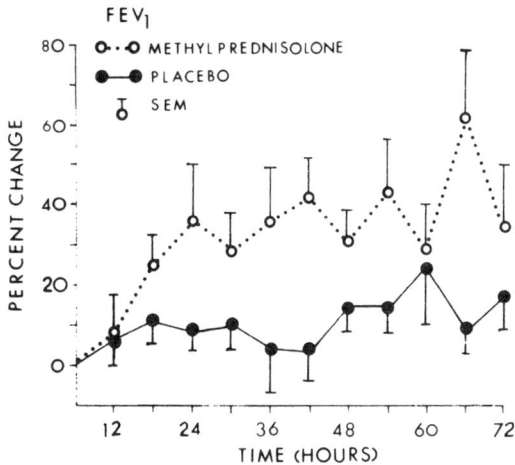

Fig. 19.3 Percentage change in forced expiratory volume in one second (FEV_1) in patients receiving methylprednisolone (open symbols) or placebo (closed symbols). Patients receiving methylprednisone had a greater improvement in airflow than did those receiving placebo. (Reproduced from reference [73].)

More recently, Emerman and colleagues performed a randomized placebo-controlled double-blind study of 96 patients presenting to a hospital emergency room with an acute exacerbation of COPD [75]. Methylprednisolone (100 mg) or placebo was given in addition to nebulized isoetharine and aminophylline. There were no differences in the rate of improvement in FEV_1 or in the rate of hospitalization between patients receiving corticosteroids or placebo. However, in this study, the duration of follow-up ranged from 2.5 to 7 hours, which is probably insufficient to detect a beneficial response to corticosteroids since these agents have a slow onset of action. In summary, although the data are limited, it seems reasonable to treat patients with exacerbations of COPD and acute respiratory failure with a course of corticosteroids.

19.4.3 INFECTION

Infection of the airway appears to be a common precipitant of acute respiratory

failure in patients with COPD. *Hemophilus influenzae* and *parainfluenzae, Streptococcus pneumoniae* and *Branhamella catarrhalis* are considered to be the most common bacterial pathogens in patients with COPD [76–79]. Less frequently, other streptococci, gram-negative enteric rods and *Staphylococcus aureus* are cultured from purulent respiratory secretions in patients with an exacerbation of COPD [77–79]. In addition, viral infections have been shown to be responsible for 20–33% of all exacerbations of COPD in two long-term studies [80,81]. This percentage may be an underestimate due to the difficulties entailed in viral isolation. Non-infectious agents may also be important but their role is difficult to quantitate. The relative importance of bacterial infection compared with viral infection or non-infectious agents in producing exacerbations has been difficult to elucidate. Patients with COPD are often chronically colonized with common bacterial pathogens. Therefore, culture of one of these organisms during an acute exacerbation does not imply that the organism is responsible for the exacerbation. However, some serologic studies have demonstrated a rise in antibody titer to *Hemophilus influenzae* or *Branhamella catarrhalis* following an exacerbation of COPD suggesting that these organisms were responsible for the exacerbation [82,83]. It is important to realize that not every episode of respiratory failure is precipitated by infection. In patients with COPD and acute respiratory failure requiring mechanical ventilation, objective evidence of distal bronchial infection (bacteria cultured from a protected brush via bronchoscopy) was observed in only 27 of 54 patients [79].

The role of antibiotics in the therapy of exacerbations of COPD remains controversial [84]. Early studies examining the effects of antibiotics did not carefully exclude patients with pneumonia nor were objective criteria used to evaluate outcome. Two carefully performed, double-blind, placebo-controlled trials have evaluated the role of antibiotics in patients with exacerbations of COPD. Nicotra and colleagues studied 40 patients who required hospitalization for an exacerbation of COPD [85]. Twenty patients received oral tetracycline for 1 week while the remainder received placebo. Patients were excluded from the study if they had a new radiographic infiltrate, fever, leukocytosis, or required mechanical ventilation. Clinical and laboratory features were similar in the antibiotic and placebo groups at study onset. At the end of the seven-day study period, there were no differences between the two groups in spirometry, arterial blood gases or physician and patient evaluation of severity of illness. Anthonisen and colleagues studied 362 exacerbations of COPD in 173 patients [86]. Patients received either a ten-day course of antibiotics (trimethoprim–sulfamethoxazole, amoxicillin or doxycycline) or placebo. Relief of symptoms within 21 days was achieved in 68% of antibiotic treated exacerbations and 55% of placebo-treated exacerbations. Peak expiratory flows recovered faster in the antibiotic treated group, although the differences were small. Treatment failures were twice as common with placebo (19%) compared with antibiotic (10%). Differences between placebo and antibiotic were greatest when a triad of symptoms – increase in dyspnea, increase in sputum volume, and sputum purulence – were observed during exacerbation; these symptoms predicted a favorable response to antibiotics.

Given this background, it seems reasonable to treat patients with COPD and acute respiratory failure with antibiotics, while recognizing that they will benefit only a minority of patients. Broad-spectrum antibiotics such as trimethoprim–sulfamethoxazole, tetracycline or amoxicillin are usually employed. The choice of antibiotic should take into account local susceptibility patterns. *Branhamella catarrhalis* is usually resistant to amoxicillin which is a potential limitation of this antibiotic choice [76]. A number of new antibiotics (amoxicillin/clavulanate, second and third generation oral cephalosporins, azithromycin, clarithromycin, ofloxacin and ciprofloxacin) have been touted as potentially useful in the treatment of exacerbations of COPD. In general, these antibiotics have a broader spectrum of activity but are more expensive. These agents have not been shown to be clinically more efficacious than older agents. It must be emphasized that this discussion pertains only to the patient without evidence of pneumonia. Patients with a parenchymal infiltrate on chest radiography and other evidence of pneumonia clearly require antibiotic therapy which should be broad spectrum in activity until an etiologic agent is identified.

19.4.4 NUTRITION

The proper role of nutrition in the management of acute respiratory failure in patients with COPD is unclear since there have been no randomized controlled prospective studies examining it in this setting [87]. Complications of either enteral nutrition or total parenteral nutrition (TPN) are frequent and can have substantial morbidity, and may even result in death. Nevertheless, pre-existing malnutrition is common in patients with COPD, particularly those in acute respiratory failure [88]. Nutritional status further deteriorates in patients requiring mechanical ventilation since these patients are unable to take food by mouth [89].

Poor nutritional status is believed to have a number of adverse effects on the respiratory system. Diaphragmatic muscle mass is less in malnourished patients. In a necropsy study, Arora and Rochester examined diaphragmatic muscle mass in patients with normal body weight who died suddenly and underweight patients who died from a variety of causes [90]. Body weight and diaphragmatic muscle mass were reduced by 30% and 40%, respectively, in the underweight patients, indicating that the diaphragm was not spared from the effects of malnutrition. In another study, Arora and Rochester found that malnourished patients without lung disease had substantially lower maximal inspiratory mouth pressures (an index of respiratory muscle strength) compared with adequately nourished patients [91]. Furthermore, in a group of malnourished surgical patients, successful nutritional repletion with total parenteral nutrition led to a 37% increase in maximal inspiratory mouth pressure [92]. Nutritional status can also affect the control of breathing. In normal volunteers, semistarvation has been shown to reduce the ventilatory response to hypoxia by 42% [93]. Immune status is also adversely affected by malnourishment. Malnourished patients have suppressed delayed cutaneous hypersensitivity and impaired T-lymphocyte transformation in response to mitogens [94]. In one study, bacterial adherence to airway cells was increased in patients with poor nutritional status [95].

In a retrospective uncontrolled study of long-term (>3 days) mechanically ventilated patients, those receiving nutritional supplementation had a significantly higher rate of weaning from mechanical ventilation (93%) than patients receiving only dextrose and water (55%) [96]. Given the potential deleterious effects of malnutrition, it is reasonable to provide nutritional support in patients who are malnourished at presentation or who are expected to require prolonged (>3 days) mechanical ventilation. The enteral route is the preferred mode of administration.

Nutritionally associated hypercapnia can occur in patients who are overzealously fed. When calories are given in excess of energy needs, lipogenesis occurs. The respiratory quotient of lipogenesis is approximately 0.8, reflecting a much greater production of CO_2 relative to O_2 consumed. In normal subjects, this increase in CO_2 production is compensated by an increase in minute ventilation, and, thus, eucapnia is maintained. However, patients with severe respiratory disease and weak respiratory muscles may not be able to sufficiently increase ventilation to prevent hypercapnia. Although the increase in CO_2 production may be of little consequence during assisted ventilation, it could impair weaning in certain patients [97].

The nutritional requirements of patients with COPD in acute respiratory failure are poorly documented. Preliminary data suggest that total caloric requirements in such patients exceeds the resting energy expenditure by 29–54% [98]. Even when this 'stress factor' is taken into account, total caloric needs are only 1663 ± 362 kcal. It has been recommended that 20% of total calories be given as protein. Since the respiratory quotient for glucose is 1.0 while it is only 0.7 for fat, CO_2 production will be slightly higher when carbohydrate rather than fat is the predominant fuel. For this reason, some authorities recommend that high concentrations of carbohydrate be avoided in patients with severe pulmonary disease. However, in the majority of patients, substitution of fat for carbohydrate has only a modest effect on CO_2 production and is of little consequence.

19.4.5 PHYSIOTHERAPY

Most patients with an exacerbation of COPD report an increase in airway secretions. Furthermore, patients with COPD and acute respiratory failure have markedly reduced expiratory flows which can impair cough effectiveness. Thus, it might seem reasonable to employ chest physical therapy to assist with secretion removal. However, a number of studies employing chest percussion and postural drainage in patients with an exacerbation of COPD were unable to show any improvement in pulmonary function or objective evidence of improved secretion removal [99,100]. Not surprisingly, chest physical therapy appears to benefit some patients with large amounts of sputum production but has no beneficial effects in those patients with scant sputum production [101,102]. Hypoxemia can significantly worsen during chest physical therapy and this deterioration in PaO_2 is most likely to occur in patients with scant sputum production [101]. Accordingly, chest physical therapy should only be considered in patients with large amounts of sputum production. Furthermore, chest physical therapy treatments should only be continued if there is clear evidence of improved secretion removal. Finally, it is prudent to monitor the patient for desaturation with a pulse oximeter during treatment and to increase oxygen flow/concentration as necessary during treatment being careful to return oxygen flow/concentration back to its original level once treatment is completed.

19.4.6 MECHANICAL VENTILATION

(a) Intubation

The majority of patients with COPD and acute respiratory failure can be managed without resort to mechanical ventilation [29]. In general, mechanical ventilation should be avoided whenever possible because patients with COPD are particularly susceptible to ventilator-associated complications. Nevertheless, a small number of patients will require ventilator therapy.

The decision of whether to institute ventilator support is a difficult one. No particular blood gas value or any other physiologic parameter serves as an absolute criterion for the institution of mechanical ventilation. Rather, the decision should be made on clinical grounds. A deteriorating mental status (confusion, obtundation, agitation) or significant cardiovascular instability are the usual indications for ventilator assistance. Patients with worsening respiratory acidosis associated with progressive 'tiredness' and increasing dyspnea despite therapy usually require mechanical ventilation

(b) Support phase

The ideal ventilator mode and settings are a matter of considerable debate. To put this problem in perspective, it is important to consider two pathophysiologic events that may occur in patients with COPD and acute respiratory failure: (1) auto-PEEP, and (2) inspiratory muscle fatigue.

(i) Auto-PEEP (syn. Intrinsic PEEP)

Patients with COPD and acute respiratory failure have severe airway obstruction and decreased pulmonary elastic recoil. Maximal expiratory flow is markedly reduced and a prolonged expiratory time is required to permit complete exhalation of inspired gas volume. These patients commonly are tachypneic and have increased ventilatory requirements. These factors result in a shortened expiratory time, so that the next inspiration starts before expiration has been completed resulting in dynamic air trapping and an alveolar pressure that remains positive at end-expiration (auto-PEEP). The resulting increase in lung volume forces the patient to breathe in the upper less compliant portion of the pressure–volume curve, thereby, increasing the elastic load to breathe. Hyperinflation forces the respiratory muscles to operate at an unfavorable position on their length–tension curve. Finally, the inspiratory muscles must generate sufficient pressure to counterbalance the positive alveolar pressure at end-expiration before inspiratory flow can begin [103]. Thus, auto-PEEP behaves like an inspiratory threshold load. The effect of dynamic hyperinflation can seriously compromise inspiratory muscle function.

Auto-PEEP may also have significant circulatory effects [104]. A high proportion of the positive alveolar pressure is transmitted to the mediastinum in patients with COPD where it can impede venous return impairing circulatory function. Dynamic hyperinflation and auto-PEEP may also increase the risk of barotrauma during mechanical ventilation.

Furthermore, during mechanical ventilation in an assist mode, auto-PEEP will surreptitiously reduce trigger sensitivity [105] (Fig. 19.4). To trigger the ventilator, the patient needs to generate a negative inspiratory pressure equivalent to the auto-PEEP level plus the sensitivity setting. This reduction in trigger sensitivity increases patient work during mechanical ventilation, which may increase patient discomfort and possibly prevent or delay the resolution of inspiratory muscle fatigue.

During mechanical ventilation, auto-PEEP can be measured by the end-expiratory port occlusion method (Fig. 19.5) [104]. With this method, the expiratory port is occluded near the time when the next inspiration is antici-

pated. With expiratory flow blocked, pressure in the ventilator tubing will equilibrate with alveolar pressure allowing the level of auto-PEEP to register on the ventilator manometer. This method is highly sensitive to the timing of occlusion and accurate measurements are most easily achieved in patients receiving controlled ventilation. Auto-PEEP can also be measured using the expiratory hold option available on some ventilators. For ventilators without an expiratory hold option, a simple method to estimate auto-PEEP has been described (Fig. 19.6) [106]. In addition, during controlled ventilation, auto-PEEP can be estimated from continuous recordings of airway pressure and flow by noting the airway pressure at which inspiratory flow begins [107].

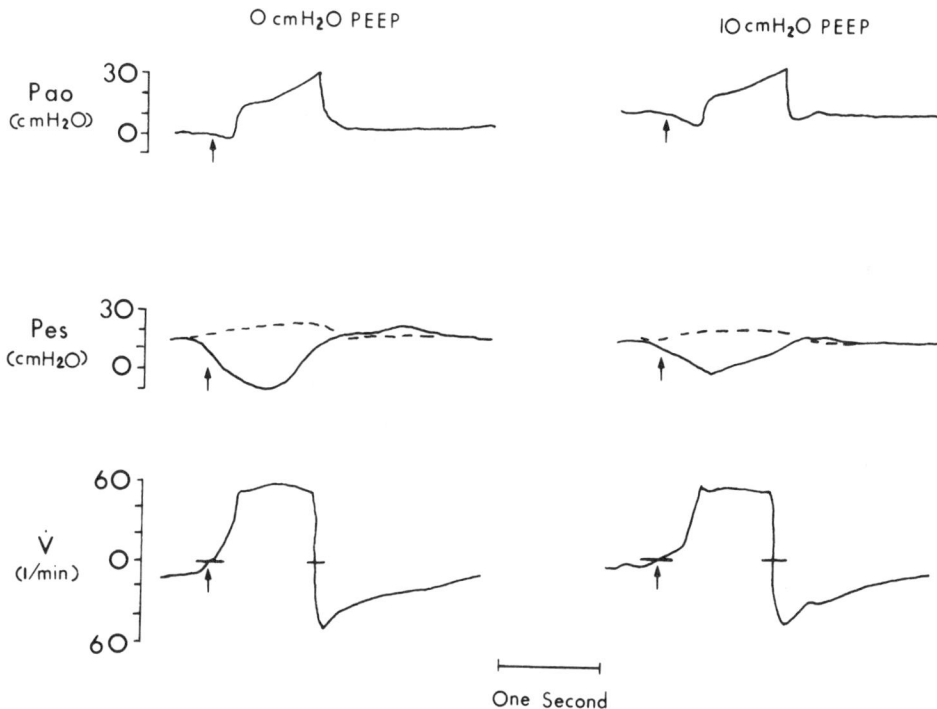

Fig. 19.4 Effect of adding external positive end-expiratory pressure (PEEP) on the effective triggering threshold pressure in 1 patient. At a PEEP of zero, a 9-cm H_2O drop in esophageal pressure (Pes) is required to lower pressure at airway opening (Pao) and trigger flow. When 10 cm H_2O of PEEP is added, inspiratory threshold pressure imposed by auto-PEEP is overcome and less subject effort is required to trigger ventilator. (Reproduced from reference [105].)

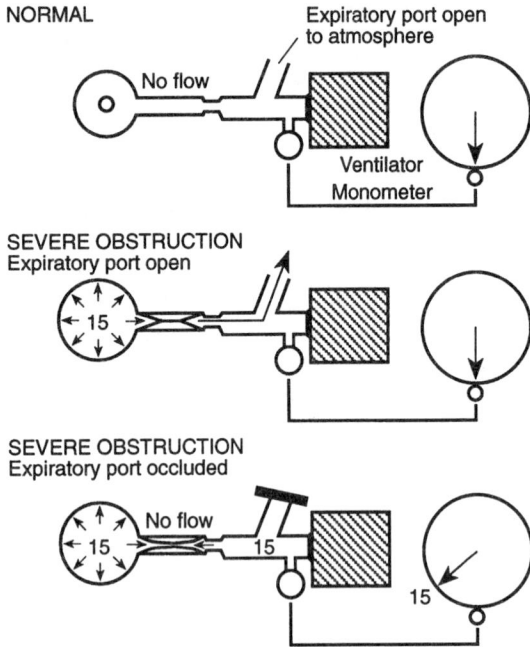

Fig. 19.5 Measurement of auto-PEEP by expiratory port occlusion. Normally (see top panel), alveolar pressure is atmospheric at the end of passive exhalation. With severe airflow obstruction (see middle panel), alveolar pressure remains elevated (in this example at 15 cmH$_2$O) and slow flow continues, even at the end of the set exhalation period. The ventilator manometer senses negligible pressure because it is open to atmosphere through large bore tubing and downstream from the site of flow limitation. With gas flow stopped by occlusion of the expiratory port at the end of the set exhalation period (see lower panel), pressure equilibrates throughout the lung-ventilator system and is displayed on the ventilator manometer. (Reproduced from reference [104].)

The occlusion methods are extremely difficult to apply in patients making spontaneous inspiratory efforts. Under these circumstances, auto-PEEP can be measured by inserting an esophageal balloon and recording esophageal pressure and inspiratory flow [108]. The amount of negative pressure required to counterbalance auto-PEEP is estimated by the change in esophageal pressure from the onset of the negative pressure swing

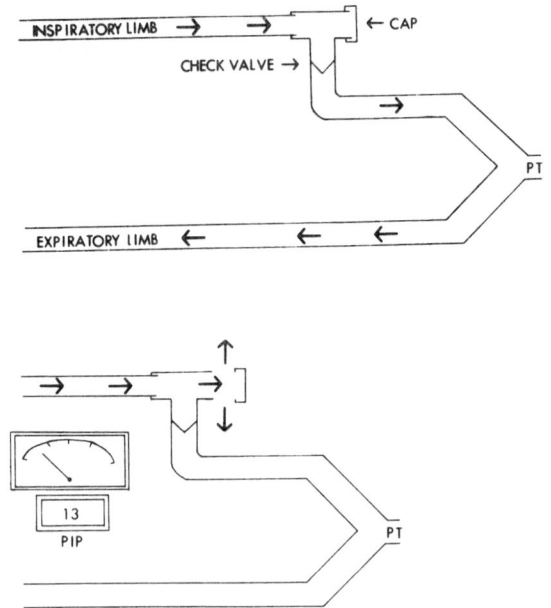

Fig. 19.6 A one way Brashi valve, a 'tee' and a cap is added to the inspiratory limb of the ventilator circuit. During exhalation the cap is removed. The next delivered tidal volume is vented to the room while the patient's lung pressure equilibrates against a closed exhalation valve. The auto-PEEP level can then be read from the ventilator digital or analog display on the ventilator manometer.

to the point at which inspiratory flow begins. For this method to be valid, the expiratory muscles must be relaxed during this time period which may not always be the case [109]. Indeed, Ninane and colleagues have measured the electrical activity of the abdominal muscles in 40 patients with COPD during resting breathing [110]. Phasic expiratory activity of the transversus abdominus was observed with every breath in 17 patients and intermittently in 11 patients. During spontaneous breathing, auto-PEEP levels measured with an esophageal balloon are lower than those obtained with the occlusion method [108].

The level of auto-PEEP is primarily dependent on the severity of airflow obstruction and the minute ventilation. Indeed, auto-

PEEP can be seen in patients without evidence of airflow obstruction if minute ventilation is sufficiently elevated [111]. Administration of sedation to decrease minute ventilation can substantially reduce the degree of dynamic hyperinflation and auto-PEEP. The machine settings chosen during mechanical ventilation can also affect the level of auto-PEEP [112]. For a given minute ventilation and tidal volume, rapid inspiratory flow rates will shorten inspiratory time and allow more time for expiration, and, thus, reduce the level of auto-PEEP [112]. Reciprocal changes in tidal volume and respiratory rate have minimal effects on end-expiratory lung volume and auto-PEEP. It is important to realize that the vast majority of patients with COPD who have an exacerbation of sufficient severity to cause acute respiratory failure will demonstrate auto-PEEP. Furthermore, the level of auto-PEEP may be quite high (>10 cmH_2O) particularly early in the patient's course [103–105,107, 112,113].

(ii) Inspiratory muscle fatigue

Although flow limitation occurs during expiration in patients with COPD, the increased work of breathing is borne primarily by the inspiratory muscles [114]. Dynamic hyperinflation puts the inspiratory muscles at a considerable disadvantage. Metabolic factors (hypocalcemia [115], hypophosphatemia [116] and hypomagnesemia [117], malnutrition and respiratory acidosis [118,119] may all decrease respiratory muscle strength and/or endurance.

Inspiratory muscle fatigue occurs when the demands imposed on the inspiratory muscles exceed their capacity. Many of the important determinants of the fatiguing process are expressed in the tension–time index. The tension–time index for the diaphragm (TTdi) is equal to mean inspiratory transdiaphragmatic pressure per breath/maximum static transdiaphragmatic pressure (Pdi/Pdi max)

times the inspiratory time/total respiratory cycle time (T_I/T_{TOT}), i.e.

$$TTdi = (Pdi/Pdi\ max) \times (T_I/T_{TOT})$$

A TTdi of >0.15–0.18 indicates a potentially fatiguing pattern of contraction [120]. Healthy subjects breathing at rest have a TTdi of 0.02. In a study of stable COPD patients, the TTdi was 0.05 (range 0.01–0.12) during resting breathing indicating a low degree of functional reserve [27]. Relatively modest alterations in breathing pattern produced an increase in TTdi above 0.20 in these patients, which invariably resulted in shifts in the power spectrum of the diaphragmatic EMG which were consistent with incipient fatigue. Based on these and other observations, it has been suspected that overt inspiratory muscle fatigue occurs in many patients with COPD who develop acute respiratory failure. Unequivocal evidence to support or refute this hypothesis is currently lacking. This uncertainty is due in large part to the lack of any simple practical method by which inspiratory muscle fatigue can be diagnosed in critically ill patients. Recently, the importance of central fatigue has been emphasized. Central fatigue can be defined as a reversible decrease in central neural drive caused by muscle overloading. Bellemare and Bigland-Ritchie found that when normal subjects breathed against a fatiguing resistive load, 50% of the ensuing force loss was due to central fatigue [121]. However, it remains unknown whether central fatigue occurs in patients with respiratory failure.

The approach to mechanical ventilation in patients with COPD and acute respiratory failure is conceptually different depending on the relative importance of fatigue. If patients develop overt peripheral muscle fatigue, then muscle rest is the rational therapy. On the other hand, if patients respond to respiratory muscle overloading by decreasing central neural respiratory output with consequent hypoventilation but no overt peripheral muscle fatigue, then muscle rest would be less likely to improve respiratory muscle performance.

(c) Ventilatory modes

Controversy exists as to the optimal mode of ventilation. This controversy is largely due to our lack of knowledge regarding the importance of overt peripheral inspiratory muscle fatigue in such patients. Marini and co-workers have shown that patients perform substantial amounts of inspiratory work during assisted mechanical ventilation [122] or synchronized intermittent mandatory ventilation [123]. In contrast, respiratory muscle work can be largely abolished during controlled mechanical ventilation if ventilator settings are adjusted appropriately [124,125]. Theoretically, if overt peripheral inspiratory muscle fatigue is present, more effective recovery should be achieved by completely resting the respiratory muscles. However, prolonged muscle inactivity may also result in muscle deconditioning and atrophy. Preliminary studies in a baboon model showed that controlled mechanical ventilation for 11 days resulted in a 46% decrease in respiratory muscle strength, a 37% decrease in respiratory muscle endurance and an increased susceptibility to inspiratory muscle fatigue [126]. Similarly, in the anesthetized rat, 48 hours of controlled mechanical ventilation resulted in a reduction in both diaphragmatic mass and *in vitro* diaphragmatic force production [127].

Unfortunately, no data are available regarding the minimum level of respiratory muscle activity required to prevent respiratory muscle deconditioning. In practice, we initiate ventilatory support in the patient with COPD and acute respiratory failure with assist-control ventilation. The settings should be carefully titrated in each patient in terms of inspiratory flow rate, tidal volume and sometimes external PEEP (to counteract the effect of auto-PEEP if this is a problem) so as to minimize patient work and discomfort. Some patients still perform considerable amounts of respiratory work, and examination of the contour of their airway pressure

waveform can be helpful in detecting these patients [124].

Pressure support is a new mode of ventilation that has become increasingly popular among clinicians [128]. Pressure support augments each spontaneous breath with a preset amount of positive pressure until the patient's inspiratory flow decreases to a system specific minimal level at which time exhalation ensues. Since the patient must initiate each breathe, an intact respiratory drive is essential. Tidal volume is determined by patient effort, the level of pressure support, and respiratory system impedance. Thus, changes in respiratory system impedance can dramatically affect the level of ventilation. Furthermore, since it is the difference between the applied positive airway pressure and alveolar pressure that drives inspiratory flow, the presence of auto-PEEP will diminish the ability of a preset level of pressure support to augment ventilation [129]. Accordingly, employment of pressure support as the sole mode of ventilator assistance may be unreliable in initiating mechanical ventilation in patients with COPD and acute respiratory failure.

(d) Ventilator settings

Although a delivered tidal volume of 10–15 ml/kg is commonly recommended, this predisposes to the development of auto-PEEP and we use a volume of 7–9 ml/kg in patients with COPD. An inspiratory flow of 60 l/min is commonly employed during ventilator assistance, but recent work in patients with COPD suggests that high inspiratory flow rates (100 l/min) improve oxygenation, possibly by increasing overall ventilation–perfusion matching, and decrease the risk of dynamic hyperinflation and auto-PEEP [112,130]. High inspiratory flow rates will also increase peak airway pressure possibly placing regions of lung served by low resistance pathways at jeopardy for overdistension (this is only likely to be a problem if the high airway pressure is transmitted to the alveolus). In order to meet patient inspiratory flow requirements reliably, inspiratory flow should be at least 5–6 times the minute ventilation requirements. If significant auto-PEEP is present, it is reasonable to increase inspiratory flow up to 100 l/min. The inspired oxygen fraction should be adjusted to maintain arterial oxygen saturation ≥90%. If the latter is being monitored by pulse oximetry, one should aim for a pulse oximeter reading of 92% rather than 90% [131].

(e) Sedation and paralysis

The patient should be sedated initially to increase patient comfort and reduce ventilatory requirements. As the underlying disease process resolves, sedation should be reduced or discontinued to facilitate weaning. Paralysis is rarely required in such patients.

(f) Role of positive end-expiratory pressure (PEEP)

PEEP is generally employed to improve oxygenation in patients with severe hypoxemia, diffuse infiltrative lung disease and reduced lung volumes. Traditionally, PEEP has been avoided in patients with COPD since adequate oxygenation is generally easy to achieve, and the patients are already hyperinflated, and, thus, there is a fear that further hyperinflation may have deleterious consequences. However, many patients with severe COPD manifest expiratory flow limitation during tidal breathing. The addition of a small amount of positive pressure downstream from the flow limiting segment will have no effect on expiratory flow or end-expiratory lung volume provided the applied pressure is less than the critical closing pressure [132]. Furthermore, the addition of PEEP will improve the effective triggering sensitivity of the ventilator, thus, reducing the amount of patient work during assisted mechanical ventilation (Fig. 19.4)

[105]. However, if too much extrinsic PEEP is added or if the patient is not flow limited, extrinsic PEEP will worsen dynamic hyperinflation with potentially detrimental consequences. Monitoring airway pressure or end-expiratory lung volume during the addition of extrinsic PEEP is helpful in identifying those patients who might benefit from this therapy [132]. If there is little change in peak and plateau pressure following the addition of extrinsic PEEP, airway collapse is likely and extrinsic PEEP may be helpful. In contrast, if peak and plateau airway pressure rise in parallel to the level of extrinsic PEEP, this suggests additional hyperinflation and extrinsic PEEP is likely to be detrimental.

Continuous positive airway pressure (CPAP) has recently been tried in COPD patients during weaning from mechanical ventilation [108]. During spontaneous breathing, auto-PEEP acts as an inspiratory threshold load. The pressure that must be generated to overcome auto-PEEP can theoretically be provided by an external CPAP device, thus, reducing the demands on the inspiratory muscles. Petrof and co-workers have shown that administration of CPAP during weaning can reduce the inspiratory work of breathing and the degree of dyspnea in patients with severe COPD [108]. Whether CPAP administration expedites weaning from mechanical ventilation in such patients remains to be determined. Furthermore, if high levels of CPAP are employed, significant additional dynamic hyperinflation could occur. It has been suggested that further dynamic hyperinflation will not occur if the level of applied CPAP is below the auto-PEEP level [108] although this has been disputed by other investigators [133,134]. Unfortunately, auto-PEEP is very difficult to measure in spontaneously breathing subjects in the absence of an esophageal balloon catheter. Thus, until further information becomes available, the routine use of CPAP during weaning is not recommended.

(g) Weaning from mechanical ventilation

Discontinuation of mechanical ventilation can be particularly difficult in the patient with COPD. The major determinant of ventilator dependency in these patients is the balance between the respiratory load and the ability of the respiratory muscles to cope with this load [135]. In contrast, oxygenation is rarely a major problem at the time that weaning is being contemplated in these patients.

Deciding the optimal time to initiate the weaning process is a controversial subject. Some physicians like to initiate weaning early in the patient's course, employing techniques like IMV, where a substantial portion of ventilation is performed spontaneously by the patient. We prefer to provide a higher level of ventilator support using assist-control ventilation, and to wean the patient using intermittent trials of spontaneous breathing, i.e. t-tube trials. However, it should be emphasized that there are no published studies that indicate the superiority of any one weaning technique over another [135].

Careful physical examination by an experienced physician is the best method of determining when a patient is ready to be weaned from the ventilator. In addition, obtaining simple physiologic indices can help in making this judgement. By indicating the earliest time that ventilatory support can be discontinued, such weaning predictors help in minimizing the duration of mechanical ventilation with its attendant risk of complications. In addition, they help in identifying patients who are likely to fail a weaning trial and, thus, cardiopulmonary and psychologic distress can be avoided, which would otherwise set the patient back in his/her clinical course.

Weaning is generally not contemplated in a patient who has difficulty with oxygenation, i.e. patients should have a PaO_2 of >60 torr while receiving an FIO_2 of ≤0.40 [135]. The patient's ventilatory capacity has been traditionally assessed by measurement of maximum inspiratory pressure (PI max), a measure of respiratory muscle strength, and minute ventilation, which reflects the patient's ventilatory requirements. Ideally, a patient should be able to generate a PI max more negative than −30 cmH_2O and have a minute ventilation of <10 l/min to be successfully weaned [136]. Unfortunately, these criteria are associated with a high rate of false positive and false negative results [137]. In a recent prospective study of weaning outcome, an index of rapid shallow breathing, viz. the frequency to tidal volume ratio, was found to be the single most accurate predictor of weaning outcome [137]. Of the patients who had a frequency/tidal volume ratio of >100 breaths/min/l, 95% failed a weaning trial, whereas 80% of the patients with lower ratios were successfully weaned (Fig. 19.7). The frequency/tidal volume ratio has a number of attractive features: it is easy to measure, it is independent of patient effort and co-operation, it appears to be quite accurate in predicting the ability to sustain ventilation, and, fortuitously, it has a 'rounded off' threshold value (100) that is easy to remember.

Management of the patient who repeatedly fails weaning trials can be very frustrating and requires considerable skill. Important factors in the management of these patients are listed in Table 19.2. A full discussion of this topic is beyond the scope of this chapter and the reader is referred elsewhere [135,138].

19.4.7 MONITORING

Patients with COPD and acute respiratory failure should ideally be admitted to an intensive care unit until their condition stabilizes. Admission to an intensive care unit will facilitate both patient monitoring and allocation of care by the nursing and respiratory therapy staff. Monitoring should be individualized for each patient. However, initially monitoring should include continuous electrocardiographic monitoring, pulse oximetry, frequent assessment of mental status, daily fluid inputs and outputs and daily patient

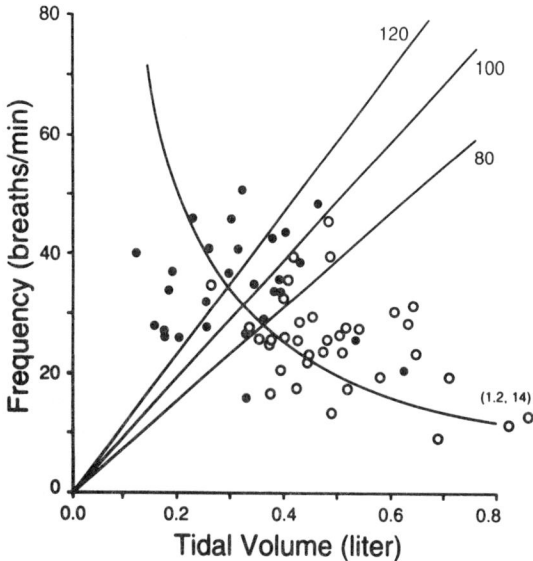

Fig. 19.7 Isopleths for the ratio of breathing frequency to tidal volume, representing different degrees of rapid shallow breathing. For the patients indicated by the points to the left of the isopleth representing 100 breaths per minute per liter, the likelihood that a weaning trial would fail was 95%, whereas for the patients indicated by the points to the right of this isopleth, the likelihood of a successful weaning outcome was 80%. The hyperbola represents a minute ventilation of 10 l/min, a criterion commonly used to predict weaning outcome; apparently this criterion was of little value in discriminating between the successfully weaned patients (open circles) and the patients in whom weaning failed (solid circles). Values for one patient (tidal volume of 1.2 liters and respiratory frequency of 14 breaths per minute) lay outside the graph. (Reproduced from reference [137].)

weights. The frequency of arterial blood gas determinations will be dependent on the patient's condition. In patients requiring mechanical ventilation, the usual ventilatory parameters should be monitored (peak and plateau airway pressure, exhaled tidal volume and minute ventilation). In addition, intrinsic PEEP should be measured as described previously. Many of the new microprocessor ventilators provide software programs that can facilitate frequent measurement of respiratory mechanics (including airway resistance and static compliance). Documentation of the accuracy of these devices in clinical practice is largely lacking. Furthermore, even if these devices measure respiratory mechanics accurately, it has not been shown that such measurements will alter patient management. More recently, commercial monitoring systems have become available that can measure the work of spontaneous breathing (requires measurement of esophageal pressure usually via a combined esophageal balloon catheter–nasogastric tube). Whether such monitoring systems will be of help in difficult to wean patients remains to be determined.

Measurement of expired CO_2 provides a non-invasive means of continuously monitoring alveolar, and, thus, arterial $PaCO_2$ [139]. In healthy subjects, end-tidal CO_2 tension ($PETCO_2$) measured as the plateau value of an exhaled sample is usually 1 torr (range up to 5 torr) less than $PaCO_2$ [140,141]. Patients with COPD and acute respiratory failure have an uneven distribution of ventilation. Because of this uneven distribution of ventilation, the capnograph shows a steadily rising expired CO_2 signal that does not reach a plateau [141]. In such patients, the $PaCO_2$–$PETCO_2$ gradient increases unpredictably by 10–20 torr or more so that $PETCO_2$ may no longer reliably reflect $PaCO_2$ [142]. Furthermore, changes in $PETCO_2$ may poorly reflect changes in $PaCO_2$ [143]. Thus, capnography cannot be used as a substitute for arterial blood gases in patients with COPD and acute respiratory failure.

In patients receiving mechanical ventilation, minute ventilation and its component parts, tidal volume and frequency are considered to be important variables that are monitored continuously. While these measurements are easily obtained in the intubated patient, problems arise in the non-intubated patient. Patients with acute respiratory failure have difficulty tolerating devices that require the use of a mouthpiece or facemask. Several

Table 19.2 Management of the patient displaying difficulty during weaning

Determine the cause of ventilator dependency
Correct correctable problems
Develop a weaning plan
Use a team approach
Psychological factors
    Inform patient of weaning plan and progress
        Provide motivation and reassurance
        Provide environmental stimulation
        Anticipate setbacks
        Consider biofeedback
Optimize pulmonary care
        Optimize ventilator settings
        Ensure optimal endotracheal tube size
        Consider tracheostomy
        Use bronchodilator therapy
        Clear secretions
        Allow respiratory muscle rest
        Provide respiratory muscle training
        Provide a bedside fan
Optimize the timing of weaning trials
Ensure adequate sleep
Use the patient's preferred posture
Ensure nutritional support
Correct abnormalities in minerals and electrolytes
Correct abnormalities in acid–base status
Optimize all aspects of general care
Encourage ambulation
Consider home mechanical ventilation

devices (magnetometer and respiratory inductive plethysmography) have been developed that measure ventilation indirectly by recording motion of the ribcage and abdomen [144]. Combined with breathing pattern analysis, this approach can provide information on the volume and timing of ventilation, the coordination of ribcage–abdominal motion and changes in end-expiratory lung volume. Disadvantages of these devices is that calibration can be tedious and volumetric accuracy is often less precise than with volume or flow sensors. Sackner and associates have recently described a simple method of calibrating the respiratory inductive plethysmograph that can provide accurate measurements of respiratory timing and ribcage–abdominal coordination, and reasonably accurate measurements of relative changes in tidal volume [145]. Evaluation of abnormalities in chest wall motion has been shown to have some predictive value during weaning from mechanical ventilation [146]. In addition, Hoffman and colleagues have shown that respiratory inductive plethysmography can be used to estimate the level of auto-PEEP during both spontaneous breathing and controlled mechanical ventilation [147]. Nevertheless, there have been no studies that have addressed whether these devices will prevent unanticipated respiratory arrest or otherwise alter patient outcome. Until such information is forthcoming, we do not advocate the routine use of these devices.

19.5 PROGNOSIS

The short-term mortality for patients with COPD in acute respiratory failure was examined in a number of studies between 1968 and 1976. An average of 28% of patients (range 22–34%) in these studies died during the acute episode [148].

In four more recent studies, mortality during an acute episode of respiratory failure ranged from 6 to 16% [22,29,149,150]. The lower mortality in these later studies is probably due, in part, to the selection of patients whose acute illness was less severe than those in prior studies. However, improvements in patient care may have also played a role. In addition, differences in the patient population studied, i.e. severity of underlying disease, age, etc. may account for the differences in mortality between studies.

Several factors are important in determining increased short-term mortality:

1. The severity of the underlying disease.
2. The severity of the precipitating illness. For example, acute respiratory failure that is brought on by a massive pulmonary embolus is likely to be associated with a higher mortality than is respiratory fail-

ure due to an exacerbation of chronic bronchitis.

3. The severity of the acute respiratory failure, as determined by a pH of less than 7.22–7.26 [21,29,151,152]. The $Paco_2$ is a much poorer predictor of mortality; probably because many of these patients have chronic hypercapnia, and, thus, the severity of the acute illness is better reflected by the degree of acidosis rather than the absolute level of $Paco_2$. The initial Pao_2 was a determinant of mortality in some studies [22,151] but not in others [21,29].

Mechanical ventilation during the acute episode does not in itself appear to be associated with increased mortality. However, there are very few data specifically addressing this issue. Many patients who require ventilatory support have severe underlying disease, and it is the severity of the disease that is primarily associated with an increase in mortality [148].

The long-term mortality for patients with COPD surviving an episode of acute respiratory failure varies from 60% or higher at one year [153] to less than 30% at two years [149]. The major factor that determines prognosis appears to be the state of the patient's underlying COPD. In fact, an episode of acute respiratory failure precipitated by an exacerbation of chronic bronchitis does not appear to affect the patient's long-term prognosis [148,149].

19.6 COMPLICATIONS OF ACUTE RESPIRATORY FAILURE

19.6.1 BAROTRAUMA

The progressive alveolar destruction that occurs in COPD may lead to the development of thin-walled subpleural blebs. Rupture of a bleb results in a pneumothorax which can cause significant pulmonary compromise due to the patient's limited pulmonary reserve. During mechanical ventilation, the incidence of pulmonary barotrauma is relatively low occurring in 1 to 8% of patients [154,155]. The frequency increases significantly in patients with ARDS [154] or necrotizing pneumonia [156], although the incidence in patients with COPD and acute respiratory failure has not been well documented. Factors that have been associated with an increased incidence of barotrauma are high peak airway pressures [154], high levels of positive end-expiratory pressure (both externally applied and auto-PEEP) [156,157] and high tidal volumes [158,159]. Animal studies have shown the importance of increases in alveolar volume in producing disruption of alveolar walls [160]. Clearly high airway pressure alone does not produce pneumothorax since normal subjects and patients do not develop pneumothorax during maximal inspiratory pressure maneuvers despite generation of very high inspiratory pressures. However, high airway pressures or PEEP commonly contribute to alveolar overdistension which is probably the major mechanism of alveolar rupture. High levels of airway pressure or PEEP tend to be more commonly found in the most severely ill patients who frequently have other factors that predispose them to barotrauma. The clinician should try to adjust ventilator settings if peak airway pressure is noted to be high (peak static airway pressure >40 cmH$_2$O) during serial monitoring. For example, a low tidal volume should help in minimizing this. Currently, there is increasing enthusiasm for the use of permissive hypercapnia in an attempt to minimize this risk [161]. Another approach that is receiving attention is the use of pressure-controlled ventilation rather than the more usual volume-controlled ventilation although satisfactorily controlled studies have not been conducted.

19.6.2 CARDIAC ARRHYTHMIAS

Cardiac arrhythmias are extremely common in patients with COPD even in the stable state. Arrhythmias include sinus tachycardia (the most common), premature atrial complexes, atrial fibrillation, multifocal atrial tachycardia, premature ventricular complexes and ventricular tachycardia. In a study of 69 patients with stable but severe COPD, 24 h ambulatory electrocardiographic monitoring revealed episodes of supraventricular tachycardia in 69% of patients, frequent premature ventricular contractions (>25/h) in 35% of patients, and non-sustained ventricular tachycardia in 22% of patients [162]. In this study, arrhythmias *per se* had no effect on mortality. Continuous electrocardiographic monitoring in hospitalized COPD patients with acute respiratory failure revealed significant arrhythmias in 11 of 16 patients [163]. In another study, routine electrocardiograms revealed significant arrhythmias in 33 of 70 patients (47%) [163]. In this study, mortality was markedly higher in patients with ventricular arrhythmias. In heterogeneous populations of patients with COPD, the presence of cardiac arrhythmias is associated with a poor prognosis with a high mortality rate over the following two years [164,165]. This finding may reflect the fact that cardiac arrhythmias are more likely in sicker patients who have more severe underlying lung disease and are more likely to succumb to their disease, or it may reflect a direct effect of the cardiac arrhythmias. Arrhythmias can result in an appreciable decrease in cardiac output which could be devastating in the acutely ill hypoxic patient. Since significant arrhythmias are often missed by routine electrocardiograms [163], continuous cardiac monitoring is important during treatment of patients with COPD and acute respiratory failure. Several factors may play a role in causing arrhythmias [166]. These factors include cor pulmonale, hypoxemia (which appears to be a weak determinant of arrhythmia), electrolyte abnormalities particularly hypokalemia, increased levels of catecholamines related to stress, coexisting ischemic heart disease, and medications.

The initial approach to cardiac arrhythmias in these patients is to identify and aggressively correct any possible metabolic abnor-

mality, i.e. hypoxemia, acidosis, alkalosis, hypokalemia, or other electrolyte abnormalities. Treatment of the underlying lung disease may be all that is required for resolution of the cardiac arrhythmias. Digoxin and theophylline levels should be checked to ensure that levels are in the appropriate therapeutic range. In particular, theophylline may contribute to the genesis of multifocal atrial tachycardia (a common rhythm disorder in patients with COPD) in some patients even at levels within the therapeutic range (16–20 mg/l) [167]. Accordingly, in the presence of multifocal atrial tachycardia, consideration should be given to lowering the dosage of aminophylline/theophylline to obtain serum levels <15 mg/l. If arrhythmias persist and cause circulatory compromise despite these measures, specific therapy should be considered. Atrial fibrillation with a rapid ventricular response can be treated with either digoxin or a calcium channel blocker. In the past, it was thought that multifocal atrial tachycardia responded only to amelioration of the underlying lung disease. However, it has recently been shown that this arrhythmia responds to treatment with verapanul, a calcium channel blocking agent, which slows the heart rate and often restores sinus rhythm [168,169]. Malignant ventricular arrhythmias should be treated according to standard regimens. There are no data that suggest that treatment of less severe ventricular arrhythmias (i.e. frequent premature ventricular contractions) with anti-arrhythmic drugs is beneficial in this patient population [170]. Given the known toxicity of most anti-arrhythmic agents, such treatment is not recommended.

19.6.3 GASTROINTESTINAL BLEEDING

Acute stress ulceration with resultant upper gastrointestinal bleeding is a well-recognized complication in patients with respiratory failure. A 20% incidence of significant gastrointestinal bleeding in patients in a respiratory ICU has been reported [171]. However, the incidence was only 9% in the patients with COPD.

Continuous enteral feeding when delivered into the stomach or proximal duodenum may reduce the risk of overt gastrointestinal bleeding in mechanically ventilated patients [172]. The mechanism for this effect is unclear. However, direct administration of substrate may improve mucosal function, thereby reducing susceptibility to acid damage. Gastric acid plays a key role in the formation of stress ulcers. Multiple studies have demonstrated that maintaining gastric pH above 4.0 reduces the incidence of overt gastrointestinal bleeding [173–175]. Accordingly, many physicians give antacids or high doses of H_2-blockers while sampling gastric contents intermittently to maintain a pH $\geq$ 4.0.

However, gastric acidity is an important natural defense mechanism in keeping the stomach sterile. Prophylactic regimens that raise intragastric pH can result in an increased growth of gram-negative bacteria in the stomach [176]. Thus, in patients receiving stress ulcer prophylaxis, the stomach may be an important reservoir of pathogenic bacteria that may retrogradely colonize the lower airways and contribute to the pathogenesis of nosocomial pneumonia. In a multivariate analysis of 233 mechanically-ventilated patients, Craven and associates found that administration of cimetidine significantly increased the risk of nosocomial pneumonia [177]. Sulcrafate is a relatively new drug that enhances gastric mucosal cytoprotective mechanisms without increasing gastric pH. A recent meta-analysis suggests that sulcrafate is as effective as antacids and possibly more effective than H_2-blockers for prophylaxis of stress ulcer bleeding [178]. In addition, sulcrafate-treated patients have lower levels of gastric colonization with gram-negative bacilli than patients receiving antacids or H_2-blockers [179]. In the aforementioned meta-analysis, a lower incidence of nosocomial pneumonia was found in patients receiving sulcrafate compared with patients receiving either antacids or H_2-blockers [178].

Thus, COPD patients with acute respiratory failure may not benefit substantially from stress ulcer prophylaxis [180], particularly if they are already being fed enterally. If stress ulcer prophylaxis is administered, sulcrafate appears to be the drug of choice at the present time (dose, 1 g every 6 hours).

19.6.4 PULMONARY EMBOLI

Pulmonary embolization has been found at autopsy in 28–51% of patients with COPD [181,182]. Whether these emboli contributed in any way to the patient's demise is unclear. However, COPD patients with acute respiratory failure have multiple risk factors for thromboembolic disease: (1) immobility and bed rest, (2) presence of right heart failure, and (3) advanced age. Since the vast majority of pulmonary emboli arise from the deep veins of the lower extremities, an estimate of the incidence of deep venous thrombosis in COPD patients with acute respiratory failure should reflect the risk of subsequent pulmonary embolus. Two studies have examined the incidence of deep venous thrombosis in decompensated patients with COPD who were sick enough to require hospital admission but did not require institution of mechanical ventilation. In a study of 45 patients, Prescott and colleagues detected 2 patients who had deep venous thrombosis on admission (4.4%) [183]. Thirty-three of these patients were followed serially with ^{125}I-labelled fibrinogen and deep venous thrombosis limited to the calf developed in 2 patients (6%). These findings reveal a surprisingly low incidence of deep venous thrombosis. In contrast, Winter and colleagues examined 29 Scottish patients with decompensated COPD using indium-111 labelled platelets [184]. Deep venous thrombosis was found in 13 patients (45%), 9 of whom had proximal vein thrombosis. The reason for the discrepancies between the two studies is not clear. Patients requiring admission to the intensive care unit and mechanical ventilation are likely to be sicker and may be at higher risk of thromboembolic disease. Significant pulmonary emboli have been observed in 20 and 27% of respiratory ICU patients at autopsy [185,186]. In the latter study only 50% of the emboli were diagnosed before death [186].

Establishing a diagnosis of pulmonary embolism is extremely difficult in patients with acute respiratory failure. Symptoms and signs are insensitive and non-specific and may reflect the underlying lung disease. Patients with COPD and acute respiratory failure are expected to have significant maldistribution of perfusion and ventilation due to their underlying lung disease. Thus, a $\dot{V}/\dot{Q}$ scan is much less helpful in this population of patients [187]. A $\dot{V}/\dot{Q}$ scan that demonstrates one or more segmental $\dot{V}/\dot{Q}$ mismatches (perfusion defect with normal ventilation) indicates a high probability of pulmonary embolism and no further diagnostic testing is required. However, the majority of patients have abnormalities of ventilation in most or all regions of the lungs rendering the scan indeterminate. Pulmonary angiograms remain the gold standard for diagnosis. However, in many medical centers, access to pulmonary angiograms is limited. Furthermore, many physicians are understandably reluctant to perform angiography in a patient with frank respiratory failure who may have a significant degree of cor pulmonale.

Since most pulmonary emboli arise from venous thrombosis in the legs it is reasonable to first evaluate the lower extremities. Impedance plethysmography is a simple test that can be performed at the bedside and is sensitive and specific for proximal vein thrombosis [188]. The presence of right heart failure may lead to bilateral false positive results. Real time, B-mode ultrasonography is a newer technique that has high sensitivity and specificity for proximal vein thrombosis in symptomatic patients [189]. If deep venous thrombosis is documented, anticoagulation is required and diagnosis of pulmonary embolism is no longer necessary. However, a negative study of the leg veins does not rule out the diagnosis of pulmonary embolism since 30% of patients with documented pulmonary embolism have negative leg studies [190]. Therefore, in patients with negative leg studies, pulmonary angiography deserves serious consideration.

Given the substantial incidence of pulmonary embolism and the difficulties in diagnosis, prophylactic therapy to prevent pulmonary embolus should be considered. Heparin in low doses (5000 units subcutaneously every 12 hours) has been shown to reduce the incidence of thromboembolic disease in medical and surgical high risk patients. Although there have been no prospective randomized studies of low-dose heparin in patients with respiratory failure, a retrospective study suggested that low-dose heparin substantially reduces the incidence of pulmonary embolism in such patients [191]. The authors recommended administration of low-dose heparin to all non-ambulatory COPD patients with acute respiratory failure in the absence of specific contraindications (i.e. known hemorrhagic diathesis, bleeding lesion, malignant hypertension, undiagnosed head injury, or severe liver disease).

19.6.5 NOSOCOMIAL PNEUMONIA

One of the most serious complications of acute respiratory failure is nosocomial pneumonia. Nosocomial pneumonia is usually caused by virulent organisms, frequently gram-negative bacilli that cause necrotizing pneumonia and may be resistant to common antibiotics. A full discussion of this topic is beyond the scope of this chapter and the reader is referred elsewhere [192]. The most common source of nosocomial pneumonia appears to be aspiration of micro-organisms that colonize the pharynx [193,194]. Critically ill patients have alterations in pharyngeal cell function that promote bacterial adherence and predispose to rapid colonization of the pharynx with hospital flora [195]. Seventy-five per cent of intensive care patients who become colonized do so within the first 72 hours [195]. A potentially preventable mode of transmission is transfer of contaminated secretions from one patient to another by medical personnel (physicians, nurses, respiratory therapists). Use of gloves during potential contact with secretions and careful handwashing between patient contacts should be mandatory practice. The stomach may also be an important reservoir of pathogenic bacteria particularly in patients receiving antacids or H_2-blockers.

The diagnosis of nosocomial pneumonia can be quite difficult. The traditional criteria used to diagnose pneumonia are (1) new or progressive pulmonary infiltrates, (2) fever, (3) leukocytosis, and (4) purulent tracheobronchial secretions. However, in the patient with COPD and acute respiratory failure, symptoms may be masked (i.e. fever may not develop while the patient is receiving high-dose steroid therapy). Furthermore, symptoms suggestive of pneumonia may have a non-infectious explanation (i.e. leukocytosis may be due to demargination of neutrophils secondary to prednisone therapy, new pulmonary infiltrates may be due to fluid overload, etc.).

The clinical diagnosis of nosocomial pneumonia particularly in the mechanically-ventilated patient has been shown to be highly imprecise. Sputum cultures cannot distinguish between airway colonization and infection. Studies utilizing invasive diagnostic methods (protected specimen brush and/or bronchoalveolar lavage with quantitative culture) have clearly shown that nosocomial pneumonia is overdiagnosed when sputum culture and clinical criteria are used for diagnosis [196,197]. Although the poor specificity of sputum culture has been well documented, the sensitivity of this technique is not well defined. Furthermore, it has not been definitively shown that invasive diagnostic methods such as the protected specimen brush or bronchoalveolar lavage with quantitative cultures

have greater sensitivity for the diagnosis of nosocomial pneumonia [197,198]. Johanson and colleagues compared invasive diagnostic methods with tracheal aspirates in anesthetized mechanically ventilated baboons [199]. The animals were sacrificed and lung tissue was cultured and these culture results were considered to be the gold standard. If a quantitative lung tissue culture of greater than $10^3/g$ tissue is considered significant, the sensitivity of bronchoalveolar lavage and tracheal aspirates were both 100% compared with 62% for the protected brush. However, the number of false positives was very high with tracheal aspirates and this false positive rate could be markedly reduced with the more invasive diagnostic methods.

The choice of empirical antibiotic therapy for nosocomial pneumonia is problematic. A study using the protected specimen brush found that 61% of isolates were gram-negative bacilli (*Pseudomonas*, *Acinetobacter* and *Proteus* were the most common gram-negative isolates), 38% were gram-positive cocci and 1% were anaerobes [200]. Initial antibiotic coverage should be broad spectrum. Once sputum culture results are available, the antibiotic spectrum can be narrowed. Many clinicians feel uncomfortable with this approach and will use invasive diagnostic methods to obtain a more precise microbiologic diagnosis [201].

19.7 SUMMARY

Correction of life-threatening hypoxemia with controlled oxygen therapy and improvement of airflow obstruction with β_2-agonists and corticosteroids are the mainstays of therapy in patients with COPD and acute respiratory failure. Most patients will respond to this therapy and mechanical ventilation can be avoided. In a minority of patients, a deteriorating mental status, cardiovascular instability, or progressive respiratory acidosis despite treatment will necessitate institution of mechanical ventilation. The majority of patients with COPD and acute respiratory failure will survive the acute episode. However, their long-term prognosis is variable and depends primarily on the severity of the underlying COPD.

REFERENCES

1. National Center for Health Statistics. Current Estimates from the National Health Interview Survey, United States 1986 Vital and Health Statistics, Series 10, No. 164 DHHS (PHS).
2. Higgins, M.W. and Thorn, T. (1989) Incidence, prevalence and mortality: intra and intercountry difference, in Hensley MJ, Saunders NA, eds. *Clinical Epidemiology of Chronic Obstructive Pulmonary Disease* (eds M.J. Hensley and N.A. Saunders), Marcel Dekker, New York, pp. 23–39.
3. Rahn, H. and Fenn, W.O. (1955) *A Graphical Analysis of Respiratory Gas Exchange.* American Physiological Society, Washington, DC.
4. Campbell, E.J.M. (1967) The J. Burns Amberson Lecture. The management of acute respiratory failure in chronic bronchitis and emphysema. *Am. Rev. Respir. Dis.,* **96,** 626–39.
5. Eldridge, F. and Gherman, C. (1968) Studies of oxygen administration in respiratory failure. *Ann. Intern. Med.,* **68,** 569–78.
6. Kilburn, K.H. (1965) Neurologic manifestations of respiratory failure. *Arch. Intern. Med.,* **116,** 409–15.
7. Westlake, E.K., Simpson, T and Kaye, M. (1955) Carbon dioxide narcosis in emphysema. *Q. J. Med.,* **24,** 155–73.
8. McNicol, M.W. and Campbell, E.J.M. (1965) Severity of respiratory failure: arterial blood gas in untreated patients. *Lancet,* **i,** 336–8.
9. Austen, F.K., Carmichael, M.W. and Adams, R.D. (1957) Neurological manifestations of chronic pulmonary insufficiency. *N. Engl. J. Med.,* **257,** 579–90.
10. Posner, J.B. and Plum, F. (1967) Spinal-fluid pH and neurologic symptoms in systemic acidosis. *N. Engl. J. Med.,* **277,** 605–13.
11. Madias, N.E. and Cohen, J.J. (1982) Respiratory acidosis, in *Acid-base,* (eds J.J. Cohen and J.P. Kassirer), Little Brown, Boston, pp. 307–49.
12. Neff, T.A. and Petty, T.L. (1972) Tolerance and survival in severe chronic hypercapnia. *Arch. Intern. Med.,* **129,** 591–6.
13. Kety, S.S. and Schmidt, C.F. (1948) The effects of altered arterial tensions of carbon dioxide and oxygen on cerebral blood flow and cerebral oxygen consumption of normal young men. *J. Clin. Invest.,* **27,** 484–92.
14. Javaheri, S. and Kazemi, H. (1987) Metabolic alkalosis and hypoventilation in humans. *Am. Rev. Respir. Dis.,* **136,** 1011–16.
15. Javaheri, S. and Mardell, E.A. (1981) Severe metabolic alkalosis: a case report. *Br. Med. J.,* **283,** 1016–17.
16. Tobin, M.J. (1989) *Essentials of Critical Care Medicine.* Churchill Livingstone, New York.
17. Aubier, M., Murciano, D. Milic-Emili, J. *et al.* (1980) Effects of the administration of O_2 on ventilation and blood gases in patients with chronic obstructive pulmonary disease during acute respiratory failure. *Am. Rev. Respir. Dis.,* **122,** 747–54.
18. Stradling, J.R. (1986) Hypercapnia during oxygen therapy in airways obstruction: a reappraisal. *Thorax,* **41,** 897–902.
19. Aubier, M., Murciano, D., Fournier, M. *et al.* (1980) Central respiratory drive in acute respiratory failure of patients with chronic obstructive pulmonary disease. *Am. Rev. Respir. Dis.,* **122,** 191–9.
20. Dunn, W.F., Nelson, S.B. and Hubmayr, R.D. (1991) Oxygen induced hypercarbia in obstructive pulmonary disease. *Am. Rev. Respir. Dis.,* **144,** 526–30.
21. Warren, P.M., Flenley, D.C., Millar, J.S. and Avery, A. (1980) Respiratory failure revisited: acute exacerbations of chronic bronchitis between 1961–68 and 1970–76. *Lancet,* **i,** 467–71.
22. Bone, R.C., Pierce, A.K. and Johnson, R.L. (1978) Controlled oxygen administration in acute respiratory failure in chronic obstructive pulmonary disease. A reappraisal. *Am. J. Med.,* **65,** 896–902.
23. Bazuaye, E.A., Stone, T.N., Corris, P.A. and Gibson, G.J. (1992) Variability of inspired oxygen concentration with nasal cannulas. *Thorax,* **47,** 609–11.
24. Tobin, M.J. (1988) Respiratory monitoring in the intensive care unit. *Am. Rev. Respir. Dis.,* **138,** 1625–42.
25. Murciano, D., Aubier, M., Bussi, S. *et al.* (1982) Comparison of esophageal, tracheal and mouth occlusion pressure in patients with chronic obstructive pulmonary disease during acute respiratory failure. *Am. Rev. Respir. Dis.,* **126,** 837–41.
26. Murciano, D., Boczkowski, J., Lecocguic, Y. *et al.* (1988) Tracheal occlusion pressure: a simple index to monitor respiratory muscle

fatigue during acute respiratory failure in patients with chronic obstructive pulmonary disease. *Ann. Intern. Med.*, **108**, 800–5.

27. Bellemare, F. and Grassino, A. (1983) Force reserve of the diaphragm in patients with chronic obstructive pulmonary disease. *J. Appl. Physiol.*, **55**, 8–15.

28. Moser, K.M., Luchsinger, P.C., Adamson, J.S. et al. (1973) Respiratory stimulation with intravenous doxapram in respiratory failure. *N. Engl. J. Med.*, **288**, 427–31.

29. Jeffrey, A.A., Warren, P.M. and Flenley, D.C. (1992) Acute hypercapnic respiratory failure in patients with chronic obstructive lung disease: risk factors and use of guidelines for management. *Thorax*, **47**, 34–40.

30. Altose, M.D. and Hudgel, D.W. (1986) The pharmacology of respiratory depressants and stimulants. *Clin. Chest Med.*, **7**, 481–94.

31. Anthonisen, N.R. and Wright, E.C. IPPB Trial Group (1986) Bronchodilator response in chronic obstructive pulmonary disease. *Am. Rev. Respir. Dis.*, **133**, 814–19.

32. Eliasson, O. and Degraff, A.C. (1985) The use of criteria for reversibility and obstruction to define patient groups for bronchodilator trials. *Am. Rev. Respir. Dis.*, **132**, 858–64.

33. Hughes, J.A., Tobin, M.J., Bellamy, D. and Hutchinson, D.C.S. (1982) Effects of ipratropium bromide and fenoterol aerosols in pulmonary emphysema. *Thorax*, **37**, 667–70.

34. Larsson, S. and Svedmyr, N. (1977) Bronchodilating effect and side effects of β_2 adrenoceptor stimulants by different modes of administration. *Am. Rev. Respir. Dis.*, **116**, 861–9.

35. Shim, C.S. and Williams, M.H. Jr. (1980) Bronchial response to oral vs. aerosol metaproterenol in asthma. *Ann. Intern. Med.*, **93**, 428–31.

36. Shim, C.S. and Williams, M.H. Jr. (1983) Bronchodilator response to oral aminophylline and terbutaline versus aerosol albuterol in patients with chronic obstructive pulmonary disease. *Am. J. Med.*, **75**, 697–701.

37. Hess, D., Horney, D. and Snyder, T. (1989) Medication-delivery performance of eight small-volume, hand-held nebulizers: Effects of diluent volume, gas flowrate and nebulizer model. *Respir. Care*, **34**, 717–23.

38. Alvine, G.F., Rodgers, P., Fitzsimmons, K.M. and Ahrens, R.C. (1992) Disposable jet nebulizers. How reliable are they? *Chest*, **101**, 316–9.

39. Jenkins, S.C., Heaton, R.W., Fulton, T.J. and Moxham, J. (1987) Comparison of domiciliary nebulized salbutamol and salbutamol from a metered-dose inhaler in stable chronic airflow limitation. *Chest*, **91**, 804–7.

40. Mestitz, H., Copland, J.M. and McDonald, C.F. (1989) Comparison of outpatient nebulized vs metered dose inhaler terbutaline in chronic airflow obstruction. *Chest*, **96**, 1237–40.

41. Newhouse, N. and Dolovich, M. (1987) Aerosol therapy: nebulizer vs metered dose inhaler. *Chest*, **91**, 799–800.

42. Jaspar, A.C., Mohsenifar, Z., Kahan, S. et al. (1987) Cost-benefit comparison of aerosol bronchodilator delivery methods in hospitalized patients. *Chest*, **91**, 614–8.

43. Turner, J.R., Corkery, K.J., Eckman, D. et al. (1988) Equivalence of continuous flow nebulizer and metered-dose inhaler with reservoir bag for treatment of acute airflow obstruction. *Chest*, **93**, 476–81.

44. Saltzman, G.A., Steele, M.T., Pribble, J.P. et al. (1989) Aerosolized metaproterenol in the treatment of asthmatics with severe airflow obstruction. Comparison of two delivery methods. *Chest*, **95**, 1017–20.

45. Summer, W., Elston, R., Tharpe, L. et al. (1989) Aerosol bronchodilator delivery methods: relative impact on pulmonary function and cost of respiratory care. *Arch. Intern. Med.*, **149**, 618–23.

46. Gay, P.C., Patel, H.G., Nelson, S.B. et al. (1991) Metered dose inhalers for bronchodilator delivery in intubated, mechanically ventilated patients. *Chest*, **99**, 66–71.

47. Fuller, H.D., Dolovich, M.B., Posmituck, G. et al. (1990) Pressurized aerosol versus jet aerosol delivery to mechanically ventilated patients: comparison of dose to the lungs. *Am. Rev. Respir. Dis.*, **141**, 440–4.

48. Gross, N.J. (1988) Ipratropium bromide. *N. Engl. J. Med.*, **319**, 486–94.

49. Taskin, D.P., Ashutosh, K. and Blacker, E.R. (1986) Comparison of anticholinergic bronchodilator ipratropium bromide with metaproterenol in chronic obstructive pulmonary disease: a 90-day multi-center study. *Am. J. Med.*, **81** (suppl. 5A), 59–68.

50. Marini, J.J. and Lakshminarayan, S. (1980) The effect of atropine inhalation in 'irreversible' chronic bronchitis. *Chest*, **77**, 591–6.

51. Braun, S.R., McKenzie, W.N., Copeland, C. et al. (1989) A comparison of the effect of ipratropium and albuterol in the treatment of

52. Gross, N.J. and Skorodin, M.S. (1984) Role of the parasympathetic system in airway obstruction due to emphysema. *N. Engl. J. Med.*, **311**, 421–5.

53. Easton, P.A., Jadue, C., Dhingra, S. and Anthonisen, N.R. (1980) A comparison of the bronchodilating effect of a beta-2 adrenergic agent (albuterol) and an anticholinergic agent (ipratropium bromide), given by aerosol alone or in sequence. *N. Engl. J. Med.*, **315**, 735–9.

54. Rebuck, A.S., Chapman, K.R., Abboud, R. *et al.* (1987) Nebulized anticholinergic and sympathomimetic treatment of asthma and chronic obstructive airways disease in the emergency room. *Am. J. Med.*, **82**, 59–64.

55. Backman, R. and Hellstrom, P-E. (1985) Fenoterol and ipratropium bromide in respiratory treatment of patients with chronic bronchitis. *Curr. Ther. Res.*, **38**, 135–40.

56. Lam, A. and Newhouse, M.T. (1990) Management of asthma and chronic airflow limitation: are methylxanthines obsolete? *Chest*, **98**, 44–52.

57. Eaton, M.L., Green, B.A., Church, T.R., *et al.* (1980) Efficacy of theophylline in 'irreversible' airflow obstruction. *Ann. Intern. Med.*, **92**, 758–61.

58. Alexander, M.L., Dull, W.L. and Kasik, J.E. (1980) Treatment of chronic obstructive pulmonary disease with orally administered theophylline: a double-blind, controlled study. *JAMA*, **244**, 2286–90.

59. Filuk, R.B., Easton, P.A. and Anthonisen, N.R. (1985) Responses to large doses of salbutamol and theophylline in patients with chronic obstructive pulmonary disease. *Am. Rev. Respir. Dis.*, **132**, 871–4.

60. Barclay, J., Whitting, B. and Addis, G.J. (1982) The influence of theophylline on maximal response to salbutamol in severe chronic obstructive pulmonary disease. *Eur. J. Clin. Pharmacol.*, **22**, 389–93.

61. Rice, K.L., Leatherman, J.W., Duane, P.G. *et al.* (1987) Aminophylline for acute exacerbations of chronic obstructive pulmonary disease. *Ann. Intern. Med.*, **107**, 305–9.

62. Powell, J.R., Vozeh, S., Hopewell, P. *et al.* (1978) Theophylline disposition in acutely ill hospitalized patients. The effect of smoking, heart failure, severe airway obstruction and pneumonia. *Am. Rev. Respir. Dis.*, **118**, 229–38.

63. Matthay, R.A., Berger, H.J., Loke, J. *et al.* (1978) Effects of aminophylline upon right and left ventricular performance in chronic obstructive pulmonary disease: noninvasive assessment by radionuclide angiocardiography. *Am. J. Med.*, **65**, 903–10.

64. Matthay, R.A., Berger, H.J., Davies, R. *et al.* (1982) Improvement in cardiac performance by oral long-acting theophylline in chronic obstructive pulmonary disease. *Am. Heart J.*, **104**, 1022–6.

65. Hooper, W.W., Slutsky, R.A., Kocienski, D.E. *et al.* (1982) Right and left ventricular response to subcutaneous terbutaline in patients with chronic obstructive pulmonary disease: Radionuclide angiographic assessment of cardiac size and function. *Am. Heart J.*, **104**, 1027–32.

66. Sigrist, S., Thomas, D., Howell, S. and Roussos, Ch. (1982) The effect of aminophylline on inspiratory muscle contractility. *Am. Rev. Respir. Dis.*, **126**, 46–50.

67. Aubier, M., DeTroyer, A., Sampson, M. *et al.* (1981) Aminophylline improves diaphragmatic contractility. *N. Engl. J. Med.*, **305**, 249–52.

68. Murciano, D., Aubier, M., Lecocguic, Y. and Pariente, R. (1984) Effects of theophylline on diaphragmatic strength and fatigue in patients with chronic obstructive pulmonary disease. *N. Engl. J. Med.*, **311**, 349–53.

69. Levy, R.D., Nava, S., Gibbons, L. and Bellemare, F. (1990) Aminophylline and human diaphragm strength *in vivo*. *J. Appl. Physiol.*, **68**, 2591–6.

70. Kongragunta, V.K., Druz, W.S and Sharp, J.T. (1988) Dyspnea and diaphragmatic fatigue in patients with chronic obstructive pulmonary disease. Responses to theophylline. *Am. Rev. Respir. Dis.*, **137**, 662–7.

71. Moxham, J., Miller, J., Wiles, C.M. *et al.* (1985) Effect of aminophylline on the human diaphragm. *Thorax*, **40**, 288–92.

72. Mador, M.J. (1990) Pharmacotherapy of the respiratory muscles. *Probl. Respir. Care*, **3**, 493–506.

73. Albert, R.K., Martin, T.R. and Lewis, S.W. (1980) Controlled clinical trial of methylprednisolone in patients with chronic bronchitis and acute respiratory insufficiency. *Ann. Intern. Med.*, **92**, 753–8.

74. Glenny, R.W. (1987) Steroids in COPD. The scripture according to Albert. *Chest*, **91**, 289–90.

75. Emerman, C.L., Connors, A.F., Lukens, T.W. *et al.* (1989) A randomized controlled trial of methylprednisolone in the emergency treatment of acute exacerbations of COPD. *Chest,* **95**, 563–7.

76. Murray, T.F. and Sethi, S. (1992) Bacterial infection in chronic obstructive pulmonary disease. *Am. Rev. Respir. Dis.,* **146**, 1067–83.

77. Chodosh, S. (1987) Acute bacterial exacerbations in bronchitis and asthma. *Am. J. Med.,* **82** (suppl. 4A), 154–63.

78. Verghese, A., Roberson, D., Kalbfleisch, J.H. and Sarubbi, F. (1990) Randomized comparative study of cefixime versus cephalexin in acute bacterial exacerbations of chronic bronchitis. *Antimicrob. Agents Chemother.,* **34**, 1041–4.

79. Fagon, J.V., Chastre, J., Trouillet, J.L. *et al.* (1990) Characterization of distal bronchial microflora during acute exacerbations of chronic bronchitis: use of the protected specimen brush technique in 54 mechanically ventilated patients. *Am. Rev. Respir. Dis.,* **142**, 1004–8.

80. Smith, C.B., Golden, C.A., Kanner, R.E. and Renzetti, A.D. (1980) Association of viral and *Mycoplasma pneumoniae* infections with acute respiratory illness in patients with chronic obstructive pulmonary disease. *Am. Rev. Respir. Dis.,* **121**, 225–32.

81. Gump, D.W., Phillips, C.A., Forsyth, B.R. *et al.* (1976) Role of infection in chronic bronchitis. *Am. Rev. Respir. Dis.,* **113**, 465–74.

82. Smith, C.B., Golden, C.A., Kanner, R.E. and Renzetti, A.D. (1976) *Haemophilus influenzae* and *Haemophilus parainfluenzae* in chronic obstructive pulmonary disease. *Lancet,* **i**, 1253–5.

83. Chapman, A.J., Musher, D.M., Johsson, S. *et al.* (1985) Development of bactericidal antibody during *Branhamella catarrhalis* infection. *J. Infect. Dis.,* **151**, 878–82.

84. Tager, I. and Speizer, F.E. (1975) Role of infection in chronic bronchitis. *N. Engl. J. Med.,* **292**, 563–71.

85. Nicotra, M.B., Rivera, M. and Awe, R.J. (1982) Antibiotic therapy of acute exacerbations of chronic bronchitis. *Ann. Intern. Med.,* **97**, 18–21.

86. Anthonisen, N.R., Manfreda, J., Warren, C.P.W. *et al.* Antibiotic therapy in exacerbations of chronic obstructive pulmonary disease. *Ann. Intern. Med.,* **106**, 196–204.

87. Koretz, R.L. (1984) Breathing and feeding. Can you have one without the other? *Chest,* **85**, 208–9.

88. Driver, A.G., McAlvey, M.T. and Smith, J.L. (1982) Nutritional assessment of patients with chronic obstructive pulmonary disease and acute respiratory failure. *Chest,* **82**, 568–71.

89. Driver, A.G. and LeBrun, M. (1980) Iatrogenic malnutrition in patients receiving ventilatory support. *JAMA,* **224**, 2195–6.

90. Arora, N.S. and Rochester, D.F. (1982) Effect of body weight and muscularity on human diaphragm muscle mass, thickness and area. *J. Appl. Physiol.,* **52**, 64–70.

91. Arora, N.S. and Rochester, D.F. (1982) Respiratory muscle strength and maximum voluntary ventilation in undernourished patients. *Am. Rev. Respir. Dis.,* **126**, 5–8.

92. Kelly, S.M., Rosa, A., Field, S. *et al.* (1984) Inspiratory muscle strength and body composition in patients receiving total parenteral nutrition therapy. *Am. Rev. Respir. Dis.,* **130**, 33–7.

93. Doekel, R.C., Zwillich, C.W., Scoggin, C.H. *et al.* (1976) Clinical semistarvation: depression of hypoxic ventilatory response. *N. Engl. J. Med.,* **295**, 358–61.

94. Martin, T.R. (1987) Relationship between malnutrition and lung infections. *Clin. Chest Med.,* **3**, 359–73.

95. Neiderman, M.S., Merrill, W.W., Ferranti, R.D. *et al.* (1984) Nutritional status and bacterial binding in the lower respiratory tract in patients with chronic tracheostomy. *Ann. Intern. Med.,* **100**, 795–800.

96. Lorca, L. and Greenbaum, D.M. (1982) Effectiveness of intensive nutritional regimes in patients who fail to wean from mechanical ventilation. *Crit. Care Med.,* **10**, 297–300.

97. Dark, D.S., Pingleton, S.K. and Kerby, G.R. (1985) Hypercapnia during weaning: a complication of nutritional support. *Chest,* **88**, 141–3.

98. Harmon, G.S. and Pingleton, S.K. (1986) Energy (calorie) requirements in mechanically ventilated COPD patients. *Am. Rev. Respir. Dis.,* **131**, 203A.

99. Jones, N.L. (1974) Physical therapy: present state of the art. *Am. Rev. Respir. Dis.,* **110**, 132–6.

100. Anthonisen, P., Riis, P. and Sodard-Andersen, T. (1964) The value of lung physiotherapy in the treatment of acute exacerbations in chronic bronchitis. *Acta Med. Scand.,* **175**, 715–9.

101. Connors, A.F., Hammon, W.E., Martin, R.J. and Rogers, R.M. (1980) Chest physical therapy. The immediate effect on oxygenation in acutely ill patients. *Chest*, **78**, 559–64.

102. Murray, J.F. (1979) The ketchup bottle method. *N. Engl. J. Med.*, **300**, 1155–7.

103. Fleury, B., Murciano, C., Talamo, C. *et al.* (1985) Work of breathing in patients with chronic obstructive pulmonary disease in acute respiratory failure. *Am. Rev. Respir. Dis.*, **131**, 816–21.

104. Pepe, P.E. and Marini, J.J. (1982) Occult positive end-expiratory pressure in mechanically ventilated patients with airflow obstruction: the auto-PEEP effect. *Am. Rev. Respir. Dis.*, **126**, 166–70.

105. Smith, T.C. and Marini, J.J. (1988) Impact of PEEP on lung mechanics and work of breathing in severe airflow obstruction. *J. Appl. Physiol.*, **65**, 1488–99.

106. Tyler, C., Cohen, N., Covington, J. and Kniebel, A. (1990) Easy determination of auto-PEEP on ventilators not equipped with an expiratory hold. *Respir. Care*, **35**, 114.

107. Rossi, A., Gottfried, S.B., Zocchi, L. *et al.* (1985) Measurement of static compliance of the total respiratory system in patients with acute respiratory failure during mechanical ventilation: the effect of intrinsic positive end-expiratory pressure. *Am. Rev. Respir. Dis.*, **131**, 672–7.

108. Petrof, B.J., Legare, M., Goldberg, P. *et al.* (1990) Continuous positive airway pressure reduces work of breathing and dyspnea during weaning from mechanical ventilation in severe chronic obstructive pulmonary disease. *Am. Rev. Respir. Dis.*, **141**, 281–9.

109. Appendini, L., Zanaboni, S., Petessio, A. *et al.* (1992) Expiratory muscle activity during application of continuous positive airway pressure (CPAP) in chronic obstructive pulmonary disease patients (COPD) with acute respiratory failure (ARF). *Am. Rev. Respir. Dis.*, **145**, 515A.

110. Ninane, V., Rypens, F., Yernault, J.C. and DeTroyer, A. (1992) Abdominal muscle use during breathing in patients with chronic airflow obstruction. *Am. Rev. Respir. Dis.*, **146**, 16–21.

111. Brown, D.G. and Pierson, D.J. (1986) Auto-PEEP is common in mechanically ventilated patients: a study of incidence, severity and detection. *Respir. Care*, **31**, 1069–74.

112. Tuxen, D.V. and Lane, S. (1987) The effects of ventilatory pattern on hyperinflation, airway pressures, and circulation in mechanical ventilation of patients with severe air-flow obstruction. *Am. Rev. Respir. Dis.*, **136**, 872–9.

113. Brogeghini, C., Brandolese, R., Poggi, R. *et al.* (1988) Respiratory mechanics during the first day of mechanical ventilation in patients with pulmonary edema and chronic airway obstruction. *Am. Rev. Respir. Dis.*, **138**, 355–61.

114. Rochester, D.F., Arora, N.S., Braun, N.M.T. and Goldberg, S.K. (1979) The respiratory muscles in chronic obstructive pulmonary disease. *Bull. Eur. Physiopath. Respir.*, **15**, 117–23.

115. Aubier, M., Viires, N., Piquet, J. *et al.* (1985) Effects of hypocalcemia on diaphragmatic strength generation. *J. Appl. Physiol.*, **58**, 2054–61.

116. Aubier, M., Murciano, D., Lecocguic, Y. *et al.* (1985) Effect of hypophosphatemia on diaphragmatic contractility in patients with acute respiratory failure. *N. Engl. J. Med.*, **313**, 420-4.

117. Molloy, D.W., Dhingra, S., Solven, F. *et al.* (1984) Hypomagnesemia and respiratory muscle power. *Am. Rev. Respir. Dis.*, **129**, 497–8.

118. Juan, G., Calverley, P., Talamo, C. *et al.* (1984) Effect of carbon dioxide on diaphragmatic function in human beings. *N. Engl. J. Med.*, **310**, 874–9.

119. Ameredes, B.T. and Clanton, T.L. (1988) Accelerated decay of inspiratory pressure during hypercapnic endurance trials in humans. *J. Appl. Physiol.*, **65**, 728–35.

120. Bellemare, F. and Grassino, A. (1982) Effect of pressure and timing of contraction on human diaphragm fatigue. *J. Appl. Physiol.*, **53**, 1190–5.

121. Bellemare, F. and Bigland-Ritchie, B. (1987) Central components of diaphragmatic fatigue assessed by phrenic nerve stimulation. *J. Appl. Physiol.*, **62**, 1307–16.

122. Marini, J.J., Rodriguez, R.M. and Lamb, V. (1986) The inspiratory workload of patient-initiated mechanical ventilation. *Am. Rev. Respir. Dis.*, **134**, 902–9.

123. Marini, J.J., Smith, T.C. and Lamb, V.J. (1988) External work output and force generation during synchronized intermittent mechanical ventilation. Effect of machine assistance on breathing effort. *Am. Rev. Respir. Dis.*, **138**, 1169–79.

124. Ward, M.E., Corbeil, C., Gibbons, W. *et al.* (1988) Optimization of respiratory muscle relaxation during mechanical ventilation. *Anesthesiology*, **69**, 29–35.

125. Henke, K.G., Arias, A., Skatrud, J.B. and Dempsey, J.A. (1988) Inhibition of inspiratory muscle activity during sleep. Chemical and nonchemical influences. *Am. Rev. Respir.*, **138**, 8–15.

126. Anzueto, A., Tobin, M.J., Moore, G. *et al.* (1987) Effect of prolonged mechanical ventilation on diaphragmatic function: a preliminary study of a baboon model. *Am. Rev. Respir. Dis.*, **135**, A201.

127. Le Bourdeiller, G., Viirer, N., Boczkowski, J. *et al.* (1994) Effects of mechanical ventilation on diaphragmatic contractile properties in rats. *Am. J. Respir. Crit, Care Med.*, **149**, 1539–44.

128. MacIntyre, N.R. (1986) Respiratory function during pressure support ventilation. *Chest*, **89**, 677–83.

129. Truwit, J.D. and Marini, J.J. (1988) Hyperinflation limits pressure control ventilation. *Chest*, **94**, 2S.

130. Connors, A.F. Jr., McCaffree, D.R. and Gray, B.A. (1981) Effect of inspiratory flow rate on gas exchange during mechanical ventilation. *Am. Rev. Respir. Dis.*, **124**, 537–43.

131. Jubran, A. and Tobin, M.J. (1990) Reliability of pulse oximetry in titrating supplemental oxygen therapy in ventilator dependent patients. *Chest*, **97**, 1420–5.

132. Tobin, M.J. and Lodato, R.F. (1989) PEEP, auto PEEP, and waterfalls. *Chest*, **96**, 449–51.

133. Gay, P.C., Rodarte, J.R. and Hubmayr, R.D. (1989) The effects of positive expiratory pressure on isovolume flow and dynamic hyperinflation in patients receiving mechanical ventilation. *Am. Rev. Respir. Dis.*, **139**, 621–6.

134. Tuxen, D.V. (1989) Detrimental effects of positive end-expiratory pressure during controlled mechanical ventilation of patients with severe airflow obstruction. *Am. Rev. Respir. Dis.*, **140**, 5–9.

135. Tobin, M.J. (1990) Weaning from mechanical ventilation, in *Current Pulmonology*, (ed. D.H. Simmons), vol. II. Year Book, Chicago, pp. 47–105.

136. Sahn, S.A. and Lakshminarayan, S. (1973) Bedside criteria for discontinuation of mechanical ventilation. *Chest*, **63**, 1002–5.

137. Yang, K.L. and Tobin, M.J. (1991) A prospective study of indexes predicting the outcome of trials of weaning from mechanical ventilation. *N. Engl. J. Med.*, **324**, 1445–50.

138. Tobin, M.J. and Yang, K. (1990) Weaning from mechanical ventilation. *Crit. Care Clinics*, **6**, 725–47.

139. Rebuck, A.S. and Chapman, K.R. (1986) Measurement and monitoring of exhaled carbon dioxide, in *Non-invasive Respiratory Monitoring*, (eds M.L. Nochomovitz and N.S. Cherniack), Churchill-Livingstone, New York, pp. 189–201.

140. Rahn, H. and Farhi, L.E. (1964) Ventilation, perfusion, and gas exchange – the V_A/Q concept, in *Handbook of Physiology* (eds W.D. Fenn and H. Rahn), Respiration, Vol. 1. Waverly Press, Baltimore, pp. 735–66.

141. Tashkin, D.P., Flick, G., Bellamy, P. and Mercurio, P. (1987) Pulmonary function, in *Diagnostic Methods in Critical Care*, (eds W.C. Shoemaker and E. Abraham), Marcel Dekker, New York, pp. 111–86.

142. Yamanaka, M.K. and Sue, D.Y. (1987) Comparison of arterial-end tidal PCO_2 difference and dead space/tidal volume ratio in respiratory failure. *Chest*, **92**, 832–5.

143. Hoffman, R.A., Krieger, B.P., Kramer, M.R. *et al.* (1989) End-tidal carbon dioxide in critically ill patients during changes in mechanical ventilation. *Am. Rev. Respir. Dis.*, **140**, 1265–8.

144. Tobin, M.J. (1986) Noninvasive evaluation of respiratory movement, in *Non-invasive Respiratory Monitoring*, (eds M.L. Nochomovitz and N.S. Cherniack), Churchill-Livingstone, New York, pp. 29–57.

145. Sackner, M.A., Watson, H., Belsito, A.S. *et al.* (1989) Calibration of respiratory inductive plethysmograph during natural breathing. *J. Appl. Physiol.*, **66**, 410–20.

146. Tobin, M.J., Guenther, S.M., Perez, W. *et al.* (1987) Konno–Mead analysis of ribcage-abdominal motion during successful and unsuccessful trials of weaning from mechanical ventilation. *Am. Rev. Respir. Dis.*, **135**, 1320–8.

147. Hoffman, R.A., Ershowsky, P. and Krieger, B.P. (1989) Determination of auto-PEEP during spontaneous and controlled ventilation by monitoring changes in end-expiratory thoracic gas volume. *Chest*, **96**, 613–6.

148. Hudson, L.D. (1987) Outcome and sequelae of acute respiratory failure, in *Acute Respiratory Failure*, (eds R.C. Bone, R.B. George and L.O. Hudson), Churchill Livingstone, New York, pp. 431–42.

149. Martin, T.R., Lewis, S.W. and Albert, R.K. (1982) The prognosis of patients with chronic obstructive pulmonary disease after hospitalization for acute respiratory failure. *Chest*, **82**, 310–4.

150. Dardes, N., Campo, S., Chiappini, M.G. *et al.* (1986) Prognosis of COPD patients after an episode of acute respiratory failure. *Eur. J. Respir. Dis.*, **69** (Suppl. 146), 377–81.

151. Asmundsson, T. and Kilburn, K.H. (1969) Survival of acute respiratory failure. A study of 239 episodes. *Ann. Intern. Med.*, **70**, 471–6.

152. Kettel, L.J., Diener, C.F., Morse, J.O., *et al.* Treatment of acute respiratory acidosis in chronic obstructive lung disease. *JAMA*, **217**, 1503–8.

153. Gottlieb, L.S. and Balchum, O.J. (1973) Course of chronic obstructive pulmonary disease following first onset of respiratory failure. *Chest*, **63**, 5–8.

154. Petersen, A.W. and Baier, H. (1983) Incidence of pulmonary barotrauma in a medical ICU. *Crit. Care Med.*, **11**, 67–9.

155. Cullen, D. and Caldera, D.L. (1979) Incidence of ventilator-induced pulmonary barotrauma in critically ill patients. *Anesthesiology*, **50**, 185–90.

156. DeLatorre, F.J., Tomasa, A., Klamburg, J. *et al.* (1977) Incidence of pneumothorax and pneumomediastinum in patients with aspiration pneumonia requiring ventilatory support. *Chest*, **72**, 141–4.

157. Zwillich, C.W., Pierson, D.J., Creagh, C.E. *et al.* (1974) Complications of assisted ventilation: a prospective study of 354 consecutive episodes. *Am. J. Med.*, **57**, 161–70.

158. Bone, R.C., Francis, P.B. and Pierce, A.K. (1975) Pulmonary barotrauma complicating positive end-expiratory pressure. *Am. Rev. Respir. Dis.*, **111**, 921.

159. Bone, R.C. (1976) Pulmonary barotrauma complicating mechanical ventilation. *Am. Rev. Respir. Dis.*, **113**, 188.

160. Schaefer, K.S., McNulty, W.P. Jr., Carey, C. and Liebow, A.A. (1958) Mechanisms in development of interstitial emphysema and air embolism on decompression from depth. *J. Appl. Physiol.*, **13**, 15–29.

161. Hickling, K.G., Henderson, S.J. and Jackson, R. (1990) Low mortality associated with low volume pressure limited ventilation with permissive hypercapnia in severe adult respiratory distress syndrome. *Intensive Care Med.*, **16**, 372–7.

162. Shih, H-T., Webb, C.R., Conway, W.A. *et al.* (1988) Frequency and significance of cardiac arrhythmias in chronic obstructive pulmonary disease. *Chest*, **94**, 44–8.

163. Holford, F.D. and Mithoefer, J.C. (1973) Cardiac arrhythmias in hospitalized patients with chronic obstructive pulmonary disease. *Am. Rev. Respir. Dis.*, **108**, 879–85.

164. Hudson, L.D., Kurt, T.L., Petty, T.L. and Genton, E. (1973) Arrhythmias associated with acute respiratory failure in patients with chronic airway obstruction. *Chest*, **63**, 661–5.

165. Khokhar, N. (1981) Cardiac arrhythmias associated with acute respiratory failure in chronic obstructive pulmonary disease. *Milit. Med.*, **146**, 856–8.

166. Brashear, R.E. (1984) Arrhythmias in patients with chronic obstructive pulmonary disease. *Med. Clin. North Am.*, **68**, 969–81.

167. Levine, J.H., Michael, J.R. and Guarnieri, T. (1985) Multifocal atrial tachycardia: a toxic effect of theophylline. *Lancet*, **i**, 12–4.

168. Salerno, D.M., Anderson, B., Sharkey, P.J. and Iber, C. (1987) Intravenous verapamil for treatment of multifocal atrial tachycardia with and without calcium pretreatment. *Ann. Intern. Med.*, **107**, 623–8.

169. Levine, J.H., Michael, J.R. and Guarnieri, T. (1985). Treatment of multifocal atrial tachycardia with verapamil. *N. Engl. J. Med.*, **312**, 21–5.

170. Pratt, C.M. (1988) Asymptomatic ventricular arrhythmias in patients with obstructive lung disease. Should they be treated? *Chest*, **94**, 2–4.

171. Harris (Pingleton), S.K., Bone, R.C. and Ruth, W.E. (1977) Gastrointestinal hemorrhage in patients in a respiratory intensive care unit. *Chest*, **72**, 301–4.

172. Pingleton, S.K. and Hadzima, S.K. (1983) Enteral alimentation and gastrointestinal bleeding in mechanically ventilated patients. *Crit. Care Med.*, **11**, 13–16.

173. Hastings, P.R., Skillman, J.J., Bushness, L.S. and Silen, W. (1978) Antacid titration in the prevention of acute gastrointestinal bleeding. *N. Engl. J. Med.*, **298**, 1041–5.

174. Khan, F., Parekh, A., Patel, S. *et al.* (1981) Results of gastric neutralization with hourly antacids and cimetidine in 320 intubated patients with respiratory failure. *Chest*, **79**, 409–12.

175. Shuman, R.B., Schuster, D.P. and Zuckerman, G.R. (1987) Prophylactic therapy for stress ulcer bleeding: a reappraisal. *Ann. Intern. Med.*, **106**, 562–7.

176. DuMoulin, G.C., Paterson, D.G., Hedley-White, J. *et al.* (1982) Aspiration of gastric bacteria in antacid-treated patients: a frequent cause of postoperative colonization of the airways. *Lancet*, **1**, 242–5.

177. Craven, D.E., Kunches, L.M., Kilinsky, V. *et al.* (1986) Risk factors for pneumonia and fatality in patients receiving continuous mechanical ventilation. *Am. Rev. Respir. Dis.*, **133**, 792–6.

178. Tryba, M. (1991) Sulcrafate versus antacids or H_2 antagonists for stress ulcer prophylaxis: a meta-analysis on efficacy and pneumonia rate. *Crit. Care Med.*, **19**, 942–9.

179. Driks, M.R., Craven, D.E., Celli, B.R. *et al.* (1987) Nosocomial pneumonia in intubated patients given sulcrafate as compared with antacids or histamine type 2 blockers. *N. Engl. J. Med.*, **317**, 376–82.

180. Wilcox, C.M. and Spenney, J.G. (1988) Stress ulcer prophylaxis in medical patients: who, what, and how much? *Am. J. Gastroenterol.*, **83**, 1199–211.

181. Baum, G.L. and Fisher, F.D. (1960) The relationship of fatal pulmonary insufficiency with cor pulmonale, right sided mural thrombi and pulmonary emboli. A preliminary report. *Am. J. Med. Sci.*, **240**, 609–12.

182. Mitchell, R.S., Silvers, G.W., Dart, G.A. *et al.* (1968) Clinical and morphologic correlations in chronic airway obstruction. *Am. Rev. Respir. Dis.*, **97**, 54–62.

183. Prescott, S.M., Richards, K.L., Tikoff, G. *et al.* (1981) Venous thromboembolism in decompensated chronic obstructive pulmonary disease. A prospective study. *Am. Rev. Respir. Dis.*, **123**, 32–6.

184. Winter, J.H., Buckler, P.W., Bautista, A.P. *et al.* (1983) Frequency of venous thrombosis in patients with an exacerbation of chronic obstructive lung disease. *Thorax*, **38**, 605–8.

185. Moser, K.M., LeMoine, J.R., Nachtwey, F.J. and Spragg, R.G. (1981) Deep venous thrombosis and pulmonary embolism, frequency in a respiratory intensive care unit. *JAMA*, **246**, 1422–4.

186. Neuhaus, A., Bentz, R.R and Weg, J.G. (1978) Pulmonary embolism in respiratory failure. *Chest*, **73**, 460–5.

187. Alderson, P.O., Biello, D.R., Sachariah, G. and Siegel, B.A. (1981) Scintigraphic detection of pulmonary embolism in patients with obstructive pulmonary disease. *Radiology*, **138**, 661–6.

188. Hull, R.D., Hirsh, J., Carter, C.J. *et al.* (1985) Diagnostic efficacy of impedance plethysmography for clinically suspected deep-vein thrombosis: a randomized trial. *Ann. Intern. Med.*, **102**, 21–8.

189. Lensing, A.W.A., Prandoni, P., Brandjes, D. *et al.* (1989) Detection of deep vein thrombosis by real-time B-mode ultrasonography. *N. Engl. J. Med.*, **320**, 342–5.

190. Hull, R.D., Hirsh, J., Carter, C.J. *et al.* (1983) Pulmonary angiography, ventilation lung scanning, and venography for clinically suspected pulmonary embolism with abnormal perfusion lung scan. *Ann. Intern. Med.*, **98**, 891–9.

191. Harris (Pingleton), S.K., Pingleton, W.W. and Ruth, W.E. (1981) Prevention of pulmonary emboli in a respiratory intensive care unit. *Chest*, **79**, 647–50.

192. Toews, G.B. (1987) Nosocomial pneumonia. *Clin. Chest Med.*, **8**, 467–79.

193. Johanson, W.G., Pierce, A.K. and Sanford, J.P. (1969) Changing pharyngeal bacterial flora of hospitalized patients: emergence of gram negative bacilli. *N. Engl. J. Med.*, **281**, 1137–40.

194. Johanson, W.G., Pierce, A.K., Sanford, J.P. and Thomas, G.D. (1972) Nosocomial respiratory infections with gram-negative bacilla: the significance of colonization of the respiratory tract. *Ann. Intern. Med.*, **77**, 701–6.

195. Johanson, W.G., Higuchi, J.H., Chaudhuri, T.R. and Woods, D.R. (1980) Bacterial adherence to epithelial cells in bacillary colonization of the respiratory tract. *Am. Rev. Respir. Dis.*, **121**, 55–63.

196. Fagon, J.Y., Chastre, J., Hance, A.J. *et al.* (1988) Detection of nosocomial lung infection in ventilated patients. Use of a protected specimen brush and quantitative culture techniques in 147 patients. *Am. Rev. Respir. Dis.*, **138**, 110–6.

197. Torres, A., De La Bellacasa, J.P., Xaubet, A. *et al.* (1989) Diagnostic value of quantitative cultures of bronchoalveolar lavage and telescoping plugged catheters in mechanically ventilated patients with bacterial pneumonia. *Am. Rev. Respir. Dis.*, **140**, 306–10.

198. Villers, D., Derrienic, M., Raffi, F. *et al.* (1985) Reliability of the bronchoscopic protected

catheter brush in intubated and ventilated patients. *Chest*, **88**, 527–30.

199. Johanson, W.G. Jr, Seidenfeld, J.J., Gomez, P. *et al.* (1988) Bacteriologic diagnosis of nosocomial pneumonia following prolonged mechanical ventilation. *Am. Rev. Respir. Dis.*, **137**, 259–64.

200. Fagon, JY., Chastre, J., Domart, Y. *et al.* (1989) Nosocomial pneumonia in patients receiving continuous mechanical ventilation. Prospective analysis of 52 episodes with use of a protected specimen brush and quantitative culture techniques. *Am. Rev. Respir. Dis.*, **139**, 877–84.

201. Meduri, G.U. (1990) Ventilator-associated pneumonia in patients with respiratory failure. A diagnostic approach. *Chest*, **97**, 1208–19.

ADDENDUM: NON-INVASIVE POSITIVE PRESSURE VENTILATION

Recently, investigators have begun to examine the role of face or nasal mask positive pressure ventilation in patients with acute respiratory failure, including patients with COPD and acute respiratory failure. Brochard and colleagues have shown that face mask positive pressure ventilation can be successfully applied to patients with exacerbations of COPD and acute respiratory failure [1]. These investigators have also presented preliminary data suggesting that mask ventilation may decrease the need for subsequent intubation in patients with exacerbations of COPD and acute respiratory failure [2]. In this latter study, patients treated with mask ventilation had a shorter hospital stay and a lower mortality than the control group who received standard therapy. A British study examining the effects of mask ventilation in patients with COPD and acute respiratory failure has also recently been published (see Chapter 10, p. 230). Clearly, considerably more study of this modality needs to be performed before the role, if any, of mask ventilation in patients with COPD and acute respiratory failure is defined.

REFERENCES

1. Brochard, L., Isabey, D., Piquet, J. *et al.* (1990) reversal of acute exacerbations of chronic obstructive lung disease by inspiratory assistance with a face mask. *N. Engl. J. Med.*, **323**, 1523–30.

2. Brochard, L., Wysocki, M., Lofaso, F. *et al.* (1993) Face mask inspiratory positive airway pressure (IPAP) for acute exacerbations of chronic respiratory insufficiency. A randomized multicenter study. *Am. Rev. Respir. Dis.*, **147**, A984.

DOMICILIARY OXYGEN THERAPY

C.B. Cooper

Something essential to life passes from the breath and once this substance is extracted air is no longer fit to breathe.

John Mayow, 1674

20.1 INTRODUCTION

One of the fundamental problems in chronic obstructive pulmonary disease is the maintenance of adequate oxygenation. Hence it is no surprise that supplementary oxygen therapy in its various forms is an important component in the treatment and rehabilitation of patients with COPD. The effects of supplementary oxygen on gas exchange within the lung are considered elsewhere (Chapter 8) as is its role in the acutely ill COPD patient (Chapter 19). This chapter will consider the physiologic effects and benefits of oxygen treatment on chronic stable COPD patients as well as some of the practical issues involved in the delivery of this important treatment.

Oxygen was discovered in the 1770s, jointly by Joseph Priestley, an English cleric, and Karl Wilhelm Scheel, a pharmacist from Sweden. John Mayow, quoted above, was one of the first scientists to appreciate its physiologic importance. Oxygen was proposed as a treatment soon after its discovery. Beddoes and Watt, in 1778, first systematically described the clinical administration and medical applications of oxygen from their experiences at the Pneumatic Institute in Clifton, Bristol. Around 1800, the therapeutic use of oxygen was virtually abandoned due to lack of proof of effectiveness in various diseases. Oxygen enjoyed a brief resurgence during the cholera epidemic of 1832 and then in the 1840s was reintroduced with the development of anesthesia.

Not until the 20th century did investigators begin a systematic study of oxygen therapy in patients with chronic pulmonary disease. In 1956, Cotes and Gilson [1] documented an increase in exercise capacity in patients with chronic lung disease using portable compressed oxygen gas cylinders. About the same time, Barach [2] reported the use of small refillable oxygen bottles for the relief of dyspnea in patients with emphysema. Campbell [3], in 1960, appreciating the fact that oxygen administration led to hypercapnia, introduced the concept of controlled oxygen therapy. The modern era of oxygen therapy gained momentum during the 1960s in Denver, Colorado, where investigation began to elucidate the beneficial effects of long-term oxygen therapy (LTOT) in patients with chronic hypoxemia.

20.2 PHYSIOLOGIC CHANGES WITH ACUTE OXYGEN THERAPY

Oxygen therapy is prescribed to correct hypoxemia and preserve vital organ function. Much of our information about the physiologic

Chronic Obstructive Pulmonary Disease. Edited by Dr P. Calverley and Professor N. Pride. Published in 1995 by Chapman & Hall, London. ISBN 0 412 46450 0

mechanisms of chronic oxygen therapy has come from the study of patients with COPD. Supplementary oxygen treatment improves oxygenation by increasing the inspired oxygen concentration (FIO_2) but the increase in arterial oxygen tension (PaO_2) which results is highly dependent on the ventilation–perfusion relationships within the lung (Chapter 8). The rise in PaO_2 is maximum when the shunt-like effect of venous admixture is least and the response becomes negligible when the effective shunt constitutes 50% or more of the cardiac output. Certain mechanisms can reduce the expected rise in PaO_2 with oxygen therapy. These include a fall in minute ventilation due to diminished respiratory drive, reversal of hypoxic pulmonary vasoconstriction which may worsen ventilation–perfusion relationships and finally absorption atelectasis. Tissue oxygen delivery (DO_2) which is the final arbiter of effective oxygen therapy, is influenced not only by PaO_2 through its effect on arterial oxygen content (CaO_2) but also by circulatory factors. Other extra pulmonary factors such as pH, arterial CaO_2 tension, ($PaCO_2$), erythrocyte levels of 2,3-diphosphoglycerate and carboxy-hemoglobin can modify CaO_2 and hence DO_2. The principal physiologic changes which result from acute oxygen treatment are both ventilatory and circulatory.

20.2.1 VENTILATORY EFFECTS

Most studies of oxygen therapy in stable advanced disease have failed to demonstrate any significant changes in resting minute ventilation [4–8]. Three studies have shown that oxygen therapy increases the dead space to tidal volume ratio (VD/VT) [8–10], by about 5% which may be due to vasodilatation in poorly ventilated areas [9]. The increase in VD/VT correlates with the fall in pulmonary artery pressure and is consistent with this explanation [10]. In addition, oxygen therapy reduces airways resistance [11] and $P_{O.1}$ and VT/Ti fall probably due to reduce respiratory drive [7,12] (Chapter 13).

The effects of oxygen therapy on minute ventilation ($\dot{V}E$) are most evident during exercise. Oxygen reduces exercise ventilation for an equivalent work rate in normal subjects [13,14] and patients with COPD [4,5,15,16]. Cotes *et al.* [5] showed that 66% oxygen reduced $\dot{V}E$ during exercise by 26% whereas Pierce *et al.* [15] showed that 40% oxygen reduced $\dot{V}E$ by 25%. The fall in $\dot{V}E$ with oxygen therapy is accompanied by a reduction in respiratory rate (fR) in both normal subjects [14] and COPD patients [7,15,16]. This reduction in $\dot{V}E$ together with the development of hypercapnia has been thought to indicate a diminished respiratory drive [15]. However, Scano *et al.* [7] found that oxygen reduces the impedance of the respiratory system during exercise resulting in lower levels of $\dot{V}E$ and mean inspiratory flow rate (VT/Ti) for a given level of respiratory drive as determined by occlusion pressure. There have been many attempts to correlate improvement in exercise tolerance with oxygen therapy with reduced mechanical demands on the respiratory muscles [7,17,18] (Chapter 9). Bye *et al.* [14] showed that 40% oxygen reduced minute ventilation and lessened EMG signs of diaphragm fatigue during exercise in normal subjects. These investigators also demonstrated similar effects in eight patients with COPD. Criner and Celli [19] showed reduced transdiaphragmatic pressures (Pdi) in COPD patients breathing 30% oxygen. At peak exercise, the contribution of abdominal pressure to Pdi was greater breathing oxygen, implying a greater contribution of the diaphragm as opposed to accessory inspiratory muscle contraction. The effects of oxygen therapy on respiratory sensation (i.e. dyspnea) are described in Section 20.4.

20.2.2 CIRCULATORY EFFECTS

Oxygen reduces resting heart rate (fc) in both normal subjects and patients with COPD [5,15] whilst fc rises when supplementary oxygen is withdrawn without any change in cardiac index [20]. Oxygen therapy can reduce cardiac output (Qc) [5,8] although no changes in left ventricular ejection fraction have been demonstrated [8]. However, the most striking circulatory effects of oxygen are on pulmonary hemodynamics. Acute oxygen administration lowers pulmonary artery pressure (Ppa) [8,21] presumably by eliminating hypoxic pulmonary vasoconstriction [22]. Conversely Ppa and pulmonary vascular resistance rise when oxygen is stopped [20].

Other circulatory effects have been identified with oxygen therapy besides alterations in pulmonary hemodynamics. Hypoxemia slows the kinetics of oxygen uptake with the onset of constant load exercise [23] and it is likely that supplemental oxygen therapy will speed oxygen uptake kinetics. Some investigators believe that chronic hypoxemia causes increased renal vascular resistance and that oxygen therapy improves renal blood flow with consequent diuresis and amelioration of fluid retention [24] but one group found that oxygen reduced renal blood flow [25].

An adequate D_{O_2} is the final arbiter of effective oxygen therapy. Normally the availability of oxygen to the lung does not influence D_{O_2}; however, a pathologic oxygen supply dependency has been described in COPD patients [26]. Kawakami *et al.* [27] studied 50 patients with COPD and showed that acute administration of oxygen increased mixed venous oxygen tension ($P\bar{v}_{O_2}$) suggesting improved oxygen delivery despite a measured reduction in cardiac index (CI). Other investigators have failed to show an increase in tissue oxygen delivery with supplementary oxygen therapy, apparently due to a concomitant fall in Q_C [28,29].

20.3 PHYSIOLOGIC CHANGES WITH CHRONIC OXYGEN THERAPY

20.3.1 EFFECTS ON PULMONARY HEMODYNAMICS

Several studies in small groups of patients conducted during the 1960s suggested that prolonged oxygen treatment could correct pulmonary hypertension induced by chronic hypoxemia as well as reduce red cell mass and increase exercise tolerance [21,30]. The practicality of ambulatory treatment was demonstrated [31] and using this method Neff and Petty reported that survival was prolonged by oxygen therapy [32]. Meanwhile, in the UK, Stark *et al.* [33,34] had begun to investigate the daily requirement of oxygen needed to reverse pulmonary hypertension. These studies led to the design of two large multicenter trials, one in the United States and one in the United Kingdom. The Nocturnal Oxygen Therapy Trial (NOTT) [35] compared two groups of patients. One group supposedly received continuous oxygen therapy (COT), although in practice, due to incomplete compliance, this averaged 17.7 hours of oxygen per day whilst the other patients were only treated with overnight oxygen therapy (12 hours per day). The Medical Research Council (MRC) study [36] compared patients receiving 15 hours of oxygen per day with a control group receiving no oxygen therapy. The patients participating in these studies had modest pulmonary hypertension at entry and had similar degrees of airflow obstruction and hypoxemia but those in the British study tended to be more hypercapnic (Table 20.1). The combined results demonstrated improved survival in patients receiving oxygen therapy. The MRC control group had an annual percentage mortality risk of 30% giving a predicted 5-year survival of only 18% which concurs with other reports of the poor prognosis in hypoxemic COPD untreated by oxygen. Fig. 20.1 shows the combined results of these trials and suggests that long-term oxygen therapy is effective in prolonging survival if given for as long as possible during each 24-hour period. In the NOTT, pulmonary hemodynamics were compared before and after 6 months of oxygen therapy [37]. Reductions in Ppa were seen during exercise in both groups and also at rest in the group receiving continuous oxygen therapy.

Table 20.1   Comparisons between the NOT trial (1980) and MRC study (1981)

	MRC Study		*NOT Trial*	
Daily duration of LTOT	0	15	12	24[a]
No. of subjects	45	42	102	101
Age (years)	57	59	66	65
FEV_1 (l)	0.7	0.7	(0.7)[b]	(0.7)[b]
FVC (l)	1.8	1.8	(1.9)[b]	(1.9)[b]
Pao_2 (kPa)	6.9	6.7	6.9	6.8
(mmHg)	52	50	52	51
$Paco_2$ (kPa)	7.2	7.3	5.9	5.7
(mmHg)	54	55	44	43
Ppa (mmHg)	34	34	29	30
PCV (%)	53	51	47	48
Annual risk (%)	29.4[c]	11.9[c]	20.6	11.9

[a] Actually about 18 hours.
[b] Derived from reported percentages of predicted values.
[c] Annual % risk as reported for men in the MRC groups.

Similar changes in pulmonary vascular resistance were observed and the same study showed that survival after 8 years was related to the decrease in mean Ppa during the first six months of treatment. Meanwhile, another report [38] showed that improved survival in

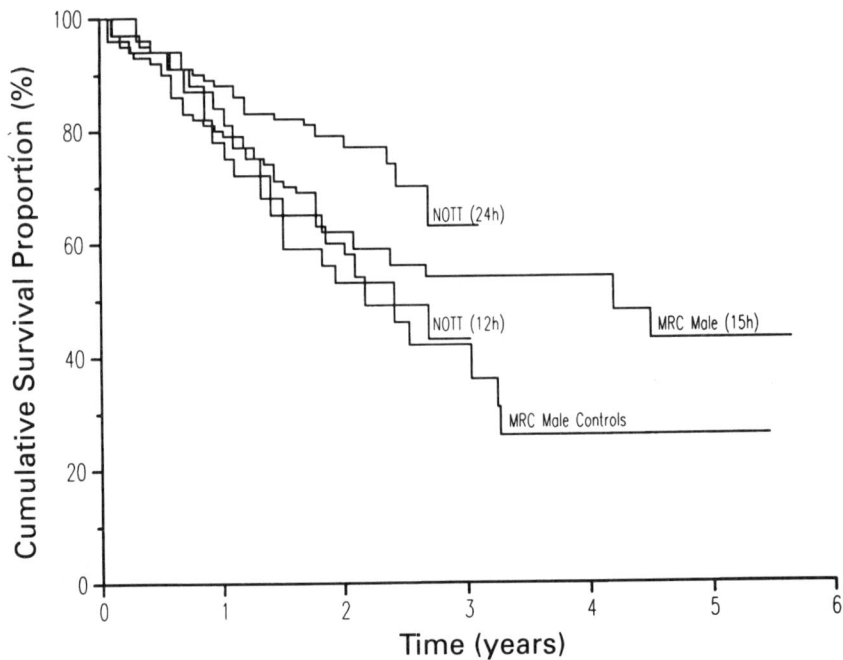

Fig. 20.1   Combined data from the Nocturnal Oxygen Therapy Trial (NOTT) [35] and the Medical Research Council (MRC) study [36]. Note that the NOTT (24 h) group also had the capability for ambulatory oxygen therapy but actually used their oxygen for only 17.7 h/day.

patients receiving LTOT was seen when Ppa fell by 5 mmHg or more.

These studies have led to the view that improved survival with oxygen results primarily from the reversal of the pulmonary hemodynamic disturbances. In the NOTT, pulmonary arterial pressures were lower after 6 months of LTOT whilst in the MRC study patients generally had higher pulmonary artery pressures at entry and these were unchanged by LTOT. Here failure of progression of pulmonary hypertension was taken to be a satisfactory therapeutic response. Weitzenblum and colleagues [39] studied pulmonary hemodynamics in 16 COPD patients with and without LTOT. An annual increase in Ppa of about 2 mmHg was observed during 47 months before LTOT began whereas during 31 months of LTOT there was a significant annual reduction in Ppa of just over 2 mmHg. The clinical significance of these small changes has yet to be determined. Fletcher and Levin demonstrated that overnight oxygen therapy can abolish nocturnal oxygen desaturation and reduce pulmonary hypertension [40]. Three studies have linked the pulmonary hemodynamic response to oxygen with prognosis in COPD patients. Ashutosh *et al.* [38] showed that a fall in Ppa of greater than 5 mmHg was associated with a better prognosis. Keller *et al.* [41] showed a significantly higher 2-year mortality in COPD patients who did not show favorable pulmonary hemodynamic changes in response to raised FIO_2. Ashutosh and Dunsky [42] studied 43 COPD patients and found that those with a fall of Ppa greater than 10 mmHg after 24 hours of 28% oxygen had better 3-year survival. However, Sliwinski *et al.* have reported that survival in a group of 46 COPD patients was not related to the effect of acute oxygen administration on Ppa [43].

Alternative explanations for improved survival should be considered because all of the reported alterations in pulmonary hemodynamics with LTOT are modest. Furthermore,

Wilkinson *et al.* [44] showed evidence of continuing pulmonary vascular disruption in a small group of patients who died of cor pulmonale despite having LTOT. Earlier studies established that mortality in COPD is related to the severity of airflow obstruction. Cooper *et al.* [45] demonstrated that FEV_1 remained the strongest predictor of survival even in patients receiving LTOT. Another study [46] by the same investigators, showed relentless deterioration in airflow obstruction despite LTOT (Fig. 20.2). Improved survival in COPD may not simply be attributable to an alteration in pulmonary hemodynamics. This may merely be an epiphenomenon and improved survival may be related to alternative physiologic changes. Closer examination of the results of the multicenter trials (Fig. 20.1) shows a distinct survival advantage in the patients receiving LTOT for about 18 hours (COT group) compared with both other treatment groups. The COT group was unique in that these patients were provided with apparatus for ambulatory oxygen therapy. Thus it is possible that they derived additional benefit from their continuing ability to exercise.

20.3.2 HEMATOLOGICAL EFFECTS

A range of hematological changes can be corrected by domiciliary oxygen therapy. Polycythemia is a physiologic adaptation to chronic hypoxemia mediated by increased erythropoietin release in response to insufficient tissue oxygen delivery. Supplementary oxygen therapy reduces both the hematocrit and the red cell mass [35,36,47] as well as erythrocyte 2,3-diphosphoglycerate levels [47]. Chronic tobacco smokers, who have increased levels of carboxyhemoglobin, are susceptible to polycythemia and less responsive to its correction by oxygen therapy [48]. One study has shown improved platelet survival time with oxygen therapy in COPD [49] although the clinical significance of this change remains unclear. The hematological

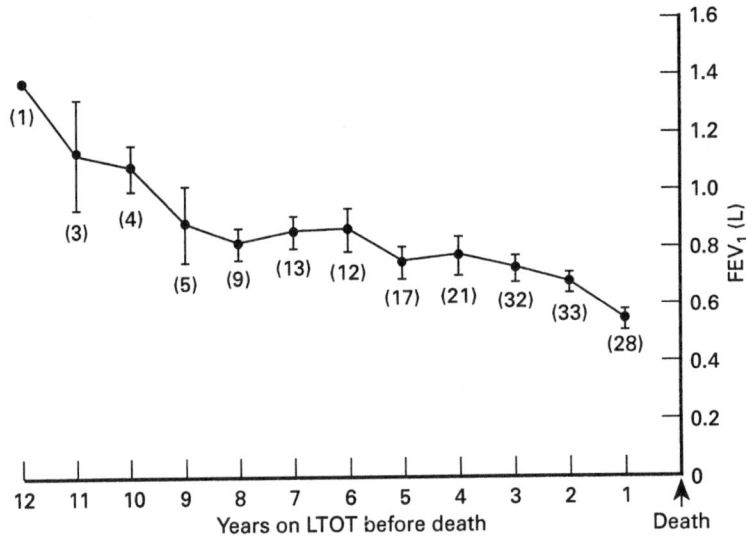

Fig. 20.2   Mean values (± SEM of FEV₁) from year to year for 37 patients having LTOT. The data are time-aligned to the point of death. The number of subjects assessed for each year prior to death is shown in parentheses.

effects of supplementary oxygen therapy might influence arterial oxygen content but the overall effect on tissue oxygen delivery will also be influenced by cardiac output, oxyhemoglobin saturation and blood viscosity.

20.3.3 NEUROPSYCHIATRIC FUNCTION

Neuropsychologic testing and life quality assessments performed in association with the NOTT showed that patients with hypoxemic COPD have disturbances of mood, personality and life quality [50]. Two short-term studies in the early 1970s demonstrated improvements in neuropsychiatric function with oxygen therapy compared with room air breathing [47,51]. One hundred and fifty COPD patients who participated in the NOTT were assessed after 6 months of LTOT and 42% showed evidence of improved cognitive function, although they reported little change in emotional status and quality of life [52]. The benefits were evident in both study groups after 6 months of therapy but only

maintained in the COT group after 12 months. These studies suggest that supplementary oxygen therapy produces selective neuropsychologic benefits in patients with chronic hypoxemia but further investigation is required to determine the impact of these changes on quality of life.

20.4 CLINICAL BENEFITS OF OXYGEN THERAPY

The clinical improvements produced by domiciliary oxygen treatment apart from prolongation of survival, are an increase in exercise capacity and a reduction in symptoms, particularly breathlessness.

20.4.1 EFFECTS ON EXERCISE CAPABILITY

Many studies have examined the effects of supplementary oxygen on exercise capability. The ability of oxygen to reduce ventilatory requirement at a given submaximal work rate has already been described. Several investigators have linked this effect to an improvement in exercise endurance in COPD patients [17,18,53–58]. The study by Raimondi *et al.* [53] showed a 30–40% increase in endurance time for constant load exercise at 70% of maximum. In the study by Bradley *et al.* [54], submaximal endurance time increased 50% at the same work rate. These investigators found a slight increase in $PaCO_2$ breathing oxygen but pH remained unchanged. Stein *et al.* [18] showed a 30% increase in treadmill endurance time breathing 30% oxygen. Similar related studies have reported an increase in walking distance [1,47,58–60]. The study by Block, Castle and Keitt [47] reported improvements in activities of daily living as well as increased treadmill distance. Several studies have reported improved maximum work rate or maximum oxygen uptake breathing oxygen in addition to improved submaximal exercise performance [15,17,18, 58]. Most studies of oxygen therapy and exercise capability have used 30–40% FIO_2. The study by Cotes and Gilson [1] was interesting in showing that 30% oxygen was almost as effective as 50% or 100% in doubling the treadmill distance. On balance, most studies of oxygen therapy during exercise have shown improvements in hypoxemic patients. However, this finding has not been universal. Longo, Moser and Luchsinga [61] showed no response in 27 COPD patients with mild hypoxemia (mean PaO_2 64 mmHg). The carefully controlled study of Lilker *et al.* [59] examined patients who had previously participated in a 12-month rehabilitation program. The improvements in walking distance were less impressive and there were no changes in dyspnea scores or maximum ventilation. Leggett and Flenley [60] reported an increased 12-minute walking distance breathing 30% oxygen but when the patients carried their oxygen apparatus, this beneficial effect was negated, possibly due to the extra weight of the oxygen bottle.

Thus the selection of patients most likely to benefit from oxygen during exercise is crucial. Davidson *et al.* [57] reported that the benefit of oxygen therapy in increasing walking distances was not related to spirometric measures or initial exercise capacity but was inversely correlated with diffusing coefficient as a percentage of the predicted value. Also these investigators noted an inverse relationship with $PaCO_2$ implying that 'pink puffers' were more likely to benefit from supplementary oxygen therapy. Although it seems intuitively likely that patients with arterial oxygen desaturation on exercise will benefit from supplementary oxygen, several studies have failed to confirm this effect [54,55,60,92]. Only one study [62] involving patients with interstitial lung disease showed definite correlation between the increase in exercise endurance time breathing oxygen and the fall in arterial oxygen saturation (SaO_2) when exercising breathing room air. Leach *et al.* [63] reported a similar correlation in patients with COPD, although the predictive value of desaturation was poor.

Earlier studies of oxygen therapy and exercise capability advocated the use of portable and domiciliary oxygen as adjunct therapy in the rehabilitation of patients with COPD [1,2,59]. Barach [2] showed that lightweight oxygen cylinders carried by patients improved exercise tolerance and reduced dyspnea. Pierce, Paez and Miller [15] specifically studied the combination of exercise training and supplementary oxygen therapy and found that exercise training imposed less physiologic stress when the patients were breathing supplementary oxygen. Woolf and Suero [64] successfully used 60% oxygen to incorporate patients in a program of rehabilitation when they had been unable to commence the program breathing room air.

20.4.2 EFFECTS ON DYSPNEA

The physiologic effects of oxygen on self-reported breathlessness have been reviewed elsewhere (Chapter 10). Early studies of oxygen treatment during exercise in COPD suggested that it reduced breathlessness [2].

In a study of 10 'pink puffers' oxygen reduced dyspnea scores during submaximal treadmill exercise and increased walking distance by 12% regardless of whether the oxygen supply was carried by an assistant or the patient [55]. Swinburn *et al.* [56] studied 5 patients with a fall in SaO_2 during exercise. Supplementary oxygen reduced submaximal levels of ventilation and breathlessness although the relationship between minute ventilation and breathlessness was unchanged. One controlled study [65] involving 20 COPD patients showed improved exercise capacity and reduced dyspnea breathing oxygen at 2 and 4 l/min compared with compressed air. These investigators also purported to show a placebo effect on walking distance and dyspnea from breathing compressed air at 3 l/min compared with room air breathing. Davidson *et al.* [57] in an elegant study of 17 COPD patients showed that higher flows of oxygen were associated with greater reductions in breathlessness during the early stages of a treadmill endurance test. One controlled study [59] did not demonstrate convincing changes in dyspnea breathing oxygen from a liquid oxygen supply compared with liquid air but these patients had already participated in a 12-month rehabilitation program. The same study also showed a placebo effect from breathing compressed air.

There is sufficient evidence from clinical trials that supplementary oxygen therapy improves exercise capability, primarily by reducing ventilatory requirement for submaximal endurance exercise at given work rates. An improvement in maximal exercise work rate or oxygen uptake does not necessarily occur. Whether there is an effect on dyspnea intensity independent of the change in ventilation is less clear. Whenever oxygen is prescribed to reduce dyspnea, it is sensible to first demonstrate some benefit using objective physiologic or psychometric measurements. Supplementary oxygen therapy might be expected to produce other symptomatic improvements including a greater willingness to exercise, improved motivation and alleviation of depression through its neuropsychologic effects, although the time course of these changes is not completely established. Improved exercise capability and enhanced activities of daily living are clearly important components of quality of life. Without adequate improvements in quality of life, the survival advantages of supplementary oxygen therapy are of questionable value.

20.5 PRACTICAL ISSUES WITH DOMICILIARY OXYGEN THERAPY

20.5.1 SELECTION OF PATIENTS

Essentially, there are three methods of providing domiciliary oxygen therapy; (a) long-term, low-dose oxygen therapy for patients with chronic respiratory failure, (b) portable oxygen therapy for exercise-related hypoxemia and breathlessness, and (c) short-burst oxygen therapy for palliation and temporary relief of symptoms.

Whatever the indication, oxygen treatment requires accurate diagnosis, if only for prognostic purposes. Other treatment must already be optimized before oxygen is introduced. This should not be done without measuring blood gas tensions breathing room air.

20.5.2 CRITERIA FOR THE PRESCRIPTION OF LTOT

Many countries in Europe, North America and Australasia have developed prescribing criteria for LTOT. These guidelines are based on the data from the NOTT and MRC study demonstrating improved survival, at least in patients with COPD taking long-term oxygen therapy. Many investigators believe that the conclusions from these data should apply to patients with other forms of chronic hypoxemic lung disease, especially those who have developed cor pulmonale. Current guidelines are shown in Table 20.2.

Table 20.2   Prescribing criteria for LTOT

United Kingdom: DHSS Drug Tariff: 1985
1.   Absolute Indications: COPD, hypoxemia, edema
         FEV_1 <1.5 l; FVC <2.0 l
         PaO_2 <55 mmHg; $PaCO_2$ >45 mmHg
         Stability demonstrated over 3 weeks
2.   As above but without edema or $PaCO_2$ >45 mmHg
3.   Palliative
Europe: Report of a SEP Task Group: 1989 [68]
1. PaO_2 <55 mmHg. 'Steady-state COPD'
2. PaO_2 55–65 mmHg with additional features as in the United States (Group 2)
3.   Restrictive disease with PaO_2 <55 mmHg
United States of America: (CMN Form HCFA-484)
1. PaO_2 ≤ 55 mmHg (room air)
         SaO_2 ≤ 88%
2. PaO_2 ≤ 59 mmHg with evidence of at least one of the following:
                  P pulmonale (>3mm in leads II, III, or aVF)
                  (pulmonary hypertension? RV hypertrophy?)
                  Dependent edema (cor pulmonale?)
                  Erythrocytosis (Hct >56%)
         CMN – Certificate of Medical Necessity
         For Group 1 – Annual update of CMN required
         For Group 2 – Revised CMN required after 3 months
Australia: Thoracic Society of Australia 1985 [71]
1. PaO_2 <56 mmHg. COPD, RVH, polycythemia, edema
2.   Desaturation <90% on exercise
3.   Refractory dyspnea associated with cardiac failure

In the United Kingdom, provisions for a new domiciliary oxygen service were originally described in the DHSS Drug Tariff in 1986 [67]. The absolute indications (Group 1) refer to patients with stable chronic obstructive pulmonary disease. This is the only patient group that has been clearly shown to have improved survival with LTOT. The British prescribing criteria recognize that an oxygen concentrator is more economic than other forms of oxygen supply and, therefore, the regulations are geared to this apparent economic benefit. These arrangements overlook the role of ambulatory oxygen therapy and the hidden economic advantages which it might hold.

In other European countries, criteria for the prescribing LTOT are influenced by political and economic factors, in particular, the method of reimbursement. Nevertheless, the general prescribing criteria for Europe are similar to those adopted in the United Kingdom and the USA [68]. These recommendations include provision for patients with restrictive pulmonary disease and PaO_2 less than 55 mmHg. Data from Sweden have shown that 67% of patients receiving LTOT have COPD [69] and the proportion is probably similar in other European countries.

Although methods of reimbursement are entirely different in the United States, the mechanisms for prescription of LTOT are just as rigorous as in Great Britain. The prescribing criteria are similar and also shown in Table 20.2. Oxygen can be prescribed based on pulse oximetry, although this is not recognized as being as reliable as direct measurement of arterial blood gas tensions. The American criteria also allow for the prescription of LTOT if the PaO_2 lies between 55 and 59 mmHg provided there are coexisting signs of end-organ dysfunction from chronic hypoxemia. Evidence of hypoxic end-organ dysfunction includes right ventricular hypertrophy, peripheral edema and erythrocytosis. Certainly it seems unusual to wait until hypoxemia is of such severity that it has caused end-organ damage before LTOT is prescribed. LTOT is prescribed in the United States using a Certificate of Medical Necessity (CMN) which is completed by the prescribing physician. For Category I patients, the CMN needs to be revised every 12 months; for Category II patients, i.e. those with a PaO_2 between 55 and 59 mmHg, the CMN must be revised after 3 months. A recent consensus conference in Washington, DC [70] addressed certain difficulties with the existing prescribing criteria in the United States. First, reimbursement is geared to oxygen flow and so the use of oxygen-conserving devices which reduce oxygen flow requirements is not encouraged by the existing reimbursement policy. Second, there is inadequate provision for LTOT prescription to unstable patients pending further evaluation. Finally, the CMN is thought to be too complex.

About the time that guidelines were being developed for the prescriptions of LTOT, Williams and Nicholl [72] conducted a community survey in the Sheffield area to assess the prevalence of chronic hypoxemia due to obstructive pulmonary disease. These investigators randomly sampled patients from general practices around the conurbation. Most patients had home spirometry and transcutaneous or direct arterial blood gas analysis. They found that 0.3% of patients sampled had hypoxemia with a PaO_2 less than 55 mmHg. Since this level of hypoxemia has been widely used as a prescribing criteria for LTOT, then it would appear that about 60 000

people in England and Wales would be eligible for this form of treatment, whilst 750 000 patients would be suitable in the USA. These estimates do not presuppose any age limits for the provision of LTOT. Actual numbers of LTOT prescriptions in these two countries are 50 000 and 800 000, although in the United Kingdom many of these patients will not strictly be taking long-term oxygen therapy. If these estimates are accurate and if the selection criteria on which they are based are accepted as appropriate, then these figures would suggest that LTOT is under-prescribed in the United Kingdom.

20.5.3 STABILITY OF CHRONIC HYPOXEMIA

During the recruitment phase of patients in the NOTT, 175 out of 409 patients initially screened (i.e. 43%) were no longer eligible for LTOT after four weeks due to spontaneous improvements in the PaO_2 to more than 55 mmHg [73]. Levi-Valensi and colleagues [74] in France, showed that 30% of stable hypoxemic patients, judged suitable for LTOT, had an increase in PaO_2 to more than 59 mmHg after 3 months of prospective monitoring without oxygen therapy. Those showing improvement could not be predicted from any measured variables such as initial pulmonary function tests. One study of patients taking LTOT has also demonstrated improvements in the baseline PaO_2 breathing room air [75]. The mechanisms of improvement in PaO_2 prior to, or during, oxygen therapy, are poorly understood and need investigation. These observations are important since LTOT is usually recommended below a critical threshold of PaO_2 and is rarely discontinued after initiation despite subsequent spontaneous improvement in PaO_2. Real dilemmas exist for the clinician in deciding when to start LTOT. In the outpatient clinic, when an initial assessment reveals hypoxemia, the patient should ideally be reassessed after four weeks of optimum medical therapy and clinical stability to obtain a more reliable baseline PaO$_2$. However, many patients are first found to be hypoxic when admitted to hospital with an acute exacerbation of COPD. The PaO$_2$ is recognized to be unstable in such patients for several weeks following acute exacerbation. However, these considerations should not necessarily preclude the initiation of LTOT. Should oxygen therapy be discontinued at the time of discharge pending re-assessment or should these patients be provided with domiciliary oxygen for a probationary period and their degree of chronic hypoxemia evaluated at a later date? Currently we do not have definite answers to these questions.

20.5.4 EFFICACY OF OXYGEN THERAPY

Domiciliary oxygen therapy needs to be individualized. Patients have different degrees of hypoxemia, respond differently to changes in FIO$_2$ and adapt in different ways to the various methods of oxygen supply and delivery. Hence, the prescription of domiciliary oxygen therapy needs to offer choices and the prescribing criteria should allow the physician to address each individual's special requirements. Generally, oxygen therapy should be adjusted to achieve an arterial oxygen tension between 70 and 90 mmHg. The oxyhemoglobin dissociation curve shows that further increases in oxygen tension will produce minimal gains in terms of arterial oxygen content as illustrated in Fig. 20.3 and the data in Table 20.3. Timms *et al.* [73] showed that adequate oxygenation is usually achieved in COPD patients using 1–3 l/min of oxygen flow via nasal cannulae. The rise in PaO$_2$ should not provoke excessive hypercapnia [76] but this is seldom a problem in clinically stable patients.

20.5.5 INDICATIONS FOR PORTABLE OXYGEN THERAPY

Demonstration of a fall in arterial oxygen saturation during exercise is a clear indication

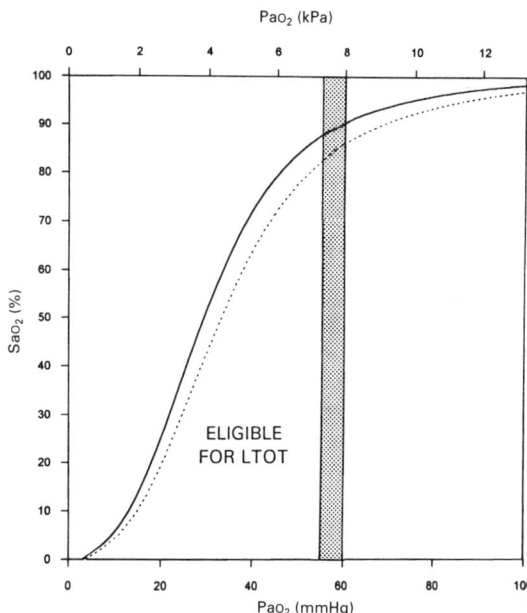

Fig. 20.3 Relationship between arterial oxygen saturation (SaO$_2$) and oxygen tension (PaO$_2$). Continuous line for PaCO$_2$ 40 mmHg, dotted line for PaCO$_2$ 50 mmHg. According to current prescribing criteria, subjects falling to the left of the shaded area are eligible for LTOT. Those within the shaded area would also be eligible in the USA if they have evidence of hypoxic organ dysfunction.

Table 20.3 Relationship between PaO$_2$, oxyhemoglobin saturation and arterial oxygen content

PaO$_2$ (mmHg)	SaO$_2$ (%)	CaO$_2$ (ml/l)
40	75	158
50	85	179
55	88	186
60	91	191
70	94	198
80	96	202
90	97	205
100	98	207

Assumptions: Solubility of O$_2$ in plasma 0.03 ml/l /mmHg; hemoglobin concentration 150 g/l; oxyhemoglobin capacity 1.39 ml/g.

for portable oxygen therapy. A treadmill test with cardiac monitoring and pulse oximetry is appropriate and a 4% fall in saturation would be adequate justification for portable oxygen therapy.

Portable oxygen therapy can improve exercise capability in patients with COPD irrespective of arterial oxygen desaturation. Furthermore, continuing physical activity has many physiologic and social advantages for the debilitated patient. The COPD patient enters a vicious cycle of declining mobility and physical deconditioning (Fig. 20.4) with increased ventilatory requirement, worsening dyspnea and further reduction in exercise capacity. Oxygen can help in breaking this vicious cycle when considered as an integral part of a comprehensive pulmonary rehabilitation program and prescribed with ambu-

latory capability. This is not to suggest that stationary oxygen supplies are ineffective but, by themselves, they cannot produce the best result in terms of rehabilitation (Chapter 21). The value of ambulatory oxygen is well recognized in the United States [77] but elsewhere prescribing criteria have focused on the improvements in survival without considering the need to maintain a patient's physical activity and quality of life. Recent changes in the prescribing regulations for cylinder and liquid oxygen in the United Kingdom have only worsened this situation. Surveys in Britain show that only one-third of patients have more than one oxygen outlet from their oxygen concentrator with obvious restrictions on their mobility. Although the more liberal guidelines in the USA allow provision of portable oxygen when patients have

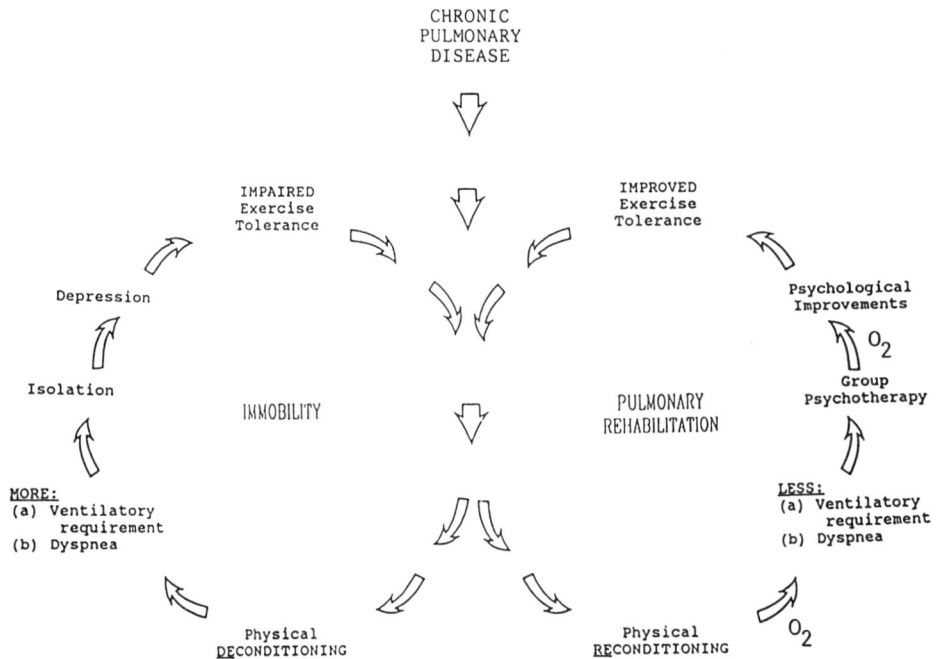

Fig. 20.4 Diagram to show the 'vicious cycle of chronic pulmonary disease' (on the left). Immobility leads to physical deconditioning, worsening symptoms, social isolation and further impairment of exercise capacity. Conversely the 'favorable cycle of pulmonary rehabilitation' (on the right) incorporates exercise and oxygen therapy to achieve physical reconditioning, improvement of symptoms, psychologic benefits and progressive improvement of exercise capacity.

exercise hypoxemia (PaO_2 less than 55 mmHg or SaO_2 less than 88%), the Medi-Care regulations restrict the patient to reimbursement for one oxygen installation only. Thus, if they have an oxygen concentrator, they must pay for portable oxygen or vice versa.

20.5.6 OTHER CONSIDERATIONS WITH LTOT

Studies have documented that about 10% of patients receiving LTOT continue to smoke tobacco [69,78]. This habit poses obvious hazards which are discussed along with other complications of oxygen therapy.

20.5.7 OXYGEN IN SPECIAL CIRCUMSTANCES

Prescribing criteria for domiciliary oxygen therapy should recognize special needs of the hypoxemic patient during sleep and travel. Patients with COPD are prone to oxygen desaturation during sleep [79,80] (Chapter 12). 'Blue bloaters' or patients predisposed to hypercapnia, seem especially vulnerable to nocturnal oxygen desaturation. Nocturnal oxygen desaturation is associated with increases in pulmonary artery pressure during hypoxemic episodes [81] which may contribute to the development of cor pulmonale [40,82,83]. Patients with nocturnal oxygen desaturation have more abnormal daytime exercise responses with greater increases in pulmonary artery pressure than do non-desaturators, reflecting their higher pulmonary vascular resistance [84]. Overnight oxygen therapy can avoid falls in oxygen saturation [81]. Calverley *et al.* [85] showed that oxygen therapy reduced the frequency of episodes of oxygen desaturation and also improved sleep quality as measured by several variables. Furthermore, abolition of nocturnal oxygen desaturation reduces cardiac dysrhythmias and prevents other electrocardiographic abnormalities which are associated with nocturnal oxygen desaturation [80]. Overnight oxygen therapy can be prescribed without an adverse rise in $PaCO_2$

[86]. A useful recommendation for COPD patients receiving domiciliary oxygen therapy is that they should increase their oxygen flow by 1 l/min during sleep.

Travel poses special problems for patients receiving domiciliary oxygen. Hypoxemia patients are at particular risk when travelling in commercial aircraft, although the incidence of death on commercial air flights is remarkably low. Commercial aircraft cabins are pressurized to be equivalent to an altitude of no greater than 8500 feet resulting in a cabin oxygen tension of around 100 mmHg. Gong *et al.* [87] proposed a hypoxia altitude simulation test (HAST) whereby patients breathe 15% oxygen in the laboratory to simulate an altitude of approximately 8000 feet. Their studies showed that problematic hypoxia at altitude could be predicted in those patients with a room air PaO_2 less than 72 mmHg. Such patients obviously need special provisions for oxygen therapy during commercial flights. Most airlines will provide supplementary oxygen but do not allow personal oxygen equipment on board. Airline travel is inadvisable for any chronically hypoxemic patient who is clinically unstable. Necessary arrangements for stable hypoxemic patients include advance contact of the airline company and a physician's letter, preferably from a pulmonary specialist, giving recommendations as to the oxygen requirements. In the USA, airlines, buses and trains are better prepared to accommodate patients receiving oxygen therapy than is currently the case in Europe.

20.6 EQUIPMENT FOR THE SUPPLY AND DELIVERY OF OXYGEN

Appropriate installation of equipment for domiciliary oxygen therapy can lead to routine use within a short time and perhaps decrease the need and the cost of hospitalization. However, to maintain mobility and quality of life, oxygen therapy must be non-restricting. The supplier of durable medical equipment has certain obligations to provide adequate patient instruction with appropriate back-up of trained staff and a 24-hour emergency service. Regular follow-up visits to the patient's home are especially helpful if hypoxemia has led to memory impairment and difficulties in compliance with the prescribed oxygen therapy. There are four alternatives for the supply of oxygen and a variety of different delivery systems which can be used in the home and each will be considered in turn. Selected specifications for oxygen supply systems are shown in Table 20.4.

20.6.1. OXYGEN SUPPLY

(a) Compressed gas cylinders

Compressed gas cylinders containing 100% oxygen are the traditional method of oxygen supply. Oxygen is stored at about 2000 psi and released through a pressure regulator which delivers about 50 psi to the patient. High pressure systems do not lend themselves to safe

transfilling within the patient's home and, therefore, regular deliveries of replenished cylinders are needed. An H-size cylinder is typically used as a stationary supply. This weighs about 70 kg and provides 6840 litres of oxygen (i.e. about 57 hours at a flow rate of 2 l/min). Oxygen from compressed gas cylinders is not as portable as liquid oxygen. An aluminum E-size cylinder, weighing about 6 kg, provides 625 litres of oxygen (i.e. 5 hours at 2 l/min) and can be towed by the patient on a purpose-built cart. Smaller C-size cylinders contain about 240 litres of oxygen and weigh only 4.5 kg. These can be carried by the patient in a nylon carrying case but provide only about 2 hours of oxygen at 2 l/min. Compressed gas cylinders need to be stored safely and protected from sources of extreme heat. Rises in temperature cause a pressure increase within the cylinders and there is the potential for explosion. Oxygen itself is neither explosive nor combustible but readily supports combustion and higher concentrations of oxygen enhance the burning speed and temperature of the flame. With 100% oxygen, plastic tubing can ignite within one second and burn with a

Table 20.4 Advantages and disadvantages of different oxygen supply systems

	Advantages	*Disadvantages*
Compressed O_2 (cylinders)	Low cost 100% O_2 High flow capability Portable (limited)	Bulky and heavy Frequent deliveries
Liquid O_2	Lightweight Portable 100% O_2	Refilling Evaporative loss Freezing Limited flows
O_2 concentrator (molecular sieve)	Low cost No refilling Safety	Fixed unit Flow limitations Electric supply Backup system Frequent maintenance
O_2 enricher (membrane separator)	Consistent O_2% Humidified output High flow capability Easy maintenance Safety	Fixed unit Lower O_2% Electric supply Backup system

flame exceeding 3000°C [88]. Oil and grease must not be allowed to contaminate the valves, regulators or connectors as this increases the fire hazard. Patients who smoke during oxygen therapy can ignite their facial hair with alarming consequences.

(b) Liquid oxygen

Liquid oxygen is a more economical means of storage than compressed gas (1 litre of liquid oxygen is equivalent to 860 litres in the gas phase). The boiling point of oxygen is –297°F, hence liquid oxygen is stored in insulated containers but at relatively low pressure. The systems need to be periodically vented to atmosphere to prevent pressure built-up and evaporative losses of oxygen can amount to about 0.5 kg/day. Apparatus weighing about 5 kg provides about 8 hours of oxygen at a flow rate of 2 l/min. One of the smallest systems, weighing 3 kg, gives a 4 hours of oxygen at 2 l/min. Liquid systems give 100% oxygen at all flow rates but the available flow rate is limited by the warming capacity of the system. Being low pressure systems, liquid oxygen does not carry major risks of explosion. However, contact with metal connectors or tubing can cause frostbite or burns. Liquid oxygen is the most expensive form of oxygen therapy but is the most portable. Although expensive, the provision of liquid oxygen has been justified in the USA if patients can make more than three journeys from home each week [89].

(c) Pressure swing adsorption molecular sieves

These electrical devices are currently the most convenient and economical means of supplying oxygen in the home [90]. Molecular sieve oxygen concentrators utilize zeolite, a synthetic aluminum silicate, which entraps gas molecules according to their size and polarity. All systems use two sieve beds alternatively in a pressure swing adsorption (PSA)

system within an intervening accumulation tank for oxygen. They are capable of producing 96% oxygen from air, since argon is also concentrated to about 4%. The major limitation of these oxygen concentrators is that they lack portability. Also, they are dependent on electricity and, therefore, a back-up oxygen supply is required for certain patients.

Molecular sieve technology has improved considerably in recent years and many reliable types of equipment are now available. The systems are limited in their flow capabilities by the size of the zeolite sieve beds. Generally, apparatus weighing 20–25 kg can produce about 90% oxygen up to flow rates of 5 l/min. Lighter and smaller systems are available, producing flow rates up to 3 l/min but clearly their flow capabilities are limited by the size of the sieve beds. Two studies have emphasized the importance of technical support and revealed malfunctions and diminished performance without frequent maintenance [91,92]. Two studies in 1985 [93,94] demonstrated a fall-off in the delivered oxygen concentration with increasing flow rates. For example, at a flow rate of 5 l/min, the systems produced only 70% oxygen but with improved technology, concentrations of 90% are now possible. A French study [95] surveyed 2414 operational oxygen concentrators in patients' homes in early 1988. Average utilization was 13–15 hours per day and the average oxygen concentration output was 92%. This study highlighted the need for regular maintenance and reported significant decreases in oxygen concentrations with increasing duration of service. Molecular sieve oxygen concentrators are reasonably safe, although their electrical and plastic components create a potential fire hazard. The author is unaware of serious safety incidents being reported with this equipment.

(d) Membrane separator oxygen enrichers

Certain complex polymer membranes are differentially permeable to oxygen and nitrogen and have the potential for use as oxygen concentrators. They work by application of a vacuum or positive pressure to one side of the polymer membrane. One system producing about 40% oxygen was compared with several molecular sieve oxygen concentrators and found to produce a satisfactory increase in arterial oxygen saturation to 91% using increased flow rates to compensate for the lower output oxygen concentration [94]. More recently, investigators in Japan have reported the use of polypropylene membrane, producing 30% oxygen from a semi-portable system weighing 4 kg and powered by a 12-volt battery. This system produced a mean increase in PaO_2 of 10 mmHg in 10 patients with chronic hypoxemia [96]. Polymer membranes also separate water vapor, producing fully saturated oxygen mixtures. The inherent humidification of these systems makes them suitable for the treatment of patients with tracheostomy, cystic fibrosis or those having transtracheal oxygen therapy. Since polymer membranes filter only molecules, they are effective barriers to foreign materials such as bacteria and other contaminants. Apparatus producing oxygen concentrations less than 50% is considerably safer than apparatus producing higher oxygen concentrations [88]. Also, membrane separators are far less complex than molecular sieve systems and require very little maintenance.

20.6.2 OXYGEN DELIVERY

Oxygen delivery systems are classified as high-flow and low-flow. With high-flow systems, the flow of gas, by itself, or with entrainment of room air, exceeds the inspiratory flow demand of the patient. With low-flow systems, this is not the case. Entrainment of room air is due to gas viscosity and not, as commonly believed, according to the Venturi or Bernouilli principles. In general, with oxygen delivery systems, steady flow is wasteful since the major benefit occurs at the beginning of inspiration. The four principal

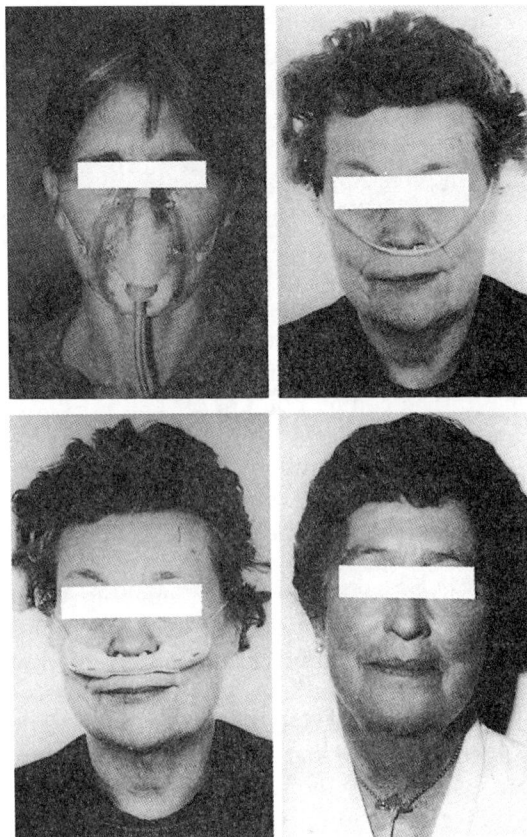

Fig. 20.5 Photographs to illustrate various methods of oxygen delivery: Face mask (top left), standard nasal cannulae (top right), nasal cannulae with a reservoir oxygen conserving device (bottom left) and transtracheal catheter (bottom right).

means of oxygen delivery are illustrated in Fig. 20.5.

(a) Face masks

A tight fitting face mask is the most efficient method of oxygen delivery but it is less well tolerated than nasal cannulae [97]. With fixed performance masks, the delivered flow usually exceeds peak inspiratory flow rate and the inspired oxygen concentration (FIO_2) can be predicted. These masks require a minimum oxygen flow rate of 4–6 l/min and are not especially suited for low FIO_2 (less than 35%). Variable performance masks use lower flow rates and are unpredictable in their inspired oxygen concentrations. With variable performance masks, a fall in minute ventilation leads to an increase in FIO_2. Variation in breathing patterns can produce large variations in FIO_2 [98] and face masks may fail in breathless patients with rapid, shallow breathing. Masks consist of a reservoir of 100–200 ml and so partial re-breathing is possible. Although masks are efficient, they make eating, communication and expectoration difficult.

(b) Nasal cannulae

Conventional nasal cannulae are the most commonly used means of oxygen delivery. They are inexpensive and relatively comfortable for the patient, allowing them to eat, sleep and communicate without encumbrance. Surprisingly, the FIO_2 is independent of whether the patient breathes through the nose or mouth [99]. There is surprisingly little exact information about the 'effective inspired oxygen concentration' with nasal cannula oxygen delivery. Certainly it seems that there is considerable variability of FIO_2, not only between different COPD patients using nasal cannulae but also from time to time in the same patient [100]. Table 20.5 shows data from two studies indicating that tracheal oxygen concentrations are lower than often assumed. Nasal cannulae are occasionally associated with complications such as dermatitis, mucosal drying and local irritation. Higher flow rates often require humidification to prevent this drying and irritation of the nasal tract. Carbon dioxide re-breathing is not a problem with nasal cannulae.

(c) Transtracheal catheter

The delivery of oxygen directly into the trachea was first described by Heimlich in 1982 [101]. The method has obvious benefits in terms of efficiency of oxygen delivery,

Table 20.5 Effective inspired oxygen concentrations

Flow (l/min)	Nasal cannulae	Transtracheal catheter
1	22.7,[a] 22.8[b]	25.0[b]
2	24.3[a]	
3	25.0,[a] 28.0[b]	34.9[b]
4	26.3[a]	
5	32.3[b]	45.2[b]

Oxygen supply ~ 100%
[a] Data from Schacter, E.N., Littner, M.R., Luddy, P. *et al.* (1980) Monitoring of oxygen delivery systems in clinical practice. *Crit. Care Med.*, 8, 405–9.
[b] Unpublished data. Cooper, C.B.

cosmesis and patient acceptance [102]. Potential advantages of transtracheal oxygen therapy (TTOT) include enhanced personal image, allowing the patients to avoid social isolation and improving their compliance. In 1986, investigators in Denver showed that TTOT was successful in patients thought to be refractory to oxygen therapy via nasal catheter or face mask delivery systems [103]. Several large groups have now reported their experience with TTOT [102,104,105,106]. Christopher *et al.* [104], studied 100 patients over a 2-year period and found patient acceptance to be 96%. This group used a 9-French catheter placed in the second or third tracheal space using a Seldinger technique. They stressed the importance of avoiding puncture of the cricothyroid membrane to reduce the incidence of dysphonia and cough. They used a stent for one week before initiating oxygen flow to reduce post-insertional cough and discomfort and thereby, supposedly, to reduce the incidence of subcutaneous emphysema. After about 6 weeks, the minitracheostomy tract is epithelialized and, by this time, the patients have been taught to remove, clean and change their catheters twice daily without the need for guide wires. Banner and Govan [107], at Harefield Hospital, reported a technique using 16 gauge angiocaths. These narrower catheters were associated with lower incidence of mucous ball formation (see below) but a higher incidence of catheter failure. Another group has reported a totally implanted system with tubing tunnelled beneath the skin to a convenient point for connection to the oxygen supply beneath the patient's clothing [108].

TTOT can reduce resting oxygen flow requirements by 25–55% compared with nasal cannula delivery [102,104,106,107]. Similar savings in terms of oxygen flow have also been reported during exercise [104] and exercise tolerance has been shown to increase with TTOT [106,109,110]. One study showed increases in walking distance despite similar patterns of arterial oxygen desaturation [110]. TTOT is associated with improved sense of taste and reduction in dyspnoea [102,107,108, 111,112]. During TTOT the trachea probably acts as an anatomical reservoir which stores oxygen during the last part of exhalation giving a high F_{IO_2} during the following inspiration. One interesting study [112] has shown that increases in oxygen flow via a transtracheal catheter caused equivalent reductions in inspired volumes at the mouth. Hence the bulk flow of oxygen into the trachea reduced inspired ventilation and might reduce the inspiratory work of the respiratory muscles.

Complications of TTOT include the formation of mucous balls (25% of cases), partially due to the drying effect of the oxygen flow directly into the trachea and also partly due to increased secretions. Hence, humidification of oxygen is needed for transtracheal use, particularly at high flow rates. The formation of mucous balls is associated with poor adherence to catheter cleaning schedules. Serious airflow obstruction has been reported due to mucous ball formation in 3 cases [106,113,114]. Other complications of TTOT with their reported incidences include cough (5–15%), superficial infection (3–7%), subcutaneous emphysema (4–10%), catheter breakage (6%), catheter dislodgement (12–22%), hemoptysis (2%) and bronchospasm (1–2%). Hoffman *et al.* [106] reported a high mortality using TTOT,

although the deaths were said to be related to underlying disease rather than the presence of the transtracheal catheter.

(d) Reservoir-conserving devices

Introduction of a small reservoir in the oxygen delivery system is an old principle which has currently regained popularity. The reservoir is intended to fill during the patient's exhalation so that more oxygen is available at the beginning of the next breath. Reservoir-conserving devices usually contain a collapsible membrane so that during the latter half of inspiration, the device serves as a simple conduit for continuing oxygen flow. The potential advantages of such systems are: (i) reduction in total oxygen requirement and, therefore, cost, and (ii) elimination of oxygen wastage during exhalation with extension of the useful operation time of various oxygen supply systems, thereby increasing their portability and range. Two types of reservoir system have been reported. The moustache reservoir (about 20 ml) is reported to reduce oxygen flow requirements by 50–75% at rest [115–117]. An alternative form of reservoir device is the pendant which hangs on the anterior chest wall and can be concealed beneath clothing [118]. This system can reduce oxygen flow requirements by 30–50% at rest [119,120] and 50–67% during exercise [117,120,121]. However, patients dislike the encumbrance of the moustache reservoir and find the pendant to be too obtrusive. The efficiency of a reservoir varies between individual patients which may reflect the degree of mouth breathing [122]. Consideration must be given to the replacement cost of the equipment because the internal membranes of a reservoir-conserving device might have a limited life span.

(e) Respiratory phased, demand or pulse oxygen delivery

These systems are increasing in popularity because of their potential for oxygen flow savings with limited supply systems such as liquid oxygen or compressed gas [123–125]. Only the gas inspired during the first 25–50% of each inspiration reaches the alveoli and is available for gas exchange, so oxygen delivery in late inspiration and throughout expiration is wasted [126]. Pulsed delivery overcomes this limitation by sensing the start of inspiration with a thermistor or pressure transducer which activates an electro-mechanical valve and releases a fixed or variable amount of oxygen as a pulse flow. The mode of operation can be varied so that the pulse of oxygen is delivered every 1, 2, 3 or 4 breaths. These systems are intricate and subject to electromechanical failure whilst rapid, shallow breathing can cause near continuous activation of the valve without oxygen conservation [122]. Humidification is seldom needed with pulsed delivery because of the reduced oxygen flow. Demand flow systems require internal batteries and there are seldom internal safety features to prevent permanent inactivation of the oxygen valve. The sensitivity of breath detection is often an issue as many systems are insufficiently sensitive to detect breathing during sleep but too sensitive to increases in ventilation, e.g. during exercise. An ideal system would allow adjustment of the sensitivity of inspiratory flow detection to compensate for these alterations in respiratory drive. Despite these difficulties, worthwhile savings have been reported in terms of oxygen flow requirements both at rest [126–128] and during exercise [129] with savings ranging from 3:1 to 7:1.

20.6.3 AVAILABLE COMBINATIONS OF OXYGEN SUPPLY AND DELIVERY SYSTEMS

Various innovative combinations of apparatus are now available, at least in the USA, for domiciliary oxygen therapy. The combination of lightweight portable oxygen supplies with oxygen-conserving devices and transtracheal oxygen delivery prolongs the useful duration of the oxygen supply and thus it is possible to obtain virtually continuous ambulatory oxygen therapy throughout the day. Lightweight portable oxygen supplies including pulse delivery devices may weigh as little as 3 kg, yet give 14 hours of oxygen flow at 2 l/min. Transtracheal oxygen delivery is clearly the most efficient and cosmetically the most acceptable method with predictably better patient compliance, but is also the most invasive method of oxygen delivery. Reservoir systems are the least expensive, simple and reliable but obviously more obtrusive and, therefore, may not be readily accepted by the patient. Demand or pulse oxygen delivery is very efficient but these systems can be subject to electromechanical failure. The combination of TTOT with pulsed oxygen flow seems especially promising in terms of reducing oxygen flow requirements [130,131]. Whilst it is now possible to provide patients with ambulatory oxygen therapy throughout the day, these systems remain expensive. However, if the continued mobility reduces hospitalization and dependency on acute medical services, such additional cost would be well worthwhile.

20.7 ADHERENCE TO PRESCRIBING CRITERIA FOR DOMICILIARY OXYGEN

Several studies in the UK have examined the adherence of the medical profession to the official guidelines. Baudouin *et al.*, [132] showed that only 43% of patients in Sheffield met the full prescribing criteria whereas Walshaw *et al.* [133] reported that 46% of patients in Liverpool had arterial oxygen tension greater than 55 mmHg breathing air. Frequent problems are the lack of demonstrable stability of chronic hypoxemia and the prescription of oxygen without prior assessment by a pulmonary specialist [132–134]. In Sheffield, 26% of patients having domiciliary oxygen therapy were not followed-up by a pulmonary physician. In Bristol, 40% of oxygen prescriptions were not initiated by pulmonary specialists and many of these patients had been inadequately investigated. In Liverpool, 44% of oxygen installations were not prescribed by a pulmonary specialist and, in many cases, too few hours of oxygen therapy were recommended.

Evidence is emerging that LTOT is prescribed too late in the natural history of the disease which causes hypoxemia. Many patients die soon after starting LTOT. McCallian and Pearce [78] noted that 50% of patients died within the first three months of LTOT and most patients prescribed oxygen were elderly and severely disabled. These observations raise several important problems. It is possible that the guidelines themselves are inappropriate and require revision. None the less, it seems that earlier referral to a pulmonary specialist may well allow earlier identification of those who need oxygen and avoidance of inappropriate prescriptions too late in the progression of the illness. Studies to resolve the optimum time of beginning this treatment are clearly needed.

20.7.1 PATIENT COMPLIANCE

Both the major multicenter trials recommend that oxygen should be used for at least 15 hours/day for maximum effect. A report from the North West Regional Health Authority in 1983 [135] examined 76 patients receiving domiciliary oxygen and found their mean usage to be 14.3 hours/day. Similar observations were made in Sheffield [92] where a later study showed that only 30 of 64 patients were using their oxygen treatment when visited at home. Two studies from France have confirmed this poor patient compliance. Vergeret *et al.* [136] showed that 38% of patients were following their prescription and taking oxygen for more than 15 hours/day, those with the most severe hypoxemia being most compliant. Prignot [137] confirmed that the duration of daily oxygen therapy was always less than that estimated by the patients but frequent home visits

improved compliance. Another study [133] used hidden clocks in oxygen concentrators and showed that only 46% of patients used their equipment for more than 15 hours/day although 79% said they did so.

There are several reasons for poor patient compliance. One obvious explanation is a lack of symptomatic improvement but patients also tend to be self-conscious of their appearance wearing equipment for oxygen therapy. Some patients have unrealistic fears of danger from the equipment which can be reduced by adequate instruction and education. Depression and memory impairment also contribute to compliance problems [136]. Two studies have shown that 10% of patients continue to smoke despite medical advice, whilst taking domiciliary oxygen [69,78]. Patient compliance can be improved by better education and more frequent home visits to monitor therapy. Oxygen therapy can be made cosmetically more acceptable and earlier prescription might remove the stigma that it is a treatment of last resort. The rehabilitative role of oxygen treatment must be stressed, pointing out the combined goals of improving longevity and quality of life.

20.8 MONITORING OXYGEN THERAPY

To be effective, oxygen therapy should achieve normal or near normal tissue oxygenation without using excessively high inspired oxygen concentrations. An adequate response to supplementary oxygen therapy has never been clearly defined, although it is clear from the oxyhemoglobin dissociation curve (Fig. 20.3) that an increase in PaO_2 to more than 80 mmHg will usually produce an oxygen saturation of over 94%. This is probably adequate for most patients as it will protect them from dramatic falls in oxygen saturation which occur on the steep portion of the dissociation curve. Greater increases in PaO_2 are unlikely to produce worthwhile changes in oxygen saturation and content as shown in Table 20.3.

20.8.1 ASSESSMENT OF OXYGENATION

Physical examination is an unreliable guide to tissue oxygenation. Peripheral cyanosis can occur due to sluggish circulation as well as a low oxyhemoglobin saturation. Central cyanosis may be detected in the presence of polycythemia even when oxygen content is normal and may be absent in anemia despite a low arterial oxygen content. It is difficult to detect in the presence of skin pigmentation. These difficulties make it necessary to assess oxygenation more directly.

(a) Arterial blood gas analysis

Arterial blood gas analysis is the gold standard for assessing oxygenation, although it is not the ideal way to judge tissue oxygen delivery. Intermittent sampling of arterial blood enables *in vitro* analysis to determine pH, PaO_2, and $PaCO_2$ using specific electrodes and commercial blood gas analysers. Technical errors can be reduced by a program of proficiency testing for blood gas laboratories [138]. Brachial or radial arteries are commonly used for sampling. When the radial artery is to be used, an Allen test should be performed to verify adequate ulnar artery perfusion of the hand prior to the procedure. Complications of arterial puncture are uncommon but pain and bruising occur in about 33% of cases especially when larger needles are used. Various intra-arterial catheters have been evaluated for continuous monitoring of arterial blood gases [139]. A fluorescent optode catheter which measures PO_2, PCO_2 and pH with reasonable accuracy and stability over 72 hours is now available for human use and is likely to find useful application in research and critical care settings [140].

(b) Pulse oximetry

Transcutaneous pulse oximetry is a readily available means of assessing arterial oxygen saturation (SaO_2). The transmission of light through the tissues is directly proportional to the oxygen saturation of the perfusing blood. Modern pulse oximeters use two wave lengths, are accurate to within 2–4% over the usual range of oxygen saturations but become less reliable below a saturation of 60% [141]. The probe is normally placed on an ear lobe or finger where the accuracy is influenced by skin pigmentation, skin perfusion and thickness as well as position and motion of the probe. Generally, the response time of pulse oximeters is adequate for most clinical purposes [142]. Pulse oximeters overestimate SaO_2 in the presence of carboxyhaemoglobin or methaemoglobin but underestimate SaO_2 if the skin is pigmented or jaundiced [143]. Pulse oximetry should not be used as a substitute for arterial blood gas analysis or as an accurate measure of PaO_2 but is useful when a rapid estimation of oxygenation is needed, e.g. during anesthesia, transportation of patients, intensive care monitoring or during bronchoscopy. Pulse oximetry can be used to titrate oxygen therapy in a hospital setting but should not be used as the only criterion for prescription.

(c) Transcutaneous oxygen tension

Heated polygraphic electrodes are available for the measurement of transcutaneous oxygen tension ($PtcO_2$). The electrodes consist of an electrolyte solution in contact with skin covered with a teflon membrane. They are maintained between 43 and 45°C to promote local hyperemia. The increased temperature also shifts the oxyhemoglobin saturation curve to the right and the PaO_2 must be corrected for this. The site of the skin electrode must be moved every 4 hours to avoid heat injury. $PtcO_2$ reflects a balance of oxygen delivery and cutaneous oxygen consumption [144] and is some 20 mmHg lower than PaO_2 [145]. Lower values of $PtcO_2$ occur in low perfusion states [146] and in peripheral vascular disease [147,148]. Inaccuracies with $PtcO_2$ measurement arise with thickened skin with superficial veins in the field of the electrode. These instruments are accurate and useful when used in neonates but more clinical experience is needed in adults to determine whether they can be reliably substituted for arterial blood gas analysis.

(d) Tissue oxygenation

None of the methods described above reliably reflects tissue oxygenation. This can be directly measured using electrode techniques but these are unlikely to have clinical applications since every tissue has its own oxygen tension characteristics and no one tissue typifies the body as a whole. Mixed venous oxygen tension ($P\bar{v}o_2$) has been proposed as an integrated value reflecting arterial oxygen saturation, hemoglobin concentration and cardiac output in relation to the whole body oxygen consumption. The assumptions about $P\bar{v}o_2$ are probably reasonable but it should be remembered that it is influenced by blood leaving organs of widely different oxygen consumptions. Thus, a low $P\bar{v}o_2$ indicates an overall problem with tissue oxygenation but a normal value cannot be taken to mean normal tissue oxygen tension in all organs. An alternative measure is the blood lactate level. Lactic acidosis develops when tissue metabolism becomes dependent on anerobic pathways implying that insufficient oxygen is available for mitochondrial metabolism. Oxygen therapy in patients with chronic lung disease reduces the lactic acidosis of exercise which is consistent with an improved tissue oxygen delivery [62].

20.9 COMPLICATIONS OF OXYGEN THERAPY

The complications of oxygen therapy can be divided into non-medical hazards and medical hazards or oxygen toxicity. Non-medical hazards have already been discussed under the section concerning equipment for domiciliary oxygen therapy. There are two principal medical hazards with oxygen therapy, the first being pulmonary oxygen toxicity and the second, hypercapnia due to alterations in respiratory control. In addition, oxygen therapy causes pulmonary vasodilatation with its potential for worsening ventilation–perfusion imbalance and also causes systemic vasoconstriction. There are certain medical hazards specifically related to breathing 100% oxygen such as absorption atelectasis due to washout of nitrogen from alveoli and also retrolental fibrodysplasia, usually noted in neonates or patients receiving hyperbaric oxygen therapy. Neither of these complications is likely to arise with domiciliary oxygen therapy since effective inspired oxygen concentrations rarely exceed 40%.

20.9.1 PULMONARY OXYGEN TOXICITY

Lavoisier, in 1785, demonstrated congestion of the lungs of guinea-pigs after breathing oxygen and, in 1878, Paul Bert firmly established that increased concentrations of oxygen can be toxic. The pathologic findings with pulmonary oxygen toxicity are non-specific, consisting of diffuse alveolar damage with capillary proliferation, hemosiderosis, interstitial fibrosis and epithelial hyperplasia [149,150]. These changes are similar to those of bronchopulmonary dysplasia in neonates. The popular explanation for pulmonary oxygen toxicity invokes a role for free radicals. Formation of singlet oxygen, hydrogen peroxide or free hydroxyl radicals in the lung might cause structural metabolic changes which ultimately lead to cell death. Type I epithelial cells are known to be particularly susceptible to oxygen-free radicals and rely on chemical defense mechanisms for protection. Animal studies have suggested that higher levels of superoxide dismutase, catalase and glutathione peroxidase might protect against pulmonary oxygen toxicity [151].

There is uncertainty about safe thresholds of inspired oxygen concentration. The toxic effects of oxygen on the pulmonary parenchyma are actually determined by the alveolar oxygen tension rather than oxygen concentrations as illustrated by experiments with astronauts who tolerated 100% oxygen for long periods when the ambient pressure was less than 1 atmosphere [152]. After breathing 100% oxygen at atmospheric pressure for a few hours, normal individuals develop an acute tracheobronchitis with substernal burning and impaired mucociliary clearance but these effects resolve quickly when they revert to breathing lower concentrations of oxygen. Breathing 75% oxygen for 24 hours does not appear to produce these symptoms whilst breathing 50% oxygen or less for up to 7 days does not impair lung function [153].

Some investigators have described an oxygen tolerance curve based on measured decreases in vital capacity [154]. Patients receiving domiciliary oxygen rarely experience inspired oxygen concentrations of more than 40% and so the risk of pulmonary oxygen toxicity is small. However, one study [155] reported that 10% of patients receiving LTOT for 6 months had histologic changes consistent with oxygen toxicity. As there is no reliable index of pulmonary oxygen toxicity and no clearly defined threshold for safe FIO_2, guidelines for oxygen prescription should aim to achieve adequate oxygenation with the minimum increase in FIO_2. In practice, this means achieving an arterial oxygen tension of between 70–90 mmHg as previously discussed.

20.9.2 HYPERCAPNIA

Oxygen inhalation might worsen ventilatory failure either by abolishing the hypoxic stimulus to breathe or reversing pulmonary hypoxic vasoconstriction. The physiologic basis of these changes is discussed elsewhere (Chapters 8, 10). Appreciation of the risk of hypercapnia during oxygen treatment led to the development of controlled oxygen therapy [3]. Table 20.6 shows typical changes

in arterial blood gas tensions with the administration of low-flow oxygen via nasal cannulae [156]. In this group of 16 stable COPD patients with oxygen flows of 2 l/min, mean arterial $PaCO_2$ increased from 55 to 61 mmHg whilst PaO_2 rose from 49 to 70 mmHg and pH changed from 7.40 to 7.37. These changes are typical for patients with COPD and illustrate several important points. First, to obtain the required increases in PaO_2 a rise in $PaCO_2$ must often be accepted. Several investigators have reported that this need not be harmful to the patient [132,136]. Neff and Petty [157] found that moderate hypercapnia associated with domiciliary oxygen therapy, was well tolerated in the long term. Indeed, $PaCO_2$ levels over 80 mmHg may be seen in some patients. However, this degree of hypercapnia usually implies that there is an additional cause for hypoventilation, e.g. sleep apnea. Another important point illustrated in Table 20.6 is that due to compensatory metabolic alkalosis in patients with chronic hypercapnia, further rises in $PaCO_2$ are usually well accommodated and the resulting change in pH is minimal. There is one potentially important advantage to be gained from hypercapnia in patients with COPD. With a higher $PaCO_2$ and correspondingly higher alveolar carbon dioxide concentration, patients can expect higher carbon dioxide outputs for a given level of alveolar ventilation. This apparent increase in efficiency of minute ventilation with more efficient elimination of carbon dioxide and hence reduced ventilatory requirement has been suggested as an adaptive mechanism in patients with chronic respiratory failure [158].

20.10 ECONOMIC CONSIDERATIONS

Unfortunately, the prescription of domiciliary oxygen therapy is burdened by economic and political considerations. Current estimates suggest that there are about 50 000 patients receiving domiciliary oxygen therapy in the UK and 60–70% of these patients have COPD.

Table 20.6 Typical arterial blood gas changes with nasal oxygen therapy

	PaO_2 (mmHg)	$PaCO_2$	pH
(mmHg)			
Room air	49	55	7.40
O_2 @ 2 l/min	70	61	7.37
O_2 @ 6 l/min	96	72	7.32

Data reproduced from [156].

About 12 000 patients have oxygen concentrators whereas roughly 40 000 patients are using compressed gas cylinders. Recent evidence suggests that domiciliary oxygen therapy is often provided as a pre-terminal or palliative measure.

20.10.1 COSTS VS BENEFITS

Domiciliary oxygen therapy is usually prescribed because it prolongs life in COPD but this is not the only goal of patient management and improvements in quality of life and the ability to perform the usual activities of daily living are equally important. From the available survival statistics, it appears that LTOT can double life expectancy [45]. The earlier prescription of LTOT will lead to more years of added life and the cost of each added year would be equivalent to one year of domiciliary oxygen therapy. This being so, it is clear that LTOT is more effective than other long-term treatments such as chronic hemodialysis or the management of complicated hypertension. Hence, the cost benefit of LTOT, at least in terms of patient survival, is probably lower than in many other chronic diseases.

A further consideration in cost benefit analysis is the improvement in neuropsychiatric function and the ability of patients to continue their normal activities of daily living. A survey of 13 500 LTOT installations in France showed that 55% of patients are able to wash unaided but that 25% never leave their homes and 25% never go on holiday [159]. Once more it must be stressed that to maintain these activities of daily living, the oxygen treatment must be non-restricting and this favors the use of portable oxygen more extensively than is the case at present. As already noted, avoidance of hospitalization by such steps will more than offset the initial costs associated with this ambulatory treatment. Oxygen-conservation techniques, can reduce the costs of therapy but the litre flow of oxygen is a relatively minor component in the overall cost and so savings from this source are relatively small. Regrettably, with domiciliary oxygen therapy, we have yet to define those patients who derive the greatest benefit in human and economic terms.

20.10.2 ACTUAL COSTS OF DOMICILIARY OXYGEN THERAPY

In the UK, cylinder oxygen therapy costs about £6500 per annum. Very few patients currently receive cylinder oxygen with ambulatory capability. The apparent costs of domiciliary oxgyen therapy from an oxygen concentrator are less. The purchase price of such devices is about £1500. However, the oxygen concentrator service is almost entirely provided by rental arrangements within nine defined Health Regions. Contracting companies appear to charge the National Health Service a rental of between £70 and £80 per month for the installation and maintenance of oxygen concentrator equipment. Although portable oxygen systems would appear to be more expensive, cost analysis rarely takes into account the full physiologic benefits and overall effects on the costs of health care. For example, maintaining patient activity and avoidance of hospitalization could account for major health care savings. The actual cost of one day in hospital is probably equivalent to the prescription of one month of oxygen therapy.

20.10.3 REIMBURSEMENT ISSUES

In most Western countries, the costs of domiciliary oxygen therapy are borne by National or Federal health care services. Unfortunately, such bureaucracies are usually concerned with cost containment and prescribing restrictions intended to contain costs often seriously limit the development of an optimal clinical service. This problem clearly exists with domiciliary oxygen therapy. In Britain, the rigidity of the domiciliary oxygen service has prevented the introduction of new technologies for oxygen supply and delivery. The range of equipment available in the UK is disappointing compared with the USA. In the New South Wales region of Australia, significant cost savings in the domiciliary oxygen therapy service were achieved by introducing central administration and withdrawal of domiciliary oxygen therapy where it was thought not to be needed [160]. A major component of these cost savings clearly came from changing patients from oxygen cylinders to oxygen concentrators. Denying patients the potential benefit of ambulatory oxygen therapy may have a detrimental effect, despite the apparent cost savings. Hence, whilst there are obvious economic gains by this strategy, the clinical impact on patients, in particular their quality of life, has not been fully evaluated.

In the USA, strict legislation governs the reinbursement for domiciliary oxygen therapy. Most LTOT is financed by the Federal government through the Medi-Care programme. Current methods of reimbursement discourage the provision of apparatus for flow savings and only cover one oxygen supply system. Thus patients with an oxygen concentrator who need an oxygen cylinder as back-up or wish to have an ambulatory capability, must meet the extra cost themselves. In the cost benefit analysis which favors the provision of oxygen concentrators rather than cylinder oxygen, hidden costs are often overlooked. These include costs of maintenance and servicing and the cost of electricity which might amount to £20 per month and, lastly, the cost of an additional back-up system as a precaution against electrical power failure. All of these factors reduce the apparent cost benefits of the molecular sieve oxygen concentrators.

20.11 FUTURE DIRECTIONS FOR OXYGEN THERAPY

The provision of domiciliary oxygen therapy is likely to change significantly in the next few years. Hopefully, this will arise from a greater appreciation of the physiologic benefits of long-term oxygen and an increased prescription to patients most in need. We must consider prescribing LTOT before the end stage of the disease is reached and studies to confirm the benefit of this approach are urgently needed. At present our treatment is akin to waiting until a patient has had a stroke before initiating antihypertensive treatment.

Careful cost-benefit analysis is needed to evaluate quality of life and the overall demands on health care services by patients with COPD. We need to examine the role of ambulatory oxygen treatment as part of programmes of pulmonary rehabilitation. Future research may well demonstrate that the combination of exercise and oxygen is of more value than simply prescribing oxygen for longer periods during the day. We need to define the effects of oxygen on aerobic capacity and to look for potentiating effects of oxygen in physical training programs for COPD patients.

The physiologic effects of transtracheal oxygen therapy deserve further investigation. It may be particularly appropriate for people with the 'overlap syndrome' of obstructive sleep apnea and COPD, whilst its effect on reducing the work of the inspiratory muscles by a reduction in inspired volume, merits further exploration.

There are clear challenges ahead in terms of the esthetics, cost and convenience of the equipment used in oxygen supply and delivery. The efficiency of the available systems of oxygen supply in relationship to newer technologies, must be evaluated. Many patients do not require 100% or near 100% oxygen supplies for a useful therapeutic effect. Once this is appreciated, then the potential for developing lightweight portable equipment is considerable. Already lightweight aluminium oxygen cylinders or reinforced plastic liquid oxygen tanks are available which, coupled with oxygen-conserving devices, provide ambulatory oxygen treatment for adequate periods during the day for most patients. Membrane technology may provide the opportunity for the development of truly portable oxygen concentrators.

There are many challenges ahead in the field of domiciliary oxygen therapy. Prescription guidelines need revision. Physiologic benefits need better definition and technologic improvements are required in the apparatus for the supply and delivery of oxygen and further research is needed to identify those patient groups in whom true cost benefits can be expected.

REFERENCES

1. Cotes, J.E. and Gilson, J.C. (1956) Effect of oxygen on exercise ability in chronic respiratory insufficiency. Use of portable apparatus. *Lancet*, **ii**, 872–6.
2. Barach, A.L. (1959) Ambulatory oxygen therapy: oxygen inhalation at home and out-of-doors. *Dis. Chest*, **35**, 229–41.
3. Campbell, E.J.M. (1960) A method of controlled oxygen administration which reduces the risk of carbon-dioxide retention. *Lancet*, **ii**, 12–14.
4. Kitchin, A.H., Lowther, C.P. and Matthews, M.B. (1961) The effects of exercise and of breathing oxygen-enriched air on the pulmonary circulation in emphysema. *Clin. Sci.*, **21**, 93–106.
5. Cotes, J.E., Pisa, Z. and Thomas, A.J. (1963) Effect of breathing oxygen upon cardiac output, heart rate, ventilation, systematic and pulmonary blood pressure in patients with chronic lung disease. *Clin. Sci.*, **25**, 305–21.
6. Holt, J.H. and Branscomb, B.V. (1965) Hemodynamic responses to controlled 100% oxygen breathing in emphysema. *J. Appl. Physiol.*, **20**, 215–20.
7. Scano, G., Van Meerhaeghe, A., Willeput, R. *et al.* (1982) Effect of oxygen on breathing during exercise in patients with chronic lung disease. *Eur. J. Respir. Dis.*, **63**, 23–30.
8. Hunt, J.M., Copeland, J., McDonald, C.F. *et al.* (1989) Cardiopulmonary response to oxygen therapy in hypoxaemic chronic airflow obstruction. *Thorax*, **44**, 930–6.
9. Lee, J. and Read, J. (1967) Effect of oxygen breathing on distribution of pulmonary blood flow in chronic obstructive lung disease. *Am. Rev. Respir. Dis.*, **96**, 1173–80.
10. Rebuck, A.S. and Vandenberg, R.A. (1973) The relationship between pulmonary arterial pressure and physiologic dead space in patients with obstructive lung disease. *Am. Rev. Respir. Dis.*, **107**, 423–8.
11. Austin, T.W., and Penman, W.B. (1967) Airway obstruction due to hypoxemia in patients with chronic lung disease. *Am. Rev. Respir. Dis.*, **95**, 567–75.
12. Grassino, A., Sorli, J., Lorange, F. *et al.* (1978) Respiratory drive and timing in chronic obstructive pulmonary disease. *Chest*, **73** (Suppl.), 290–3.
13. Wasserman, K., Whipp, B.J., Casaburi, R. *et al.* (1979) Ventilatory control during exercise in man. *Bull. Eur. Physiopathol. Respir.*, **15**, 27–51.
14. Bye, P.T.P., Esau, S.A., Walley, K.E. *et al.* (1984) Ventilatory muscles during exercise in air and oxygen in normal men. *J. Appl. Physiol.*, **56**, 464–71.
15. Pierce, A.K., Paez, P.N. and Miller, W.F. (1965) Exercise training with the aid of a portable oxygen supply in patients with emphysema. *Am. Rev. Respir. Dis.*, **91**, 653–9.
16. Bye, P.T.P., Esau, S.A., Levy, R.D. *et al.* (1985) Ventilatory muscle function during exercise in air and oxygen in patients with chronic airflow limitation. *Am. Rev. Respir. Dis.*, **132**, 236–40.
17. Vyas, M.N., Banister, E.W., Morton, J.W. *et al.* (1971) Response to exercise in patients with chronic airway obstruction. II. Effects of breathing 40 percent oxygen. *Am. Rev. Respir. Dis.*, **103**, 401–12.
18. Stein, D.A., Bradley, B.L. and Miller, W.C. (1982) Mechanisms of oxygen effects on exercise in patients with chronic obstructive pulmonary disease. *Chest*, **81**, 6–10.

19. Criner, G.J. and Celli, B.R. (1987) Ventilatory muscle recruitment in exercise with O_2 in obstructed patients with mild hypoxemia. *J. Appl. Physiol.*, **63**, 195–200.

20. Selinger, S.R., Kennedy, T.P., Buescher, P. *et al.* (1987) Effects of removing oxygen from patients with chronic obstructive pulmonary disease. *Am. Rev. Respir. Dis.*, **136**, 85–91.

21. Abraham, A.S., Cole, R.B. and Bishop, J.M. (1968) Reversal of pulmonary hypertension by prolonged oxygen administration to patients with chronic bronchitis. *Circ. Res.*, **23**, 147–57.

22. Abraham, A.S., Hedworth-Whitty, R.B. and Bishop, J.M. (1967) Effects of acute hypoxia and hypervolemia singly and together, upon the pulmonary circulation in patients with chronic bronchitis. *Clin. Sci.*, **33**, 371–80.

23. Springer, C., Barstow, T.J., Wasserman, K. and Cooper, D.M. (1991) Oxygen uptake and heart rate responses during hypoxic exercise in children and adults. *Med. Sci. Sports Exerc.*, **23**, 71–9.

24. Baudouin, S.V., Bott, J., Ward, A. *et al.* (1992) Short term effect of oxygen on renal hemodynamics in patients with chronic obstructive airways disease. *Thorax*, **47**, 550–4.

25. Aber, G.M., Harris, A.M. and Bishop, J.M. (1964) The effect of acute changes in inspired oxygen concentration on cardiac, respiratory and renal function in patients with chronic obstructive airways disease. *Clin. Sci.*, **26**, 133–43.

26. Brent, B.N., Matthay, R.A., Mahler, D.A. *et al.* (1984) Relationship between oxygen uptake and oxygen transport in stable patients with chronic obstructive pulmonary disease. *Am. Rev. Respir. Dis.*, **129**, 682–6.

27. Kawakami, Y., Kishi, F., Yamamoto, H. and Miyamoto, K. (1983) Relation of oxygen delivery, mixed venous oxygenation and pulmonary hemodynamics to prognosis in chronic obstructive pulmonary disease. *N. Engl. J. Med.*, **308**, 1045–9.

28. Degaute, J-P., Domenighetti, G., Naeije, R. *et al.* (1981) Oxygen delivery in acute exacerbation of chronic obstructive pulmonary disease. Effects of controlled oxygen therapy. *Am. Rev. Respir. Dis.*, **124**, 26–30.

29. Corriveau, M.L., Rosen, B.J. and Dolan, G.F. (1989) Oxygen transport and oxygen consumption during supplemental oxygen administration in patients with chronic obstructive pulmonary disease. *Am. J. Med.*, **87**, 633–7.

30. Levine, B.E., Bigelow, D.V., Hamstra, R.D. *et al.* (1967) The role of long-term continuous oxygen administration in patients with chronic airway obstruction with hypoxemia. *Ann. Intern. Med.*, **66**, 639–50.

31. Petty, T.L. and Finigan, M.M. (1968) The clinical evaluation of prolonged ambulatory oxygen therapy in patients with chronic airway obstruction. *Am. J. Med.*, **45**, 242–52.

32. Neff, T.A. and Petty, T.L. (1970) Long-term continuous oxygen therapy in chronic airway obstruction: Mortality in relationship to cor pulmonale, hypoxia and hypercapnia. *Ann. Intern. Med.*, **72**, 621–6.

33. Stark, R.D., Finnegan, P. and Bishop, J.M. (1972) Daily requirement of oxygen to reverse pulmonary hypertension in patients with chronic bronchitis. *Br. Med. J.*, **3**, 724–8.

34. Stark, R.D., Finnegan, P. and Bishop, J.M. (1973) Long-term domiciliary oxygen in chronic bronchitis with pulmonary hypertension. *Br. Med. J.*, **3**, 467–70.

35. Nocturnal Oxygen Therapy Trial Group (1980) Continuous or nocturnal oxygen therapy in hypoxemic chronic obstructive lung disease. *Ann. Intern. Med.*, **93**, 391–8.

36. Medical Research Council Working Party (1981) Long term domiciliary oxygen therapy in chronic hypoxic cor pulmonale complicating chronic bronchitis and emphysema. *Lancet*, **i**, 681–6.

37. Timms, R.M., Khaja, F.U., Williams, G.W. *et al.* (1985) Hemodynamic response to oxygen therapy in chronic obstructive pulmonary disease. *Ann. Intern. Med.*, **102**, 29–36.

38. Ashutosh, K., Mead, G. and Dunksy, M. (1983) Early effects of oxygen administration and prognosis in chronic obstructive pulmonary disease and cor pulmonale. *Am. Rev. Respir. Dis.*, **127**, 399–404.

39. Weitzenblum, E., Sautegeau, A., Ehrhart, M. *et al.* (1985) Long-term oxygen therapy can reverse the progression of pulmonary hypertension in patients with chronic obstructive pulmonary disease. *Am. Rev. Respir. Dis.*, **131**, 493–8.

40. Fletcher, E.C. and Levin, D.C. (1984) Cardiopulmonary hemodynamics during sleep in subjects with chronic obstructive pulmonary disease. The effect of short- and-long term oxygen. *Chest*, **85**, 6–14.

41. Keller, R., Ragaz, A. and Borer, P. (1985) Predictors for early mortality in patients with

long-term oxygen home therapy. *Respiration*, **48**, 216–21.

42. Ashutosh, K. and Dunsky, M. (1987) Noninvasive tests for responsiveness of pulmonary hypertension to oxygen. Prediction of survival in patients with chronic obstructive lung disease and cor pulmonale. *Chest*, **92**, 393–9.

43. Sliwinski, P., Hawrylkiewicz, I., Goreca, D. and Zielinski, J. (1992) Acute effects of oxygen on pulmonary arterial pressure does not predict survival on long-term oxygen therapy in chronic obstructive pulmonary disease. *Am. Rev. Respir. Dis.*, **146**, 665–9.

44. Wilkinson, M., Langhorne, C.A., Heath, D. *et al.* (1988) A pathophysiological study of 10 cases of hypoxic cor pulmonale. *Q. J. Med.*, **249**, 65–85.

45. Cooper, C.B., Waterhouse, J. and Howard, P. (1987) Twelve year clinical study of patients with hypoxic cor pulmonale given long term domiciliary oxygen therapy. *Thorax*, **42**, 105–10.

46. Cooper, C.B. and Howard, P. (1991) An analysis of sequential physiologic changes in hypoxic cor pulmonale during long-term oxygen therapy. *Chest*, **100**, 76–80.

47. Block, A.J., Castle, J.R. and Keitt, A.S. (1974) Chronic oxygen therapy. Treatment of chronic obstructive pulmonary disease at sea level. *Chest*, **65**, 279–88.

48. Calverley, P.M.A., Leggett, R.J., McElderry, L. and Flenley, D.C. (1982) Cigarette smoking and secondary polycythemia in hypoxic cor pulmonale. *Am. Rev. Respir. Dis.*, **125**, 507–10.

49. Johnson, T.S., Ellis, J.H. Jr and Steel, P.P. (1978) Improvement in platelet survival time with oxygen in patients with chronic obstructive airway disease. *Am. Rev. Respir. Dis.*, **117**, 255–7.

50. Grant, I., Heaton, R.K., McSweeney, A.J. *et al.* (1982) Neuropsychologic findings in hypoxemic chronic obstructive pulmonary disease. *Arch. Intern. Med.*, **142**, 1470–6.

51. Krop, H.D., Block, A.J. and Cohen, E. (1973) Neuropsychologic effects of continuous oxygen therapy in chronic obstructive pulmonary disease. *Chest*, **64**, 317–22.

52. Heaton, R.K., Grant, I., McSweeney, A.J. *et al.* (1983) Psychologic effects of continuous and nocturnal oygen therapy in hypoxemic chronic obstructive pulmonary disease. *Arch. Intern. Med.*, **143**, 1941–7.

53. Raimondi, A.C., Edwards, R.H.T., Denison, D.M. *et al.* (1970) Exercise tolerance breathing a low density gas mixture, 35% oxygen and air in patients with chronic obstructive bronchitis. *Clin. Sci.*, **39**, 675–85.

54. Bradley, B.L., Garner, A.E., Billiu, D. *et al.* (1978) Oxygen-assisted exercise in chronic obstructive lung disease. *Am. Rev. Respir. Dis.*, **118**, 239–43.

55. Woodcock, A.A., Gross, E.R. and Geddes, D.M. (1981) Oxygen relieves breathlessness in 'pink puffers'. *Lancet*, **i**, 907–9.

56. Swinburn, C.R., Wakefield, J.M. and Jones, P.W. (1984) Relationship between ventilation and breathlessness during exercise in chronic obstructive airways disease is not altered by prevention of hypoxemia. *Clin. Sci.*, **67**, 515–9.

57. Davidson, A.C., Leach, R., George, R.J.D. and Geddes, D.M. (1988) Supplemental oxygen and exercise ability in chronic obstructive airways disease. *Thorax*, **43**, 965–71.

58. Zack, M.B. and Palange, A.V. (1985) Oxygen supplemented exercise of ventilatory and non-ventilatory muscles in pulmonary rehabilitation. *Chest*, **88**, 669–75.

59. Lilker, E.S., Karnick, A. and Lerner, L. (1975) Portable oxygen in chronic obstructive lung disease with hypoxemia and cor pulmonale. A controlled double-blind crossover study. *Chest*, **68**, 236–41.

60. Leggett, R.J.E. and Flenley, D.C. (1977) Portable oxgyen and exercise tolerance in patients with chronic hypoxic cor pulmonale. *Br. Med. J.*, **2**, 84–6.

61. Longo, A.M., Moser, K.M. and Luchsinger, P.C. (1971) The role of oxygen therapy in the rehabilitation of patients with chronic obstructive pulmonary disease. *Am. Rev. Respir. Dis.*, **103**, 690–7.

62. Bye, P.T.P., Anderson, A.S.D., Woolcock, A.J. *et al.* (1982) Bicycle endurance performance of patients with interstitial lung disease breathing air and oxygen. *Am. Rev. Respir. Dis.*, **126**, 1005–12.

63. Leach, R.M., Davidson, A.C., Chinn, S. *et al.* (1992) Portable liquid oxygen and exercise ability in severe respiratory disability. *Thorax*, **47**, 781–9.

64. Woolf, C.R. and Suero, J.T. (1969) Alterations in lung mechanics and gas exchange following training in chronic obstructive lung disease. *Dis. Chest*, **55**, 37–44.

65. Waterhouse, J.C. and Howard, P. (1983) Breathlessness and portable oxygen in chronic obstructive airways disease. *Thorax*, **38**, 302–6.

66. The Drug Tariff (1986) Introduction of oxygen concentrators to the domiciliary oxygen therapy service. Department of Health and Social Security, London, (Publication #FPN 398).

67. Home oxygen – still room for improvement (1990) *Drug. Ther. Bull.*, **28**, 99–100.

68. Report of a SEP Task Group (1989) Recommendations for long term oxygen therapy (LTOT). *Eur. Respir. J.*, **2**, 160–4.

69. Strom, K. and Boe, J. (1989) A national register for long-term oxygen therapy in chronic hypoxia: preliminary results. *Eur. Respir. J.*, **1**, 952–8.

70. Conference Report (1990) New problems in supply, reimbursement, and certification of medical necessity for long-term therapy. *Am. Rev. Respir. Dis.*, **142**, 721–4.

71. Breslin, A.B.X., Colebatch, H.J.H., Engel, L. *et al.* (1985) Domiciliary oxygen treatment. *Med. J. Aust.*, **142**, 508–10.

72. Williams, B.T. and Nicholl, J.P. (1985) Prevalence of hypoxaemic chronic obstructive lung disease with reference to long-term oxygen therapy. *Lancet*, **ii**, 369–72.

73. Timms, R.M., Kvale, P.A., Anthonisen, N.R. *et al.* (1981) Selection of patients with chronic obstructive pulmonary disease for long-term oxygen therapy. *JAMA*, **245**, 2514–6.

74. Levi-Valensi, P., Weitzenblum, E., Pedinielli, J-L. *et al.* (1986) Three-month follow-up of arterial blood gas determinations in candidates for long-term oxygen therapy. A multicentric study. *Am. Rev. Respir. Dis.*, **133**, 547–51.

75. O'Donahue, W.J. Jr (1991) Effect of oxygen therapy on increasing arterial oxygen tension in hypoxemic patients with stable chronic obstructive pulmonary disease while breathing ambient air. *Chest*, **100**, 968–72.

76. Stretton, T.B. (1985) Provision of long term oxygen therapy. *Thorax*, **40**, 801–5.

77. Conference Report (1988) Further recommendations for prescribing and supplying long-term oxygen therapy. *Am. Rev. Respir. Dis.*, **138**, 745–7.

78. McCallion, J. and Pearce, S.J. (1988) Oxygen concentrators: which patients are being treated and are the DHSS guidelines being followed? *Thorax*, **44**, 859P (Abstract).

79. Douglas, N.J., Calverley, P.M.A., Leggett, R.J.E. *et al.* (1979) Transient hypoxemia during sleep in chronic bronchitis and emphysema. *Lancet*, **i**, 1–4.

80. Tirlapur, V.G. and Mir, M.A. (1982) Nocturnal hypoxemia and associated electrocardiographic changes in patients with chronic obstructive airways disease. *N. Engl. J. Med.*, **306**, 125–30.

81. Boysen, P.G., Block, A.J., Wynne, J.W. *et al.* (1979) Nocturnal pulmonary hypertension in patients with chronic obstructive pulmonary disease. *Chest*, **76**, 536–42.

82. DeMarco, F.J., Wynne, J.W., Block, A.J. *et al.* (1981) Oxygen desaturation during sleep as a determinant of the 'blue and bloated' syndrome. *Chest*, **79**, 621–5.

83. Levi-Valensi, P., Weitzenblum, E., Rida, Z. *et al.* (1992) Sleep-related oxgyen desaturation and daytime pulmonary haemodynamics in COPD patients. *Eur. Respir. J.*, **5**, 301–7.

84. Fletcher, E.C., Luckett, R.A., Miller, T. *et al.* (1989) Exercise hemodynamics and gas exchange in patients with chronic obstructive pulmonary disease, sleep desaturation and a daytime PaO_2 above 60 mmHg. *Am. Rev. Respir. Dis.*, **140**, 1237–45.

85. Calverley, P.M.A., Brezinova, V., Douglas, N.J. *et al.* (1982) The effect of oxygenation on sleep quality in chronic bronchitis and emphysema. *Am. Rev. Respir. Dis.*, **126**, 206–10.

86. Goldstein, R.S., Rancharan, V., Bowes, G. *et al.* (1984) Effect of supplemental nocturnal oxygen on gas exchange in patients with severe obstructive lung disease. *N. Engl. J. Med.*, **310**, 425–9.

87. Gong, H., Tashkin, D.P., Lee, E.Y. *et al.* (1984) Hypoxia-altitude simulation test. Evaluation of patients with chronic airway obstruction. *Am. Rev. Respir. Dis.*, **130**, 980–6.

88. West, G.A. and Primeau, P. (1983) Nonmedical hazards of long-term oxygen therapy. *Respir. Care*, **28**, 906–12.

89. McDonald, G.J. (1983) Long-term oxygen therapy delivery systems. *Respir. Care*, **28**, 898–905.

90. Lowson, K.V., Drummond, M.F. and Bishop, J.M. (1981) Costing new services: Long-term domiciliary oxygen therapy. *Lancet*, **i**, 1146–9.

91. Bongard, J.P., Pahud, C. and DeHaller, R. (1989) Insufficient oxygen concentration obtained at domiciliary controls of eighteen concentrators. *Eur. Respir. J.*, **2**, 280–2.

92. Evans, T.W., Waterhouse, J. and Howard, P. (1983) Clinical experience with the oxygen concentrator. *Br. Med. J.*, **287**, 459–61.

93. Johns, D.P., Rochford, P.D. and Streeton, J.A. (1985) Evaluation of six oxgyen concentrators. *Thorax*, **40**, 806–10.

94. Gould, G.A., Scott, W., Hayhurst, M.D. and Flenley, D.C. (1985) Technical and clinical assessment of oxygen concentrators. *Thorax*, **40**, 811–6.

95. Sous-Commission Technique ANTADIR (1991) Home controls of a sample of 2414 oxygen concentrators. *Eur. Respir. J.*, **4**, 227–31.

96. Akutsu, T., Ishihara, J., Wakai, Y. *et al.* (1990) Development and clinical application of a portable oxygen concentrator. *Frontiers Med. Biol. Eng.*, **2**, 293–301.

97. Green, I.D. (1967) Choice of method for administration of oxygen. *Br. Med. J.*, **3**, 593–6.

98. Leigh, J.M. (1970) Variation in performance of oxygen therapy devices. *Anesthesia*, **25**, 210–22.

99. Gould, G.A., Forsyth, I.S. and Flenley, D.C. (1986) Comparison of two oxygen conserving nasal prong systems and the effects of nose and mouth breathing. *Thorax*, **41**, 808–9.

100. Bazuaye, E.A., Stone, T.N., Corris, P.A. and Gibson, A.J. (1992) Variability of inspired oxygen concentration with nasal cannulas. *Thorax*, **47**, 609–11.

101. Heimlich, H.J. (1982) Respiratory rehabilitation with transtracheal oxygen system. *Ann. Otol. Rhinol. Laryngol.*, **91**, 643–7.

102. Heimlich, H.J. and Carr, G.C. (1985) Transtracheal catheter technique for pulmonary rehabilitation. *Ann. Otol. Rhinol. Laryngol.*, **94**, 502–4.

103. Christopher, K.L., Spofford, B.T., Brannin, P.K. *et al.* (1986) Transtracheal oxygen therapy for refractory hypoxemia. *JAMA*, **256**, 494–7.

104. Christopher, K.L., Spofford, B.T., Petrun, M.D. *et al.* (1987) A program for transtracheal oxygen delivery. Assessment of safety and efficacy. *Ann. Intern. Med.*, **107**, 802–8.

105. Walsh, D.A. and Govan, J.R. (1990) Long term continuous domiciliary oxygen therapy by transtracheal catheter. *Thorax*, **45**, 478–81.

106. Hoffman, L.A., Johnson, J.T., Wesmiller, S.W., *et al.* (1991) Transtracheal delivery of oxygen: efficacy and safety for long-term continuous therapy. *Ann. Otol. Rhinol. Laryngol.*, **100**, 108–15.

107. Banner, N.R. and Govan, J.R. (1986) Long term transtracheal oxygen delivery through microcatheter in patients with hypoxaemia due to chronic obstructive airways disease. *Br. Med. J.*, **293**, 111–4.

108. Johnson, L.P. and Cary, J.M. (1987) The implanted intratracheal oxygen catheter. *Surg. Gynecol. Obstet.*, **165**, 75–6.

109. Bloom, B.S., Daniel, J.M., Wiseman, M. *et al.* (1989) Transtracheal oxygen delivery and patients with chronic obstructive pulmonary disease. *Respir. Med.*, **83**, 281–8.

110. Wesmiller, S.W., Hoffman, L.A., Sciurba, F.C. *et al.* (1990) Exercise tolerance during nasal cannula and transtracheal oxygen delivery. *Am. Rev. Respir. Dis.*, **141**, 789–91.

111. Hoffman, L.A., Dauber, J.H., Ferson, P.F. *et al.* (1987) Patient response to transtracheal oxygen delivery. *Am. Rev. Respir. Dis.*, **135**, 153–6.

112. Couser, J.I. Jr and Make, B.J. (1989) Transtracheal oxygen decreases inspired minute ventilation. *Am. Rev. Respir. Dis.*, **139**, 627–31.

113. Fletcher, E.C., Nickeson, D. and Costarangos-Galarza, C. (1988) Endotracheal mass resulting from a transtracheal oxygen catheter. *Chest*, **93**, 438–9.

114. Adamo, J.P., Mehta, A.C., Stelmach, K. *et al.* (1990) The Cleveland Clinic's initial experience with transtracheal oxygen therapy. *Respir. Care*, **35**, 153–60.

115. Tiep, B.L., Nicotra, B., Carter, R. *et al.* (1984) Evaluation of low-flow oxygen-conserving nasal cannula. *Am. Rev. Respir. Dis.*, **130**, 500–2.

116. Moore-Gillon, J.C., George, R.J.D. and Geddes, D.M. (1985) An oxygen conserving nasal cannula. *Thorax*, **40**, 817–9.

117. Soffer, M., Tashkin, D.P., Shapiro, B.J., *et al.* (1985) Conservation of oxygen supply using a reservoir nasal cannula in hypoxemic patients at rest and during exercise. *Chest*, **88**, 663–8.

118. Tiep, B.L., Belman, M.J., Mittman, C. *et al.* (1985) A new pendant storage oxygen-conserving nasal cannula. *Chest*, **87**, 381–3.

119. Gonzales, S.C., Huntington, D., Romo, R. and Light, R.W. (1986) Efficacy of the Oxymizer Pendant in reducing oxygen requirements of hypoxemic patients. *Respir. Care*, **31**, 681–8.

120. Claiborne, R.A., Paynter, D.E., Dutt, A.K. *et al.* (1987) Evaluation of the use of an oxygen

conservation device in long-term oxygen therapy. *Am. Rev. Respir. Dis.*, **136**, 1095–8.

121. Carter, R., Williams, J.S., Berry, J. *et al* (1986) Evaluation of the pendant oxygen-conserving nasal cannula during exercise. *Chest*, **89**, 806–10.

122. Gould, G.A., Hayhurst, M.D., Scott, W. and Flenley, D.C. (1985) Clinical assessment of oxygen conserving devices in chronic bronchitis and emphysema. *Thorax*, **40**, 820–4.

123. Cotes, J.E. (1963) Continuous versus intermittent administration of oxygen during exercise to patients with chronic lung disease. *Lancet*, **i**, 1075–7.

124. Pflug, A.E., Cheney, F.W. Jr, and Butler, J. (1972) Evaluation of an intermittent oxygen flow system. *Am. Rev. Respir. Dis.*, **105**, 449–52.

125. Auerbach, D., Flick, M.R. and Block, A.J. (1978) A new cannula system using intermittent-demand nasal flow. *Chest*, **74**, 39–43.

126. Tiep, B.L., Nicotra, N.B., Carter, P.R. *et al.* (1985) Low-concentration oxygen therapy via a demand oxygen delivery system. *Chest*, **87**, 636–8.

127. Mecikalski, M. and Shigeoka, J.W. (1984) A demand valve conserves oxgyen in subjects with chronic obstructive pulmonary disease. *Chest*, **86**, 667–70.

128. Winter, R.J.D., George, R.J.D., Moore-Gillon, J.C. *et al.* (1984) Inspiration-phased oxygen delivery. *Lancet*, **i**, 1371–2.

129. Tiep, B.L., Carter, R., Nicotra, B. *et al.* (1987) Demand oxygen delivery during exercise. *Chest*, **91**, 15–20.

130. Leger, P., Gerard, M. and Robert, D. (1986) Simultaneous use of a pulsed dose demand valve (PDV) with a transtracheal catheter (TTC): an optimal O_2 saving for long term O_2 therapy. *Am. Rev. Respir. Dis.*, **133**, 350 (abstract).

131. Tiep, B.L., Christopher, K.L., Spofford, B.T. *et al.* (1990) Pulsed nasal and transtracheal oxygen delivery. *Chest*, **97**, 364–8.

132. Baudouin, S.V., Waterhouse, J.C., Tahtamouni, T. *et al.* (1990) Long term domiciliary oxygen treatment for chronic respiratory failure reviewed. *Thorax*, **45**, 195–8.

133. Walshaw, M.J., Lim, R., Evans, C.C. *et al.* (1988) Prescription of oxygen concentrators for long-term oxygen treatment: reassessment in one district. *Br. Med. J.*, **297**, 1030–2.

134. Dilworth, J.P., Higgs, C.M.B., Jones, P.A. *et al.* (1989) Prescription of oxygen concentrators: adherence to published guidelines. *Thorax*, **44**, 576–8.

135. North Western Regional Health Authority (1983) Pilot development of domiciliary oxygen concentrators. Report No. 4/9/176. Manchester, North Western Regional Health Authority.

136. Vergeret, G., Tunon de Lara, M., Douvier, J.J. *et al.* (1986) Compliance of COPD patients with long term oxygen therapy. *Eur. J. Respir. Dis.*, **69** (Suppl.146), 421–5.

137. Prignot, J. (1987) Home monitoring of patients on long-term oxygen therapy. *Bull. Int. Union Tuberc. Lung Dis.*, **62**, 33–4.

138. Hansen, J.E. (1982) Participant responses to blood gas proficiency testing reports. *Chest*, **101**, 1240–4.

139. Bromberg, P.A., Lewis, B.F. (1980) Monitoring oxygen therapy. *Am. Rev. Respir. Dis.*, **122**, 55–9.

140. Shapiro, B.A. (1992) *In-vivo* monitoring of arterial blood gases and pH. *Respir. Care*, **37**, 165–9.

141. Hannhart, B., Haberer, J-P., Saumier, C. *et al.* (1991) Accuracy and precision of fourteen pulse oximeters. *Eur. Resp. J.*, **4**, 115–9.

142. Saunders, N.A., Powles, A.C.P. and Rebuck, A.S. (1976) Ear oximetry: accuracy and practicability in the assessment of arterial oxygenation. *Am. Rev. Respir. Dis.*, **113**, 745–9.

143. Chaudhary, B.A. and Burki, N.K. (1978) Ear oximetry in clinical practice. *Am. Rev. Respir. Dis.*, **117**, 173–5.

144. Wyss, C.R., Matsen, F.A., King, R.V. *et al.* (1981) Dependence of trans-cutaneous oxygen tension on local arterial-venous pressure gradient in normal subjects. *Clin. Sci.*, **60**, 499–506.

145. Gothgen, I. and Jacobsen, E. (1978) Transcutaneous oxygen tension measurement I. Age variation and reproducibility. *Acta Anaesthesiol. Scand.*, Suppl. **67**, 66–70.

146. Peabody, J.L., Willis, M.M., Gregory, G.A. *et al.* (1978) Clinical limitations and advantages of transcutaneous oxygen electrodes. *Acta Anaesthesiol Scand.*, Suppl. **68**, 76–82.

147. Dowd, G.S.E., Linge, K. and Bentley, G. (1982) Transcutaneous PO_2 measurement in skin ischemia. *Lancet*, **i**, 48.

148. Wyss, C.R., Matsen, F.A., Simmons, C.W. *et al.* (1984) Transcutaneous oxygen tension

measurements on limbs of diabetic and non diabetic patients with peripheral vascular disease. *Surgery*, **95**, 339–46.

149. Pratt, P.C. (1965) The reaction of the human lung to enriched oxygen atmosphere. *Ann. NY Acad. Sci.*, **121**, 809–22.

150. Pratt, P.C. (1974) Pathology of pulmonary oxygen toxicity. *Am. Rev. Respir. Dis.*, **110**, 51–7.

151. White, C.W., Avraham, K.B., Stanley, P.F. *et al.* (1991) Transgenic mice with expression of elevated copper-zinc superoxide dismutase in the lungs are resistant to pulmonary oxygen toxicity. *J. Clin. Invest.*, **87**, 2162–8.

152. Morgan, T.E. Jr, Cutler, R.G., Shaw, E.G. *et al.* (1963) Physiologic effect of exposure to increased oxygen tension at 5 psia. *Aerospace Med.*, **34**, 720–6.

153. Sevitt, S. (1974) Diffuse and focal oxygen pneumonitis: A preliminary report on the threshold of pulmonary oxygen toxicity in man. *J. Clin. Pathol.*, **27**, 21–30.

154. Welch, B.E., Morgan, T.E. Jr and Clamann, H.G. (1963) Time-concentration effects in relation to oxygen toxicity in man. *Fed. Proc.*, **22**, 1053–6.

155. Petty, T.L., Stanford, R.E. and Neff, T.A. (1971) Continuous oxygen therapy in chronic airway obstruction: Observations on possible oxygen toxicity and survival. *Ann. Intern. Med.*, **75**, 361–7.

156. Nolte, D. (1976) Nutzen und Gefahren der Sauerstoff-therapie bei chronischer Atemin-suffizienz. *Wien. Med. Wochenschr.*, **126**, 325–9.

157. Neff, T.A. and Petty, T.L. (1972) Tolerance and survival in severe chronic hypercapnia. *Arch. Intern. Med.*, **129**, 591–6.

158. Barach, A.L. (1974) Hypercapnia in chronic obstructive lung disease – an adaptive response to low-flow oxygen therapy. *Chest*, **66**, 112–3.

159. Muir, J.F. and Laumonier, F. (1990) Living conditions of serious chronic insufficiency patients treated at home on oxygen therapy or assisted ventilation. *Lung*, **168** (suppl.) 489–94.

160. McKeon, J.L., Saunders, N.A. and Murree-Allen, K. (1987) Domiciliary oxygen: rationalization of supply in the Hunter region from 1982–1986. *Med. J. Aust.*, **146**, 73–8.

C.J. Clark

Pulmonary rehabilitation has been defined [1] as the 'art of medical practice where an individually tailored, multidisciplinary program is formulated which through accurate diagnosis, therapy, emotional support and education, stabilizes or reverses both the physio- and psychopathology of pulmonary diseases and attempts to return the patient to the highest possible functional capacity allowed by his pulmonary handicap and overall life situation.' This global definition indicates the potential difficulties involved in the evaluation of the efficacy of rehabilitation treatment. There is tacit recognition that:

1. diagnosis is a component of pulmonary rehabilitation hopefully leading to improved patient characterization before treatment,
2. treatment requirements will vary between individuals,
3. the program is a process using existing treatments, and designed to integrate together the various components which have proven efficacy, and finally
4. at best the patient will remain handicapped by his illness.

This chapter will provide a current perspective on the principles of pulmonary rehabilitation, the type of patient for whom it is proposed, its various components including the required infrastructure and finally evidence that any or all of these components provide benefit.

COPD is a frustrating illness not only for patients, who may suffer considerable psychopathology [2] but also for their physicians whose medical treatment has only partial success in alleviating symptoms and improving functional capacity. Not only are mortality rates high [3] but so is the level of morbidity and this is responsible for a high proportion of health care costs in different countries [4]. In a recent historical perspective, Petty [5] has traced the roots of pulmonary rehabilitation from the period when tuberculosis was prevalent and required prolonged convalescence to the pioneering contributions from Drs Barach and Haas, whose personal clinical observations led them to believe that a systematic program of physical exercise and breathing training could improve exercise tolerance and general wellbeing, not only in patients with tuberculosis but also emphysema. Subsequently a consensus view was published [6] on the use of systematized care for patients with COPD and then the scientific basis for inpatient therapy was reviewed [7]. Over the past decade individual contributors have published their experience with a variety of programs and now there is an increasing interest in pulmonary rehabilitation with the development of improved methodologies for measurement of exercise performance

Chronic Obstructive Pulmonary Disease. Edited by Dr P. Calverley and Professor N. Pride. Published in 1995 by Chapman & Hall, London. ISBN 0 412 46450 0

respiratory muscle function, sleep studies and subjective measures such as breathlessness, anxiety and depression and quality of life.

21.1 COMPONENTS OF A COMPREHENSIVE REHABILITATION PROGRAM

Recent European [8] and North American [9] guidelines recommend that all of the components listed in Table 21.1 should be systematically considered within a pulmonary rehabilitation program. The strength of the scientific rationale for each component is variable. Several aspects such as oxygen therapy and respiratory muscle training are addressed in detail elsewhere (Chapters 9, 20) and will be mentioned here only briefly in the context of their potential contribution to the outcome of rehabilitation programs.

I will not attempt to prioritize individual components and an alternative to the inclusion of all of these in setting up a rehabilitation program [9a], is to consider how much of the contents of Table 21.1 is already included in existing routine medical services. Pulmonary rehabilitation should be viewed as an adjunct and not an alternative to routine respiratory care.

21.1.1 EXERCISE TRAINING

The rationale for exercise training in pulmonary rehabilitation is that the 'condition of exercise is not a mere variant of the condition of rest, it is the essence of the machine' [10]. There are essentially two different practical strategies for exercise rehabilitation, depending on the patient under consideration. The first approach attempts to improve cardiorespiratory fitness by aerobic (continuous and rhythmic) exercise of 20–30 min duration at least 3 times a week [11]. The type of activity is not critical but the exercise intensity should increase oxygen uptake to a level commensurate with a 'training effect' on both heart (i.e. improving stroke volume) and peripheral muscle (i.e. increasing oxygen extraction) [12]. There remains controversy regarding the suitability of this (aerobic) approach in COPD patients. It has been suggested [13] that these patients would be unable to achieve the required training effect through inability to tolerate exercise at the critical training intensity because of breathlessness [14]. However, Casaburi and colleagues have shown that specific subgroups of patients (generally those with mild to moderate exercise limit-

Table 21.1 Components of a pulmonary rehabilitation program [9]

Pharmacological therapy: Bronchodilators, anti-allergics, corticosteroids, antibiotics, immunization (e.g. influenza)
Education: Pathophysiology, use of peak flow meter, use of drugs, including their administration side-effects, avoidance of aggravating stimuli, cessation of smoking, family education
Physical therapy: Breathing retraining, relaxation techniques, mobilization exercises, postural drainage, vibration, coughing
Exercise conditioning: Endurance training, interval training, improvement of mechanical skills, desensitization to dyspnea, training in activities of daily life
Occupational therapy: Ergonomics, vocational therapy
Psychosocial support: Psychological counselling, psychopharmacological agents, group therapy, support of family, sexual counselling
Follow-up treatment: Visiting nurses, general practitioners, patient organizations, 'refresher' courses
Oxygen therapy: If necessary
Nutritional therapy: If necessary
Respiratory muscles: Inspiratory muscle training, active expiration, resting respiratory muscles, ventilator weaning

---

The relative importance of these components varies depending on the patient under consideration, i.e. not all are applicable to every patient in pulmonary rehabilitation programmes.

ation but including the more severely disabled patients who can reach a lactic 'threshold') can develop these physiologic adaptations resulting in substantial reductions of minute ventilation at equivalent submaximal workloads following training [15, 16]. This group recommends the use of exercise testing to identify those COPD patients who can reach this threshold and then train them at this level of exercise intensity.

The second approach applies to patients who cannot sustain sufficient exercise to improve aerobic fitness because of breathlessness; they need to improve mobility and stamina, rather than achieve physiologic 'fitness' targets [17]. An important component of perceived exertion in these patients is the sense of discomfort and fatigue in exercising muscle caused by enforced periods of inactivity in any patient with chronic illness [18]. Suboptimal conditioning of muscle is common and this has been described as the 'cycle of deconditioning' present in any excessively sedentary individual. Adaptations resulting from chronic dynamic exercise of individual muscles consist of increased oxygen extraction through muscle fibre hypertrophy, increased mitochondrial volume and capillary blood supply [19]. Jones and colleagues [20] showed twice the average intensity of leg discomfort in COPD patients at maximal exercise as compared with normal subjects at the same exercise intensity, although breathlessness remained the major limiting factor. Skeletal muscle fatigue has been demonstrated in patients with COPD using EMG fatigue criteria [21] and static strength of peripheral skeletal muscle may be significantly lower in patients with airflow limitation presumably because of deconditioning [22]. A number of programs have simply provided regular exercise sessions where the patient works at the maximal tolerable ventilatory limit and have shown considerable benefit in improving mobility [17].

An alternative approach to rhythmic, repetitive whole body exercise has been specific muscle training. In one study [23] a standard weightlifting program for both upper and lower limb muscles with isotonic repetitions at 60% of maximal muscle capacity produced improved muscle strength. Endurance time during cycling at 80% of maximum workload also increased by 73% with no change in control subjects. There were also significant improvements in daily breathlessness and 'mastery' of daily living activities. Another study used a program more suitable for the home environment requiring no gymnasium facilities, i.e. relying on isotonic muscle repetitions carefully designed so as not to exceed the maximum capacity of individual patients, following an initial hospital assessment [24]. Marked improvements in muscle strength and endurance plus overall exercise tolerance as measured by endurance time during steady state treadmill walking were observed.

(a) Upper limb exercise training

In patients with COPD the stabilizing effect of the shoulder girdle is important to offset the mechanical disadvantage of hyperinflation to the respiratory muscles. This may be lost during work involving the upper extremities resulting in dyssynchronous breathing [25, 26]. Breathlessness is therefore often pronounced during such activities [25] producing greater limitation than during leg exercise at equivalent 'whole body' work. Current approaches to upper limb training exercises have included cycle ergometry with varying resistances, unsupported arm exercise, raising a ball with the arms above the horizontal, passing a bean bag over the head and isotonic exercises, i.e. repeated muscle contractions using standard multi-gym facilities [27,28]. Session duration, the number per week and the length of the program require to be approximately the same as those for lower body training [29,30]. These studies have shown no change in respiratory muscle function despite which improvements in upper limb endurance were demonstrated.

(b) Exercise rehabilitation in the presence of arterial blood gas abnormalities during exercise

These patients form a subgroup for whom there are no guidelines for rehabilitation programs. Carefully supervised exercise conditioning with oxygen supplementation in a hospital gymnasium setting would seem to be an appropriate approach to the management of those patients who develop hypoxemia during exercise. These individuals cannot usually be predicted from resting measurements of pulmonary function or gas exchange [31,32]. While there are no published data documenting the effects of supplemental oxygen on exercise rehabilitation outcomes, a number of studies have demonstrated improvement in exercise tolerance during oxygen use compared with air even in non-hypoxemic patients [33,34,35,36]. The magnitude of this effect is often small and idiosyncratic, restricted to individual patients rather than a predictable group effect. The best rationale for oxygen use in rehabilitation at present would be to ensure that exercise prescription is safe, i.e. to rule out the potential for cardiac events secondary to severe arterial oxygen desaturation during exercise. This is, however, an assumption as there are no data currently available regarding the prevalence of adverse cardiac events during exercise in COPD. Resting hypercapnia should not be considered a contraindication to pulmonary rehabilitation. One study of patients with resting hypercapnia showed improved exercise tolerance of a similar magnitude to a parallel group of eucapnic patients after pulmonary rehabilitation, without adverse effects [37].

(c) Specific components designed to alleviate ventilatory limitation during exercise

Two strategies to reduce ventilatory limitation during exercise have recently been investigated; respiratory muscle training and ventilatory-assist devices.

(i) Respiratory muscle training

There has been a recent shift in research emphasis from attempts to train respiratory muscle using overload techniques (i.e. performance of work beyond a critical level) to improve exercise tolerance in COPD [38] towards the potential role of periodic rest in the reduction of incipient muscle fatigue [39]. Despite a major emphasis on the possible benefits of respiratory muscle training [40] its failure to consistently produce favourable results has been highlighted in a recent meta-analysis [41] and this is probably related to multiple factors such as patient selection, specific methods for respiratory muscle training and continuing doubt as to the role of respiratory muscle fatigue in ventilatory limitation in COPD [42,43]. This topic is considered in further detail elsewhere (Chapter 9). However, two studies support the use of resistive inspiratory loading during pulmonary rehabilitation [44,45]. Both studies showed a reduction in breathlessness and one [44] showed improved ventilatory muscle strength, endurance and exercise capacity. The clinical relevance of these small changes is uncertain. There is a need for further longitudinal controlled studies, closely monitoring breathing strategy to ensure that the ventilatory muscles are appropriately and progressively loaded. Meantime, since rehabilitation treatment of many kinds may induce a component of respiratory muscle training [46] it is logical to include simple measurements such as P_I max and P_E max to monitor any global improvements in respiratory muscle function which may accrue.

(ii) Ventilatory assistance during exercise

Continuous positive airway pressure (CPAP) has been used recently during exercise in patients with severe COPD. Expiratory flow rates during tidal breathing in such patients are close to or equal to the maximum expiratory flow–volume relationship [47,48]. COPD patients can increase expiratory flow rates during exercise through dynamic hyper-inflation [49] but this is offset by an increase in inspiratory work since tidal volume operates in a less compliant range of the pressure–volume relationship and initiation of inspiration requires additional inspiratory pressure to overcome increased elastic recoil of the respiratory system [50]. This 'intrinsic PEEP' has been reported in COPD patients during exercise [51,52]. The application of continuous positive airway pressure (CPAP) may counterbalance increased recoil pressure at end-expiration and thus reduce dyspnea and work of breathing as seen during weaning from mechanical ventilation [53]. A recent study [54] showed that the application of approximately 10 cmH_2O of CPAP during exercise significantly improved breathlessness in 5 of 8 patients studied. The 3 remaining subjects experienced a deterioration in breathlessness. Transdiaphragmatic pressure measurements showed a complicated picture but suggested that the relief of breathlessness was related to a reduction in time-integrals of esophageal and diaphragmatic pressures whereas in the patients with deterioration excessive abdominal muscle recruitment was occurring as shown by increases in the pressure–time integral of gastric pressure.

In another study [55] CPAP improved breathlessness during exercise in 8 COPD patients and continuous positive inspiratory pressure; unloading of the inspiratory muscles appeared to be the predominant mechanism as opposed to effects on dynamic compression during expiration because continuous positive expiratory pressure alone did not relieve breathlessness. The magnitude of the improved exercise endurance appeared potentially clinically relevant, increasing tolerance of submaximal exercise at approximately 70% of maximum work capacity from approximately 6 to 9 min. Further work is required to determine the role of this form of treatment in pulmonary rehabilitation, either to provide ventilatory assistance during exercise training or, if mobile devices are feasible to improve daily exercise performance in severely limited patients. The role of CPAP currently remains as a research tool.

21.1.2 CONTROLLED BREATHING TECHNIQUES

Controlled breathing techniques attempt to diminish breathlessness by training patients to breath in an efficient and comfortable fashion. Over 30 years ago Barach and Miller [56,57] recognized that COPD patients could reduce breathlessness by consciously altering their breathing patterns. The goals of controlled breathing techniques have been defined [58] as: (a) to restore the diaphragm to a more normal position and function, (b) to decrease the respiratory rate by employing a breathing pattern that diminishes air trapping and improves the respiratory duty cycle, (c) to diminish the work of breathing, and (d) to reduce dyspnea and allay patient anxiety.

Pursed-lip breathing is usually the easiest breathing technique to learn. A number of authors have observed a substantial increase in tidal volume with reduced respiratory rate and minute ventilation both at rest and during exercise. Those patients with the greatest reduction in breathlessness demonstrated the largest changes in breathing pattern [58]. Pursed-lip breathing at rest has been demonstrated to reduce arterial P_{CO_2} and improve P_{O_2} at rest [59]. The physiologic responses to pursed-lip breathing have been investigated. Functional residual capacity decreases insignificantly and therefore improved breathlessness cannot be due to the effects of diminished end-expiratory lung volume on length–tension relationships of the diaphragm [60, 61].

Pursed-lip breathing has been simulated employing an apparatus including a rubber stopper with a small orifice to mimic the technique. Those subjects who experienced spontaneous relief of dyspnea during pursed-lip breathing were found to have significantly greater reduction in non-elastic expiratory resistance when they used the artificial system leading the authors to conclude that pursed-lip breathing was likely to lessen dynamic airways collapse. There is no evidence that reduction in breathlessness is due to diminution of the work of breathing [62] and indeed a recent study has shown a substantial increase in the inspiratory work of breathing in 12 patients with chronic airways obstruction [63]. These authors examined the effects of the technique on respiratory muscle function for the first time, and showed that at rest pursed-lip breathing shifted a major portion of inspiratory work from the diaphragm to rib cage muscles, as manifested by transdiaphragmatic pressure changes, i.e. a decrease in positive P_{ab} and a more negative P_{pb} during inspiration while the technique was employed during expiration. It is possible therefore that this change in the distribution of work across the respiratory muscles contributes to a reduction in dyspnea.

Recent work has also clarified the effect of various postures on respiratory muscle function and suggests that improved mechanical efficiency of the diaphragm may be responsible for relief of dyspnea and the physiologic benefit seen particularly with leaning forward and head down (Trendelenburg) postures [64]. In particular the 'leaning forward' position during exercise may be helpful in view of the recent finding [65] that dyspnea was diminished and exercise tolerance improved during walking in the leaning forward posture, in COPD patients who had developed paradoxical diaphragm motion during exercise in the upright position.

Diaphragmatic breathing exercises attempt to enhance diaphragmatic function through improved positioning of the diaphragm as distinct from ventilatory muscle strength training which attempts to improve respiratory muscle strength and endurance. The technique is very simple. The patient lies supine or tilted by 15° in the head down position. The patient's dominant hand is placed on the upper abdomen and the other hand on the upper anterior chest wall to allow monitoring of an inspiratory outward motion of the abdomen while minimizing chest excursions. A conscious effort is made to employ only the diaphragm during inspiration and to maximize abdominal protrusion. The anterior abdominal wall muscles are consciously contracted during inspiration and can also be contracted during expiration to displace the diaphragm to a more cephalad position. The same exercises are repeated while sitting and later standing in a forward leaning posture once mastered lying down.

The exercises are considered most helpful for patients with severe hyperventilation. In addition to the clinical benefit of reduction in breathlessness there are reports of significantly improved lung function in individual patients [66,67,68] although which patients will respond cannot be predicted in advance. A change in breathing pattern with increased tidal volume and a reduction in respiratory rate has been reported [69]. Although in theory regional changes in chest wall configuration should follow training in diaphragmatic breathing, three studies have failed to demonstrate any redistribution of ventilation in a comparison of diaphragmatic and conventional breathing [70]. Furthermore, a study of the effects of diaphragmatic breathing on thoracoabdominal motion in COPD has suggested increased distortion of rib cage and abdominal compartments away from the normal relaxation characteristics, which represents less mechanically efficient breathing and a theoretical increase in the work of breathing [71]. The overall benefits therefore have not been established and the technique though widely recommended for inclusion in pulmonary rehabilitation remains unvalidated.

21.1.3 NUTRITIONAL REQUIREMENTS

Malnutrition is an important clinical problem in patients with COPD [72]. The prevalence is highest in patients with severe airway obstruction [73, 74], and features of emphysema such as hyperinflation and low diffusing capacity [75]. Although there is no universally accepted definition of malnutrition, patients weighing less than 90% of ideal body weight are generally considered to be malnourished. Common measurements in nutritional assessment which aid the diagnosis of malnutrition are summarized in Table 21.2. Malnutrition has been shown to be associated with increased mortality in COPD. In a study of factors affecting prognosis in emphysema, cor pulmonale and weight loss were identified as the two significant clinical signs associated with higher mortality [76]. Several factors may contribute to this poor prognosis including loss of diaphragm weight [77] and global respiratory muscle function as measured by P_{Imax} and P_{Emax} [78, 79]. Malnutrition may adversely affect prognosis through loss of connective tissue proteins [80] and predisposition to increased infections through diminution of respiratory defence mechanisms such as phagocytic activity [81]. The idea of nutritional support appears logical though its contribution to improved outcome including quality of life, exercise capacity and prognosis remains to be established.

Resting energy expenditure in patients with stable chronic obstructive airways disease is usually elevated by between 10% and 20% [81–84] and this contrasts with the adaptive reduction in metabolic rate usually observed in other causes of malnutrition. However, despite this higher resting energy expenditure, total energy expenditure over 24 hours is often normal [85] and probably due to spontaneously reduced physical activity compensating for resting hypermetabolism. It therefore remains unclear whether poor nutritional status in COPD can be attributed to a state of hypermetabolism as is usually assumed. Several studies have assessed the effect of nutritional support [86–90], but mean weight gain only averaged between 2 and 4.5 kg. Despite intensive energy supplementation more than 30% above the usual intake amounting to more than 45 kcal/kg/day, improvements in peripheral and respiratory muscle performance and exercise capacity were small. P_{Imax} increased on average by 13 cmH$_2$O. These studies were short term lasting between 2 and 4 weeks but even in the one [87] which lasted 9 months the weight gain was lost once the patients returned to their usual diet. Failure seemed due both to the inability of patients to supplement energy intake sufficiently without spontaneous reduction in their other sources of usual energy intake and to high levels of intolerance of supplemental formulas.

The composition of supplementation diets requires consideration because theoretical consideration suggests that carbohydrate-based diets may be deleterious to COPD patients. When the energy sources shift from fat to carbohydrates the CO_2 production and RQ increase producing increased ventilatory demands, although hypercapnia has been demonstrated during weaning from mechan-

Table 21.2 Common measurements in nutritional assessment

Variable	Significance
(Current weight) – (usual weight)	Trend in nutritional status
Body weight (% ideal body weight)	Global nutritional assessment
Body mass index (kg/m^2)	Global nutritional assessment
Skinfold thickness	Fat mass
Midarm muscle circumference	Muscle mass
(Body weight) – (fat mass)	Fat-free mass
Bioelectrical impedance	Fat-free mass

Taken from Fitting, J. Nutrition in COPD *Eur. Respir. Rev.* 1991, 1:6, 511–519 ?[75a].

ical ventilation in patients with COPD [91]. Carbohydrates appear considerably less harmful when taken orally by ambulatory patients. One study assessed the effect of low, moderate and high carbohydrate diets in hypercapnic ambulatory COPD patients and found little increase in minute ventilation [92]. While low-carbohydrate, high-fat supplements may be preferable in patients with acute respiratory failure, their role in stable ambulatory patients has not been established. Furthermore, patients can often only tolerate a diet of traditional composition with carbohydrate intake at least 50% of the total. These avoid satiety and bloating and this has led to counselling strategies to counteract the effect of symptoms on food intake (Table 21.3).

21.1.4 HEALTH EDUCATION

Optimal medical practice should always include adequate explanations of the nature of the underlying disease process and the rationale for proposed treatment. However, in the busy outpatient clinic time for such an approach is often not available. Pulmonary rehabilitation programs provide an alternative setting and indeed the success of the program is likely to require the understanding and co-operation, not only of the patient but also of the family.

A check list of areas of education that may be helpful for patients is given in Table 21.4. There are, however, very limited data regarding the effects of such educational programs. Studies which have examined individual program components have shown that patients can learn to understand their disease better [93]. However, a recent controlled study of the effect of an education program showed a disappointing lack of impact on symptoms, physiologic function, mental or social function, in 213 patients who completed the education program versus 325 patients who acted as controls [94] although 'health locus of control' improved suggesting an increased patient belief that they could control their own health. Another study evaluating a comprehensive education program dealing with psychosocial aspects of COPD demonstrated improved knowledge of COPD but no impact on daily function including quality of life [95].

Although the primary role of education appears to help patients better understand their illness thereby obtaining optimal compliance with treatment, and achievement of realistic goals [96], evidence that these outcomes occur is still required.

21.2 PATIENT SELECTION FOR REHABILITATION PROGRAMS

There are no general guidelines for patient selection for pulmonary rehabilitation since any patient with symptomatic chronic lung disease is a potential candidate. We have however recently described [9a] a method of selection using clinical, lung function and exercise evaluation which allows streamlining of the patients according to ability. Each aspect of pulmonary rehabilitation imposes an intensive requirement on a limited infrastructure namely professional staff time and facilities, particularly access to hospital or other gymnasiums. The outpatient chest clinic acts as a filter, carefully referring patients on the basis of availability of places in the rehabilitation program. The most suitable patients recognize they have some impairment or disability related to the disease and are motivated to be active participants in their own care to improve their health status [97]. Patients with mild to moderate disease are often considered to be coping adequately and therein lies a paradox. Such patients often find their COPD frustrating and disabling precisely because of their expectations of continuing in demanding jobs and their desire to live a normal life, whereas more severely disabled patients often have different, generally lower, expectations. The former, however, stand to gain most, particularly from exercise rehabilitation which should not be reserved

Table 21.3 Summary of symptoms and counselling strategies for nutritional therapy in chronic obstructive pulmonary disease

Complaint	Estimated frequency (%)	Recommendations
Anorexia	73	Eat high-calorie food first
		Have favorite foods available
		Try more frequent meals and snacks throughout the day
		Push yourself to eat
		Add margarine, butter, mayonnaise, sauces, and gravies to diet to add calories
Early satiety	87	Eat high-calorie foods first
		Limit liquid consumption during meal; sip liquids 1 h after meals
		Eat cold foods first, as they can give less of a sense of fullness than hot foods
Dyspnea	73	Rest before meals
		Use bronchodilators before meals
		Use secretion clearance strategies if indicated
		Eat more slowly
		Use pursed-lip breathing between bites
		Use tripod position for meals
		Have readily prepared meals available for periods of increased shortness of breath
		Physician should evaluate for meal desaturation; refer patient for oxygen evaluation if necessary
Fatigue	60	Rest before meals
		Have readily prepared meals available for periods of increased fatigue or illness
		Try to eat larger meals in periods of less fatigue
Bloating	80	Treat shortness of breath early to prevent the swallowing of air
		Eat smaller, more frequent meals
		Avoid rushed meals
		Avoid gas-forming foods (individual to patient)
Constipation	50	Incorporate exercise as tolerated
		Eat high-fiber foods and drink adequate quantities of fluids
		Physician should determine the need for a stool softener
Dental problems	30	Eat soft, high-calorie foods
		Facilitate use of dental services as appropriate

From Donahoe, M. and Rogers, R.M. (1990) Nutritional assessment and support in chronic obstructive pulmonary disease. *Clin. Chest Med.*, 11, 499.

Table 21.4   Areas of education which may be helpful for patients

---

Normal anatomy and physiology of the lungs and heart
Types of lung disease and other conditions that affect the function of the lungs
Abnormal anatomy and physiology associated with pulmonary disorders
Types of medical tests that will be performed, procedures for testing, and interpretation and significance
    of the results
Medications: drug actions, description of products, desired beneficial effects, side effects, techniques of
    self-administration, and methods to assist patients to remember to take the medication
Breathing exercises, including whether to perform them at rest, during exercise, or during recovery from
    exercise or stress
Energy conservation techniques associated with activities of daily living
Relaxation techniques and methods to reduce stress
Emotional aspects of chronic disease
Nutrition and fluid intake
Causes of shortness of breath
Role of exercise and physical fitness
Recognizing problems associated with their disease: infection, hypercapnia, hypoxia
How to treat symptoms
Who to call for problems

From Burns, M. (1986) Pulmonary Rehabilitation, in *Clin. Chest Med., 7*, 4th ed., Saunders, Philadelphia.

for patients with end stage chronic lung disease.

Pulmonary rehabilitation therefore requires identification of different outcomes for these disparate groups with features such as nutritional assessment, determination of oxygen requirements, and psychosocial functioning being particularly relevant to the most severely disabled patients, for whom exercise training is not a realistic option. For the remainder of the COPD population where exercise training is possible, inclusion in one of the two different strategies for exercise rehabilitation requires additional assessment. There is wide *inter*subject variability with respect to lung function and mobility, and furthermore an illness such as COPD is dynamic, i.e. subject to intercurrent exacerbations which produce *intra*subject variability.

We determine the exercise requirements for individual patients by assessment using basic lung function and progressive incremental exercise testing [97] followed by a further assessment by the program physiotherapist of the patient's ability to participate in a particular program on a 'trial and error' basis

[9a]. There is no one accurate physiologic measure of disability and prediction formulas suffer from wide confidence intervals [98,99] limiting their role in this particular situation. A realistic evaluation of the factors likely to influence adherence of the patient (i.e. the extent to which individuals follow treatment recommendations) is also required and includes motivation, the extent of disability, the frequency of intercurrent exacerbations of disease, external socioeconomic factors, work commitments and travel requirements.

Non-compliance rates are not only high among patients with chronic conditions, but particularly where therapy involves lifestyle modification and exercise (as do rehabilitation programs) [100,101]. It is therefore important to remember the adage that for 'exercise to be habitual it should be easily accessible and without adverse sequelae.' Ideally it should also be dynamic, interesting, fun and varied [102].

Finally, it is important to note with regard to selection for exercise programs that following selection, in our experience patients with broadly similar disability should be grouped together within programs. To maintain the individual approach a program physiotherapist normally can only manage groups of approximately 8–10 patients per session and widely varying levels of disability can reinforce negative attitudes to their disease amongst the more severely disabled.

21.3 EVIDENCE FOR IMPROVEMENT AFTER PULMONARY REHABILITATION

Most studies evaluating exercise performance after rehabilitation have used either progressive incremental exercise testing in the laboratory setting, timed walking tests, e.g. the 6-minute or 12-minute walk test, and most recently the shuttle test [103] which has a component of imposed 'pacing' (Chapter 13). All of these tests measure maximal exercise capacity. The shuttle test consists of walking between two cones at a rate determined by an auditory signal which increases with time until the patient can no longer tolerate exercise. An additional method of exercise assessment consists of the measurement of endurance time and/or endurance work during steady state exercise usually on a treadmill or bicycle. This has the additional advantage of providing an index of the likely effects of rehabilitation treatment on the tolerance of daily activities. Guidelines for evaluating the results of pulmonary rehabilitation have recently been published [96] and the results of the various programs have also been extensively tabulated [17].

Although many of these reports did not include control data, virtually all showed patient improvement of a clinically relevant magnitude in peak work rate, maximum oxygen consumption, timed walk tests or endurance time. The studies which contained control groups confirm the impression that rehabilitation using a wide range of programs results in considerable improvement in maximum exercise tolerance.

In one study for example [104] regular stair climbing at home for 3 months led to a 16% increase in Vo_2 max and a 23% increase in

maximum workload in the treatment group (as compared with a 12% and 4% decrease in the same measures in the control group). Another study [105] showed that attention to rehabilitation techniques, such as breathing control even without exercise training, improved maximum exercise tolerance during bicycle ergometry. Important subjective improvements included an increase in the performance of activities of daily living [104,106–108] and a reduction in symptoms such as breathlessness during exercise [106].

Most of the studies which used timed walking tests showed a clinically relevant improvement in the distance walked after treatment, e.g. a 42% increase was observed in one uncontrolled study of 24 patients undergoing supervised exercise for 3 months [109]. A 51% increase was reported in another study of 63 patients [110] and a 6% increase was noted in a controlled study of 28 patients compared with a 2% decrease in control subjects [104].

Improvements in endurance time have been reported, of a magnitude greater than anticipated from improvements in maximal exercise level. For example, one study of 63 patients [110] showed no improvement in peak work rate or oxygen consumption but did demonstrate a 57% increase in endurance time. Another study [111] evaluating 15 patients for 6 weeks showed a doubling of endurance time with no increase in peak work rate. Contributory factors to this outcome include an improved strategy for performance of steady-state work and peripheral, skeletal muscle conditioning.

21.3.1 THE EFFECTS OF TREATMENT ON 'QUALITY OF LIFE' MEASURES

There is an increasing interest in the development of instruments for 'quality of life' measurement, which have validity and are sufficiently practical to be useful in monitoring the effects of pulmonary rehabilitation. The required components of such instruments have recently been reviewed [2]. McSweeny gives a definition of quality of life that encompasses

1. emotional functioning,
2. social role functioning,
3. the ability to perform daily living activities, and
4. the ability to participate in enjoyable activities.

This approach requires a generic global assessment as distinct from quality of life instruments which are disease specific and measure the impact of a particular symptom such as breathlessness. Current examples of both kinds of instruments are given in Table 21.5. Studies using these methods have improved symptom scores, performance of activities of daily living, psychosocial factors (e.g. mood) and general well-being [108, 112–114] and these benefits are measurable several years after rehabilitation. The emphasis on global assessment is likely to increase as psychosocial interventions are incorporated into multimodal pulmonary rehabilitation [115]. One carefully designed, randomized controlled study [114] has shown highly beneficial changes in quality of life measures when a behavioral intervention program was used in addition to regular exercise. Psychiatric morbidity frequently occurs in COPD patients [116] although the exact prevalence has not been accurately established.

Screening instruments for evaluation have been recommended [117] in addition to quality of life measurement in order to expedite psychiatric advice for those patients who show evidence of psychopathology. This can be very advantageous as pre-rehabilitation psychologic status as distinct from physiologic measures of disability can determine the response to the program. Specific techniques such as relaxation training [118] and meditation [119] have improved exercise tolerance and recovery after exertion in randomized clinical trials. Perhaps one of the most

beneficial functions of the rehabilitation 'process' is to direct some additional energy and thought beyond the traditional goals of symptom treatment towards these additional quality of life and psychosocial issues.

21.3.2 THE EFFECTS OF PULMONARY REHABILITATION ON SURVIVAL

There is encouraging evidence that the comprehensive care provided by pulmonary rehabilitation can improve survival. In one study [120] the survival at 5 years of 252 patients was 20% greater than that of a comparison group of patients with COPD attending a routine outpatient clinic. Another study of 182 patients [121] found a 17% better survival rate at 10 years than that expected from the mortality figures of comparable patients with COPD. There are other similar reports of improved survival compared with life expectancy data [122]. It is not possible to determine which specific components of the program were responsible for improved survival as such information would require large patient groups to allow subgroup analysis, evaluation over a number of years, and adequate contrast groups. There has been no multicenter evaluation of a comprehensive standardized rehabilitation program to date. However, such an approach has been used to demonstrate improved life expectancy with a single treatment (long-term oxygen therapy) and to demonstrate which patients are most likely to benefit from such treatment [123].

21.4 COST BENEFIT ANALYSIS

The impact of COPD on health care in Europe is probably similar to that in the United States, where an age-adjusted COPD mortality of 1.4% per year is rising with a correspondingly increased economic impact (e.g. 4.55 billion dollars in the 1970s, 26 billion dollars in the 1980s). This has prompted an analysis of the potential benefits of com-

Table 21.5 Selected HRQL instruments used in patients with chronic obstructive pulmonary disease (COPD)

Instrument	Domains and dimensions examined	Length	Administration	Reproducible, valid and responsive
Generic:				
Sickness impact profile (SIP)	Physical: ambulation, mobility, body care. Social: general well being, work/social role performance, social support and participation, global social function, personal relationships, and global emotional functioning	136 items (30 min)	Self-administered	Reproducibility, validity and responsiveness well demonstrated
Medical outcomes study (MOS)	Functioning: physical, role, and social. Well being: mental health, health perceptions, and bodily pain	20 items (3 min)	Self-administered	Reproducibility, validity well demonstrated; responsiveness in COPD not well studied
Quality of well being (QWB)	Mobility: access to modes of transportation. Physical: limits to activity. Social: limits to activity. Symptoms: review of systems	50 items (12 min)	Trained interviewer administered	Reproducible and valid; responsiveness in COPD not well demonstrated
Nottingham health profile (NHP)	Health: energy, pain, emotional reactions, sleep, social isolation, physical mobility. Life functioning: employment, relationships, personal life, sex, hobbies, vacations, housework	45 items (10 min)	Self-administered	Reproducible and valid; responsiveness in COPD not well demonstrated
COPD specific:				
Chronic respiratory disease questionnaire (CRDQ)	Dyspnoea, fatigue, mastery over disease, emotional dysfunction	20 items (20 min)	Trained interviewer administered	Reproducible,; validity and responsiveness well demonstrated
St George's respiratory questionnaire (SGRQ)	Symptoms: cough, sputum, wheeze, breathlessness. Activity: physical functioning, housework, hobbies. Impact on daily life: social and emotional impact	76 items (? min)	Self-administered	Reproducibility, validity and responsiveness well demonstrated
Oxygen cost diagram (OCD)	Single vertical line to be marked in location to indicate degree of disability caused by dyspnoea	1 item (< 5 min)	Self-administered	Intermediate reproducibility and validity. Not as responsive as SGRQ
Baseline dyspnoea index (BDI)	Functional impairment, magnitude of task evoking dyspnoea, magnitude of effort evoking dyspnoea	3 indices with four grades (< 5 min)	Trained interviewer administered	Reproducibility, validity and responsiveness well demonstrated

Source: Curtis J.R., Deyo R.A., Hudson L.D. (1994) Health related quality of life among patients with chronic obstructive pulmonary disease. *Thorax;* **49:** 162–170

prehensive rehabilitation programs in reducing the economic impact on health care resources. One study [124] compared the effects of pulmonary rehabilitation programs with the benefits which have been demonstrated for other types of health care programs such as hypertension screening and renal dialysis and showed that significant cost savings can accrue from pulmonary rehabilitation as compared with routine medical management.

Other authors have used reduction in days spent in hospital as an indication of cost effectiveness. Petty reported a 38% decrease in total hospital days from 868 days to 542 days for 85 patients, one year after conclusion of pulmonary rehabilitation [125]. Similarly Johnson [126] reported a 55% decrease in hospital days for 96 patients over a similar period. A further study [127] has shown a marked reduction in the number of repeat admissions in a group of 24 patients in the year after pulmonary rehabilitation (5 admissions compared with 30 in the previous year). Two other studies [126, 128] reported a similar average decrease in hospital stay per patient/year of 20 and 21 days respectively including the cost of pulmonary rehabilitation in the cost benefit analysis with the conclusion that there had been highly significant net cost savings. Long-term benefits have been demonstrated over periods of 4 years [129] (73% reduction in hospitalizations in the first year and 61% in the fourth for the 44 patients who survived, and 8 years [130]). In the latter case only 8% of the rehabilitation group required sheltered care as compared with 17% of the comparison group. Although a number of factors may have influenced these outcomes, the available data support the view that pulmonary rehabilitation programs are not only very beneficial to the individual but offer cost-effective therapy for COPD in general.

21.5 SUMMARY

The current resurgence of interest in pulmonary rehabilitation for patients with COPD suggests some optimism that this frustrating and debilitating illness can be ameliorated by approaches extending beyond simple pharmacologic management of the underlying disease process. The challenge is two-fold: first to supply comprehensive care to the millions of patients suffering from COPD and secondly to advance the scientific basis for pulmonary rehabilitation in order to enhance its applications.

While the comprehensive nature of pulmonary rehabilitation may seem daunting to interested physicians, the organization can be shared by adopting a cooperative approach to treatment with related health professionals in a multidisciplinary setting.

ACKNOWLEDGEMENTS

I am greatly indebted to my secretary, Mrs Ann Glen for her careful help, in the preparation of this manuscript.

REFERENCES

1. Petty, T.L. (1977) Pulmonary rehabilitation. *Respir. Care*, **22**, 68–77.
2. McSweeny, J. (1988) Quality of life in COPD, in *Chronic Obstructive Pulmonary Disease: A Behavioural Perspective. Lung Biology in Health and Disease*, (eds J. McSweeny and I. Grant), Vol. 36, Marcel Dekker, New York.
3. World Health Organization (1977) *Manual of the International Classification of Diseases, Injuries and Causes of Death*, World Health Organization, Geneva.
4. Higgins, M. (1993) Epidemiology of obstructive pulmonary disease, in *Principles and Practice of Pulmonary Rehabilitation*, (eds R. Casaburi and T. Petty), Saunders, Philadelphia.
5. Petty, T.L. (1993) Pulmonary rehabilitation: a personal historical perspective, in *Principles and Practice of Pulmonary Rehabilitation*, (eds R. Casaburi and T. Petty), Saunders, Philadelphia.
6. Hodgkin, J.E., Balchum, O.J., Kass, I. *et al.* (1975) Chronic obstructive airways diseases. Current concepts in diagnosis and comprehensive care. *JAMA*, **232**, 1243–60.

7. Proceedings of the Conference on the Scientific Basis of Respiratory Therapy (1974) *Am. Rev. Respir. Dis.*, **110**, 51–202.

8. European Respiratory Society Rehabilitation and Chronic Care Scientific Group (1991). Pulmonary rehabilitation in chronic obstructive pulmonary disease (COPD) with recommendations for its use. *Eur. Respir. Rev.*, Review No. 6, 1–568.

9. Make, B.J. (1986) Pulmonary Rehabilitation, in: *Clin. Chest Med.*, **7**, 4th ed., Saunders, Philadelphia.

9a. Clark, C.J. (1994) Setting up a pulmonary rehabilitation programme. *Thorax*, **49**, 270–78.

10. Barcroft, J. (1934) *Features in the Architecture of Physiological Function*, Cambridge University Press, Cambridge, England.

11. American College of Sports Medicine (1980) *Guidelines for Graded Exercise Testing and Exercise Prescription*, 2nd edn, Lea & Febiger, Philadelphia.

12. Astrand, P.O. and Rodahl, K (1977) *Textbook of Work Physiology*, 2nd edn, McGraw-Hill, New York.

13. Belman, M.J. (1986) Exercise in chronic obstructive pulmonary disease. *Clin. Chest Med.*, **7**, 585–97.

14. Wasserman, K., Hansen, J.E., Sue, D.Y. and Whipp, B.J. (1987) *Principles of Exercise Testing and Interpretation*, Lea & Febiger, Philadelphia, p. 52.

15. Casaburi, R., Patessio, A., Loli, F. *et al.* (1991) Reductions in exercise lactic acidosis and ventilation as a result of exercise training in patients with obstructive lung disease. *Am. Rev. Respir. Dis.*, **143**, 9–18.

16. Casaburi, R. and Wasserman, K. (1986) Exercise training in pulmonary rehabilitation. *N. Engl. J. Med.*, **314**, 1509–11.

17. Casaburi, R. and Petty, T. (eds) (1993) Exercise training in chronic obstructive lung disease, in *Principles and Practice of Pulmonary Rehabilitation*, Saunders, Philadelphia.

18. Clausen, J.P. (1976) Circulatory adjustments to dynamic exercise and effect of physical training in normal subjects and patients with coronary artery disease. *Prog. Cardiovasc. Dis.*, **18**, 459–95.

19. Holloszy, J.O. (1976) Adaptations of muscular tissue to training. *Prog. Cardiovasc. Dis.*, **18**, 445–58.

20. Jones, N.L. Kearon, M.C. and Leblanc, P. *et al.* (1989) Symptoms limiting activity in chronic airflow limitation. *Am. Rev. Respir. Dis.*, **139**, A319.

21. Guell, R., Gimenez, M. and Marchand, M. (1989) Dyspnoea, pain in the legs and quadriceps electro-myographic fatigue at maximal exercise in patients with chronic airway obstruction. *Eur. Respir. J.*, Suppl. **2**, 385s.

22. Allard, C., Jones, N.L. and Killian, K. J. (1989) Static peripheral skeletal muscle strength and exercise capacity in patients with chronic airflow limitation. *Am. Rev. Respir. Dis.* **138**, A90.

23. Simpson, K., Killian, K., McCartney, N. *et al.* (1992) Randomised control trial of weight-lifting exercise in patients with chronic airflow limitation. *Thorax*, **47**, 70–5.

24. Mackay, E., Cochrane, L.M. and Clark, C.J. (1992) The effects of sequential isolated muscle training on peripheral muscle conditioning and exercise tolerance in patients with COPD. *Eur. Respir. J.*, **5** (Suppl. 15): 30S.

25. Celli, B.R., Rassulo, J. and Make, B.J. (1986) Dyssynchronous breathing during arm but not leg exercise in patients with chronic airflow obstruction. *N. Engl. J. Med.*, **314**, 1485–90.

26. Criner, G.J. and Celli, B.R. (1988) Effect of unsupported arm exercise on ventilatory muscle recruitment in patients with severe chronic airflow obstruction. *Am. Rev. Respir. Dis.* **138**, 856–61.

27. Ries, A.L., Ellis, B. and Hawkins, R.W. (1988) Upper extremity exercise training in chronic obstructive pulmonary disease. *Chest*, **93**, 688–92.

28. Lake, F.R., Henderson, K., Briffa, T. *et al.* (1990) Upper-limb and lower-limb exercise training in patients with chronic airflow obstruction. *Chest*, **97**, 1077–82.

29. Franklin, B.A. (1985) Exercise testing, training and arm ergometry. *Sports Med.*, **2**, 100–19.

30. Franklin, B.A. (1989) Aerobic exercise training programs for the upper body. *Med. Sci. Sports Exerc.*, **21**, S141–S148.

31. Sue, D.Y., Oren, A., Hansen, J.E. and Wasserman, K. (1987) Diffusing capacity for carbon monoxide as a predictor of gas exchange during exercise. *N. Engl. J. Med.*, **316**, 1301–6.

32. Ries, A.L., Farrow, J.T. and Clausen, J.L. (1988) Pulmonary function tests cannot predict exercise-induced hypoxemia in chronic obstructive pulmonary disease. *Chest*, **93**, 454–9.

33. Zack, M.B. and Palange, A.V. (1985) Oxygen supplemented exercise of ventilatory and

nonventilatory muscles in pulmonary rehabilitation. *Chest*, **88**, 669–74.

34. Cotes, J.E. and Gilson, J.C. (1956) Effect of oxygen on exercise ability in chronic respiratory insufficiency: Use of portable apparatus. *Lancet*, **1**, 872–6.

35. Woodcock, A.A., Gross, E.R. and Geddes, D.M. (1981) Oxygen relieves breathlessness in 'pink puffers'. *Lancet*, **i**, 907–9.

36. Stein, D.A., Bradley, B.L. and Miller, W.C. (1982) Mechanisms of oxygen effects on exercise in patients with chronic obstructive pulmonary disease. *Chest*, **81**, 6–10.

37. Foster, S., Lopez, D. and Thomas, H.M. (1988) Pulmonary rehabilitation in COPD patients with elevated PCO_2. *Am. Rev. Respir. Dis.*, **138**, 1519–23.

38. Pardy, R.L., Reid, D.W. and Belman, M.J. (1988) Respiratory muscle training. *Clin. Chest Med.*, **9**, 287–96.

39. Rochester, D.F. (1988) Does respiratory muscle rest relieve fatigue or incipient failure? *Am. Rev. Respir. Dis.*, **138**, 516–7.

40. Grassino, A. (1989) Inspiratory muscle training in COPD patients. *Eur. Respir. J.*, Suppl. 2, 581s–586s.

41. Smith, K., Cook, D., Guyatt, G.H. *et al.* (1992) Respiratory muscle training in chronic airflow limitation: a meta-analysis. *Am. Rev. Respir. Dis.*, **145**, 533–9.

42. Moxham, J. (1990) Respiratory muscle fatigue, mechanisms, evaluation and therapy. *Br. J. Anaesth.*, **65**, 43–53.

43. Laroche, C.M., Moxham, J. and Green, M. (1989) Respiratory muscle weakness and fatigue. *Q. J. Med.*, **71**, 373–97.

44. Dekhuijzen, P.N., Folgering, H.T. and van Herwaarden, C. L. (1991) Target-flow inspiratory muscle training during pulmonary rehabilitation in patients with COPD. *Chest*, **99**, 128–33.

45. Harver, A., Mahler, D.A. and Daubenspeck, J.A. (1989) Targeted inspiratory muscle training improves respiratory muscle function and reduces dyspnoea in patients with chronic obstructive disease. *Ann. Intern. Med.*, **111**, 117–24.

46. Black, L.F. and Hyatt, R.E. (1969) Maximal respiratory pressures: Normal values and relationship to age and sex. *Am. Rev. Respir. Dis.*, **99**, 696–702.

47. Grimby, G. and Stiksa, J. (1970) Flow-volume curves and breathing patterns during exercise

in patients with obstructive lung disease. *Scand. J. Clin. Lab. Invest.*, **25**, 303–13.

48. Potter, W.A., Olafsson, S. and Hyatt, R.E. (1971) Ventilatory mechanics and expiratory flow limitation during exercise in patients with obstructive lung disease. *J. Clin. Invest.*, **50**, 910–9.

49. Stubbing, D.G., Pengelly, L.D., Morse, J.L.C. and Jones, N. (1980) Pulmonary mechanics during exercise in subjects with chronic airflow obstruction. *J. Appl. Physiol.*, **49**, 511–5.

50. Younes, M. (1989) Load responses, dyspnoea and respiratory failure. *Chest*, **3**, 595–685.

51. Fleury, B., Murciano, C., Talamo, C. *et al.* (1985) Work of breathing in patients with chronic obstructive pulmonary disease in acute respiratory failure. *Am. Rev. Respir. Dis.*, **131**, 822–7.

52. Haluszka, J., Chartrand, D.A., Grassino, A.E. *et al.* (1990) Intrinsic PEEP and arterial PCO_2 in stable patients with chronic obstructive pulmonary disease. *Am. Rev. Respir. Dis.*, **141**, 1194–7.

53. Smith, T.C. and Marini, J.J. (1988) Impact of PEEP on lung mechanics and work of breathing in severe airflow obstruction. *J. Appl. Physiol.*, **65**, 1488–99.

54. Petrof, B.J., Calderini, E. and Gottfried, S.B. (1990) Effect of CPAP on respiratory effort and dyspnoea during exercise in COPD. *J. Appl. Physiol.*, **69**, 179–88.

55. O'Donnell, D.E., Sanii, R., Gresinecht, G. *et al.* (1988) Effect of continuous positive airway pressure on respiratory sensation in patients with chronic obstructive pulmonary disease during submaximal exercise. *Am. Rev. Respir. Dis.*, **138**, 1185–91.

56. Barach, A.L. (1955) Breathing exercises in pulmonary emphysema and allied chronic respiratory disease. *Arch. Phys. Med. Rehab.*, **36**, 379–90.

57. Miller, W.F. (1954) A physiologic evaluation of the effects of diaphragmatic breathing training in patients with chronic pulmonary emphysema. *Am. J. Med.*, **17**, 471–7.

58. Faling, J.L. (1993) Controlled breathing techniques and chest physical therapy in chronic obstructive pulmonary disease and allied conditions, in *Principles and Practice of Pulmonary Rehabilitation*, (eds R. Casaburi and T. Petty), Saunders, Philadelphia.

59. Mueller, R.E., Petty, T.L. and Filley, G.F. (1970) Ventilation and arterial blood gas

changes induced by pursed lip breathing. *J. Appl. Physiol.*, **28**, 784–9.

60. Thoman, R.L., Stoker, G.L. and Ross, J.C. (1966) The efficacy of pursed-lips breathing in patients with chronic obstructive pulmonary disease. *Am. Rev. Respir. Dis.*, **93**, 100–5.

61. Ingram, R.H. Jr and Schilder, D.P. (1967) Effect of pursed lips expiration on the pulmonary pressure-flow relationship in obstructive lung disease. *Am. Rev. Respir. Dis.*, **96**, 381–7.

62. Tiep, B.L., Burns, M., Kao, D. *et al.* (1986). Pursed lips breathing training using ear oximetry. *Chest*, **90**, 218–21.

63. Roa, J., Epstein, S., Breslin, E. *et al.* (1991) Work of breathing and ventilatory muscle recruitment during pursed lip breathing in patients with chronic airway obstruction. *Am. Rev. Respir. Dis.*, **143**, A77.

64. Sharp, J.T., Drutz, W.S., Moisan, T. *et al.* (1980) Postural relief of dyspnea in severe chronic obstructive pulmonary disease. *Am. Rev. Respir. Dis.*, **122**, 201–11.

65. Delgado, H.R., Braun, SR., Skatrud, J. B. *et al.* (1982) Chest wall and abdominal motion during exercise in patients with chronic obstructive pulmonary disease. *Am. Rev. Respir. Dis.*, **126**, 200–5.

66. Miller, W.F. (1958) Physical therapeutic measures in the treatment of chronic bronchopulmonary disorders: Methods for breathing training. *Am. J. Med.* **24**, 929–40.

67. Sinclair, J.D. (1955) The effect of breathing exercises in pulmonary emphysema. *Thorax*, **10**, 246–9.

68. McNeil, R.S. and McKenzie, J.M. (1955) An assessment of the value of breathing exercises in chronic bronchitis and asthma. *Thorax*, **10**, 250–2.

69. Willeput, R., Vachaudez, J.P., Lenders, D. *et al.* (1983) Thoracoabdominal motion during chest physiotherapy in patients affected by chronic obstructive lung disease. *Respiration*, **44**, 204–14.

70. Brach, B.B., Chao, R.P., Sgroi, V.L. *et al.* (1977) Xenon washout patterns during diaphragmatic breathing. Studies in normal persons and patients with chronic obstructive pulmonary disease. *Chest*, **71**, 735–9.

71. Sackner, M.A., Gonzalez, H.F., Jenouri, G. and Rodriguez, M. (1984) Effects of abdominal and thoracic breathing on breathing pattern components in normal subjects and in patients with chronic obstructive pulmonary disease. *Am. Rev. Respir. Dis.*, **130**, 584–7.

72. Wilson, D.O., Rogers, R.M., Hoffman, R.M. (1985) Nutrition and chronic lung disease. *Am. Rev. Respir. Dis.*, **132**, 1347–65.

73. Burrows, B., Niden, A. H., Barclay, W. R. and Kasik, J.E. (1964) Chronic obstructive lung disease. II. Relationship of clinical and physiological findings to the severity of airways obstruction. *Am. Rev. Respir. Dis.*, **91**, 665–78.

74. Renzetti, A.D., McClement, J.H. and Litt, B.D. (1966) The veterans administration cooperative study of pulmonary function. III. Mortality in relation to respiratory function in chronic obstructive pulmonary disease. *Am. J. Med.*, **41**, 115–29.

75. Wilson, D.O., Rogers, R.M., Wright, E.C. and Anthonisen, N. R. (1989) Body weight in chronic obstructive pulmonary disease. The National Institutes of Health intermittent positive-pressure breathing trial. *Am. Rev. Respir. Dis.*, **139**, 1435–8.

76. Boushy, S.F., Adhikari, P.K., Sakamoto, A. and Lewis, B. M. (1964) Factors affecting prognosis in emphysema. *Dis. Chest*, **45**, 402–11.

77. Thurlbeck, M.M., (1978) Diaphragm and body weight in emphysema. *Thorax*, **33**, 483–7.

78. Rochester, D.F. and Braun, N.M.T. (1985) Determinants of maximal inspiratory pressure in chronic obstructive pulmonary disease. *Am. Rev. Respir. Dis.*, **132**, 42–7.

79. Donahoe, M., Rogers, R.M., Wilson, D.O. and Pennock, B. E. (1989) Oxygen consumption of the respiratory muscles in normal and in malnourished patients with chronic obstructive pulmonary disease. *Am. Rev. Respir. Dis.*, **140**, 385–91.

80. Sahebjami, H. (1986) Nutrition and the pulmonary parenchyma. *Clin. Chest Med.*, **7**, 111–26.

81. Shennib, H., Chu-Jeng Chiu R., Mulder, D.S. and Lough, J.O. (1984) Depression and delayed recovery of alveolar macrophage function during starvation and refeeding. *Surg. Gynecol. Obstet.*, **158**, 535–40.

82. Goldstein, S.A., Thomashow, B.M., Kvetan, V. *et al.* (1988) Nitrogen and energy relationships in malnourished patients with emphysema. *Am. Rev. Respir. Dis.*, **138**, 636–44.

83. Fitting, J.W., Frascarolo, Ph., Jequier, E. and Leuenberger, Ph. (1989) Energy expenditure and rib cage-abdominal motion in chronic

obstructive pulmonary disease. *Eur. Respir. J.*, **2**, 840–5.

84. Wilson, D.O., Donahoe, M., Rogers, R.M. and Pennock, B.E. (1990) Metabolic rate and weight loss in chronic obstructive lung disease. *J. Parenter. Enteral Nutr.*, **14L**, 7–11.

85. Hugli, O., Schutz, Y., Leuenberger, Ph. and Fitting, J.W. (1991) The daily energy expenditure of COPD patients in confined and free-living conditions. *Am. Rev. Respir. Dis.*, **143**, A453.

86. Lewis, M.I., Belman, M.J. and Door-Uyemura, L. (1987) Nutritional supplementation in ambulatory patients with chronic obstructive pulmonary disease. *Am. Rev. Respir. Dis.*, **135**, 1062–8.

87. Knowles, J.B., Fairbairn, M.S., Wiggs, B.J. *et al.* (1988) Dietary supplementation and respiratory muscle performance in patients with COPD. *Chest*, **93**, 977–83.

88. Efthimiou, J., Fleming, J., Gomes, C. and Spiro, S.G. (1988) The effect of supplementary oral nutrition in poorly nourished patients with chronic obstructive pulmonary disease. *Am. Rev. Respir. Dis.*, **137**, 1075–82.

89. Otte, K.F., Ahlburg, P., D'Amore, F. and Stellfield, M. (1989) Nutritional repletion in malnourished patients with emphysema. *J. Parenter. Enteral Nutr.*, **13**, 152–6.

90. Whittaker, J.S., Ryan, C.F., Buckley, P.A. and Road, J.R. (1990) The effects of refeeding on peripheral and respiratory muscle function in malnourished chronic obstructive pulmonary disease patients. *Am. Rev. Respir. Dis.*, **142**, 283–8.

91. Covelli, H.D., Waylon Black, J., Olsen, M.S. and Beekman, J.F. (1981) Respiratory failure precipitated by high carbohydrate loads. *Ann. Intern. Med.*, **95**, 579–81.

92. Angelillo, V.A., Bedi, S., Durfee, D. *et al.* (1985) Effects of low and high carbohydrate feedings in ambulatory patients with chronic obstructive pulmonary disease and chronic hypercapnia. *Ann. Intern. Med.*, **103**, 883–5.

93. Neish, C.M. and Hopp, J.W. (1988) The role of education in pulmonary rehabilitation. *J. Cardiopulmonary Rehabil.*, **11**, 439–41.

94. Howland, J., Nelson, E.C., Barlow, P.B. *et al.* (1986) Chronic obstructive airway disease: impact of health education. *Chest*, **90**, 233–8.

95. Askikaga, T., Vacek, P.M. and Lewis, S.O. (1980) Evaluation of a community-based education programme for individuals with chronic obstructive pulmonary disease. *J. Rehabil. Res. Dev.*, **46**, 23–7.

96. Kaplan, R.M., Eakin, E.G. and Ries, A.L. (1993) Psychosocial issues in the rehabilitation of patients with chronic obstructive pulmonary disease, in *Principles and Practice of Pulmonary Rehabilitation*, (eds. R. Casaburi and T. Petty), Saunders, Philadelphia.

97. Clark, C.J. (1993) Evaluating the results of pulmonary rehabilitation treatment, in *Principles and Practice of Pulmonary Rehabilitation*, (eds. R. Casaburi and T. Petty), Saunders, Philadelphia.

98. Jones, P.W., Baveystock, C.M. and Littlejohns, P. (1989) Relationships between general health measured with the sickness impact profile and respiratory symptoms, physiological measures and mood in patients with chronic airflow limitation. *Am. Rev. Respir. Dis.*, **140**, 1538–43.

99. Cotes, J.E., Bishop, J.M., Capel, L.H. *et al.* (1981) Disabling chest disease; prevention and care: a report of the Royal College of Physicians by the College Committee on Thoracic Medicine. *J. R. Coll. Physicians Lond.*, **15**, 69–87.

100. Sackett, D.L. (1976) The magnitude of compliance and non-compliance, in *Compliance with Therapeutic Regimens*, (eds D.L. Sackett and R.B. Haynes). John Hopkins University Press, Baltimore.

101. Carmody, T., Senner, J., Malineau, M. and Matarazzo, G. (1980) Physical exercise rehabilitation: long term dropout rate in cardiac patients. *J. Behav. Med.*, **3**, 163–8.

102. Larson, E.B. and Bruce, R.A. (1987) Health benefits of exercise in an aging society. *Arch. Intern. Med.*, **147**, 353–6.

103. Singh, S.J., Morgan, M.D.L., Scott, S. *et al.* (1992) Development of a shuttle walking test of disability in patients with chronic airways obstructive. *Thorax*, **47**, 1019–24.

104. McGavin, C.R., Gupta, S.P., Lloyd, E.L. and McHardy, J.R. (1977) Physical rehabilitation of chronic bronchitis; Results of a controlled trial of exercises in the home. *Thorax*, **32**, 307–11.

105. Ambrosino, N., Paggiaro, P.L., Macchi, M. *et al.* (1981) A study of short-term effect of rehabilitative therapy in chronic obstructive pulmonary disease. *Respiration*, **41**, 40–4.

106. Booker, H.A. (1984) Exercise training and breathing control in patients with chronic airflow limitation. *Physiotherapy*, **70**, 258–60.

107. Sinclair, D.J.M. and Ingram, C.G. (1980) Controlled trial of supervised exercise training in chronic bronchitis. *Br. Med. J.*, **280**, 519–21.

108. Cockroft, A., Bagnall, P., Heslop, A. *et al.* (1987) Controlled trial of respiratory health worker visiting patients with chronic respiratory disability. *Br. Med. J.*, **294**, 225–8.

109. Tydeman, D.E., Chandler, A.R., Graveling, B.M. *et al.* (1984) An investigation into the effects of exercise tolerance training on patients with chronic airways obstruction. *Physiotherapy*, **70**, 261–4.

110. Zack, M.B. and Palange, A.V. (1985) Oxygen supplemented exercise of ventilatory and nonventilatory muscles in pulmonary rehabilitation. *Chest*, **88**, 669–75.

111. Mohsenifar, Z., Horak, D., Brown, H.V. and Koerner, S. K. (1983) Sensitive indices of improvement in a pulmonary rehabilitation programme. *Chest*, **83**, 189–92.

112. Mall, R.W. and Medeiros, M. (1989) Objective evaluation of results of a pulmonary rehabilitation programme in a community hospital. *Chest*, **94**, 1156–60.

113. Bebout, D.E., Hodgkin, J.E., Zorn, E.G. *et al.* (1983) Clinical and physiological outcomes of a university-hospital pulmonary rehabilitation programme. *Respir. Care*, **28**, 1468–73.

114. Atkins, C.J., Kaplan, R.M., Timms, R.M. *et al.* (1984) Behavioral exercise programmes in the management of chronic obstructive pulmonary disease. *J. Consult. Clin. Psychol.*, **52**, 591–603.

115. Dudley, D.L., Glaser, E. M., Jorgenson, B.N. and Logan, D.L. (1980) Psychosocial concomitants to rehabilitation in chronic obstructive pulmonary disease. Part 2. Psychosocial treatment. *Chest*, **77**, 544–684.

116. Krop, H.D., Block, A.J. and Cohen, E. (1973) Neuropsychologic effects of continuous oxygen therapy in chronic obstructive pulmonary disease. *Chest*, **64**, 317–22.

117. Williams, S.J. (1989) Chronic respiratory illness and disability: a critical review of the psychosocial literature. *Soc. Sci. Med.*, **28**, 791–803.

118. Renfroe, K.L. (1988) Effect of progressive relaxation on dypnoea and state anxiety patients with chronic obstructive pulmonary disease. *Heart Lung*, **17**, 408–13.

119. Tandon, M.K. (1978) Adjunct treament with yoga in chronic severe airways obstruction. *Thorax*, **33**, 514–7.

120. Haas, A. and Cardon, H. (1969) Rehabilitation in chronic obstructive pulmonary disease: a 5 year study of 252 patients. *Med. Clin. North Am.*, **53**, 593–606.

121. Sahn, S.A., Nett, L.M. and Petty, T.L. (1980) Ten year follow-up of a comprehensive rehabilitation programme for severe COPD. *Chest*, **77**, 311–4.

122. Anthonisen, N.R., Wright, E.C. and Hodgkin, J.E. (1986) Prognosis in chronic obstructive pulmonary disease. *Am. Rev. Respir. Dis.*, **133**, 14–20.

123. Nocturnal Oxygen Therapy Trial Group. (1980) Continuous or nocturnal oxygen therapy in hypoxaemic chronic obstructive lung disease. *Ann. Intern. Med.*, **93**, 391–8.

124. Toevs, C.D., Kaplan, R.M. and Atkins, C.J. (1984) The costs and effects of behavioral programs in chronic obstructive pulmonary disease. *Med. Care*, **22**, 1088–1100.

125. Petty, T.L., Neff, L.M., Finigan, M.M. *et al.* (1969) A comprehensive care programme for chronic airways obstruction: methods and preliminary evaluation of symptomatic and functional improvement. *Ann. Intern. Med.*, **70**, 1109–20.

126. Johnson, H.R., Tanzi, F., Balchum, O.J. *et al.* (1980) Inpatient comprehensive pulmonary rehabilitation in severe COPD. *Respir. Ther.*, May/June, 15–19.

127. Agle, D.P. Baum, G.L., Chester, E.H. and Wendt, M. (1973) Multidiscipline treatment of chronic pulmonary insufficiency: 1. Psychologic aspects of rehabilitation. *Psychosom. Med.*, **35**, 41–9.

128. Alpert, J.S., Bass, H., Szucs, M.M. *et al.* (1975) Effects of physical training on hemodynamics and pulmonary function at rest and during exercise in patients with chronic obstructive pulmonary disease. *Chest*, **66**, 647–51.

129. Hudson, L.D., Tyler, M.L. and Petty, T.L. (1976) Hospitalisation needs during an outpatient rehabilitation programme for severe chronic airway obstruction. *Chest*, **70**, 606–10.

130. Haas, A. and Cardon, H. (1969) Rehabilitation in chronic obstructive pulmonary disease: a 5 year study of 252 male patients. *Med. Clin. North Am.*, **53**, 593–606.

BULLOUS LUNG DISEASE

22

M.D.L. Morgan

Many of the mechanical and physiologic properties of the lung are determined by its complex honeycomb structure. The lung parenchyma is formed by a matrix of millions of air-containing spaces of roughly equal size. The interdependence of these units is reflected in the uniform distribution of elastic forces throughout the lung which support the smaller airways and maintain their patency. In most forms of chronic obstructive lung disease the destructive pathology is relatively uniformly distributed. Occasionally one part of the lung is affected preferentially leading to the development of parenchymal destruction and the formation of a large abnormal airspace within the lung. If the space exceeds the confining powers of interdependence it will develop mechanical and elastic properies of its own which may interfere with the function of the remainder of the lung. Such is the case in bullous lung disease where large, redundant spaces may develop within the lung and compromise its function. These bullae usually occur in association with generalized emphysema but can can coexist with normal lung. In comparison to other forms of chronic obstructive lung disease, bulla formation is not very common. However, it is important because it offers one of the very few opportunities for surgical correction of lung disease which results in functional improvement. For this reason the assessment of such patients has to be more detailed so that the surgical opportunity can be exploited. This chapter will examine the nature of bullous lung disease and its presentation. It will also describe the methods of assessment for surgery and the details of outcome.

22.1 DEFINITION

There is a confusion of terms which describe abnormal large airspaces within the lung. Often the nomenclature has been used loosely and descriptions of cavities, cysts, bullae and blebs have been used interchangeably. For the purpose of this chapter we will define them precisely [1].

Cyst: This is a generic term which describes an abnormal airspace between 1 cm^3 and several liters in size. Congenital cysts arising from the tracheobronchial tree are lined by ciliated epithelium. Acquired cysts, including cavities, bullae and pneumatoceles, lack an epithelial lining and arise as a result of local injury.

Cavity: An acquired cyst with a non-epithelial lining but a wall which is thicker than 3 mm. Such a space usually arises following pulmonary infection or fibrosis.

Bleb: A small, but immediately subpleural collection of air external to the internal elastic layer of the visceral pleura. Such spaces are prone to rupture and lead to spontaneous pneumothorax.

Chronic Obstructive Pulmonary Disease. Edited by Dr P. Calverley and Professor N. Pride. Published in 1995 by Chapman & Hall, London. ISBN 0 412 46450 0

Bulla: An acquired air-filled space within the lung parenchyma larger than 1 cm^3 which has an oval or round shape and characteristically thin walls of minimal thickness.

The term pneumatocele is often synonymous with a bulla and also results from tissue lysis. However, it is usually reserved for small postinfective cysts in conditions such as staphylococcal pneumonia which are likely to recover spontaneously. Acquired cysts are more likely to be called bullae if they are associated with airway obstruction. The co-existence of bullae and emphysematous obstructive airway disease is known as bullous lung disease. This chapter is concerned primarily with the latter since the presence of large bullae may worsen symptoms of airway obstruction but at the same time offer an opportunity for therapy.

22.2 STRUCTURE AND PATHOLOGY

Bullae develop from a region of local pulmonary destruction which does not always have to be emphysematous. The local destruction can arise from degenerative, lytic or traumatic causes. Bullae have been described in association with tuberculosis, sarcoidosis, AIDS and trauma amongst others [2,3,4]. In approximately 20% of cases the surrounding lung is seen to be normal but the majority of cases are associated with emphysema and chronic airway obstruction [5]. The size and the structure of emphysematous bullae are variable but their appearance has been classified by Reid according to the size and position of the region of destruction [6]. Type 1 bullae are characterized by mushroom-like expansion into the pleural space. In this case the epicenter of parenchymal damage is close to the pleural surface and the external wall of the bulla is stretched pleura with a narrow neck connecting the bulla to the lung. A type 2 bulla has less pleural surface and a broader neck which merges into emphysematous lung. The type 3 bulla is deep within the lung and has no pleural

reflection. Although these three forms of bulla can be distinguished they probably do not signify a difference in etiology rather than an indication of the anatomic site of origin which results in their different appearances.

The macroscopic appearance of bullae is usually spheroid or lobular. The cavity, containing air, may be septate and contain fibrous bands which are the remnants of stretched fibrous tissue and blood vessels. The thin lining of the cysts is not epithelial but derived from alveolar pneumocytes and is relatively avascular [6,7]. Contrary to some theories of origin the floor of bullae does not contain a single feeding airway (Plate 1, p. 544). In most cases the bulla floor merges imperceptibly into the alveolar ducts and alveolae of adjacent lung, though sometimes the alveolar septa may form a funnel at the base.

22.3 ORIGIN AND DEVELOPMENT OF EMPHYSEMATOUS BULLAE

The development of symptomatic dyspnea in a patient with bullous disease is usually associated with the radiologic progression of the bulla and apparent reduction in the volume of surrounding normal lung. One obvious explanation for this appearance would be the gradual development of relative positive pressure within the bulla which compresses surrounding lung or prevents its expansion. The belief has developed that bullae form in a region of local weakness which is simultaneously supplied by airways that have a valvular structure which allows gas to enter but impedes its exit. This attractive hypothesis explains the development of a bulla and also provides a rationale for surgery by the release of compressed lung and this mechanism is therefore still widely believed to be responsible. The logic of this explanation does not, however, stand up to detailed scrutiny and the physical evidence that exists does not support the compression theory.

The presence of a valvular obstruction within the feeding airways is a prerequisite for the development of a large pressurized cyst. Histologic features of such valves were described by Hayashi as cited by Head and Avery in 1949 [8,9]. More recent and detailed histologic examination of the junctional areas between bullae and normal lung do not confirm their presence [6,7]. There may be some areas of ill-defined fibrosis but most bullae have widely patent communications with adjacent lung or simply merge with it. Even assuming that such valvular obstructions exist it is difficult to see how the bulla can fill under pressure during normal breathing. This 'bicycle pump' theory of development requires that gas will enter an area of high pressure rather than distend more compliant lung. This is difficult to conceive but it is possible that the bullous space may be enlarged during cough or expiration.

Evidence against a compression theory can also be obtained from changes in volume, pressure and gas content within a bulla during spontaneous ventilation. The measurement of bulla volume by CT in full inspiration and expiration allows an estimate of the bulla vital capacity. A large bulla itself may contain up to 4 l of gas but the volume change during a breath is usually less than 8% of the bulla vital capacity. The volume change is in the appropriate direction, i.e. larger on inspiration. Most bullae do not therefore contribute significantly to gas exchange but do fill and empty synchronously with the rest of the lung. This feature would not be compatible with expiratory filling of a cyst under pressure.

Direct measurement of the pressure within bullae has been made at operation or percutaneously by some surgeons [7,10]. Interestingly the pressures have been very similar to expected pleural pressure (−11 cm H_2O during tidal breathing and −27 cm H_2O at TLC). When intrabulla pressure has been measured simultaneously with pleural pressure the two signals have similar amplitudes

and are in phase. This confirms that bullae are subject to the same pressure changes during spontaneous inspiration as the rest of the lung. Surgeons are aware that a bulla readily presents itself at thoracotomy and understandably gives the impression of containing gas under pressure. Direct measurement of intrabulla pressure has also been made during IPPV when the airway pressure is transmitted with slight attenuation to the bulla. However, continued observation in one case demonstrated the development of PEEP within the bullae which would give the bulla the appearance of being under tension when the chest is opened [7]. Under these artificial circumstances of IPPV the intrabulla pressure may be suprapleural.

The content of the gas within bullae has been examined by taking samples from direct puncture. Kaltreider and Fray reported that the oxygen and carbon dioxide content of bullae were similar to that found in mixed venous blood [10]. They also examined the wash-in of acetylene which was minimal. Gas sampling experiments have been repeated recently by examination of the O_2 and CO_2 tensions within bullae before and during hyperoxygenation [7]. The bulla P_{O_2} and P_{CO_2} were identical to the expected alveolar values. During oxygen wash-in the P_{O_2} rose at a rate which was slower than the rise in arterial P_{O_2} and did not reach equilibrium over the study period. These experiments suggest that bullae are large spaces which do ventilate slowly but probably do not contribute significantly to gas exchange. The large, relatively avascular, internal surface area permits gas equilibrium to the level of mixed venous blood.

Although the physiologic behaviour of bullae can be characterized there is still some difficulty in understanding how they arise and take their shape. Some light can be shed on this problem by examining the mechanical properties of a bulla independently from the whole lung. In 1962, Ting examined the pressure–volume characteristics of both a bulla and its adjoining lung [11]. He discovered that the bulla was initially very compliant and filled easily and rapidly. However, once it was full it behaved like a paper bag with non-compliant walls and therefore does not really have any elasticity (Fig. 22.1).

Superimposition of the P–V curve of the adjoining lung highlights the major difference in the elastic properties. If the lung and the bulla are subject to similar pleural pressures on inspiration the bulla will be completely full almost before the lung has begun to inflate. This suggests that under normal conditions of tidal breathing the bulla may be permanently inflated as the lung fills and empties.

These observations about the behavior of bullae suggest an alternative hypothesis for their generation. It is no longer necessary to invoke the presence of valvular obstruction and preferential inflation. The bulla may exist purely because of the breakdown of the forces of interdependence. If degeneration occurs in an unbalanced fashion in a region of lung it may initially be contained by a redistribution of forces throughout the lung. If this mechanism for damage limitation fails then the lung matrix may simply retract from the space and form a bulla. Effectively the bulla then becomes functionally external to the lung and behaves as a pneumothorax. The retraction of tissue away from the space would explain the development of the spheroid shape and the bulla would then cause symptoms by behaving as a space-occupying lesion. The lung surrounding the bulla may retract and collapse but need not be compressed. There would be an associated reduction in elastic recoil pressure and attempts to compensate for this would result in symptomatic hyperinflation. The rationale for surgery still exists but is likely to be successful because it repairs the elastic matrix of the lung rather than relieving compression (Fig. 22.2).

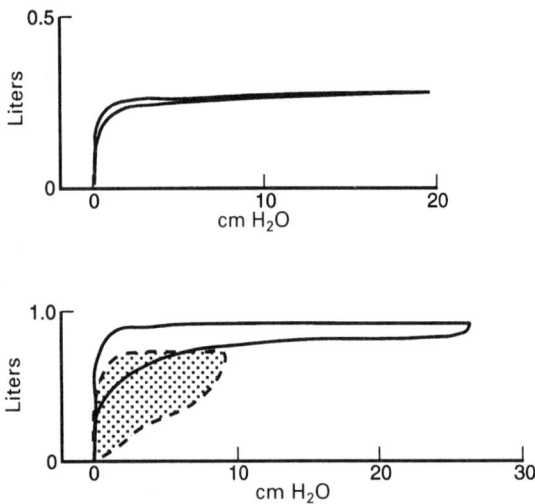

22.4 CLINICAL FEATURES AND PHYSIOLOGY

Exertional dyspnea is the usual presenting feature of bullous lung disease. There are no qualitative features which distinguish the symptom from associated emphysema but it is likely to occur at lower age than would be expected. Sometimes the bulla is a chance finding on the radiograph or associated with minimal disturbance. Less commonly the bulla may rupture and present with a pneumothorax which may be difficult to manage without surgery. Occasionally a bulla may be misinterpreted as a pneumothorax in a breathless patient and a chest drain inserted directly into the cavity. Another unusual presentation is with coincidental infection within the bulla. The subsequent radiographic appearance of a spheroid abscess may be recognized, especially if the walls become thickened by inflammatory tissue. Sometimes bullae will resolve spontaneously following infection. Clinical examination of the patient

Fig. 22.1 Schematic P–V curves of bulla and adjacent lung taken from Ting (1963). The pressure–volume curves from two excised bullae demonstrate that they are extremely compliant until full, i.e. they behave like paper bags. The P–V characteristics of adjacent lung (shaded) removed at surgery in the lower panel shows that the bulla will always be inflated fully over the range of tidal breathing.

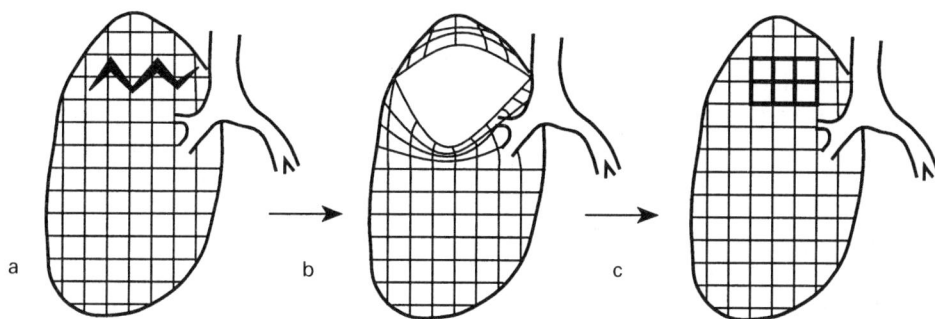

Fig. 22.2 A schematic view of the possible evolution of bullae. If a local defect occurs in the lung matrix (a) then the elastic properties of the lung may make it recoil and create a spherical space (b). The rationale for surgery should then be to reconstruct the lung matrix rather than to remove a space occupying bulla (c).

with a large bulla will often demonstrate asymmetric hyperinflation and reduction of chest wall expansion. The percussion note may also be resonant but this feature cannot be relied upon if the bulla is not superficial.

Like the presentation, the physiologic picture may be non-specific and can be confused by the associated chronic obstructive lung disease [12,13,14]. There is almost invariably some degree of airway obstruction with a reduction in FEV_1 and FEV_1/FVC. This may reflect concomitant emphysema or can be accounted for entirely by a loss of pulmonary elastic recoil which accompanies large bullae [15]. There is always some degree of hyperinflation, more so of RV and FRC than TLC. Since most bullae do not ventilate in the course of tidal breathing there is discrepancy between the plethysmographic TLC and helium dilution TLC or V_A. The volume of trapped gas measured this way is an estimate of the volume of the bulla but does not correlate particularly well with postoperative improvement [13]. Gas exchange is usually impaired and manifest by hypoxia or reduced T_{LCO}. The K_{CO} is useful when the bulla is non-ventilating as it is likely to reflect the quality of the non-bullous lung and may help to make a decision regarding surgery. Incremental exercise performance is reduced in a pattern associated with ventilatory limit-

ation and a high heart rate reserve as in other patients with COPD [16]. There may also be a greater dyspnea/$\dot{V}O_2$ gradient on exercise but this has not been compared directly [17]. None of these features can identify bullous disease distinctly, though in comparison with generalized emphysema there is hyperinflation and gas trapping with relative preservation of carbon monoxide transfer.

Occasionally a bulla may ventilate significantly during tidal breathing and exert its detrimental influence as a source of increased dead space. This is extremely unusual in patients with emphysematous bullae but is more common in other cystic conditions [18]. If it is present it may be recognized by lack of gas trapping, high $\dot{V}E/\dot{V}O_2$ on exercise, and hypercapnia.

22.5 RADIOLOGICAL APPEARANCE AND IMAGING

Bullae may be clearly identified on the plain postero-anterior or lateral radiograph as round or oval hyperlucent areas with thin curvilinear boundaries [19] (Fig. 22.3). Septal lines may traverse the bulla and this feature helps to distinguish it from a pneumothorax. Incidental evidence of the effect of the bulla on surrounding lung may be visible as displacement of the fissures, mediastinum or

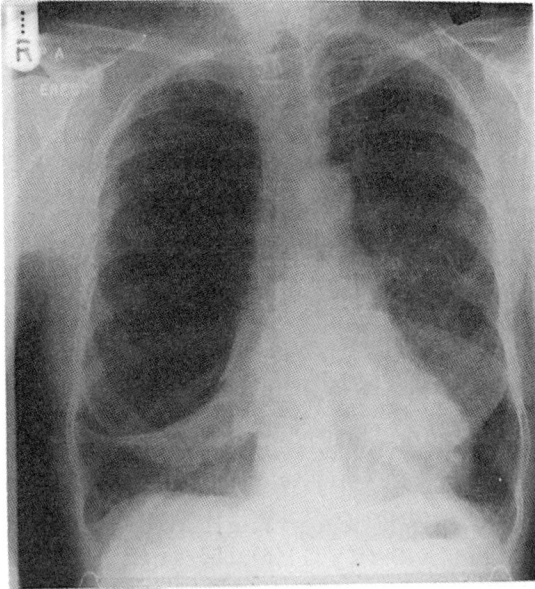

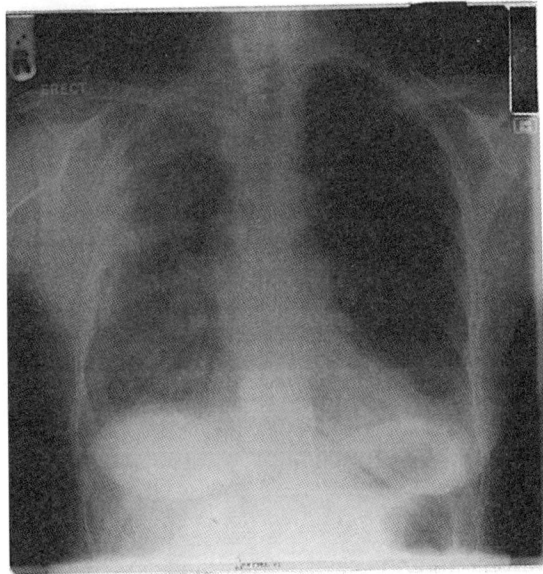

Fig. 22.3 Chest radiograph of patient with bullous disease. (a) There is an obvious large bulla in the right lung with collapsed lung below and against the mediastinum. There are a few septal lines which traverse the bulla. There is also bullous change in the top of the left lung. (b) One week after uneventful surgery the right lung has fully expanded.

diaphragm. The appearance of a bulla on plain radiograph may be specific but significant bullae may go unrecognized for several reasons.

The development of computed tomography of the lung has been invaluable in aiding the definition of bullae and their distinction from pulmonary emphysema [19–22]. The reasons for lack of sensitivity of the plain radiograph are obvious when the lung is imaged in the transverse plane. Bullae seldom occupy the whole thickness of the thorax and some lung is usually interspersed between the chest wall and the bulla (Fig. 22.4). This reduces the chances of definite identification on the plain film when it is obvious on the CT. The plain radiograph will also hide bullae when they are paramediastinal or in the posterior costophrenic sinus. CT displays the internal structure of the bulla – whether it is unilocular or contains septa – but it has not yet been used to predict the pathologic classification, though this could be anticipated. With CT it is possible to estimate the volume of a bulla by measuring and summing the area of bulla in each slice [13]. This technique can be developed by measuring the volume in inspiration and expiration to assess ventilation, which cannot be assessed by the change in area of the bulla in a single slice since a bulla can distort considerably during a breath though its volume may not change (see also chapter 14).

Other imaging techniques such as isotope scanning, bronchography and angiography have been applied to bullous lung disease. These tests have had more relevance to the assessment of the non-bullous lung prior to surgery rather than the description of the bulla itself.

22.6 ASSESSMENT FOR SURGERY

The assessment of suitability for surgery is central to the interest that bullous lung disease holds for clinicians. A few patients with severe airflow obstruction and dis-

(a)

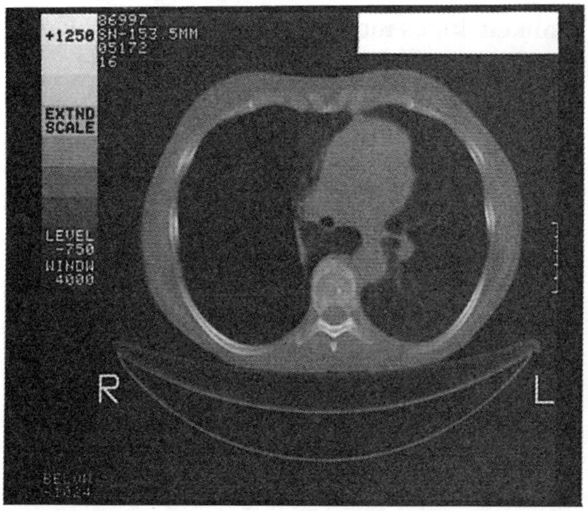

(b)

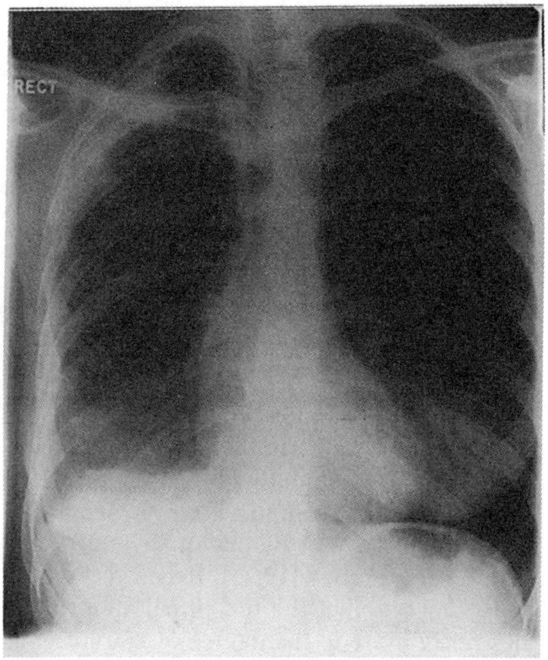

(c)

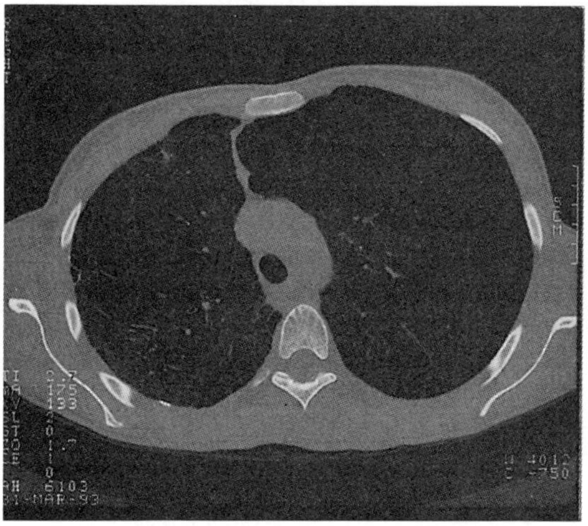

Fig. 22.4 (a) CT scan of the thorax from the patient in Fig. 22.4. This confirms the presence of a large bulla in the right lung. Sometimes the adjacent lung which in this case is flattened against the mediastinum may lie anteriorly or posteriorly and blur the definition of the bulla on the plain radiograph. The opposite lung contains small areas of parenchymal destruction but no major area amenable to surgery. (b) The chest radiograph from another patient suggests a bulla in the left upper lung. In this case the CT (c) uncovers the presence of bilateral destructive emphysema which is worse on the left. There is no surgical opportunity in this case.

abling breathlessness may have their lives transformed by operation. Unfortunately the wrong patient selection may have disastrous consequences. The ability to make more detailed functional assessments now makes the decision easier and opens the possibility of surgery to patients with minimal symptoms. It is probably still unreasonable to offer surgery to patients with asymptomatic bullae since some risk is present. However, they should be followed-up until symptomatic.

In patients with dyspnea the best surgical results will be in young patients with large bullae, minimal airway obstruction and normal surrounding lung. The definition of these patients has never really been difficult. The problem has been to identify which patients with chronic airflow limitation would benefit from bullectomy. In the past the inability to identify bullae and assess the non-bullous lung has led to some proscriptive statements about the likelihood of success. In patients with bullae less than 50% of the hemithorax, FEV_1 <1 l, hypercapnia or significant sputum production was considered to carry a high risk of failure. Prior to the use of CT, other techniques such as bronchography, pulmonary angiography, endobronchial lung function and ventilation–perfusion isotope scanning have been used to improve the accuracy of judgement.

The situation has been improved considerably by the introduction of computed tomography. The technique will describe the size and anatomy of the bulla and also describe the quality of surrounding lung. The presence and degree of surrounding emphysema can be judged by eye or by one of several visual scoring techniques [19,23]. Recent CT evidence suggests that the functional abnormalities relate more to the degree of emphysema in the non-bullous lung and not to the bulla itself [24]. The surgeon is therefore in a position to make an accurate assessment prior to operation and decide on the most appropriate technique. Some judgement is still required if the bulla is relatively small and surrounded by emphysematous lung. The improvement

following removal of a bulla of 500 ml or less in a patient with associated emphysema is unlikely to balance the surgical damage. Even with CT some doubts will remain concerning the ability of the non-bullous lung to expand following bulla removal. Pulmonary angiography may be used to demonstrate preserved vasculature in the collapsed lung which would suggest that it is capable of a recovery of function. Quantitative isotope scanning has been promoted as a useful investigation but rigorous assessment of the predictive value of the technique has not been undertaken. Scans obtained before and after surgery may demonstrate retained perfusion in the collapsed peribullous lung which improves after operation [25]. However, good results can still be obtained in patients with poor scan perfusion in the surrounding collapsed lung. There appears to be no technique which will predict whether the surrounding lung will expand and function though in most cases it seems to do so. Other hopeful methods such as bronchospirometry and bronchoscopic inert gas techniques have also proved disappointing. This is not really surprising in view of our knowledge of the ventilatory behavior of the bulla and surrounding lung. If gas does not enter these

Table 22.1 Indicators of surgical outcome

Good	Neutral	Poor
Large bulla size (>1 l)	FEV_1	Bulla volume <1 l (1/3 hemithorax)
Unilocular appearance on CT	Hypercapnia	Multiple or locular bullae
Demonstration of crowded airways or vessels in adjacent lung (any technique)	Hypoxemia	Generalized emphysema
Lack of generalized emphysema on CT	Operative technique	Lobectomy
Preserved KCO		Sputum production Bronchiectasis

Presentation of those features which are thought to be associated with surgical outcome. The 'good' features when present are likely to be related to a good symptomatic and functional improvement. 'Neutral' features are those attributes that do not appear to effect the functional outcome. Obviously the risk of surgery is greater in patients with low FEV_1 or respiratory failure but the physiologic outcome may be good if the indications are correct. 'Poor' indicators are those factors which make surgery difficult or unlikely to be successful.

regions the effect will not be recorded and lung function tests therefore generally describe the state of the non-bullous lung. The detailed description of pulmonary function and exercise performance prior to surgery should not determine whether the patient is suitable for surgery. It will, however, help to grade the risk and assess the improvement. Other general factors such as smoking behavior, sputum production, obesity and psychologic determination are as important as with other forms of surgery (Table 22.1).

Occasionally surgery may help patients with large ventilating bullae that act as dead space. Features which alert the clinician to this situation include excessive dyspnea, hypercapnia and high VD/VT on exercise. Under these circumstances the ventilation may be confirmed by $\dot{V}A/\dot{Q}$ scanning.

22.7 SURGICAL TREATMENT OF EMPHYSEMA

Radical surgical treatment of pulmonary emphysema has been the subject of experiment over the past few decades [26]. Transplantation which was initially thought to be impractical has developed into an effective form of treatment (Chapter 23). Other forms of surgery for generalized emphysema such as lobectomy have not been as successful and ideas about the effective surgical management of emphysematous bullae have developed. Many procedures have been described to remove bullae. These include excision and plication, wedge resection, marsupialization and intracavitary drainage [5]. Most surgeons do not have extensive experience at dealing with bullae because they are unusual. However, the exact nature of the surgery may not be too important and improved knowledge about the behavior of bullae helps guide surgical principles. First, it is illogical to remove any functioning tissue and operations should aim to preserve as much non-bullous lung as possible. Lobectomy and pneumonectomy must be avoided,

if at all possible. However, there may be circumstances where that is unavoidable, particularly when there are large ventilating cysts [18]. The other expectation of surgery is to restore the elastic integrity of the lung by removing the space and repairing the defect in the lung matrix and allowing the collapsed lung to expand. In concept this is more like darning a ladder in a stocking than excising an expanding cyst. Successful surgery should therefore aim to obliterate the bullous space with as little disruption as possible.

Most operations are performed through a conventional lateral thoracotomy but bilateral bullae can be simultaneously approached through median sternotomy [27,28]. Recently, more superficial bullae have been approached by thoracoscopy and coagulated by laser [29]. Bullae with large pleural surfaces and narrow necks can be excised with plication or oversewing of the stalks. Larger, deeper, bullae will need to be opened and excised along the base. The base is a potential source of air leak and must therefore be closed carefully by suture, staple or teflon strip [30].

An alternative to thoracotomy is percutaneous intracavitary drainage. This was originally described by Monaldi for the treatment of tuberculosis and later modified for emphysematous bullae by MacArthur [31,32]. In this procedure a balloon catheter is inserted directly in to the bulla after pleurodesis is achieved by purse string suture and talc. Prolonged suction is continued after surgery to appose the walls of the bulla and effect collapse of the space. This operation can be performed under local anesthetic in poor risk patients but can be used routinely [33]. It will be interesting to see in future how this procedure compares with thoracoscopic surgery.

22.8 THE RESULTS OF SURGERY

Unlike most forms of thoracic surgery, bullectomy can improve pulmonary function and produce dramatic results almost immediately following operation. Obviously there is an operative risk to patients with very poor preoperative lung function who may not survive. Those patients who have successful surgery can expect a short-term improvement in symptoms and physiology while the long-term effects may be determined by the subsequent behavior of the underlying lung disease.

The immediate consequences of surgery for bullous lung disease have been studied by several authors [13,24,34–39]. It is not a common procedure and most surgical series are relatively small and collected over a number of years. The average cardiothoracic center may have three or four cases per year. In most instances the risk of operation appears to be acceptable. The perioperative mortality in the published series ranges from 0 to 20%, but the deaths include patients with very poor preoperative function and incidental unavoidable complications. The postoperative improvement in symptoms and function is variable and depends upon the overall preoperative function, the size of the bulla and the condition of the surrounding lung. The best functional results occur in patients with minimal symptoms and nearly normal lung function tests. Patients with bullae less than about 1 l in volume, poor overall function and widespread emphysema probably show insufficient improvement to justify the operation [39]. This does not seem a very strong argument for performing surgery but real gains can be obtained for patients with disabling disease who fall between these categories. As patients with lung disease progress, the functional deterioration may go unnoticed for a long time before it impacts on everyday life. When a patient is severely disabled by airway obstruction even modest improvements in pulmonary function can have a dramatic effect on the quality of life.

Benefit from surgery may be detectable even during the course of the operation as the collapsed lung re-expands and gas exchange recovers. In the short term after surgery, improvements can be expected in airway function with average gains of 20% in FEV_1, FVC, and sGAW. All series report reductions in plethysmographic lung volumes and gas trapping which are in proportion with the size of the bulla. This relationship is not exact however, perhaps because the effects of surgical techniques such as Monaldi drainage do not always ablate the bulla entirely. The changes in elastic recoil pressure have not been measured often and the results are not consistent [15,34]. There are no predictable changes in blood gases or carbon monoxide transfer though improvements have been noted, particularly in bad cases. These laboratory changes are translated into symptomatic improvements which are reflected in reduction of dyspnea scores and better exercise performance. The latter shows improvements in $\dot{V}O_2$, workload and reduction in $\dot{V}E/\dot{V}O_2$. The beneficial improvement in functional capacity may be considerable. Some of this improvement may be accounted for by a reduction in dyspnea/$\dot{V}O_2$ and dyspnea threshold which makes exercise more comfortable [17].

Although these changes can be expected from a population of patients with bullous disease it is quite difficult to predict the postoperative improvement from any preoperative measurements. A recent attempt to develop predictive correlations for preoperative tests suggest that the FEV_1 (% predicted) and the slope of phase III of the single-breath nitrogen washout curve offer the best guess [40]. These two measurements presumably reflect the quality of the non-bullous lung. Nevertheless the correlation was not sufficiently high to be of value in an individual case. Such unpredictability of the degree of improvement highlights the lack of sensitivity of lung function tests alone to predict outcome. There is no single test which is useful, but comprehensive tests of function and performance have validity as objective baseline measurements and perhaps as estimates of operative risk. Bullous lung disease has attracted scientific interest over the past few decades but there are still many unanswered questions. It is still not

Table 22.2 Series of surgical outcomes

	No.	Assessment	Outcome	Postoperative Mortality	Follow-up	FEV_1 (pre-post) mean (l)
Foreman et al. 1968 [25]	13	CXR Lung function Isotope scan	Lung function Isotope scan	0%	2–127 months	1.23–1.72
Pride et al. 1973 [34]	18	CXR (insp&exp) Lung function $\dot{V}/\dot{Q}$scan	Lung function	5.5%	6–9 months	1.04–1.30
Fitzgerald et al. 1974 [35]	84	CXR Lung function Various imaging	Lung function	2.4%	1–20 years (mean 7.3 years)	1.09–1.79
Potgeiter et al. 1981 [36]	21	CXR Lung function Bronchograms	Lung function	9.5%	n/a	1.29–1.92
Morgan et al. 1986 [13]	12	CXR Lung function CT scan	Lung function	0%	2–12 months	1.01–1.53
Connolly and Wilson 1989 [38]	19	CXR Lung function Various imaging	Lung function	0%	3–22 years	anecdotal
Nicholadze 1992 [39]	46	CXR Lung function CT scan	Lung function	0%	1/2weeks–2/5 years	2.1–2.0 2.1–2.6

Comparison of some of the series of surgical intervention in bullous lung disease. Many of the data are not comparable in terms of outcome or studied at similar times. None of the studies directly compare one mode of prediction with another, though informal comparisons are often made in discussion.

possible to give clear advice about the timing or appropriateness of surgery other than in generalization. There is a lack of objectivity with regard to the recommendations that relate to the correct investigations to determine surgical outcome. The fundamental comparative studies of different methods of preoperative investigation, for example isotope vs CT scans, have not yet been done. This is understandably difficult because bullae are relatively uncommon and it would take time in a major center to collect sufficient cases. As a consequence, prediction of surgical success is based upon the limited amount of data that is available and the experience or prejudice of the clinician.

Investigators of the long-term effects of surgery are agreed about the consequences. There have now been several examinations of function from 4 to 23 years after operation and one fear about surgery has been dispelled [35,41,42]. Once removed, giant bullae do not seem to recur and surgery is not a catalyst for the development of further bullae. The immediate improvement of function following operation seems to be maintained. The subsequent rate of deterioration is related to the condition of the remaining lung and varies from stability to an annual decline of FEV_1 which is similar to other patients with chronic obstructive lung disease. Those patients who continue to smoke following surgery have a more rapid decline in function than those who do not [42].

22.9 CONCLUSIONS

In summary, bullous lung disease is an unusual variant of chronic obstructive lung disease which has important surgical opportunities for treatment. Large bullae may develop alongside normal lung or any grade of generalized emphysema. Current evidence suggests that bullae originate from a region of local degeneration which becomes a space from which the remainder of the lung retracts. Both the bulla and the lung are subject to similar pleural pressure changes but their mechanical properties determine different behaviors. Most bullae ventilate slowly and do not contribute to tidal ventilation or gas exchange. They produce symptoms by acting as a space occupying mass which forces hyperinflation as a compensation. The hyperinflation may not be effective enough to maintain elastic recoil and prevent airway narrowing in adjacent lung.

The principal aim of surgery should be to ablate the abnormal space and restore elastic integrity to the whole lung. Several surgical operations have been developed to achieve this purpose with the ability to conserve as much functioning tissue as possible. The assessment of suitable patients for surgery will always have a subjective element and physiologic tests alone do not allow the correct decision to be made when lung function is poor. The development of pulmonary imaging has revolutionized assessment. It is now possible to define and measure the dimensions of the bulla and to judge the quality of the surrounding lung. This not only identifies the presence of an operable bulla but also may recommend a specific procedure. It should now be possible to give serious consideration to surgery to all patients with bullae larger than 1 l irrespective of the presence of additional obstructive lung disease. The complication rate of surgery, which is already acceptable, should become even lower with the development of minimally invasive surgical techniques. The patient with bullous disease should be considered fortunate enough to have a form of chronic obstructive lung disease for which surgery can offer long-term benefit.

REFERENCES

1. CIBA Guest Symposium (1959) *Thorax*, **14**, 286–99.
2. Freundlich, I.M. (1981) *Pulmonary Masses, Cysts and Cavities*, Year Book, Chicago.
3. Packe, G.E., Ayres, J.G., Citron, K.M. and Stableforth, D.E. (1986) Large lung bullae in sarcoidosis. *Thorax*, **41**, 792–7.
4. Kuhlman, J.E., Knowles, M.C., Fishman, E.K. and Seigelman, S.S. (1989) Premature bullous pulmonary damage in AIDS: CT diagnosis. *Radiology*, **173**, 23–26.
5. Klingman, R.R., Angelillo, V.A. and DeMeester, T.R. (1991) Cystic and bullous lung disease. *Ann. Thorac. Surg.*, **52**, 576–80.
6. Reid, R. (1967) *The Pathology of Emphysema*, Lloyd-Luke.
7. Morgan, M.D.L., Edwards, C.W., Morris, J. and Matthews, H.R. (1989) Origin and behaviour of emphysematous bullae. *Thorax*, **44**, 533–8.
8. Hayashi, J. (1914) Ueber totlichen pneumothorax durch infarckt und emphysema. *Frankfurt Ztschr. Pathol.*, **16**, 1–16.
9. Head, J.R. and Avery, E.E. (1949) Intracavitatory suction (Monaldi) in the treatment of emphysematous bullae and blebs. *J. Thorac. Cardiovasc. Surg.*, **18**, 761–76.
10. Kaltreider. N.L. and Fray, W.W. (1939) Pathological physiology of pulmonary cysts and bullae. *Am. J. Med. Sci.*, **197**, 62–77.
11. Ting, E.Y., Klopstock, R. and Lyons, H.A. (1963) Mechanical properties of pulmonary cysts and bullae. *Am. Rev. Respir. Dis.*, **87**, 538–44.
12. Pride, N.B., Hugh-Jones, P., O'Brien, E.N. and Smith, L.A. (1970) Changes in lung function following the surgical treatment of bullous emphysema. *Q. J. Med.*, **39**, 49–69.
13. Morgan, M.D.L., Denison, D.M. and Strickland, B. (1986) Value of computed tomography for selecting patients with bullous lung disease for surgery. *Thorax*, **41**, 855–62.
14. Wade, J.F., Mortenson, R. and Irvin, C.G. (1991) Physiologic evaluation of bullous emphysema. *Chest*, **100**, 1151–4.
15. Gelb, A.F., Gold, W.M. and Nadel, J.A. (1973) Mechanisms limiting airflow in bullous lung disease. *Am. Rev. Respir. Dis.*, **107**, 571–8.
16. Wasserman, K., Hansen, S. and Whipp, B. (1987) *Principles of Exercise Testing and Interpretation*. Lea and Francis.
17. Teramoto, S., Fukuchi, Y., Nagase, T. *et al.* (1992) Quantitative assessment of dyspnea

during exercise before and after bullectomy for giant bulla. *Chest*, **102**, 1362–6.

18. Bateman, E.D., Westerman, D.E., Hewitson, R.P. and Ferguson, A.D. (1981) Pneumonectomy for massive ventilated lung cysts. *Thorax*, **36**, 554–6.

19. Sanders, C. (1991) The radiographic diagnosis of emphysema. *Radiol. Clin. North Am.*, **29**, 1019–30.

20. Morgan, M.D.L. and Strickland, B. (1984) Computed tomography in the assessment of bullous lung disease. *Br. J. Dis. Chest*, **78**, 10–25.

21. Carr, D.H. and Pride, N.B. (1984) Computed tomography in preoperative assessment of bullous emphysema. *Clin. Radiol.*, **35**, 43–5.

22. Fiore, D., Biondetti, P.R., Sartori, F. and Calabro, F. (1982) The role of computed tomography in the evaluation of bullous lung disease. *J. Comput. Tomogr.*, **6**(1), 105–8.

23. Morgan, M.D.L. (1992) The detection and quantification of pulmonary emphysema by computed tomography. *Thorax*, **47**, 1001–4.

24. Gould, G.A., Redpath, A.T., Ryan, M. *et al.* Parenchymal emphysema measured by CT lung density correlates with lung function in patients with bullous disease. *Eur. Respir. J.*, **6**, 698–704.

25. Foreman, S., Weil, H., Duke, R. *et al.* (1968) Bullous disease of the lung. *Ann. Intern. Med.*, **69**, 757–67.

26. Gaensler, E.A., Cogell, D.W., Knudson, R.J. *et al.* (1983) Surgical management of emphysema. *Clin. Chest Med.*, **4**, 443–63.

27. Cooper, J.D., Nelems, J.M. and Pearson, F.G. (1978) Extended indications for median sternotomy in patients requiring pulmonary resection. *Ann. Thorac. Surg.*, **26**, 413–20.

28. Iwa, T., Watanabe, Y. and Fukatani, G. (1981) Simultaneous bilateral operations for bullous emphysema by median sternotomy. *J. Thorac. Cardiovasc. Surg.*, **81**, 732–7.

29. Wakabayashi, A., Brenner, M., Kayaleh, R.A. *et al.* (1991) Thorascopic carbon dioxide laser treatment of bullous emphysema. *Lancet*, **337**, 881–3.

30. Parmar, J.H., Hubbard, W.G. and Mathews, H.R.W. (1987) Teflon strip pneumostasis for excision of giant emphysematous bullae. *Thorax*, **42**, 144–8.

31. Monaldi, V. (1947) Endocavitary aspiration: its practical applications. *Tubercle*, **28**, 223–8.

32. MacArthur, A.M. and Fountain, S.W. (1977) Intracavitary suction and drainage in the treatment of emphysematous bullae. *Thorax*, **32**, 668–72.

33. Venn, G.E., Williams, P.R. and Goldstraw, P. (1988) Intracavitary drainage for bullous emphysematous lung disease: experience with the Brompton technique. *Thorax*, **43**, 998–1002.

34. Pride, N.B., Barter, C.E. and Hugh-Jones P. (1973) The ventilation of bullae and the effect of their removal on thoracic gas volumes and tests of over-all pulmonary function. *Am. Rev. Respir. Dis.*, **107**, 83–98.

35. Fitzgerald, M.X., Keelan, P.J., Cugell, D.W. and Gaensler, E.A. (1974) Long-term results of surgery for bullous emphysema. *J. Thorac. Cardiovasc. Surg.*, **68**, 566–87.

36. Potgeiter, P.D., Benatar, S.R., Hewitson, R.P. and Ferguson, A.D. (1981) Surgical treatment of bullous lung disease. *Thorax*, **36**, 885–90.

37. Laros, C.D., Gelissen, M.D., Bergstein, P.G.M. *et al.* (1980) Bullectomy for giant bullae in emphysema. *J. Thorac. Cardiovasc. Surg.*, **91**, 63–70.

38. Connolly, J.E. and Wilson, A. (1989) The current status of surgery for bullous emphysema. *J. Thorac. Cardiovasc. Surg.*, **97**, 351–61.

39. Nicholadze, G.D. (1992) Functional results of surgery for bullous emphysema. *Chest*, **101**, 119–22.

40. Ohta, M., Nakahara, K., Yasumitsu, T. *et al.* (1992) Prediction of postoperative performance status in patients with giant bullae. *Chest*, **101**, 668–73.

41. Pearson, M.G. and Ogilvie, C. (1983) Surgical treatment of emphysematous bullae: late outcome. *Thorax*, **38**, 134–37.

42. Hughes, J.A., Macarthur, A.M., Hutchison, D.C.S. and Hugh–Jones, P. (1984) Long term changes in lung function after surgical treatment of bullous emphysema in smokers and ex-smokers. *Thorax*, **39**, 140–42.

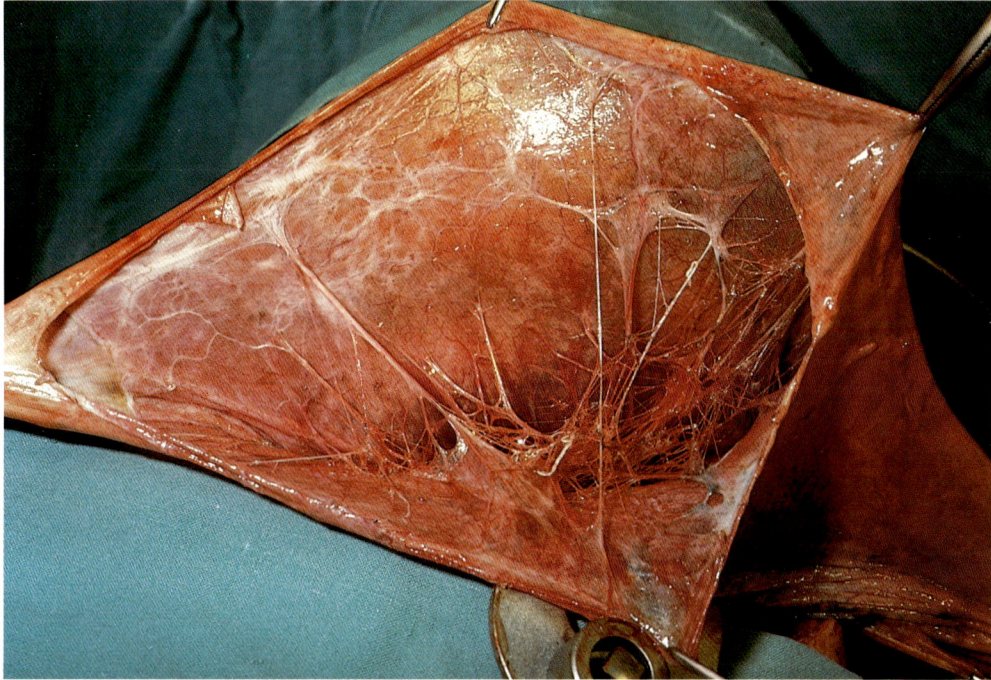

(a)

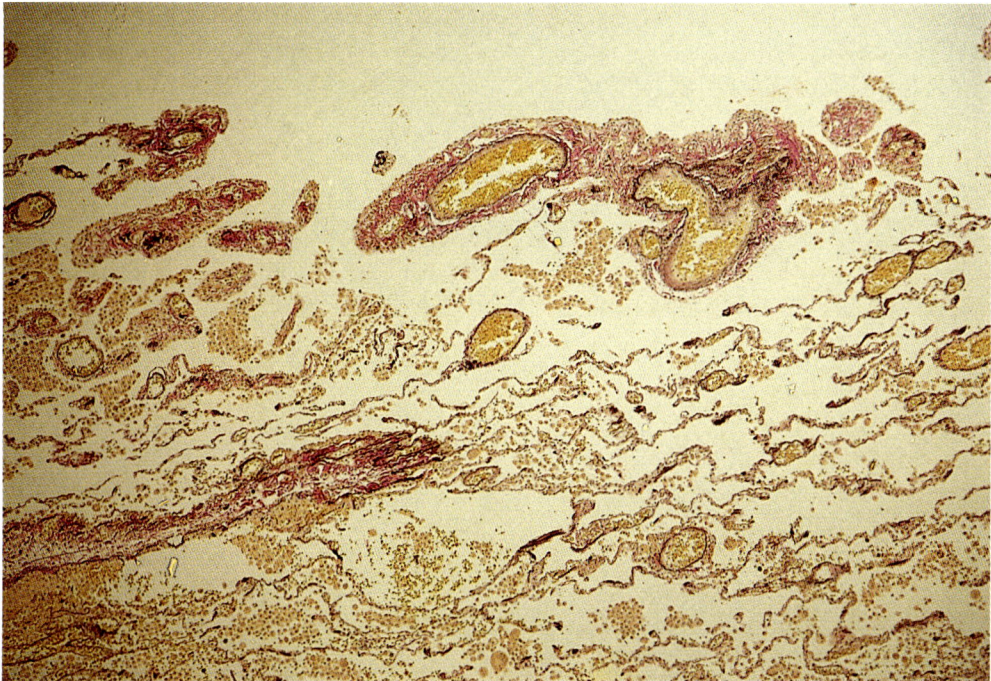

(b)

Plate 1 Photograph of bulla floor (a) and photomicrograph of the histology of junctional area (b). When they are opened at surgery the bullae contain thin septa. The floor of this bulla also has widely patent openings which communicate with the feeding airways. Microscopy of the junctional area does not demonstrate any physical valvular mechanism. The alveolar spaces simply merge into the bulla cavity at the top of the picture. (copyright).

LUNG TRANSPLANTATION

P. Corris

23.1 INTRODUCTION

The modern era for lung transplantation began in 1981 when Bruce Reitz and colleagues from Stanford University introduced heart lung transplantation for patients with pulmonary vascular disease [1]. Indications for combined heart and lung transplants (HLT) were subsequently widened to include various pulmonary conditions [2]. Survival rates were good and in marked contrast with results obtained for single lung transplantation over the preceding 25 years [3]. The success of HLT was based on reliable healing of the tracheal anastomosis compared with the bronchial anastomotic breakdown seen frequently following single lung transplantation (SLT). This reliable healing reflected a good blood supply to the proximal donor trachea via donor coronary artery/bronchial artery anastomoses, in contrast to the lack of blood supplied to the proximal donor bronchus following transplantation of a single lung. The lack of success with SLT was also based on both poor selection of potential recipients, some of whom were septic and had multi-organ failure, and the apparently insuperable problems of rejection and infection.

It was realized that many patients undergoing HLT, however, received a new heart unnecessarily. After a period of research, success was reported with SLT in patients with fibrosing lung disease by the Toronto Group in 1986 [4].

Important potential factors were careful patient selection, restoration of a viable blood supply to the bronchial anastomosis by wrapping it with a pedicle of greater omentum and the introduction of cyclosporin A as the principal immunosuppressant. It has been shown subsequently that the bronchial anastomosis does not require a wrap of omentum for reliable healing and very few centers now perform this procedure although the UK Harefield Group are now carrying out direct revascularization of donor bronchial artery to ensure good blood supply to the donor bronchus.

In 1988 the double lung transplant operation (DLT) using an *en bloc* transplantation of both lungs with a tracheal anastomosis was introduced by Patterson and colleagues [5]. However, this procedure was accompanied by much more frequent problems with airway healing than the HLT operation [6]. In addition, the operation was, if anything, more complex than HLT and the extensive mediastinal dissection frequently led to denervation of the recipient's native heart. Bleeding was at least as great a problem as that for HLT, and by 1989 the procedure as originally described has been largely abandoned. Noirclerc [7] provided the solution to the problem of airway healing by performing two separate bronchial anastomoses, since as

Chronic Obstructive Pulmonary Disease. Edited by Dr P. Calverley and Professor N. Pride. Published in 1995 by Chapman & Hall, London. ISBN 0 412 46450 0

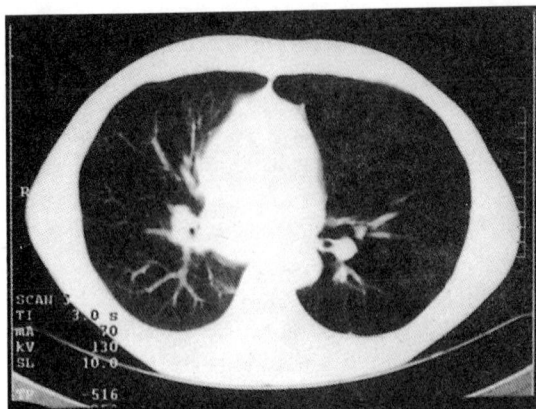

Fig. 23.1 CT Scan following right single lung transplant in a patient with emphysema. There is a marked contrast between the vascularity and density of lung parenchyma between the transplanted normal right lung and emphysematous left lung.

in SLT, the donor bronchus is better vascularized initially if the anastomosis is close to the lung parenchyma. This concept was further developed by Pasque [8] with the bilateral sequential lung transplant. As its name implies, two separated lungs are implanted with separate hilar anastomoses (each of bronchus, pulmonary artery and left atrial cuff). The heart and mediastinum are left largely undisturbed. The incision is a transverse bilateral thoracotomy, dividing the sternum horizontally. In contrast to HLT, SLT and bilateral sequential lung transplantation do not in general require cardiopulmonary bypass with associated anticoagulation.

23.2 EVOLUTION OF LUNG TRANSPLANTATION IN COPD

It was originally believed that patients with end-stage COPD were not suitable for SLT. Objections to SLT for emphysema arose because of perceived problems with the native lung, which would be ventilated during a period of positive-pressure ventilation leading to air trapping, subsequent mediastinal shift and compression of the transplanted lung.

Since perfusion would be directed towards the transplanted lung because of expected lower pulmonary vascular resistance, ventilation perfusion ($\dot{V}_A/\dot{Q}$) imbalance would result. These considerations proved to be more than theory and experience in the early 1970s demonstrated that severe ventilation perfusion imbalance and hyperinflation of the native lung actually occurred [9,10]. Therefore patients with emphysema including those with inherited α_1-antitrypsin deficiency were initially treated with combined HLT. Moreover the successful results in patients with α_1-antitrypsin deficiency showed that such patients could undergo transplant procedures and retain normal lung function in the first 12–18 months without replacement therapy [11]. The shortfall in donor heart lung blocks led to the introduction of the *en bloc* double lung transplant for emphysema but as previously noted this operation was associated with tracheal anastomotic complications in 50% of patients and quickly lost favor. Successful introduction of single lung transplantation for patients with fibrosing lung disease led to re-examination of this procedure for patients with emphysema since techniques of donor lung preservation and surgical technique had improved dramatically from those methods used in the early 1970s.

After a preliminary report of successful SLT for emphysema by Mal and co-workers [12] in France in 1989, the Washington Lung Transplant Group cautiously embarked on a program of SLT in patients with emphysema and demonstrated the utility and safety of this procedure in carefully selected patients [13]. Although the mechanics of the native lung remain the same, improvements in patient selection, lung preservation and anesthetic management have contributed to the success. Subsequent experience from other groups including our own have demonstrated the potential problem of residual infection in the native lung [14]. Moreover, most patients with large bilateral bullae may still show evidence of gross hyperinflation of the native lung in the

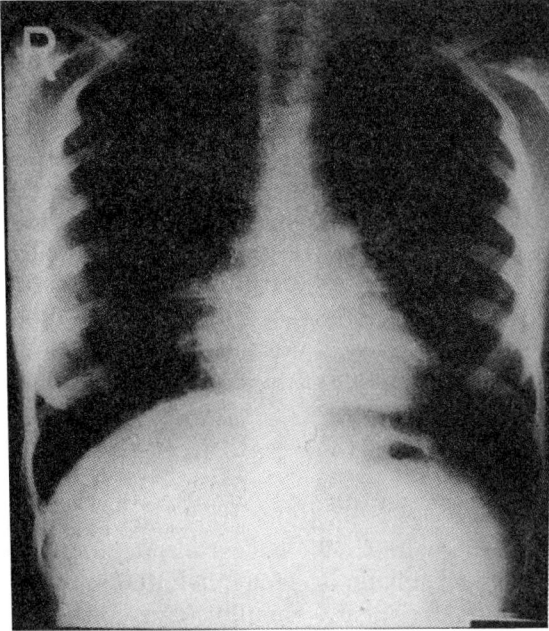

Fig. 23.2 Chest radiograph of patient following bilateral sequential lung transplantation.

plantation of heart and lungs or both lungs alone, with an upper age limit of 60 years for transplantation of single lung. The higher age limit for single lung reflects the increased availability of suitable single lungs.

23.3.2 DISABILITY/LIFE EXPECTANCY

Transplantation is usually considered for a patient when estimated life expectancy is less than 18 months. Clearly in COPD it is difficult to make an accurate prediction of survival. However, estimates are based on current level of lung function, the rate of decline over previous years and the date of onset of cor pulmonale. In Newcastle the first 25 patients with emphysema accepted for transplantation had a mean FEV_1 of 22% predicted, a mean vital capacity of 48% predicted and a mean diffusing capacity for carbon monoxide by the single breath method of 29% predicted values.

23.3.3 NUTRITIONAL STATE

Many patients reaching the end stage of chronic pulmonary disease suffer from cachexia and malnutrition [16]. All recipients lose weight in the first week following transplantation and severe preoperative nutritional deficiency leads to an inability to withstand the rigors of the postoperative period, increasing susceptibility to infection and poor wound healing. Obesity, on the other hand, increases surgical risk, predisposing to atelectasis and impairing postoperative mobility which is essential following lung transplantation. Ideally recipients should be within 15 kg of their ideal body weight. There is an increased mortality in adult patients whose body weight is less than 40 kg. The early unsuccessful transplant recipients were all bed bound and the majority of transplant centres now require that recipients are capable of self-care and able to participate in gentle exercise rehabilitation to maintain muscle bulk and physical fitness.

early postoperative period after SLT and thus the bilateral sequential lung transplant was successfully applied to patients with emphysema who were not suitable for SLT [15].

There is now reasonable agreement about technical approaches to transplantation for COPD, in particular emphysema where experience is greatest. Those patients with no history of recurrent pulmonary sepsis and no evidence of large bilateral bullae are suitable for consideration of SLT. Those patients with frequent pulmonary sepsis or marked bullous disease may be considered for HLT or bilateral sequential lung transplantation, with the latter procedure being increasingly used as the procedure of choice.

23.3 INDICATIONS, CONSIDERATIONS AND CRITERIA FOR LUNG TRANSPLANTATION

23.3.1 AGE

The shortfall in suitable donor organs leads to an upper age limit of 50 years for trans-

23.3.4 INFECTION

Localized sepsis preoperatively may lead to severe systemic infection postoperatively because of the need for immunosuppressive therapy. Extrapulmonary sepsis therefore mitigates against successful transplantation. Patients with recurrent or persistent pulmonary infection are not suitable for SLT. Oral hygiene is important and all patients should have any dental sepsis eradicated preoperatively. The presence of an aspergilloma is a contraindication to any form of lung transplant. Removal of the lung containing an aspergilloma is likely to result in seeding of the pleural space with *Aspergillus* leading to fungal empyema. Removal of the contralateral lung for single lung transplant leaves the aspergilloma *in situ* and subsequent immunosuppression inevitably will lead to disseminated *Aspergillus* infection.

23.3.5 PREVIOUS SURGERY

There is a risk of life-threatening hemorrhage when the native lungs are removed if there are pleural scars or adhesions. Clearly there is a gradation of risk from scarring due to previous open lung biopsy via a limited thoracotomy to previous total pleurectomy and the latter is regarded as a contraindication for HLT. This has important consequences for the management of pneumothorax in potential recipients with emphysema. If pleurodesis is required, surgeons should be advised to perform limited anterior pleurodesis. The use of the anti-fibrinolytic aprotinin during transplant surgery reduces bleeding in patients who have undergone previous thoracotomy [17], and the recent development of bilateral sequential lung transplantation via a transverse bilateral thoracotomy allows the surgeon much better access to the pleural space than is afforded by a sternotomy. In this regard the bilateral sequential lung transplantation has advantages over the original HLT.

23.3.6 SYSTEMIC CORTICOSTERIODS

Although early lung transplant programs insisted on patients being weaned from corticosteroids, this proved very difficult to achieve in practice, particularly in patients with COPD. More recent experience in Newcastle has shown that bronchial anastomoses are at no greater risks in patients receiving up to 20 mg of prednisolone a day compared with those on no prednisolone [18] providing there is no evidence of steroid-induced thinning of the skin, osteoporosis or myopathy.

23.3.7 CARDIAC DISEASE

Patients with COPD under consideration for SLT or bilateral sequential lung transplantation ideally should have sufficient preservation of right ventricular function to allow single lung anesthesia, obviating the need for cardiopulmonary bypass. The right ventricle has a very great capacity to show improved function after successful surgery when pulmonary vascular resistance falls to normal and the Toronto Group have successfully performed a single lung transplant in a patient with a right ventricular ejection fraction of only 12%, although the mean right ventricular ejection fractions of a series of patients reported by this group were 31% and 38% for their SLT and DLT candidates respectively [19]. We have shown that following SLT for pulmonary fibrosis, pulmonary vascular resistance, pulmonary artery pressure and right ventricular performance returned to normal even when markedly abnormal preoperatively [20]. The presence of cor pulmonale complicating COPD is not a contraindication for successful SLT.

23.3.8 PSYCHOLOGIC FACTORS

There is no procedure in medicine which provides more stress for recipients and family than lung transplantation. The process begins

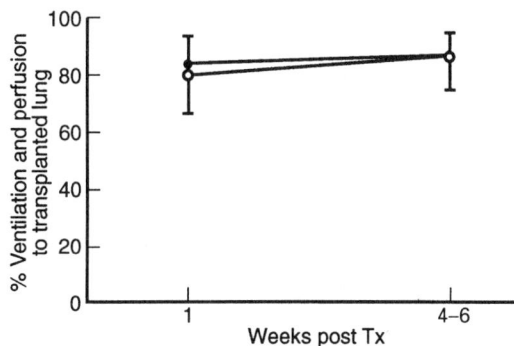

Fig. 23.3 Results of quantitative ventilation and perfusion scanning in the first six patients undergoing single lung transplantation for emphysema. The results show immediate and sustained preferential ventilation and perfusion to the transplanted lung.

from the time of initial referral and lasts until postoperative rehabilitation is complete. Any potential recipient must be well motivated and want a lung transplant, be able to cope and have demonstrated a willingness to comply. A supportive family or circle of close friends is essential. Underlying psychiatric illness, abuse of alcohol or drugs including cigarettes constitute contraindications.

23.3.9 PRESENCE OF OTHER MAJOR ORGAN DYSFUNCTION

Good renal and hepatic function are essential particularly in view of cyclosporin toxicity [21]. A creatinine clearance of over 50 ml/min is required. Only minor abnormalities of liver function are acceptable. This is clearly of importance in patients with α_1-antitrypsin deficiency who may have abnormalities of hepatic function as a result of their disease. The presence of portal hypertension would preclude consideration of lung transplantation alone. Type I diabetes mellitus if well-controlled no longer rules out transplantation.

23.4 MATCHING DONOR TO RECIPIENT

Donor matching is based on ABO compatability and size by calculating the predicted total lung capacity (TLC) of both donor and recipient using height, age and sex. There is no direct measurement of donor lung TLC. In patients with COPD who have much greater lung capacities than predicted, it is preferable to give larger lungs than predicted as above, particularly if carrying out SLT. The size discrepancy between the transplanted lung and hemithorax commonly prevents sealing of any parenchymal leak which if present may lead to pneumothoraces persisting for several days. The chest wall remains compliant, and in practice is observed to change shape in the first few days after transplantation. A screening lymphocytotoxic cross-match using recipient serum and a banked pool of lymphocytes is carried out in all potential recipients accepted for transplantation to exclude the presence of pre-formed antibodies. Direct cross-match with lymphocytes from a potential donor is only carried out prospectively when this screening test is positive. Wherever possible donor and recipient are matched for cytomegalovirus (CMV) status. If a CMV-negative recipient receives a CMV-positive organ, serious CMV infection can be ameliorated by giving prophylactic CMV hyperimmunoglobulin [22].

23.5 POSTOPERATIVE COMPLICATIONS AND FOLLOW-UP

23.5.1 IMMUNOSUPPRESSION AND POSTOPERATIVE MANAGEMENT

Most patients are extubated within 36 hours of surgery and then begin an active programme of mobilization. Fluid intake is restricted in the early postoperative period with diuresis encouraged to avoid accumulation of fluid in the lungs. Prophylactic antibiotics in the form of flucloxacillin and metronidazole are given for the first five days

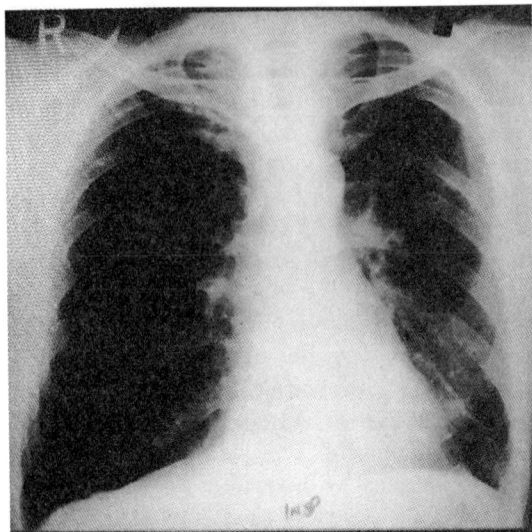

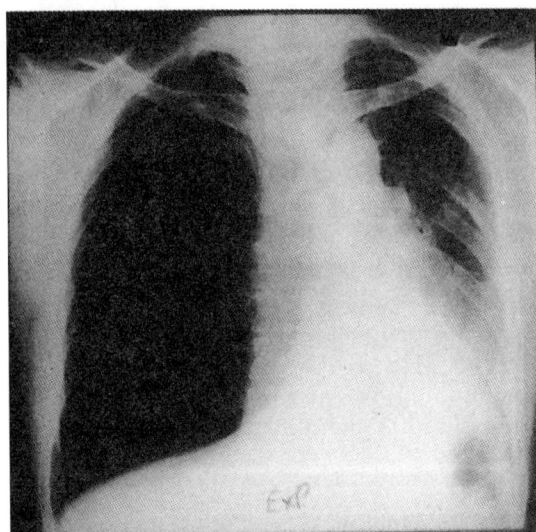

Fig. 23.4a,b 4a) Inspiratory, 4b) expiratory films following left single lung transplantation. Note the mediastinal shift towards the transplanted lung which occurs during expiration.

and the donor lungs are lavaged with samples sent to microbiology, prior to implantation so that appropriate antibiotics may be started early to cover 'donor acquired' pulmonary sepsis. At present patients receive azathioprine, rabbit antithymocyte globulin,

methylprednisolone and cyclosporin during the immediate postoperative period. Antithymocyte globulin is stopped after three days and methylprednisolone substituted by oral prednisolone at a rapidly tailing dose to a maintenance of 0.1 mg/kg. If patients have no evidence of lung rejection at six months maintenance steroids are withdrawn. Rejection episodes are treated with pulsed methylprednisolone 10 mg/kg i.v. for three days followed by augmented oral prednisolone for one month.

23.5.2 ASSESSMENT OF GRAFT FUNCTION

Over the first few postoperative days analysis of blood gases and examination of chest radiographs are used to monitor graft function. Thereafter chest radiographs are performed daily for approximately one week and lung function is monitored by continuous oximetry, daily spirometry and regular measurement of lung volumes and diffusing capacity. Patients undergoing single lung transplantation for COPD undergo a ventilation perfusion scan in the first week to ensure good perfusion and ventilation to the newly transplanted lung. In patients with emphysema there is both early preferential ventilation and perfusion to the transplanted lung unlike the situation following single lung transplantation for pulmonary fibrosis when preferential ventilation appears to lag behind preferential perfusion by about three weeks [23]. The principal problem in the management of lung transplant patients is that clinically it is impossible to separate opportunist infections of the lung from lung rejection. Both complications can present with identical respiratory symptoms and identical respiratory physical signs. A chest radiograph is also unhelpful since pulmonary infiltrates may be common to both and in the early postoperative period may also occur as a result of reimplantation injury. Moreover the chest radiograph may be entirely normal in patients experiencing acute rejection. This is particularly true in the first month after transplantation. During most episodes of acute rejection and infection the FEV$_1$ and diffusing capacity show a sustained fall of greater than 10% and thus unlike other solid organ transplant patients graft function following lung transplantation can be monitored with ease.

A diagnosis of rejection is currently based on transbronchial lung biopsy using alligator forceps under radiologic screening [24]. The principal morphologic changes found in acute rejection are perivascular infiltrates which may extend into alveolar septa at the later stages of rejection. Additionally bronchial tissue may also show evidence of a lymphocytic infiltrate. It is our practice to carry out three or four biopsies from each lobe of one lung since rejection may be patchy and the use of multiple biopsies from multiple lobes affords a greater chance of positive diagnosis. Moreover opportunist infection and rejection may coexist. In a series reported from Papworth Hospital just under 25% of the biopsies performed in the face of a deteriorating clinical condition or a reduction in lung function showed the presence of both infection and rejection. For this reason bronchoalveolar lavage is routinely combined with transbronchial biopsy and lavage fluid submitted for both viral culture, monoclonal staining for *Pneumocystis* and routine culture for bacteria and fungi. In Newcastle, as part of a series of prospective studies trying to determine the etiology of obliterative bronchiolitis we carry out routine surveillance transbronchial lung biopsies on all patients at a week, a month, three months, six months, 12 months and thereafter on an annual basis.

23.5.3 RESULTS

Providing patients are appropriately selected the results of HLT, SLT and bilateral sequential single lung transplantation are good [11,13,15, 25]. Approximately 10–15% of recipients will die in the first few weeks following transplantation generally due to problems with

poor lung preservation leading to diffuse alveolar damage, sepsis or both. The one-year survival for centers in the UK lies between 68 and 75%, with a three-year survival of 55–60%. The most important complications leading to death comprise opportunist infections and the development of obliterative bronchiolitis (OB). Current data suggest approximately 30% of patients surviving the perioperative period will subsequently develop OB within 5 years of their transplant. This leads in the majority of cases to a progressive deterioration in lung function unresponsive to medical therapy and the ultimate progression to respiratory failure, death or consideration of retransplantation after 6–12 months.

Functional results in survivors measured in terms of FEV$_1$ and exercise performance are good although better after HLT and bilateral sequential lung transplant compared with SLT alone [15]. Results one year following transplantation show a mean FEV$_1$ of 50% predicted following single lung transplant and 70% predicted values following sequential bilateral lung transplant. However, all patients should expect restoration of normal lifestyle with little or no functional restriction during normal activities of daily living. Exercise data from Newcastle comparing the six-minute walking distances and maximum oxygen consumption during an incremental symptom-limited exercise test show that in patients with emphysema all patients return to a normal six-minute walking distance of 600 metres or greater by one year with no evidence of desaturation on exercise. The maximum oxygen consumption is significantly greater in HLT and bilateral sequential lung transplants compared to single lung transplantation alone. However, maximum oxygen during the symptom-limited test remains at around 50% predicted for a given subject in the first year probably due to decompensation on account of the pretransplant disability.

After SLT for COPD the transplanted lung receives approximately 80% of total ventilation and perfusion over the first year. As one would predict the flow volume curve after SLT for emphysema shows a two compartment pattern, the initial high flow originating from the transplanted lung and the subsequent 'tail' of low flow from the native lung. Lung function, computed tomographic scans and transbronchial lung biopsies have revealed normal results in patients up to five years after transplantation indicating the potential for prolonged survival in patients who do not develop OB.

23.5.4 LONG-TERM COMPLICATIONS

(a) Obliterative bronchiolitis

This process may be defined physiologically by the development of progressive irreversible airflow obstruction unresponsive to augmented steroids [26]. Pathology shows obliteration of bronchioles, the lumens of which are filled by organizing fibrin associated with fibroblasts and mononuclear cells. Immunohistology has revealed that the walls of the bronchioles are infiltrated by CD8 lymphocytes [27]. The small bronchioles are left as fibrous bands extending out to the pleura with associated dilatation and bronchiectasis of proximal airways. Vascular sclerosis affecting both pulmonary arteries and pulmonary veins may also be seen in conjunction with obliterative bronchiolitis. Current evidence suggests that the development of obliterative bronchiolitis is related to the incidence and severity of rejection occuring in the first 6–12 months following transplantation and it is the presence of persisting rejection after six months which is probably most important. More recent evidence from Newcastle has demonstrated a clear relationship between the presence of organizing pneumonia and the subsequent development of obliterative bronchiolitis.

The disease usually results in a progressive loss of function due to airflow obstruction over a 6–12 month period leading to respiratory failure and death. However, a few patients appear to 'stabilize' with evidence of inactive OB on biopsy and an attenuation of the loss in FEV_1. Some patients with OB have demonstrated a clinical response to increased immunosuppression [28]. Continued research aims to identify those patients at risk of this most important complication at an early stage when augmented immunosuppression may be successful in preventing irreversible bronchiolar obliteration.

(b) Lymphoproliferative disorders

The association between immunosuppression and lymphoproliferative disorders has been well recognized and the most common form affects the B cell lineage resulting in B cell non-Hodgkin's lymphoma. These lymphomas are usually associated with the Epstein–Barr virus. Normal lymphatic tissue has been found within lung transplant parenchyma itself as well as in lymph nodes and spleen and the lymphoma usually responds to a reduction in the level of immunosuppression (particularly cyclosporin) and the administration of high dose acyclovir.

23.5.5 DISEASE RECURRENCE

So far there is no evidence that patients with COPD including those with α_1-antitrypsin deficiency and emphysema, have developed recurrence of their original disease. All transplant centers regard the cessation of smoking as an absolute requirement for acceptance onto the active waiting list and thus providing that recipients do not take up smoking again it should reduce the potential risks.

23.6 CONCLUSIONS

Lung transplantation now offers an effective therapy for patients with end-stage COPD. Debate remains as to which operation patients with COPD and particularly emphysema are most suited but in practice well chosen recipients, without the presence of frequent pulmonary sepsis or bilateral bullae appear to do well with single lung transplantation. Patients with these complications do as well with bilateral sequential single lung transplants as HLT. The major problems facing lung transplantation at this time comprise a shortfall in suitable donor organs compared to the number of potential recipients and for this reason we do not advocate that patients on the active waiting list should be intubated for chronic ventilation. In the early postoperative period opportunist infection and graft rejection remain major problems and in the long term obliterative bronchiolitis will affect approximately 30% of patients leading to potential graft failure. There is much current research aimed at reducing this figure and certainly patients with COPD who have received lung transplants and remain free of this complication enjoy an excellent standard of life with normal or near normal restoration of activity and good prospects of prolonged survival.

REFERENCES

1. Reitz, B.A., Wallwork, J., Hunt, S.A. *et al.* (1982) Heart lung transplantation: a successful therapy for patients with pulmonary vascular disease. *N. Engl. J. Med.,* **306**, 557–63.
2. Penketh, A., Higenbottam, T., Hakim, M. and Wallwork, J. (1987) Heart and lung transplantation in patients with end stage lung disease. *Br. Med. J.,* **295**, 311–4.
3. Wildevuuer, C.R.H. and Benfield, J.R. (1979) A review of 23 lung transplantations by 20 surgeons. *Ann. Thorac. Surg.,* **9**, 489–515.
4. Toronto Lung Transplant Group (1986) Unilateral transplant for pulmonary fibrosis. *N. Engl. J. Med.,* **314**, 1140–45.
5. Patterson, G.A., Cooper, J.D., Goldman, B. *et al.* (1988) Technique of successful clinical double lung transplantation. *Ann. Thorac. Surg.,* **45**, 626–33.
6. Patterson, G.A., Todd, T.R., Cooper, J.D. *et al.* (1990) Airway complications following double lung transplantation. *J. Thorac. Cardiovasc. Surg.,* **99**, 14–21.
7. Noirclerc, M.J., Metras, D., Vaillant, A. *et al.* (1990) Bilateral bronchial anastomosis in double lung and heart lung transplantations. *Eur. J. Cardiothorac. Surg.,* **4**, 314–7.
8. Pasque, M.K., Cooper, J.D., Kaiser, L.R. *et al.* (1990) Improved technique for bilateral lung transplantations: rationale and initial clinical experience. *Ann. Thorac. Surg.,* **49**, 785–91.
9. Stevens, P.M., Johnson, P.C., Bell, R.L. *et al.* (1970) Regional ventilation and perfusion after lung transplantations in patients with emphysema. *N. Engl. J. Med.,* **282**, 245–9.
10. Vanderhoeft, R.J., Roemans, P., Nemry, C. *et al.* (1974) Left lung transplantation in a patient with emphysema. *Arch. Surg.,* **103**, 505–9.
11 Khaghani, A., Banner, N., Ozdogan, E. *et al.* (1991) Medium term results of combined heart and lung transplantation for emphysema. *J. Heart Lung Transplant.,* **10**, 15–21.
12. Mal, H., Andreassin, B., Fabrice, P. *et al.* (1989) Unilateral lung transplantations in end stage pulmonary emphysema. *Am. Rev. Respir. Dis.,* **26**, 704–6.
13. Kaiser, L.R., Cooper, J.D., Trulock, E.P. *et al.* (1991) The evolution of single lung transplantation for emphysema. *J. Thorac. Cardiovasc. Surg.,* **102**, 333–41.
14. Colquhoun, I.W., Gascoigne, A.D., Gould, F.K. *et al.* (1991) Native pulmonary sepsis following single lung transplantation. *Transplantation,* **52**, 931–3.
15. Kaiser, L.R., Pasque, M.K., Trulock, E.P. *et al.* (1991) Bilateral sequential lung transplantations: the procedure of choice for double lung replacement. *Ann. Thorac. Surg.,* **52**, 438–446.
16. Hunter, A.M.B., Carey, M.A. and Larsh, H.W. (1981) The nutritional status of patients with chronic obstructive pulmonary disease. *Am. Rev. Respir. Dis.,* **124**, 376–81.
17. Bidstrup, B.P., Royston, D., Supsford, R.W. and Taylor, K.M. (1989) Reduction in blood loss and blood use after cardiopulmonary bypass with high dose Aprotinin. *J. Thorac. Cardiovasc. Surg.,* **93**, 364–72.
18. Colquhoun, I.W., Gascoigne, A.D., Au, J. *et al.* (1994) Airway complications following pulmonary transplantation. *Ann. Thorac. Surg.,* (in press).
19. Morrison, D.L., Maurer, J.R. and Grossman, R.F. (1990) Preoperative assessment for lung transplantation clinics. *Chest Med.,* **2**, 207–15.
20. Doig, J.C., Richens, D., Corris, P.A. *et al.* (1991) Resolution of pulmonary hypertension after

single lung transplantation. *Br. Heart J.*, **66**, 431–4.

21. Bennett, W.M. and Pulliam, J.P. (1983) Cyclosporine nephrotoxicity. *Ann. Intern. Med.*, **99**, 851–4.

22. Gould, F.K., Freeman, R., Taylor, C.E. *et al.* (1994). Prophylaxis and management of cytomegalovirus pneumonitis following pulmonary transplantation. *J. Heart Lung Transplant.*, (in press).

23. McCleod, A.T., Stone, T.N., Hawkins, T. *et al.* (1989) Ventilation perfusion relationships after single lung transplantation for pulmonary fibrosis. *Am. Rev. Respir. Dis.*, **139**, A265.

24. Higenbottam, T., Stuart, S., Penketh, A. and Wallwork, J. (1988) Transbronchial lung biopsy for the diagnosis of rejection in heart lung transplant recipients. *Transplantation*, **46**, 532–9.

25. Yacoub, M., Khaghani, A., Theodoropoulos, S. *et al.* (1991) Single lung transplantation for obstructive airways disease. *Transpl. Proc.*, **23**, 1213–4.

26. Scott, J.P., Higenbottam, T.W., Sharples, C. *et al.* (1991) Risk factors for obliterative bronchiolitis in heart lung transplant recipients. *Transplantation*, **51**, 813–7.

27. Milne, D.S., Gascoigne, A.D., Wilkes, J. *et al.* The immunohistological features of obliterative bronchiolitis

28. Glanville, A.R., Baldwin, J.C., Burke, C.M. *et al.* (1987) Obliterative bronchiolitis after heart lung transplantation: apparent arrest by augmented immunosuppression. *Ann. Intern. Med.*, **107**, 300–4.

INDEX

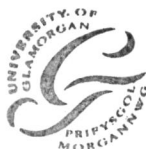